New Insights into Neuropathic Pain

New Insights into Neuropathic Pain

Editor: Vin Lopez

FOSTER ACADEMICS

www.fosteracademics.com

www.fosteracademics.com

FOSTER ACADEMICS

Cataloging-in-Publication Data

New insights into neuropathic pain / edited by Vin Lopez.
p. cm.
Includes bibliographical references and index.
ISBN 978-1-63242-559-1
1. Central pain. 2. Nervous system. 3. Neuralgia. I. Lopez, Vin.
RC368 .N49 2018
616.047 2--dc23

Foster Academics,
118-35 Queens Blvd., Suite 400,
Forest Hills, NY 11375, USA

ISBN 978-1-63242-559-1 (Hardback)

Printed and bound in China.

Contents

Preface

It is often said that books are a boon to mankind. They document every progress and pass on the knowledge from one generation to the other. They play a crucial role in our lives. Thus I was both excited and nervous while editing this book. I was pleased by the thought of being able to make a mark but I was also nervous to do it right because the future of students depends upon it. Hence, I took a few months to research further into the discipline, revise my knowledge and also explore some more aspects. Post this process, I begun with the editing of this book.

Neuropathic pain is a specific kind of pain that is caused when somatosensory nervous system is damaged. The symptoms include sensations of shocks, stabbings, itching, numbness, etc. These abnormal sensations are known as dysesthesia. There are three primary types of neuropathic pain- peripheral neuropathic pain, mixed neuropathic pain and central neuropathic pain. This book unravels the recent studies in the field of medical science related to neuropathic pain and its cause and treatment. Different approaches, evaluations, methodologies and advanced studies on this field have been included in it. The book will serve as a reference to a broad spectrum of readers.

I thank my publisher with all my heart for considering me worthy of this unparalleled opportunity and for showing unwavering faith in my skills. I would also like to thank the editorial team who worked closely with me at every step and contributed immensely towards the successful completion of this book. Last but not the least, I wish to thank my friends and colleagues for their support.

Editor

LASSBio-1135: A Dual TRPV1 Antagonist and Anti-TNF-Alpha Compound Orally Effective in Models of Inflammatory and Neuropathic Pain

Cleverton K. F. Lima[1], Rafael M. Silva[2], Renata B. Lacerda[3], Bruna L. R. Santos[1], Rafaela V. Silva[1], Luciana S. Amaral[2], Luís E. M. Quintas[2], Carlos A. M. Fraga[2,3], Eliezer J. Barreiro[3], Marília Z. P. Guimaraes[2], Ana L. P. Miranda[1]*

1 Laboratório de Estudos em Farmacologia Experimental (LEFEx), Faculdade de Farmácia, Universidade Federal do Rio de Janeiro, Rio de Janeiro, RJ, Brazil, **2** Instituto de Ciências Biomédicas, Universidade Federal do Rio de Janeiro, Rio de Janeiro, RJ, Brazil, **3** Laboratório de Avaliação e Síntese de Substâncias Bioativas (LASSBio), Faculdade de Farmácia, Universidade Federal do Rio de Janeiro, Rio de Janeiro, RJ, Brazil

Abstract

LASSBio-1135 is an imidazo[1,2-a]pyridine derivative with high efficacy in screening models of nociception and inflammation, presumed as a weak COX-2 inhibitor. In order to tease out its mechanism of action, we investigated others possible target for LASSBio-1135, such as TNF-α and TRPV1, to better characterize it as a multitarget compound useful in the treatment of chronic pain. TRPV1 modulation was assessed in TRPV1-expressing Xenopus oocytes against capsaicin and low pH-induced current. Modulation of TNF-α production was evaluated in culture of macrophages stimulated with LPS. *In vivo* efficacy of LASSBio-1135 was investigated in carrageenan and partial sciatic ligation-induced thermal hyperalgesia and mechanical allodynia. Corroborating its previous demonstration of efficacy in a model of capsaicin-induced hyperalgesia, LASSBio-1135 blocks capsaicin-elicited currents in a non-competitive way with an IC_{50} of 580 nM as well as low pH-induced current at 50 μM. As an additional action, LASSBio-1135 inhibited TNF-α release in these cells stimulated by LPS with an IC_{50} of 546 nM by reducing p38 MAPK phosphorilation. Oral administration of 100 $\mu mol.Kg^{-1}$ LASSBio-1135 markedly reduced thermal hyperalgesia induced by carrageenan, however at 10 $\mu mol.Kg^{-1}$ only a partial reduction was observed at the 4th h. Neutrophil recruitment and TNF-α production after carrageenan stimulus was also inhibited by the treatment with LASSBio-1135. Modulating TRPV1 and TNF-α production, two key therapeutic targets of neuropathic pain, 100 $\mu mol.Kg^{-1}$ LASSBio-1135 was orally efficacious in reversing thermal hyperalgesia and mechanical allodynia produced by partial sciatic ligation 7–11 days after surgery without provoking hyperthermia, a common side effect of TRPV1 antagonists. In conclusion LASSBio-1135, besides being a weak COX-2 inhibitor, is a non-competitive TRPV1 antagonist and a TNF-α inhibitor. As a multitarget compound, LASSBio-1135 is orally efficacious in a model of neuropathic pain without presenting hyperthermia.

Editor: Michael Costigan, Boston Children's Hospital and Harvard Medical School, United States of America

Funding: This work was supported by Coordenação de Aperfeiçoamento de Pessoal de Nível Superior (BR), Conselho Nacional de Desenvolvimento Científico e Tecnológico (BR), Fundação de Amparo à Pesquisa do Estado do Rio de Janeiro (BR), and Instituto Nacional de Ciência e Tecnologia em Fármacos e Medicamentos (BR). The funders had no role in study design, data collection and analysis, decision to publish, or preparation of the manuscript.

Competing Interests: The authors have declared that no competing interests exist.

* E-mail: analu@pharma.ufrj.br

Introduction

The pharmacological treatment of patients with chronic pain is a current challenge, since existing drugs have little efficacy and present serious side effects. The two major types of chronic pain, inflammatory and neuropathic pain, are mostly treated with drugs that alleviate the symptoms without affecting the underlying disease, such as nonsteroidal and steroidal anti-inflammatory drugs, opioids, antidepressants, and anticonvulsants, depending on the nature of pain. Controlling the inflammatory response is essential not only in inflammatory chronic pain, as pointed by recent studies that have shown the role of inflammation in the development of neuropathic pain and consequently have supported new therapeutic approaches that target immune response [1].

LASSBio-1135 belongs to a series of imidazo[1,2-*a*]pyridine derivatives designed as dual inhibitors of p38 mitogen-activated protein kinase (p38 MAPK) and cyclooxigenase-2 (COX-2) based on the structures of SB203580 (p38 MAPK inhibitor) and celecoxib (COX-2 selective inhibitor) [2]. The *in vivo* pharmacological screening for anti-inflammatory and antinociceptive activities pointed out this compound as one of the most prominent of the series, since LASSBio-1135 reduced the carrageenan-induced paw edema and it completely abrogated capsaicin-induced thermal hyperalgesia. However, *in vitro* studies regarding its mechanism of action derivative showed that it did not inhibit p38 MAPK activity as planned, but it inhibited weakly COX-2 activity, reducing TXB_2 production in whole blood stimulated with lipopolysaccharide (LPS) ($IC_{50} = 18{,}5$ μM) [2]. Therefore, the robust *in vivo* actions of this compound were not consistent with the meager *in vitro* activities, suggesting that other mechanisms might be involved in these actions.

LASSBio-1135 high efficacy in capsaicin-induced hyperalgesia could indicate the transient receptor potential vanilloid receptor type 1(TRPV1) as a possible target. TRPV1 is a nonselective cation channel expressed in subtypes of nociceptive neurons that is activated by physical or chemical stimuli, including capsaicin (CAP), heat, protons and endogenous cannabinoids (CB) [3;4]. Recent studies have described that TRPV1 activation is essential for the establishment of inflammation and pain in models of arthritis, showing that the expression of this receptor is increased, contributing to enhanced thermal sensitivity [5;6;7]. In addition to its effects on inflammatory pain, TRPV1 also contributes to neuropathic pain, as its expression is up-regulated in uninjured and down-regulated in injured fibers after partial nerve injury, and its blockade reduces pain sensitivity in nerve injury models [8;9]. Interestingly, Chen *et al.* [10] showed recently that TRPV1 plays a role in spinal cord glial activation after partial nerve injury and consequently this channel may also modulate glial activation during neuropathic pain and arthritis. Thus, several TRPV1 antagonists have been developed as a useful pharmacological alternative to treat chronic pain, some of them reaching clinical trials, however most studies were discontinued due to the main side effect presented in humans: hyperthermia [11].

The inflammatory mediators produced by immune cells, such as cytokines and chemokines, play essential roles in the development of inflammatory and neuropathic pain, acting both in the peripheral and in the central nervous system (CNS). Among the cytokines, it is well known that tumor necrosis factor alpha (TNF-α) is released by immune, immune-like glial and glial cells, in the context of inflammatory and neuropathic pain [12]. TNF-α emerges as another target for LASSBio-1135 action, since it was designed as a p38 MAPK inhibitor. As mentioned previously, LASSBio-1135 does not inhibit directly p38 MAPK activity as predicted, however its structure has the imidazo-pyridine moiety present in several inhibitors of the signaling pathways involved in TNF-α production [13], which supports the idea of TNF-α modulation. Several lines of evidence have demonstrated that TNF-α contributes to the degeneration of the injured nerve and to sensitize the primary afferents neurons directly, or indirectly through the induction of other mediators [14;15;16]. In the dorsal root ganglion (DRG), TNF-α induces the macrophage recruitment after adjuvant-induced arthritis and nerve injury. It also modulates TTX-resistant Na^+ channels, by mechanisms that are p38 MAPK activation-dependent, and sensitizes TRPV1 [17;18;19;20]. Furthermore, it has been observed that TNF-α produced by glial cells in the dorsal horn of the spinal cord may also sensitize these neurons, changing their sensitivity [21]. Hence, anti-TNF-α therapies have successfully been evaluated in animal models of neuropathic and inflammatory pain [22].

Here, we show that LASSBio-1135 acts as a multitarget compound, inhibiting TNF-α production both *in vitro* and *in vivo*, and inhibiting TRPV1 currents *in vitro*, actions that could explain the diminished inflammatory and nociceptive responses in models of inflammatory and neuropathic pain. In addition, these LASSBio-1135 antinociceptive effects were present in doses in which the animals did not develop hyperthermia, the main side effect of classical TRPV1 antagonists.

Methods

All procedures involving animals were carried out under the approval by the Comissão de Ética no Uso de Animais from the Federal University of Rio de Janeiro (CEUA-UFRJ; FARM-ACIA04) and were in accordance with international guidelines. In experiments with animals, mice and rats of both sexes from the Faculty of Pharmacy breeding unity were used and at the end of the experiments animals were euthanized in CO_2 chamber.

Materials

The rat TRPV1 clone was a generous gift from Dr. David Julius. Drugs used in this study were purchased from the following sources: capsaicin (Alexis or Sigma), dimethylsulfoxide (DMSO) (Sigma or Vetec), arabic gum (Sigma), carrageenan (Cialgas), ketamine (Syntec), xylazine (König), RPMI 1640 (Sigma), Lipopolysaccharide (LPS) from *E. coli* (Sigma), Thioglycollate (Sigma), foetal bovine serum (FBS) (Gibco), ELISA Kit for TNF-α (BD Bioscience). LASSBio-1135 was synthesized in our laboratory as described before [2].

Oocyte Preparation and Electrophysiology

Oocytes expressing TRPV1 were obtained as described previously [23]. Briefly, adult *Xenopus laevis* female frogs were anaesthetized with tricaine and part of the ovary was surgically removed. The removed tissues was placed in a saline solution containing (in mM) 96 NaCl, 2 KCl, 5 $MgCl_2$, 5 HEPES at pH 7.6, and were then treated with collagenase (Type 1, 0.8 $mg.ml^{-1}$, Worthington) to remove the follicular membrane. Oocytes were injected with approximately 2.0 ng of rat TRPV1 cRNA obtained with mMESSAGE mMACHINE T7 (Ambion), by using a nanoliter injector. Oocytes were maintained in ND-96 (in mM: 96 NaCl, 2 KCl, 1.8 $CaCl_2$, 1 $MgCl_2$, 5 HEPES) supplemented with 40 $\mu g.ml^{-1}$ gentamicin for 5–7 days before analysis. For recording, oocytes were placed in a small chamber under continuous superfusion with ND-96 (without gentamicin), at a flow rate of approximately 1 $ml.min^{-1}$, and the same solution was used to dilute the test compounds, except when acidic pH was applied. In the latter case, the solution used was composed of (in mM): 96 NaCl, 2 KCl, 1 $MgCl_2$, 0.1 $CaCl_2$ and 5 sodium acetate, pH 5.5. Two electrode voltage-clamp recordings were obtained at room temperature (20–22°C) under a holding potential of −60 mV, using Geneclamp 500 amplifier (Axon Instruments). Electrodes were obtained on a horizontal puller (P-97, Sutter) aiming to achieve a final resistance of 0.6–1.2 MΩ and were filled with 3 M KCl. Recordings were digitized with a MacLab A/D converter (AD Instruments) at 100 Hz and digitally filtered at 2 Hz (low pass). Drug stock solutions were made in ethanol (capsaicin) or DMSO (LASSBio-1135) and were diluted in ND-96 just before the experiments, in a way that final ethanol and DMSO concentrations did not exceed 0.1% and 0.2%, respectively, and appropriate controls were tested. The solutions were exchanged via a programmable solenoid pinch valve controller (AutoMate Scientific Inc.) and were generally applied in 45-second pulses. Each pulse of LASSBio-1135 in admixture with other agents was immediately preceded by LASSBio-1135 alone in the same concentration, to allow drug equilibration. As a control, we performed an experiment with 3 consecutive applications of CAP.

LPS-induced TNF-α Production in Cultures of Mice Peritoneal Macrophages

BALBc mice were stimulated with 3% thyoglicollate (1 ml per mouse; i.p.) and 3 days later the peritoneal cavity was washed with RPMI 1640 and the peritoneal macrophages were plated onto 96-wells plates (30,000 cells per well) and allowed to adhere for 1 hour at 37°C in a humidified 5% CO_2 atmosphere [30]. Subsequently, the wells were rinsed once with sterile phosphate buffer saline (PBS) and then it was added RPMI 1640 supplemented with 10%

foetal bovine serum, streptomycin and penicillin (50 U.ml^{-1}). Then macrophages were incubated with the vehicle or compounds for 1 hour, followed by stimulation with LPS (100 ng.ml^{-1}) for 24 hours [27], after which the supernatants were collected to measure TNF-α production by ELISA.

Cell Viability: MTT Assay

Cell viability was evaluated using (3-(4,5-dimethylthiazol-2-yl)-2,5-diphenyltetrazolium bromide (MTT) assay in culture of macrophages. Briefly, murine peritoneal macrophages were obtained and cultivated as described above. After 18 h of stimuli with LPS was add 20 μl of MTT solution (5 mg.ml^{-1}) and allowed the cells to incubate for 4 h. At the end, it was add 200 μl of DMSO to dissolve formazan and the absorbance was read at 532 nm.

Western Blot Analysis

Immunoblotting was performed with lysates from cultured peritoneal macrophages obtained as described above but plated on 6-wells plates (3.500.000 cells per well). After 1 h of LPS stimuli, cells were lysed with lysis buffer (1% Triton, 20 mM Tris pH 7.6, 1 mM EDTA, 150 mM NaCl, 1 mM NaF, 1 mM $NaVO_3$) containing a protease inhibitors cocktail (Sigma). Aliquots of macrophages lysates containing 30 μg of proteins in each well were subjected to electrophoresis in 10% SDS-polyacrilamide gels (Bio-Rad, Miniproteam) and transferred to nitrocellulose membranes (Bio-Rad). The membranes were then blocked with 5% non-fat milk solution in TBS buffer (25 mM Tris pH 7.6, 0.2 M NaCl) and incubated overnight at 4°C with a primary antibody against phospho-p38 MAPK (1:1000) or total p38 MAPK (1:1000) (both from Cell Signalling). The blots were incubated for 1 h with HRP-conjugated secondary antibody (1:5000) (Santa Cruz) at room temperature and then revealed with ECL solution (Thermo Scientific) for 2 min following exposition to Hyperfilm (Amersham Biosciences). The same blot was first immunoreacted with phospho-p38 MAPK, following by stripping with glycine at pH 2.0 and then the incubation procedure was repeated with total p38 MAPK antibody.

Carrageenan-induced Hyperalgesia Assay

The systemic anti-hyperalgesic activity of LASSBio-1135 in a model of inflammatory pain was evaluated using carrageenan-induced thermal hyperalgesia assay. LASSBio-1135 was orally administered (100 μmol.kg^{-1} or 10 μmol.kg^{-1}; 0.1 ml.20 g^{-1}) as a suspension in 5% arabic gum in saline (vehicle). Control animals received an equal volume of vehicle. One hour later, the animals were injected with either 0.1 ml of 1% carrageenan solution in saline or sterile saline (NaCl 0.9%), into the subplantar surface of the right hind paws. The thermal hyperalgesia was determined using the modified hot-plate test [24]. Rats were placed individually on a hot plate with the temperature set at 51°C. The withdrawal latency response of the challenged paw was determined at 0, 30, 60, 120, 180, and 240 min post-challenge.

Myeloperoxidase Activity

The myeloperoxidase (MPO) activity assay was performed to evaluate the leukocyte recruitment to the injured plantar tissue after carrageenan challenge [25;26]. The plantar tissue of the hind paw was harvested 4 h after carrageenan or saline i.pl. 0.9% injection and kept at −80°C until the day of the experiment. At the day of the experiment, samples were weighed and adjusted to 50 mgml^{-1} with 50 mM K_2HPO_4 buffer (pH 6.0) containing 0.5% of hexadecyl trimethylammonium bromide, following by homogenization using a Turrax (T18) for 2 min at 22,000 rpm and centrifuged at 13,000 rpm for 4 min. The supernatants were collected and aliquots of 100 μl were added to 96 well-plates together with 100 μl of development solution containing 0.167 mg.ml^{-1} of O-dianisidine dihydrochloride (OPD) and 0.015% hydrogen peroxide. The MPO activity was measured using a spectrophotometer at 450 nm (TP-reader). A standard curve of neutrophils, obtained from rats bone marrows, was used to compare with MPO activity obtained in the samples.

TNF-α Quantification

TNF-α quantification in injured paw was performed in skin tissues samples harvested 4 h after challenge with carrageenan or saline. Skin tissues samples were homogenised in PBS containing protease inhibitor cocktail (Sigma), centrifuged at 13.000 rpm at 4°C for 15 min, the supernatant was collected and TNF-α production was evaluated by ELISA kit (BD Bioscinese).

Neuropathic Pain Model

The anti-hyperalgesic and anti-allodynic activities of LASSBio-1135 in chronic neuropathic pain model was investigated using the partial sciatic ligation (PSL) assay described by Seltzer *et al.* [28]. Experiments were performed with adult Swiss mice of both sexes weighing from 20 to 30 g. Surgical procedures were performed under ketamine (100 mg.Kg^{-1}; i.p.) and xylazine (20 mg.Kg^{-1}; i.p.) anaesthesia. First, a small incision was made on the left hind leg and then the sciatic nerve ligation was made by tying a knot positioned between the last third or half of the dorsal portion of the nerve, using absorbable 4.0 silk. In sham-operated animals the nerve was exposed without ligation. The withdrawal responses were determined before surgery and after a hypernociceptive thermal stimulus caused by a radiant heat light source (Ugo Basile) positioned directly on the plantar surface of the left hind paw for thermal stimuli and using calibrated Von Frey filaments. LASSBio-1135 was administered orally at a dose of 100 μmol.Kg^{-1} once a day starting at day 5 and ending at day 13. The withdrawal latency of the left hind paw was recorded 5, 7, 9, 11 and 13 days after sciatic ligation and always one hour after the administration of LASSBio-1135 or vehicle (5% arabic gum).

Hargreaves Test

Baseline thermal latency was evaluated using Hargreaves test. LASSBio-1135 at 100 μmol.Kg^{-1} or vehicle were orally administered and evaluation of thermal sensitivity was performed using a radiant heat light source (Ugo Basile) positioned directly on the plantar surface of the left hind paw. The withdrawal latency was evaluated 1, 2, 3, 4 and 6 h after administration of LASSBio-1135 or vehicle.

Temperature Measurements

LASSBio-1135 was evaluated in its ability to change body temperature, using the animals submitted to PSL. Animals had their rectal temperature measured with a digital thermometer (sensitivity 0.1°C) before surgery and each day after 5 days later, when LASSBio-1135 treatment began, always 1 h after administration of the compound (100 μmol.Kg^{-1}; 0.1 ml.20 g^{-1}) or vehicle.

Statistical Analyses

Peak amplitudes of digitized current traces were measured with Chart software. Results were expressed as mean ± SEM and compared with appropriate control groups. Data were statistically analyzed by the Students *t* test, One-way and Two-way ANOVA

(Dunnett post-test and Bonferroni post-test) for a significance level of $p<0.05$. When appropriate, the IC_{50} values (*i.e.* the concentration able to inhibit 50% of the maximum effect observed) were determined by non-linear regression using GraphPad Prism software v. 5.0.

Results

LASSBio-1135 Inhibits Capsaicin- pH 5.5-elicited Currents in Xenopus Oocytes Expressing TRPV1

As previously shown by our group in a pharmacological screening, LASSBio-1135 was orally effective in completely reducing hyperalgesia induced by capsaicin, suggesting the possibility of TRPV1 modulation [2]. To investigate whether LASSBio-1135 could modulate TRPV1 activity, *Xenopus* oocytes were injected with TRPV1 cRNA and electrophysiological recordings were performed. Firstly, oocytes were challenged with submaximal 1 μM capsaicin (CAP), then followed by CAP with co-administration of LASSBio-1135 at 5 μM. The co-application of LASSBio-1135 reduced the CAP current approximately by half which is completely reversed by final application of CAP (Figure 1A). As a control, three consecutive application of CAP do not promote desensitization phenomenon of TRPV1 in our conditions (Figure S1). LASSBio-1135 co-administration inhibited CAP-evoked currents in a concentration-dependent manner (Figure 1B, $IC_{50} = 580$ nM), however it is observed only a partial reversibility at higher concentrations. Next we asked whether LASSBio-1135 would also interfere with other modalities of TRPV1 activation, particularly the acidic pH, which is found in inflammatory conditions. Similarly to what observed with CAP stimulation, LASSBio-1135 at 50 μM also reduced proton-evoked currents (Figure 1C). Hence, these results suggest that this new compound might act as an antagonist of the TRPV1 receptor.

Next, to get an idea of the nature of the LASSBio-1135 antagonist effect on TRPV1, we treated oocytes with increasing concentrations of CAP with or without 5 μM LASSBio-1135. As can be observed in figure 1D, there was only a slight shift in the CAP EC_{50} in the presence of LASSBio-1135 compared with CAP alone (0.37 to 0.47 μM). However, more interestingly, in the presence of LASSBio-1135 the concentration-response curve of CAP did not reach the maximal effect (CAP = 100%; CAP+ LASSBio-1135 = 59±19%). These results suggest that LASSBio-1135 might be a non-competitive TRPV1 antagonist.

LASSBio-1135 Inhibits TNF-α Production in LPS-stimulated Murine Peritoneal Macrophage by Reducing p38 MAPK Activation

LASSBio-1135 has the structural scaffold of many compounds which interfere with several proteins kinases involved in TNF-α production, raising up the possibility of immune modulation. In order to investigate this hypothesis and attribute immune modulation to LASSBio-1135 mechanism of action we evaluated whether this compound reduces TNF-α release in inflammatory cells. Murine peritoneal macrophages were stimulated with 100 $ng.ml^{-1}$ of LPS for 24 h to induce TNF-α production. Macrophages produced a large amount of TNF-α in response to LPS which was reduced with previous incubation of increasing concentrations of LASSBio-1135 (Figure 2A), thus presenting a concentration-dependent inhibition (Figure 2B, $IC_{50} = 642$ nM). Moreover, LASSBio-1135 only interferes significantly with cell viability in concentrations higher than 100 μM, as shown by MTT assay (Figure 2C).

In an attempt to confirm that LASSBio-1135 could inhibit TNF-α production by interfering with signalling pathways we decided to investigate if its action could involve modulation of p38 MAPK upstream signalling pathway, since it does not inhibit p38 activity [2]. For this purpose, murine peritoneal macrophages, previously treated with different concentrations of LASSBio-1135, were stimulated with LPS and the cell lysates were submitted to immunoblotting for phosphorylated p38 [29]. LPS rapidly induced the phosphorylation of p38 MAPK compared to the unstimulated group and the cell treatment with LASSBio-1135 reduced the activation of this protein kinase in a concentration-dependent manner (Figure 2D).

LASSBio-1135 Inhibits Thermal Hyperalgesia Induced by Carrageenan Reducing TNF-α Production and Neutrophils Recruitment

The therapeutic efficacy of LASSBio-1135 as an anti-inflammatory compound *in vivo* was proved in model of paw inflammation induced by carrageenan, however its efficacy as anti-hyperalgesic was evaluated only after capsaicin stimulation. Having demonstrated that LASSBio-1135 modulate neuronal activation by TRPV1 antagonism and immune activity by interfering with TNF-α production, we decided to investigate its efficacy to alleviate thermal hyperalgesia response in a model of inflammatory pain. Then, we used the carrageenan-induced thermal hyperalgesia assay, where we proceeded the prior administration of two doses of LASSBio-1135 (p.o.) at 100 $\mu mol.Kg^{-1}$ and 10 $\mu mol.Kg^{-1}$, which previously proved effective [2], followed by the i.pl. injection of carrageenan 1h later. At 100 $\mu mol.Kg^{-1}$, LASSBio-1135 totally abrogated the thermal hyperalgesia since one hour after the challenge with carrageenan, while at 10 $\mu mol.Kg^{-1}$ a significant reduction is observed only four hours after challenge (Figure 3A) (Baseline values: Vehicle = 12.1 s±0.4; LASSBio-1135 10 $\mu mol.Kg^{-1}$ = 10.4 s±0.6; LASSBio-1135 100 $\mu mol.Kg^{-1}$ = 12.9 s±0.7).

TNF-α is one of the cytokines released during carrageenan-induced inflammation and it is responsible for sensitizing primary afferent nociceptor as well as for orchestrating inflammatory response recruiting leukocytes [26]. As a TNF-α inhibitor *in vitro*, we investigated whether LASSBio-1135 could reduce hyperalgesia by hampering TNF-α production and then the recruitment of neutrophils. The injured paws were harvested and neutrophil recruitment was evaluated by the MPO-assay. Both doses of LASSBio-1135 reduced the cell recruitment in agreement with the results of hyperalgesia at the 4th h (Figures 3A and 3B). Regarding the TNF-α production, both doses of LASSBio-1135 at 100 $\mu mol.Kg^{-1}$ and at 10 $\mu mol.Kg^{-1}$ reduce this cytokine production in the injured paw. As observed for neutrophil recruitment, LASSBio-1135 strongly reduced TNF-α production, keeping the concentration similar to the saline treated animals (Figure 3C).

LASSBio-1135 Reduces the Thermal Hyperalgesia and Mechanical Allodynia in Model of Neuropathic Pain

Considering the activity presented by LASSBio-1135 against TRPV1 and TNF-α, two relevant targets for the treatment of neuropathic pain based on the modification of this disease, and the efficacy presented by this compound in models of acute and inflammatory pain we decided to investigate if the oral treatment with LASSBio-1135 is effective in model of neuropathic pain induced by partial sciatic ligation. Then, 5 days after the surgery to establish nerve injury we started the daily treatment with the dose of 100 $\mu mol.Kg^{-1}$ of LASSBio-1135 (p.o.), which was the most effective dose in pain assays as described above, or vehicle. The evaluation of thermal (Baseline values: Sham = 9.9 s±0.5; Vehi-

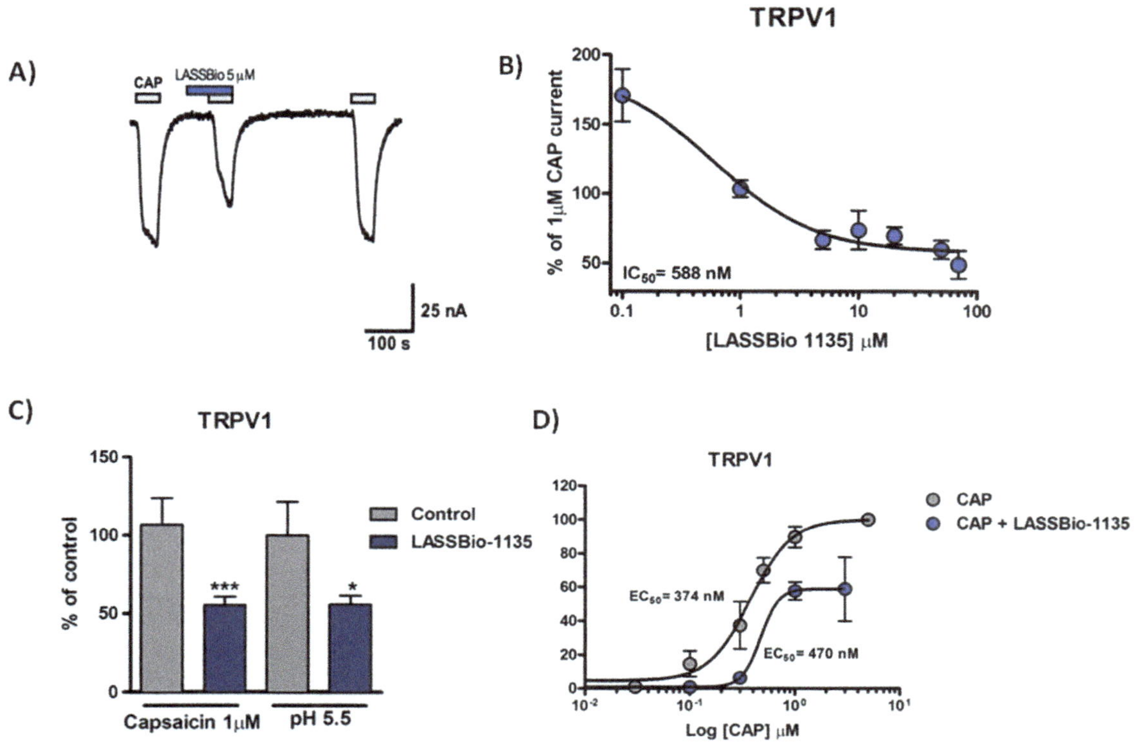

Figure 1. LASSBio-1135 is a non-competitive TRPV1 antagonist. A) Representative recordings of inhibition produced by LASSBio-1135 at 5 µM of 1 µM capsaicin currents in TRPV1-expressing oocyte. B) Concentration-response curve of LASSBio-1135 against 1 µM capsaicin, normalized by 10 µM capsaicin applied at the end of recording. Estimated IC_{50} was 588 nM (*n* = 5–8 oocytes per concentration). C) Quantification of peak currents in capsaicin and pH 5.5 in the presence or absence of LASSBio-1135 at 50 µM, normalized by the response to capsaicin or pH 5.5 applied at the end of recording (*n* = 6 per group). Results were analyzed using Student *t* test (*n* = 6 oocytes per group, *p<0.05 compared to control group). D) Concentration-response curves of capsaicin and capsaicin plus 5 µM of LASSBio-1135 in TRPV1 currents. Estimated EC_{50} for capsaicin were 374 nM and 470 nM, alone and in the presence of LASSBio-1135, respectively (*n* = 5–6 oocytes in each curve). IC_{50} e EC_{50} values were determined by non-linear regression using GraphPad Prism software.

cle = 10.2 s±0.6; LASSBio-1135 = 11.0 s±0.8) or mechanical allodynia was performed in every other day. In the first day of treatment it was not observed any change in thermal sensitivity or mechanical allodynia of injured mice compared to the vehicle group (Figure 4A and 4B). However, at the 7th day post-ligation, i.e. after 3 days of treatment with LASSBio-1135, it started to be effective reducing in thermal hyperalgesia and mechanical allodynia, however it was more efficacious in reducing thermal sensitivity, where the delta of latency was similar to the sham operated mice (Δ of latency: Sham = 0.5±0.2 s; LASSBio-1135 = −0.5±0.9 s), than in reducing mechanical allodynia, where it was observer only a partial decrease in mechanical sensitivity. The anti-hyperalgesic activity of LASSBio-1135 was slightly reduced in thermal hyperalgesia and it was unaffected in mechanical allodynia, however it remained effective until the 7th day of treatment (n = 6–8 animals, *p<0,05) (Figure 4A and 4B). Also, we did not observe any changes in baseline thermal sensitivity (Figure 4C).

The Long-term Treatment with LASSBio-1135 did not Promote Hyperthermia

Classical TRPV1 antagonists promote increase in body temperature, except those which inhibit CAP-induced currents but not proton and heat activation [30;31]. Thus, to prove that LASSBIo-1135 is efficacious without presenting this main side effect, we also verified the rectal temperature of mice submitted to the nerve injury and daily treated with vehicle or LASSBio-1135 (100 µmol.Kg^{-1}, p.o.). Sham and vehicle treated animals did not show changes in body temperature during the days of test performance (Figure 5). Fortunately, the treatment with LASSBio-1135 did not increase significantly the body temperature of the mice, despite of promoting a slightly increase in the temperature (Δ of temperature = 0.13±0.19°C) when it starts to be effective as an anti-hyperalgesic activity (at the 7th day post-ligation). This change is not statistically significant and it is not as high as that verified for the treatment with classical TRPV1 antagonists [32].

Discussion and Conclusions

There is growing body of evidence showing that therapeutic alternatives which control neuronal activity and immune activation might be useful in the management of chronic pain [23;33;34]. Here, we have reported that LASSBio-1135, an imidazo[1,2-*a*]pyridine derivative previously described as an analgesic and anti-inflammatory prototype inhibitor of COX-2 [2], modulates neuronal activity by antagonizing TRPV1 and immune activation by inhibiting TNF-α production. Beside this *in vitro* characterization, LASSBio-1135 was evaluated *in vivo* showing efficacy in models of acute inflammatory pain and neuropathic pain.

The search for clarifying LASSBio-1135 mechanism of action raised due to intriguingly discrepancy between its efficacy observed

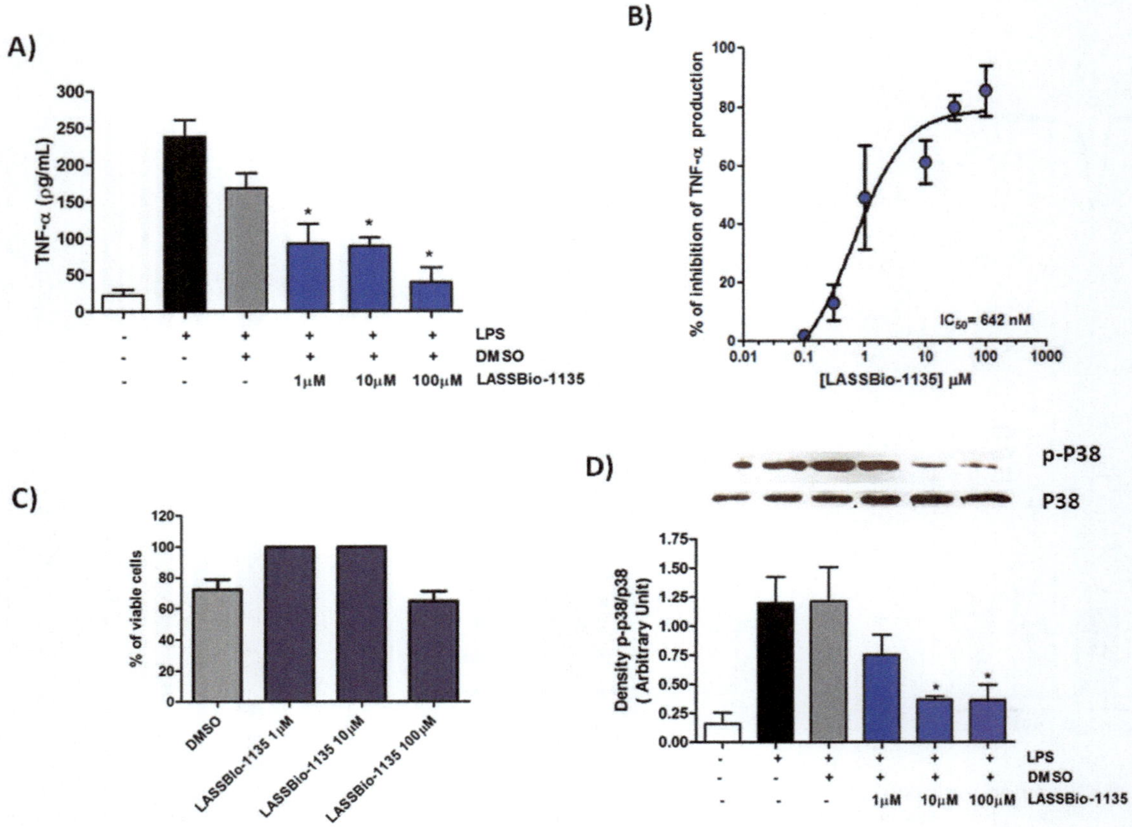

Figure 2. LASSBio-1135 inhibits TNF-α production in murine macrophages stimulated with LPS by blockade of p38 MAPK signaling pathway. A) Representative graph showing that LASSBio-1135 inhibits TNF-α release by macrophages stimulated with LPS (100 ng.ml^{-1}) at three different concentrations. Results were analyzed using One-way ANOVA followed by Dunnett post-test ($n = 3$–4 experiments per group, *$p < 0.05$ compared to DMSO group). B) Concentration-response curve of LASSBio-1135. The IC_{50} estimated was 642 nM ($n = 3$–4 experiments per concentration). D) LASSBio-1135 interferes with cell viability only at 100 μM. Results were analyzed using One-way ANOVA followed by Dunnett post-test ($n = 3$–4 experiments per group, *$p < 0.05$ compared to DMSO group) C) LASSBio-1135 reduces p38 MAPK activation induced by LPS in a concentration-dependent fashion. Results were analyzed using One-way ANOVA followed by Dunnett post-test ($n = 3$ experiments per group, *$p < 0.05$ compared to DMSO group).

in vivo studies and its poor *in vitro* effects. The anti-hyperalgesic efficacy presented previously by oral administration of LASSBio-1135 in capsaicin-induced thermal hyperalgesia, a model where classical anti-inflammatory inhibitors of COX as celecoxib are ineffective, strongly suggested that this compound might modulate targets other than COX-2 [2], such as TRPV1. In agreement with this effect, LASSBio-1135 antagonizes TRPV1 expressed in oocytes of *X. laevis* by non-competitive mechanisms. COX inhibitory effect of LASSBio-1135 did not interfere with its action against TRPV1 observed in oocytes from *X. laevis*, since it is known that these cells express only COX-1 constitutively, which is not inhibited by LASSBio-1135 [45].

The modulation of TRPV1 channels has been suggested as a relevant target to manage painful conditions and many efforts have driven the search to find new antagonists of this receptor. TRPV1 antagonists have long been designed and successfully evaluated in models of inflammatory and neuropathic pain, being able to reduce pain-associated symptoms such as thermal hyperalgesia and even mechanical allodynia through modulation of TRPV1 in the CNS [31]. The majority were developed as competitive antagonists based on the structure of two potent TRPV1 agonists, capsaicin and resiniferatoxin (RTX), interacting with the vannilloid binding pocket antagonizing TRPV1 activation by capsaicin and protons. Meanwhile only a few compounds have been reported as non-competitive antagonists but studies with representatives of this class, such as DD161515 which presents a similar potency to LASSBio-1135, suggest the existence of a different receptor site from the CAP binding site [35]. These findings support the idea that the interaction of LASSBio-1135 with TRPV1 might not be dependent on the vanilloid binding pocket, since it blocks TRPV1 non-competitively.

In addition to neuronal activity modulation, it has been reported that the development of both inflammatory and neuropathic pain depend on the action of immune cells [36;17]. These cells orchestrate the inflammatory response producing chemokines, lipids mediators and cytokines, mainly the TNF-α. Recent works have pointed out the specific role of TNF-α in the development of mechanical hyperalgesia in models of arthritis [17] and in the development of neuropathic pain. The up-regulation of TNF-α production was described in the DRG of animals submitted to spinal nerve ligation [36]. Then, compounds that dampen immune cells activation, inhibiting TNF-α production could be useful to treat these two types of chronic pain. We have previously demonstrated that LASSBio-1135 reduces inflammatory response induced by carrageenan, firstly by weakly inhibiting COX-2 and now we show that this compound may also play this

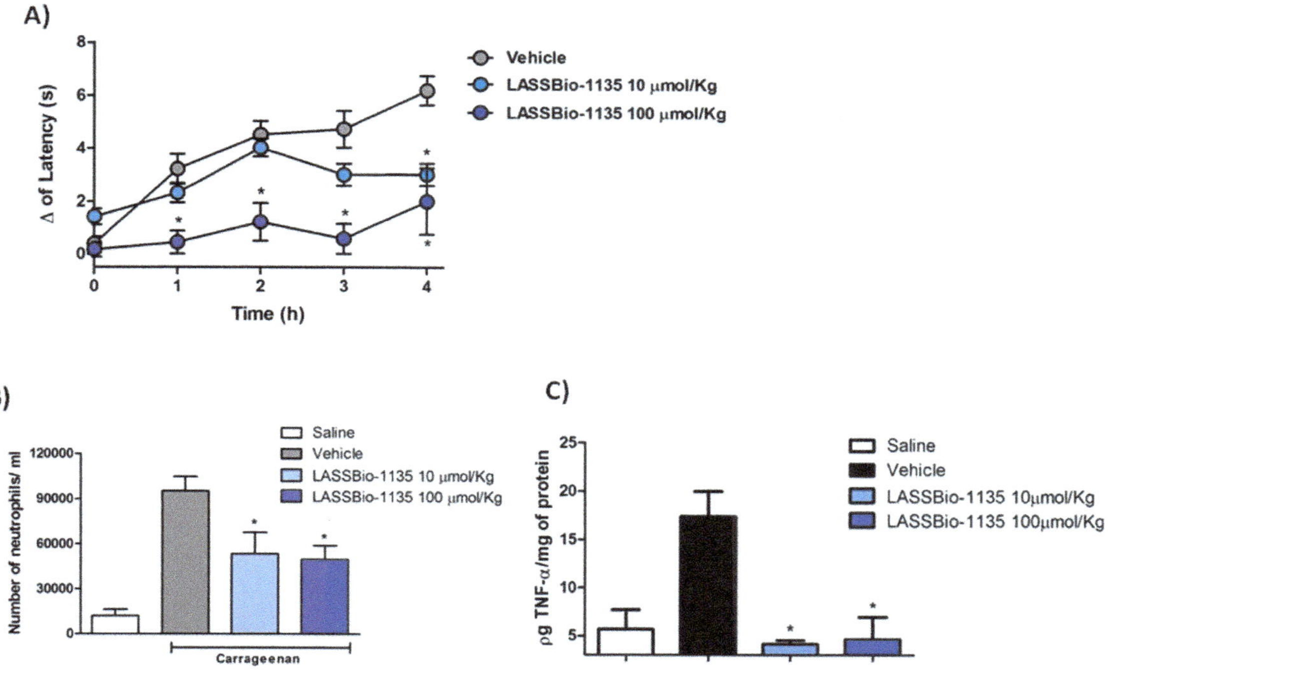

Figure 3. LASSBio-1135 inhibits carrageenan-induced thermal hyperalgesia by reducing TNF-α production and neutrophils infiltration in the injured paw. A) Oral pre-treatment with LASSBio-1135 at 10 and 100 µmol.Kg^{-1} 1 hour before carrageenan injection into the paw, reduces thermal hyperalgesia at different time points.Results were analyzed using Two-way ANOVA followed by Bonferroni post-test. ($n = 6$–8 animals per group, *$p<0.05$ compared to vehicle group). B) 4 hours after stimulus with carrageenan paws were removed and neutrophils migration was quantified by MPO activity. LASSBio-1135 treatment also reduces neutrophils migration Results were analyzed using One-way ANOVA followed by Dunnett post-test ($n = 4$ animals per group, *$p<0.05$ compared to vehicle group). C) The same tissue samples were used to quantify TNF-α production. LASSBio-1135 oral treatment with 10 µmol.Kg^{-1} and 100 µmol.Kg^{-1} also reduced TNF-α production in the injured paw Results were analyzed using One-way ANOVA followed by Dunnett post-test ($n = 3$–4 animals per group, *$p<0.05$ compared to vehicle group).

action by inhibiting directly TNF-α production by immune cells. TNF-α inhibitory effect is independent of TRPV1 antagonism and of COX inhibition, since macrophages and others immune cells do not express TRPV1 and many COX inhibitors, such as Celecoxib and Etoricoxib, do not interfere directly with TNF-α production in isolated macrophages (Unpublished data). In fact, as we observed a higher potency for TNF-α inhibition in macrophages ($IC_{50} = 642$ nM) and TRPV1 antagonism (588 nM) compared to COX-2 inhibition ($IC_{50} = 18.5$ µM), this might mainly drive the *in vivo* anti–inflammatory effects reported for LASSBio-1135.

The signaling pathways involved in TNF-α production by immune cells involves the activation of MAPK cascade, especially p38 MAPK [29;37]. The activation of p38 MAPK in both immune cells and in neuronal cells is implicated in most of the modulatories actions of TNF-α during inflammation and pain [38;39]. It has been demonstrated that activation of p38 MAPK is related to the TNF-α-mediated bone destruction during arthritis in animal models and the treatment with p38 MAPK inhibitors is able to reduce TNF-α production controlling the inflammatory response [40;41]. Thus, LASSBio-1135 inhibited TNF-α production by interfering in the activation of p38 MAPK either inhibiting directly its activation or interfering in the upstream signalling pathway, which means that this compound probably interferes in intracellular signalling to reduce cytokine production. This hypothesis is supported by the scaffold present in LASSBio-1135 molecular structure. The imidazo-pyridine group is present in some inhibitors of protein kinases involved in MAPK signalling pathways, due to its affinity to bind in their ATP pocket [18]. The modulation of p38 MAPK signalling pathway could also control the expression of inflammatory mediators other than TNF-α, such as IL-1β and COX-2, which were not evaluated here and contribute to inflammatory and nociceptive response.

Multi-targeted Therapy to Manager Chronic Pain

Current therapies to treat patients with chronic pain, such as arthritis-associated pain and several forms of neuropathic pain, consist in using single therapies or some combined therapies which are mostly unsuccessful. Trying to surpass this obstacle, new approaches have been tested to alleviate pain using drug combination or even using multi-target compounds. For instance, the combination of celecoxib, a COX-2 inhibitor, and pregabalin, a calcium-channel blocker, is more efficacious than the monotherapy with either compound alone to treat chronic low-back pain [42]. Similarly, Tributino *et al.* [26] showed that the multi-target compound LASSBio-881, a TRPV1 antagonist which is also CB-ligand and COX inhibitor, is effective in models of chronic pain. LASSBio-1135 may control inflammatory and neuropathic pain through the *in vivo* modulation of immune response and neuronal activity, demonstrated by its effectiveness in reducing inflammatory pain induced by carrageenan dampening TNF-α production and neutrophil migration as well as reducing hyperalgesia induced by nerve injury.

It is not completely clear how TRPV1 activation modulates the inflammatory response, one of the hypotheses resides on the fact that TRPV1 activation drives neurogenic inflammation. In consonance with that, it was shown reduced leukocyte recruitment and bone damage in animal model of arthritis using TRPV1-knockout mice. Conversely animals submitted to inflammatory

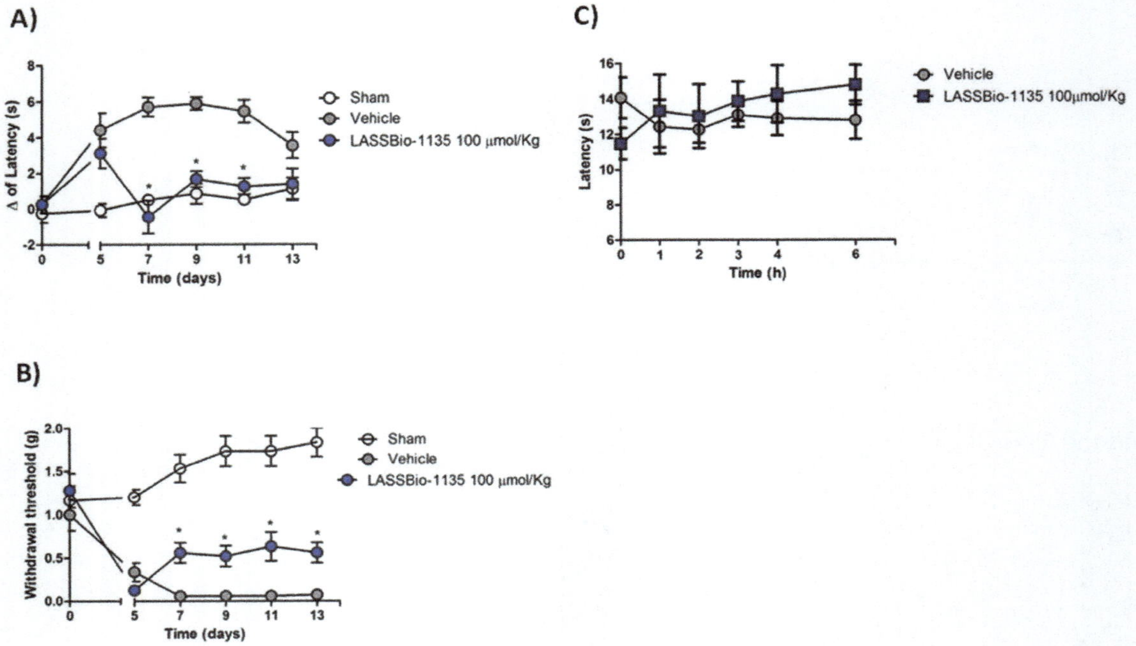

Figure 4. LASSBio-1135 is orally effective in reducing thermal and mechanical hypersensitivity induced by partial sciatic ligation. A) LASSBio-1135 (100 µmol.Kg^{-1}; p.o.) inhibits thermal hyperalgesia induced by a radiant heat light source. Delta (Δ) of latency was obtained by comparing times of withdrawal before and after surgery. B) LASSBio-1135 (100 µmol.Kg^{-1}; p.o.) also inhibits mechanical allodynia induced by Von Frey filaments. The compound was daily administered from day 5 until day 13 after surgery, 1 hour before evaluation of thermal and mechanical hypersensitivity. The withdrawal responses were determined beginning 5 days after the surgery. C) LASSBio-1135 (100 µmol.Kg^{-1}; p.o.) did not affect baseline thermal sensibility induced by a radiant heat light source. Compound or vehicle were administered and evaluation of thermal sensitivity was performed at subsequent 1, 2, 3, 4 and 6 h. Results are expressed as mean ± SEM and analysed using Two-way ANOVA followed by Bonferroni post-test (*n* = 6–8 animals; *$p < 0.05$ compared to vehicle group).

challenge and treated with TRPV1 agonist reduced the production of cytokines [7;43]. However this direct TRPV1 effect in inflammatory response is not enough to explain LASSBio-1135 effect in inflammatory pain model, since we described that this compound also inhibited directly TNF-α in macrophage culture, cells that do not express TRPV1 and strongly drive inflammatory response, with a similar potency as that to antagonize TRPV1 (TNF-α $IC_{50} = 642$ nM, TRPV1 $IC_{50} = 580$ nM) [5;43]. Thus, LASSBio-1135 likely hampered carrageenan-induced hyperalgesia through both mechanisms: reduction of TNF-α production in immune cells and reduction of neuronal activity by antagonizing TRPV1, mainly at higher doses. This effect is dose-dependent, because the higher efficacy was observed only at 100 µmol.Kg^{-1}, even 1 h after treatment, however at 10 µmol.Kg^{-1} was only observed a late effect, which could suggest that at this dose does not occur modulation of both systems.

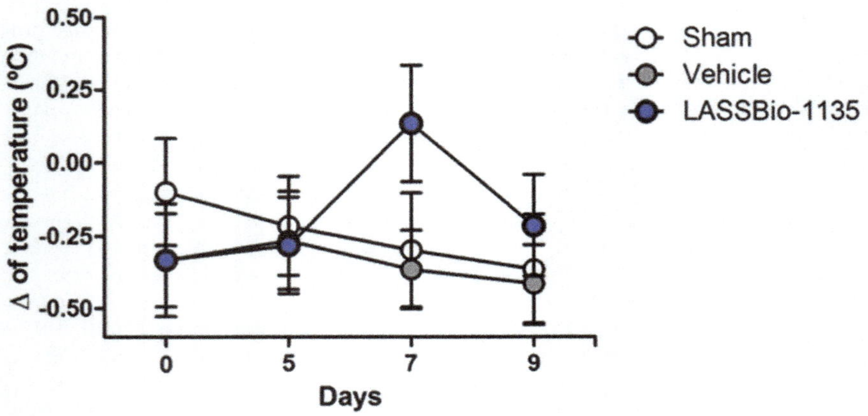

Figure 5. LASSBio-1135 chronic treatment did not promote hyperthermia. Animals submitted to partial sciatic ligation and daily treated with vehicle or LASSBio-1135 (100 µmol.Kg^{-1}, p.o.) had their rectal temperature measured 1 hour after compound administration. Delta (Δ) of temperature was obtained comparing the measures of temperature obtained before and after surgery. Results are expressed as mean ± SEM (*n* = 6–8 animals).

Similar to inflammatory pain, neuropathic pain also requires immune activation for its development and maintenance. Thus, therapies which control only neuronal activity are not successful in modifying the disease, alleviating only the symptoms (for review [33]). LASSBio-1135 can control targets involved in neuronal and immune activities with the same potency, enhancing its potential applicability in the treatment of neuropathic pain. Even though the treatment was not effective at the first day of treatment, continuous treatment showed to be efficacious, which might reflect either erratic bioavailability or that the effect depends mostly on TNF-α reduction which would take longer to modify the disease. Overall, we suggest that the long-term treatment with LASSBio-1135 during peripheral nerve injury alleviates hyperalgesia by controlling neuronal excitability while modifying the disease by hampering immune activation.

LASSBio-1135 and the Risks of Being a Multi-targeted Compound

One concern regarding the therapeutic use of multi-targeted compound is the risks of side effects due to their promiscuity. Considering this issue, we investigated the main possible side effects due to the treatment with LASSBio-1135. Clinical trials with TRPV1 antagonists proved their efficacy as analgesics, however they have pointed out hyperthermia as the main undesirable effect of this compounds class [44]. Fortunately, the long-term treatment with LASSBio-1135 did not promote any change in body temperature of mice (Figure 5). This effect could be explained by its multi-targeted characteristic, since at the dose of 100 μmol.Kg^{-1} LASSBio-1135 could counterbalance the hyperthermic effect of the TRPV1 blockage by inhibiting COX-2 (IC_{50} = 18.5 μM), which is known to be involved in regulation of body temperature [2]. We also evaluated if LASSBio-1135 interferes in thermal sensitivity in uninjured mice which did not happen (unpublished data). During long-term treatment with LASSBio-1135 we did not observe change in body weight or behaviour, such as hypolocomotion. Hence, the lack of the commonly observed major side effects for TRPV1 antagonists makes LASSBio-1135 an attractive lead compound with therapeutic potential.

In conclusion, we described here the efficacy of a new multi-targeted compound in models of inflammatory and neuropathic pain. We suggest that the inhibition of targets such as TNF-α, TRPV1 and COX-2 at similar magnitude order contributes to the high efficacy of LASSBio-1135 as well as for reducing the side effects related to interferences in these targets. Our findings suggest that LASSBio-1135 may be a multi-targeted drug prototype to treat chronic pain.

Supporting Information

Figure S1 Effect of consecutives applications of CAP in TRPV1-expressing oocytes. Representative recordings of three subsequent applications of CAP at 1 μM.

Acknowledgments

The authors are grateful to Joselina Calixto for all technical assistance.

Author Contributions

Conceived and designed the experiments: CKFL MZPG ALPM. Performed the experiments: CKFL RMS RBL BLRS RVS LSA. Analyzed the data: CKFL LEMQ MZPG ALPM. Contributed reagents/materials/analysis tools: RBL LEMQ EJB CAMF MZPG. Wrote the paper: CKFL MZPG ALPM. Designed and synthesized LASSBio-1135: RBL EJB CAMF.

References

1. Austin PJ, Moalem-Taylor G (2010) The neuro-immune balance in neuropathic pain: involvement of inflammatory immune cells, immune-like glial cells and cytokines. J Neuroimmunol 229: 26–50.
2. Lacerda RB, Lima CKF, Louback LS, Romeiro NC, Miranda ALP, et al. (2009) Discovery of novel analgesic and anti-inflammatory 3-arylamine-imidazo[1,2-a]pyridine symbiotic prototypes. Bioorg Med Chem 17(1): 74–84.
3. Caterina MJ, Schumacher MA, Tominaga M, Rosen TA, Levine JD, et al. (1997) The capsaicin receptor: a heat-activated ion channel in the pain pathway. Nature 389: 816–824.
4. Zygmunt PM, Petersson J, Andersson DA, Chuang H, Sorgard M, et al. (1999) Vanilloid receptors on sensory nerves mediate the vasodilator action of anandamide. Nature 400: 452–457.
5. Szabó A, Helyes Z, Sándor K, Bite A, Pintér E, et al. (2005) Role of transient receptor potential vanilloid 1 receptors in adjuvant-induced chronic arthritis: in vivo study using gene-deficient mice. J Pharmacol Exp Ther 314(1): 111–119.
6. Carlton SM, Coggeshall RE (2001) Peripheral capsaicin receptors increase in the inflamed rat hindpaw: a possible mechanism for peripheral sensitization. Neurosci Lett 310: 53–56.
7. Keeble J, Russell F, Curtis B, Starr A, Pinter E, et al. (2005) Involvement of Transient Receptor Potential Vanilloid 1 in the Vascular and Hyperalgesic Components of Joint Inflammation. Arthritis & Rrheumatism 52(10): 3248–3256.
8. Hudson LJ, Bevan S, Wotherspoon G, Gentry C, Fox A, et al. (2001) VR1 protein expression increases in undamaged DRG neurons after partial nerve injury. Eur J Neurosci 13: 2105–2114.
9. Walker KM, Urban L, Medhurst SJ, Patel S, Panesar M, et al. (2003) The VR1 antagonist capsazepine reverses mechanical hyperalgesia in models of inflammatory and neuropathic pain. J Pharmacol Exp Ther 304: 56–62.
10. Chen Y, Willcockson HH, Valtschanof JG (2009) Influence of the vanilloid receptor TRPV1 on the activation of spinal cord glia in mouse models of pain. Exp Neuro 220(2): 383–390.
11. Gunthorpe MJ, Chizh BA (2009) Clinical development of TRPV1 antagonists: targeting a pivotal point in the pain pathway. Drug Discov Today 14(1–2): 56–67.
12. Leung L, Cahill CM (2010) TNF-alpha and neuropathic pain-a review. J Neuroinflammation 7: 27.
13. Gaestel M, Katlyarov A, Kracht M (2009) Targeting innate immunity protein kinase signaling in inflammation. Nat Rev Drug Discov 8: 480–499.
14. George A, Buehl A, Sommer C (2005) Tumor necrosis factor receptor 1 and 2 proteins are differentially regulated during Wallerian degeneration of mouse sciatic nerve. Exp Neurol 192: 163–166.
15. Cunha FQ, Poole S, Lorenzetti BB, Ferreira SH (1992) The pivotal role of tumour necrosis factor alpha in the development of inflammatory hyperalgesia. Br J Pharmacol 107: 660–664.
16. Cunha TM, Verri WA Jr, Silva JS, Poole S, Cunha FQ, et al. (2005) A cascade of cytokines mediates mechanical inflammatory hyperalgesia in mice. Proc Natl Acad Sci USA. 102(5): 1755–1760.
17. von Banchet GS, Boettger MK, Fischer N, Gajda M, Bräuer M, et al. (2009) Experimental arthritis causes tumor necrosis factor-a-dependent infiltration of macrophages into rat dorsal root ganglia which correlates with pain-related behavior Pain 145: 151–159.
18. Wei XH, Zang Y, Wu CY, Xu JT, Xin WJ, et al. (2007) Peri-sciatic administration of recombinant rat TNF-alpha induces mechanical allodynia via upregulation of TNF-alpha in dorsal root ganglia and in spinal dorsal horn: the role of NF-kappa B pathway. Exp Neurol 205(2): 471–84.
19. Jin X, Gereau RW 4th (2006) Acute p38-mediated modulation of tetrodotoxin-resistant sodium channels in mouse sensory neurons by tumor necrosis factor-alpha. J Neurosci 26: 246–255.
20. Nicol GD, Lopshire JC, Pafford CM (1997) Tumor necrosis factor enhances the capsaicin sensitivity of rat sensory neurons. J Neurosci 17: 975–982.
21. Kawasaki Y, Zhang L, Cheng JK, Ji RR (2008) Cytokine mechanisms of central sensitization: distinct and overlapping role of interleukin-1b, interleukin-6, and tumor necrosis factor-α in regulating synaptic and neuronal activity in the superficial spinal cord. J Neurosci 28: 5189–5194.
22. Watkins LR, Maier SF (2004) Targeting glia to control clinical pain: an idea whose time has come. Drug Discov Today Ther Strat 1: 83–88.
23. Tributino JLM, Santos MLH, Mesquita CM, Lima CKF, Silva LL, et al. (2010) LASSBio-881: an N-acylhydrazone transient receptor potential vanilloid subfamily type 1 antagonist orally effective against the hyperalgesia induced by capsaicin or partial sciatic ligation. Br J Pharmacol 159: 1716–1723.
24. Lavich TR, Cordeiro RS, Silva PM, Martins MA (2005) A novel hot-plate test sensitive to hyperalgesic stimuli and non-opioid analgesics. Braz J Med Biol Res 38(3): 445–51.

25. Bradley PP, Priebat DA, Christensen RD, Rothstein G (1982) Measurement of cutaneous inflammation: estimation of neutrophils content with an enzyme marker. J Invest Dermatol 78: 206–209.
26. Cunha TM, Verri WA Jr, Schivo IR, Napimoga MH, Parada CA, et al. (2008) Crucial role of neutrophils in the development of mechanical inflammatory hyperalgesia. J Leukocyte Biol 83(4): 824–832.
27. Gallily R, Yamin A, Waksmann Y, Ovadia H, Weidenfeld J, et al. (1997) Protection against septic shock and suppression of tumor necrosis factor alpha and nitric oxide production by dexanabinol (HU-211), a nonpsychotropic cannabinoid. J Pharmacol Exp Ther 283: 918–924.
28. Seltzer Z, Dubner R, Shir Y (1990) A novel behavioral model of neuropathic pain disorders produced in rats by partial sciatic nerve injury. Pain 43: 245–250.
29. Ulevitch RJ, Tobias PS (1995) Receptor-dependent mechanisms of cell stimulation by bacterial endotoxin. Annu Rev Immunol 13: 437–57.
30. Lehto SG, Tamir R, Deng H, Klionsky L, Kuang R, et al. (2008) Antihyperalgesic effects of (R,E)-N-(2-Hydroxy-2,3-dihydro-1H-inden-4-yl)-3-(2-(piperidin-1-yl)-4-(trifluoromethyl)phenyl)-acrylamide (AMG8562), a novel transient receptor potential vanilloid type 1 modulator that does not cause hyperthermia in rats. J Pharmacol Exp Ther 326: 218–229.
31. Watabiki T, Kiso T, Tsukamoto M, Aoki T, Matsuoka N (2011) Intrathecal administration of AS1928370, a transient receptor potential vanilloid 1 antagonist, attenuates mechanical allodynia in a mouse model of neuropathic pain. Biol Pharm Bull 34(7): 1105–8.
32. Blum CA, Caldwell T, Zheng X, Bakthavatchalam R, Capitosti S, et al. (2010) Discovery of novel 6,6-heterocycles as transient receptor potential vanilloid (TRPV1) antagonists. J Med Chem 53(8): 3330–48.
33. Scholz J, Woolf CJ (2007) The neuropathic pain triad: neurons, immune cells and glia. Nat Neurosci 10(11): 1361–8.
34. Ledeboer A, Hutchinson MR, Watkins LR, Johnson KW (2007) Ibudilast (AV-411): a new class therapeutic candidate for neuropathic pain and opioid withdrawal syndromes. Expert Opin Investig Drugs 16: 935–950.
35. García-Martínez C, Humet M, Planells-Cases R, Gomis A, Caprini M, et al. (2002) Attenuation of thermal nociception and hyperalgesia by VR1 blockers. Proc Natl Acad Sci USA 99(4): 2374–2379.
36. Dubový P, Jancálek R, Klusáková I, Svízenská I, Pejchalová K (2006) Intra- and extraneuronal changes of immunofluorescence staining for TNF-alpha and TNFR1 in the dorsal root ganglia of rat peripheral neuropathic pain models. Cell Mol Neurobiol 26(7–8): 1205–17.
37. Hambleton J, Weinsteint SI, Lemt L, DeFranco AI (1996) Activation of c-Jun N-terminal kinase in bacterial lipopolysaccharide-stimulated macrophages. Proc Natl Acad Sci USA 93: 2774–2778.
38. Lee JC, Laydon JT, McDonnell PC, Gallagher TF, Kumar S, et al. (1994) A protein kinase involved in the regulation of inflammatory cytokine biosynthesis. Nature 372: 739–746.
39. Miller RJ, Jung H, Bhangoo SK, White FA (2009) Cytokine and Chemokine Regulation of Sensory Neuron Function. Handb Exp Pharmacol 194: 417–449.
40. Badger AM, Bradbeer JN, Votta B, Lee JC, Adams JL, et al. (1996) Pharmacological profile of SB203580, a selective inhibitor of cytokine suppressive binding protein/p38 kinase, in animal models of arthritis, bone resorption, endotoxin shock and immune function. J Pharmacol Exp Ther 279: 1453–1461.
41. Zwerina J, Hayer S, Redlich K, Bobacz K, Kollias G, et al. (2006) Activation of p38MAPK is a key step in tumor necrosis factor-mediated inflammatory bone destruction. Arthritis Rheum 54: 463–472.
42. Romanò CL, Romanò D, Bonora C, Mineo G (2009) Pregabalin, celecoxib, and their combination for treatment of chronic low-back pain. J Orthopaed Traumatol 10: 185–191.
43. Tsuji F, Murai M, Oki K, Seki I, Ueda K, et al. (2010) Transient receptor potential vanilloid 1 agonists as candidates for anti-inflammatory and immunomodulatory agents. Eur J Pharmacol 627: 332–339.
44. Wong GY, Gavva NR (2009) Therapeutic potential of vanilloid receptor TRPV1 agonists and antagonists as analgesics: Recent advances and setbacks. Brain Res Rev 60(1): 267–77.
45. Sena J, Liu Z (2008) Expression of cyclooxygenase genes and production of prostaglandins during ovulation in the ovarian follicles of Xenopus laevis. Gen Comp Endocrinol 157(2): 165–73

2

Inhibition of Fatty Acid Binding Proteins Elevates Brain Anandamide Levels and Produces Analgesia

Martin Kaczocha[1]*, Mario J. Rebecchi[1], Brian P. Ralph[2], Yu-Han Gary Teng[3], William T. Berger[3], William Galbavy[1], Matthew W. Elmes[2], Sherrye T. Glaser[4], Liqun Wang[2], Robert C. Rizzo[5], Dale G. Deutsch[2], Iwao Ojima[3]

1 Department of Anesthesiology, Stony Brook University, Stony Brook, New York, United States of America, **2** Department of Biochemistry and Cell Biology, Stony Brook University, Stony Brook, New York, United States of America, **3** Department of Chemistry and the Institute of Chemical Biology and Drug Discovery, Stony Brook University, Stony Brook, New York, United States of America, **4** Department of Biological Sciences, Kingsborough Community College, Brooklyn, New York, United States of America, **5** Department of Applied Mathematics and Statistics, Stony Brook University, Stony Brook, New York, United States of America

Abstract

The endocannabinoid anandamide (AEA) is an antinociceptive lipid that is inactivated through cellular uptake and subsequent catabolism by fatty acid amide hydrolase (FAAH). Fatty acid binding proteins (FABPs) are intracellular carriers that deliver AEA and related N-acylethanolamines (NAEs) to FAAH for hydrolysis. The mammalian brain expresses three FABP subtypes: FABP3, FABP5, and FABP7. Recent work from our group has revealed that pharmacological inhibition of FABPs reduces inflammatory pain in mice. The goal of the current work was to explore the effects of FABP inhibition upon nociception in diverse models of pain. We developed inhibitors with differential affinities for FABPs to elucidate the subtype(s) that contributes to the antinociceptive effects of FABP inhibitors. Inhibition of FABPs reduced nociception associated with inflammatory, visceral, and neuropathic pain. The antinociceptive effects of FABP inhibitors mirrored their affinities for FABP5, while binding to FABP3 and FABP7 was not a predictor of *in vivo* efficacy. The antinociceptive effects of FABP inhibitors were mediated by cannabinoid receptor 1 (CB_1) and peroxisome proliferator-activated receptor alpha (PPARα) and FABP inhibition elevated brain levels of AEA, providing the first direct evidence that FABPs regulate brain endocannabinoid tone. These results highlight FABPs as novel targets for the development of analgesic and anti-inflammatory therapeutics.

Editor: Theodore John Price, University of Arizona, United States of America

Funding: This work was supported by National Institutes of Health grants DA035923, DA032232, and DA016419. The funders had no role in study design, data collection and analysis, decision to publish, or preparation of the manuscript.

Competing Interests: Stony Brook University has filed a patent on behalf of MK, WTB, RCR, DGD, and IO covering the compounds described in this manuscript. US Provisional Application 61/674,108: α and γ-Truxillic Acid Derivatives and Pharmaceutical Compositions Thereof. There are no further patents, products in development or marketed products to declare.

* E-mail: Martin.Kaczocha@Stonybrook.edu

Introduction

Fatty acid binding proteins (FABPs) comprise a family of small cytoplasmic lipid transport proteins [1]. FABPs are expressed in numerous tissues, including the central and peripheral nervous systems [2–6] and bind to a subset of endogenous ligands including fatty acids, retinoic acid, and N-acylethanolamines (NAEs) [7–10]. The endocannabinoid anandamide (AEA) is an NAE that activates cannabinoid receptors (CB) while palmitoylethanolamide (PEA) and oleoylethanolamide (OEA) signal through nuclear peroxisome proliferator-activated receptor alpha (PPARα) [11–13].

FABPs regulate a plethora of physiological processes including lipid metabolism, neurite outgrowth, inflammation, sleep, and neuronal signaling [14–20]. Consequently, modulation of FABP function may hold therapeutic promise for the treatment of diverse disorders. Indeed, genetic or pharmacological inhibition of FABPs protects against atherosclerosis, diet induced obesity, experimental autoimmune encephalomyelitis and ameliorates dyslipidemias [20–22]. These effects are mediated through distinct targets including kinases, PPAR gamma, and through attenuation of pro-inflammatory cytokine release [20,23–25].

We have previously demonstrated that FABP5 and FABP7 are capable of binding to NAEs including AEA and OEA and regulate their signaling and catabolism by fatty acid amide hydrolase (FAAH), the principal NAE hydrolyzing enzyme in mice [8,9,26]. Previous work has established that inhibition of FAAH potentiates NAE signaling at CB_1, CB_2, and PPARα receptors and produces antinociceptive and anti-inflammatory effects in models of visceral, inflammatory, and neuropathic pain [26–29]. Similar effects are observed following inhibition of monoacylglycerol lipase, the major enzyme that hydrolyzes the endocannabinoid 2-arachidonoylglycerol (2-AG) [30]. These data indicate that targeting endocannabinoids and NAEs may offer a therapeutic avenue for the treatment of pain and inflammation.

Recently, we developed a novel α-truxillic acid-based FABP inhibitor termed SBFI26 and demonstrated that pharmacological FABP inhibition reduced nociception and inflammation in the formalin and carrageenan models of pain [31]. Here, we evaluate three new analogs based on SBFI26 to determine how inhibition across FABP3, FABP5, and FABP7 would reduce nociception associated with models of visceral, inflammatory, and neuropathic pain. Furthermore, we examined the role of CB and PPARα receptors in these processes and determined whether FABP inhibition elevates NAE and endocannabinoid levels in mouse brain.

Materials and Methods

Ethics Statement

The experiments conducted herein conform to the National Institutes of Health Guidelines for the Care and Use of Laboratory Animals and were approved by the Stony Brook University Institutional Animal Care and Use Committee (IACUC #2011-1834).

Chemicals

12-NBD-stearate [12-*N*-methyl-(7-nitrobenz-2-oxa-1,3-diazo) aminostearicacid] was from Avanti Polar Lipids (Alabaster, AL). PEA, d_4-PEA, OEA, d_2-OEA, 2-AG and d_5-2-AG were from Cayman Chemical (Ann Arbor, MI). AEA and d_4-AEA were from R&D systems. [^{14}C]AEA (arachidonoyl-[1-^{14}C]ethanolamide, 60 mCi/mmol) was provided by the Drug Supply Program at the National Institute on Drug Abuse while [^{3}H]2-oleoylglycerol ([^{3}H]2-OG) was purchased from Perkin Elmer. Acetonitrile, chloroform, and methanol were of the highest possible purity and were obtained from Fisher Scientific.

Synthesis of SBFI26, SBFI50, SBFI60, and SBFI62

Synthesis of SBFI26 (alpha-2,4-diphenylcyclobutane-1,3-dicarboxylic acid mono-1-naphthyl ester). Alpha-truxillic acid (297 mg, 1.0 mmol) was suspended in thionyl chloride (3 mL), and one drop of DMF was added to the suspension. The reaction mixture was heated to reflux for 3 h. The excess thionyl chloride and DMF was removed *in vacuo* and truxillic acyl chloride was obtained, which was used directly in the subsequent reaction. To the solution of truxillic acyl chloride in THF (10 mL) was added drop wise the solution of 1-naphthol (120 mg, 0.84 mmol) in THF (5 mL) and pyridine (0.5 mL), and the reaction mixture was heated to reflux for 3 h. The reaction was quenched with addition of water (2 mL). The resulted solution was diluted with ethyl acetate (15 mL) and the aqueous layer was separated. The organic layer was dried over $MgSO_4$ and concentrated *in vacuo*. The crude product was purified by flashed column chromatography on silica gel using ethyl acetate/hexanes (10% → 25%) as eluent to afford alpha-truxillic acid mono-1-naphthyl ester as white solid (202 mg, 57%): m.p.: 192–193 °C; ^{1}H NMR (300 MHz, $(CD_3)_2CO$) δ 4.15 (dd, J = 10.4, 7.0 Hz, 1H), 4.56 (dd, J = 10.4, 7.0 Hz, 1H), 4.75–4.68 (m, 2H), 6.42 (d, J = 7.5 Hz, 1H), 7.65–7.24 (m, 15H), 7.72 (d, J = 8.2 Hz, 1H); ^{13}C NMR (300 MHz, $(CD_3)_2CO$) δ 41.650, 42.119, 45.416, 46.766, 117.932, 121.361, 125.251, 125.678, 126.270, 126.724, 126.849, 126.921, 127.396, 127.629, 127.826, 128.245, 128.271, 128.490, 128.754, 129.055, 134.473, 139.456, 170.680, 172.139; HRMS (ES) m/z calculated for $C_{28}H_{22}O_4$ + NH_4 $(M + NH_4)^+$: 440.1862, found 440.1856 (Δ -1.2 ppm).

Synthesis of SBFI50 (alpha-2,4-diphenylcyclobutane-1,3-dicarboxylic acid mono-2-naphthyl ester). Alpha-truxillic acid (297 mg, 1.0 mmol) was suspended in thionyl chloride (3 mL), and one drop of DMF was added to the suspension. The reaction mixture was heated to reflux for 3 h. The excess thionyl chloride and DMF was removed *in vacuo* and truxillic acyl chloride was obtained, which was used directly in the subsequent reaction. To the solution of truxillic acyl chloride in THF (10 mL) was added drop wise the solution of 2-naphthol (115 mg, 0.80 mmol) in THF (5 mL) and pyridine (0.5 mL), and the reaction mixture was heated to reflux for 3 h. The reaction was quenched with addition of water (2 mL). The resulted solution was diluted with ethyl acetate (15 mL) and the aqueous layer was separated. The organic layer was dried over $MgSO_4$ and concentrated *in vacuo*. The crude product was purified by flashed column chromatography on silica gel using ethyl acetate/hexanes (10% → 25%) as eluent to afford alpha-truxillic acid mono-2-naphthyl ester as white solid (175 mg, 52%): m.p.: 204–206 °C; ^{1}H NMR (300 MHz, $(CD_3)_2CO$) δ 4.15 (dd, J = 10.6, 7.2 Hz, 1H), 4.34 (dd, J = 10.6, 7.2 Hz, 1H), 4.71–4.58 (m, 2H), 6.58 (d, J = 8.8 Hz, 1H), 6.84 (s, 1H), 7.61–7.26 (m, 12H), 7.78–7.70 (m, 2H), 7.86 (d, J = 8.0 Hz, 1H); ^{13}C NMR (300 MHz, $(CD_3)_2CO$) δ 41.295, 42.022, 46.043, 46.768, 118.430, 121.305, 125.596, 126.457, 126.909, 127.250, 127.294, 127.635, 127.808, 128.184, 128.264, 128,606, 128.870, 131.389, 133.634, 139.244, 139.349, 148.374, 170.656, 172.154; HRMS (ES) m/z calculated for $C_{28}H_{22}O_4$ + NH_4 $(M + NH_4)^+$: 440.1864, found 440.1856 (Δ -1.8 ppm).

Synthesis of SBFI60 (alpha-2,4-diphenylcyclobutane-1,3-dicarboxylic acid mono-1-naphthyl amide). Alpha-truxillic acid (150 mg, 0.51 mmol) was suspended in thionyl chloride (3 mL), and one drop of DMF was added to the suspension. The reaction mixture was heated to reflux for 3 h. The excess thionyl chloride and DMF was removed *in vacuo* and truxillic acyl chloride was obtained, which was used directly in the subsequent reaction. To the solution of truxillic acyl chloride in THF (10 mL) was added dropwise the solution of naphthyl-1-amine (36 mg, 0.25 mmol) in THF (5 mL) and pyridine (0.2 mL), and the reaction mixture was heated to reflux for 3 h. The reaction was quenched with addition of 1 M HCl solution (2 mL). The resulted solution was diluted with ethyl acetate (15 mL) and the aqueous layer was separated. The organic layer was dried over $MgSO_4$ and concentrated *in vacuo*. The crude product was crystallized from ethyl acetate to afford alpha-truxillic acid mono-1-naphthyl amide as white solid (72 mg, 68%): m.p.: 198–200 °C; ^{1}H NMR (300 MHz, $(CD_3)_2SO$) δ 3.95 (dd, J = 10.4, 6.6 Hz, 1H), 4.20 (dd, J = 10.4, 6.6 Hz, 1H), 4.44 (m, 2H), 7.07 (d, J = 7.4 Hz, 1H), 7.24–7.47 (m, 14H), 7.65 (d, J = 8.1 Hz, 1H), 7.83 (d, J = 8.1 Hz, 1H), 9.81 (s, 1H), 12.11 (s, 1H); ^{13}C NMR (300 MHz, $(CD_3)_2SO$) δ 40.834, 42.202, 46.384, 47.840, 122.251, 123.442, 125.652, 125.756, 125.972, 126.280, 127.102, 127.166, 128.093, 128.211, 128.374, 128.435, 128.606, 128.701, 133.841, 133.950, 139.780, 140.511, 170.419, 173.592; HRMS (ES) m/z calculated for $C_{28}H_{23}NO_3$ + NH_4 $(M + NH_4)^+$: 440.1862, found 440.1856 (Δ -1.2 ppm).

Synthesis of SBFI62 (2,4-diphenylcyclobutane-1,3-dicarboxylic acid di-1-naphthyl amide). Alpha-truxillic acid (50 mg, 0.17 mmol) was suspended in thionyl chloride (1.5 mL), and one drop of DMF was added to the suspension. The reaction mixture was heated to reflux for 3 h. The excess thionyl chloride and DMF was removed *in vacuo* and truxillic acyl chloride was obtained, which was used directly in the subsequent reaction. To the solution of truxillic acyl chloride in THF (10 mL) was added dropwise the solution of naphthyl-1-amine (48 mg, 0.34 mmol) in THF (3 mL) and pyridine (0.2 mL), and the reaction mixture was heated to reflux for 3 h. The reaction was quenched with addition of 1 M HCl solution (2 mL). The resulted solution was diluted with ethyl acetate (15 mL) and the aqueous layer was separated. The organic layer was dried over $MgSO_4$ and concentrated *in vacuo*. The crude product was crystallized from ethyl acetate to afford alpha-truxillic acid di-1-naphthyl amide as white solid (75 mg, 82%): m.p.: >240 °C; ^{1}H NMR (300 MHz, $(CD_3)_2SO$) δ 4.34 (t, J = 7.74 Hz, 2H), 4.65 (t, J = 7.74 Hz, 2H), 7.09 (d, J = 7.4 Hz, 2H), 7.25–7.55 (m, 18H), 7.67 (d, J = 8.1 Hz, 2H),

7.83 (d, *J* = 8.1 Hz, 2H) 9.87 (s, 2H); ^{13}C NMR (300 MHz, $(CD_3)_2SO$) δ 41.358, 47.665, 122.340, 123.526, 125.656, 125.783, 125.972, 126.286, 127.155, 128.205, 128.473, 128.624, 128.674, 133.972, 140.425, 170.654; HRMS (ES) m/z calculated for $C_{38}H_{30}N_2O_2$ + H $(M+H)^+$:547.2386, found 547.2386 (Δ 0 ppm).

Drugs

SBFI26, SBFI50, SBFI60, and SBFI62 were synthesized as described above. Rimonabant, SR144528, PF-3845, and naloxone were kindly provided by the Drug Supply Program at the National Institute on Drug Abuse. GW6471 was from Sigma. All drugs were injected in a volume of 10 μl/g body weight.

Energy Scoring of SB-FI compounds with FABPs

Molecular mechanics-based interaction energy scores were computed using DOCK version 6.6. An energy grid for FABP7 (PDB: 1FE3) was previously generated with 6–9 Lennard-Jones exponents and at 0.3 Å resolution and re-docking of SBFI26 was performed [31] using the standard DOCK flexible ligand (FLX) protocol [32]. Additional target FABPs – FABP5 (PDB: 1B56), and FABP3 (PDB: 3RSW) – were aligned to FABP7 in UCSF Chimera [33] using protein backbone alpha-carbons resulting in RMSDs of 0.95 Å for FABP5 and 0.96 Å for FABP3, suggesting an overall good alignment. Structures and mol2 files of the α-truxillic acid analogs SBFI50, SBFI60, and SBFI62 were created from SBFI26 in UCSF Chimera preserving the binding pose from initial docking to the FABP7 grid. All four SB-FI ligands were then energy-minimized in each FABP pocket using parameters consistent with the DOCK rigid ligand (RGD) protocol [32]. Energy minimizations were performed in Cartesian space and with 6–12 Lennard-Jones exponents [34]. All calculations were performed on a Dell PowerEdge T110 server running Ubuntu version 12.04 and using an Intel quad-core CPU in the Rizzo laboratory (Dept. of Applied Mathematics and Statistics, Stony Brook University).

Binding of Inhibitors to FABPs

Inhibitory constant (K_i) values were elucidated utilizing NBD-stearate fluorescence displacement as described previously [9,31]. The tests were performed in 96-well plates containing inhibitors (0.1 – 50.0 μM), FABP, and NBD-stearate. Fluorescence intensity was measured with a FLUOstar OPTIMA spectrofluorometer with excitation and emission wavelengths of 460 and 544 nm, respectively. K_i values were derived from nonlinear regression analysis using the equation $K_i = IC_{50}/(1+([\text{NBD-stearate}]/K_d))$. Respective K_d values of 0.18, 0.16, and 0.22 μM for NBD-stearate with FABP3, FABP5, and FABP7 were determined previously [9].

Enzyme Assays

AEA and 2-OG hydrolysis was determined using modified protocols to those described previously [8,35]. Mice were injected with inhibitors (20 mg/kg, i.p.) and the brains and livers were harvested 60 min later. The tissue homogenates were subsequently incubated with 30 μM [^{14}C]AEA or 10 μM [^{3}H]2-OG for 30 min. Reactions were stopped with two volumes of chloroform:methanol (1:1) and the methanol phase was counted using a Beckman LS6500 scintillation counter.

Cytotoxicity

Cytotoxicity of the FABP inhibitors SBFI26 and BMS309403 were examined using the MTT [3-(4,5-dimethylthiazol-2-yl)-2,5 diphenyl tetrazolium bromide] colorimetric assay. HeLa cells were seeded into 96-well plates (15,000 cells/well) and incubated for 24 hours at 37°C in DMEM supplemented with 10% FBS, penicillin (100 U/mL) and streptomycin (100 μg/mL). The cells were subsequently washed with PBS and treated with serum-free DMEM containing 10 nM to 1 mM SBFI26, BMS309403, or 5 mM hydrogen peroxide as a positive control. Following a 24 hr incubation, the cells were washed with PBS and treated with MTT (0.5 mg/mL in PBS) for 4 hrs. The cells were subsequently solubilized using DMSO and the absorbance was read at 562 nm in a microplate reader.

Animals

Male C57Bl/6 mice (22–30 g, Taconic Farms) or male Fischer 344 rats (250–350 g, Taconic Farms) were used for all experiments. The animals were group housed at room temperature and kept on a 12:12 hour light:dark cycle with *ad libitum* access to water and food. The animals were habituated to the experimental room for one day before testing and at least two hours before each experiment. All experiments were approved by the Stony Brook University Institutional Animal Care and Use Committee. Unless otherwise stated, animals were euthanized with CO_2 and subsequently decapitated. The experimenter was blinded to the treatment condition of each animal.

Carrageenan-induced Paw Edema and Thermal Hyperalgesia

Paw edema was induced by injecting 1% λ-carrageenan (20 μl, in sterile saline) into the plantar surface of the left hind paw using a 30 gauge needle attached to a glass syringe (Hamilton Company). Paw diameters were measured before carrageenan injection and 4 or 24 hours after injection using digital electronic calipers (Fisher) and expressed to the nearest ± 0.01 mm. SBFI26, SBFI50, SBFI60, and SBFI62 were dissolved in DMSO:cremophor-EL:saline (4% DMSO:10% Cremophor-EL) and administered (20 mg/kg, i.p.) 60 min prior to injection of carrageenan. Receptor antagonists were injected 10 min before the inhibitors. Rimonabant and SR144528 (3 mg/kg, i.p.) were dissolved in ethanol:cremophor-EL:saline (1:1:18) while GW6471 (4 mg/kg, i.p.) was dissolved in DMSO:cremophor-EL:saline (2% DMSO:5% Cremophor-EL). Edema is reported as the change in paw diameter at 24 hr compared to the baseline. Thermal hyperalgesia was measured using the Hargreaves plantar apparatus (Ugo Basile) as previously reported [31].

Formalin Test

Mice were habituated to the observation chamber (Plexiglas box, 25 cm×25 cm×25 cm) for 30 min prior to formalin injection. Mice were administered FABP inhibitors 60 min prior to formalin. The animals subsequently received an injection of formalin (2.5% in saline, 20 μl) into the plantar surface of the right hind paw using a 30 gauge needle and were immediately placed back into the observation chamber and nocifensive behavior (time spent licking or biting the paw) was recorded for 60 min. Nocifensive behavior was scored during the first phase (0–5 min) and the second phase (~15–45 min) of the formalin test.

Acetic acid-induced Writhing

Mice were acclimated to the laboratory environment for at least two hours and were habituated to the testing chamber for 30 min prior to acetic acid challenge. SBFI26, SBFI50, SBFI60, and SBFI62 (20 mg/kg) were administered via the subcutaneous route 60 min before acetic acid. Rimonabant, SR144528, GW6471, and naloxone were given 10 min before the inhibitors via the subcutaneous route. The mice subsequently received an i.p.

injection of acetic acid (0.6% in sterile saline, 10 μl/g) and were placed in observation chambers. Abdominal stretches (marked by extension of the body and hind limbs) were counted for 20 min starting at 5 min post-injection.

Locomotor Activity

Mice received injections of SBFI26 (20 mg/kg, i.p.) and 60 min later were placed in an observation chamber (46×25×20 cm) demarcated with 7×7 cm grids. Locomotor activity was recorded for 5 min by a video camera suspended above the chamber and subsequently scored by an observer blinded to the treatment conditions. A grid crossing was scored when both hind legs of the animal crossed the border of each grid square.

Rectal temperature

Rectal temperature was measured at baseline and 90 min following vehicle or drug administration, by inserting a thermocouple probe 1.5 cm into the rectum and the temperature was read using a thermocouple meter (Kent Scientific).

Rat neuropathic pain model

Male Fisher 344 rats were habituated and pre-injury evoked responses were obtained. The Hargreaves test was used to assess thermal hyperalgesia [36]. Briefly, plexiglass enclosures were set atop a plexiglass platform and infrared source set at 50% power located under the platform was used as the heat stimulus (Ugo Basile). A 200 mW, 535 nm diode laser was mounted in an adjustable stand placed beneath the plexiglass platform, and was used as an alternative heat stimulus for some of the animals in this study. The latency time to hind paw lift during heating of the plantar surface was recorded. Five recordings were obtained on each hind paw with at least 2 min rest between measurements. The maximum time for exposure to the infrared or diode laser source was 30.5 s to avoid any possible tissue injury. For mechanical threshold measurements, the animal enclosures rested on a screen with mesh of 0.5 cm spacing. Following acclimation, an electronic von Frey Anesthesiometer (IITC Life Sciences) was applied with increasing pressure to the plantar surface of the hind paw until the animals lifted the hind paw. The number of grams of force applied by the probe to induce withdrawal was recorded. Five recordings were obtained on each hind paw with at least 3 min between measurements. For CCI surgeries, our procedure closely followed that reported previously [37]. Briefly, each animal received an i.p. injection of ketamine/xylazine (75 mg/kg and 10 mg/kg, respectively). The hind leg was surgically prepped and the anesthetized animal placed prone on an sterile towel over a heating pad. The temperature was monitored rectally. A skin incision was made mid-thigh with a medium curved scalpel and then scissors were used to expose the sciatic nerve. Approximately 1 cm of the main trunk proximal to the trifuraction was isolated and 4 strands of 4-0 chromic gut were tied around the nerve ~ 1 mm apart under magnification. In a modification of the original method, a 2-0 prolene strand was placed between the nerve and the gut to which the suture was tightened. The prolene strand was then removed. This prevented over tightening and reduced subsequent motor paralysis. The muscle layers were then reopposed and sutured, and surgical staples were used to close the skin. On post-injury days 7 through 10, heat and mechanical measurements were obained for the ipsilateral hindpaw of each CCI animal. Immediately following the post-injury measurements, animals were randomized and received i.p. injections of vehicle or 20 mg/kg SBI26 (DMSO:cremophor:sterile saline 1:1:2 by volume). Up to 0.8 ml of drug or vehicle was injected. The observer was blinded as to administration of drug or vehicle. Thermal and mechanical measurements were performed at 1 and 4 h post-injection. Data were normalized to pre-injury baseline measurements for each animal.

Pharmacokinetics

Mice were injected with SBFI26 (20 mg/kg, i.p.) and were subsequently rapidly euthanized by decapitation at the indicated time points. The brain was rapidly removed and submerged in liquid nitrogen while the blood was collected into a K_2-EDTA collection tube (Fisher). Plasma was isolated by centrifugation of the blood and 50 μl of the plasma was combined with 150 μl acetonitrile and centrifuged to remove the resulting protein pellet. Subsequently, 50 μl of water was added to 50 μl of the supernatant and 10 μl was injected for analysis into a Thermo TSQ Quantum Access Triple Quadrupole mass spectrometer (ThermoFisher). LC separation was achieved on a Luna C18 (150×2 mm) column. Mobile phase A consisted of 100% H_20 while mobile phase B was composed of 100% acetonitrile. The flow rate was 200 μl/min. A linear gradient was used and started at 50% B for 2 min, then ramped to 100% B in 8 min., with a 2 min hold at 100% B. The system was then equilibrated at 50% B for a cycle time of 20 min. The mass spectrometer was operated in the negative ion mode with the high voltage set at −3.5 kV. The sheath pressure was 20 and the capillary was set to 270 °C. Multiple reaction monitoring (MRM) was used with the transition *m/z* 421 to 277 at 29 eV as the quantitation channel, while *m/z* 421 to 205 at 17 eV was employed as a conformation channel. SBFI26 quantification was performed using an external calibration curve.

Lipid Quantification

Quantification of endogenous NAEs and 2-AG were performed as previously described with minor modifications [30]. Mice were rapidly euthanized by decapitation and their brains flash frozen in liquid nitrogen. The brains were subsequently thawed, weighed, and homogenized in 8 ml of 2:1:1 $CHCl_3$:MeOH:Tris (50 mM, pH 8) in the presence of 4 ng d_4-PEA, 4 ng d_2-OEA, 400 pg d_4-AEA, and 40 ng d_5-2-AG. Following centrifugation at 4°C, the organic layer was removed and brought up to 8 ml with the same buffer and centrifuged again. The resulting organic layer was dried down with argon and resuspended with 100 μl of 2:1 $CHCl_3$:MeOH and 10 μl was injected into the Thermo TSQ Quantum Access Triple Quadropole mass spectrometer. LC separation was achieved on a Gemini C18 (50×2 mm×5 μm) equipped with a Gemini C18 SecurityGuard precolumn (4 mm length ×2 mm internal diameter). Mobile phase A consisted of 95:5% v:v H_20:MeOH while mobile phase B was composed of 60:35:5 v:v:v *i*-PrOH:MeOH:H_2O and quantification was performed in the positive ion mode with the voltage set at 4 kV. 0.1% formic acid was added to assist in ionization. The sheath pressure was 30 and the capillary was set at 270 °C. The flow rate was 100 μl/min. The gradient started at 0% B and increased to 100% B over 15 min followed by an isocratic gradient of 100% B for 10 min, and was equilibrated for 15 min at 0% B.

PPARα Transactivation Assay

PPARα activation was performed in HeLa cells as previously described [9].

Statistical Analysis

Behavioral data are presented as means ± S.E.M. of at least 6 animals per group. Statistical significance between vehicle, inhibitor, and antagonist groups was determined using one-way

ANOVA followed by Dunnett or Tukey post hoc analysis as appropriate. For CCI measurements, the data were analyzed using repeated measured ANOVA followed by Tukey post hoc analysis. In all cases, differences of $p<0.05$ were considered significant.

Results

Design and *in vitro* Evaluation of FABP Inhibitors

The mammalian central nervous system expresses FABP3, FABP5, and FABP7 [38]. In a recent publication [31], we showed that pharmacological inhibition of FABPs with SBFI26, a compound with a high affinity for FABP5 and FABP7 reduced nociception in the formalin and carrageenan models of pain. To begin identifying the FABP subtypes mediating such antinociceptive effects, we designed three novel analogs of SBFI26 termed SBFI50, SBFI60, and SBFI62 (Fig. 1A), that display differential binding to FABP5 and FABP7. As an additional objective, the inhibitors were designed to exhibit limited binding to FABP3 because ablation of this protein has been previously shown to contribute to age-related cardiac hypertrophy [39].

SBFI50 was designed as a regioisomer of SBFI26 by coupling a 2-naphthol group with α-truxillic acid (Fig. 1A). In SBFI60, the ester bond between the α-truxillic acid and the naphthyl group of SBFI26 was replaced with an amide bond using naphthyl-1-amine. Computational analysis through energy-minimization suggested that although these three related inhibitors could be accommodated in the different FABP pockets as suggested by similar binding geometries (Fig. 1B), they would all possess higher affinities for FABP7 relative to FABP5 or FABP3 (Table 1). Encouragingly, these computational predictions showed a strong correlation (Figure 1C) with experimentally measured binding affinities (Table 2), suggesting the atomistic models employed in these studies can be used to explore different structure activity relationship series to optimize inhibitor potency.

Overall, compared to SBFI26, SBFI50 and SBFI60 possessed lower experimental affinities for FABP5, retained high affinities for FABP7, and were equally poor inhibitors of FABP3 (Table 2). Unexpectedly, SBFI60 proved to be an extremely weak inhibitor of FABP3 (K_i>10 μM), suggesting that this compound may represent a novel scaffold for the design of future FABP5 and FABP7 selective inhibitors. An additional inhibitor, a dinaphthylamide analog of SBFI60 termed SBFI62 was also evaluated. Here, both of the carboxylic acids of α-truxillic acid were fully functionalized (Fig. 1A). Because SBFI62 lacks the free carboxylate previously determined to be important for interaction affinity [31], it was expected to exhibit low affinity across the FABP3, FABP5, and FABP7 series. A series of energy minimizations for this analog revealed that the added bulkier naphthylamide group would not allow for a conserved binding geometry shared by the other three inhibitors tested, which would similarly suggest lower affinity (data not shown). Indeed, when tested experimentally, SBFI62 showed much lower binding affinity for FABP5 and especially for FABP7 (Table 2).

FABP Inhibitors Produce Antinociceptive Effects

The antinociceptive effects of the FABP inhibitors were examined using diverse models of nociception. In the carrageenan model of inflammatory pain, SBFI26 and SBFI50 (20 mg/kg, i.p.) reduced thermal hyperalgesia and paw edema while SBFI60 and SBFI62 were without effect (Fig. 2A). In the formalin model of inflammatory pain, SBFI26, SBFI50, and SBFI60 reduced the first phase of nociception while SBFI26 also reduced the second phase (Fig. 2B). Similar to the carrageenan model, SBFI62 was without effect. The antinociceptive effects of FABP inhibitors were also examined using the acetic acid writhing model of visceral pain. SBFI26 significantly reduced writhing induced by acetic acid while SBFI50, SBFI60, and SBFI62 were without effect (Fig. 2C). A dose response analysis revealed that SBFI26 exhibited near maximal efficacy at a dose of 20 mg/kg and increasing the dose did not significantly enhance the antinociceptive effects of this compound (Fig. 2D).

CB_1 and PPARα Receptors Mediate the Antinociceptive Effects of FABP Inhibitors

To examine the mechanism(s) mediating the analgesic effects of FABP inhibitors, mice were pretreated with the CB_1 antagonist rimonabant, the CB_2 antagonist SR144528, the PPARα antagonist GW6471, or the opioid receptor antagonist naloxone. Treatment of mice with rimonabant completely blocked the antinociceptive effects of SBFI26 in the acetic acid test (Fig. 2E), indicating that CB_1 receptors mediate the effects of SBFI26. Rimonabant also blocked the antinociceptive effects of the FAAH inhibitor PF-3845, which is known to produce CB_1-mediated analgesia by potentiating AEA signaling [40]. The antinociceptive effects of SBFI26 were also blocked by the PPARα antagonist

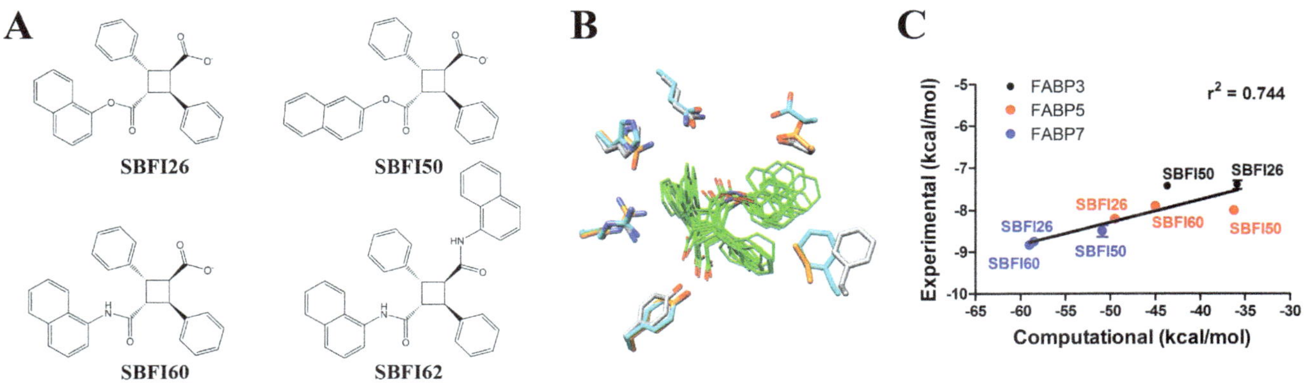

Figure 1. Structures and binding affinities of FABP inhibitors. (A) Chemical structures of FABP inhibitors. (B) Superimposed models of SBFI26, SBFI50, and SBFI60 in the binding pockets of FABP3, FABP5, and FABP7 reveal similar binding geometries. Amino acids lining the binding pockets are shown with teal, gold, and grey representing FABP3, FABP5, and FABP7, respectively. (C) Correlation between binding affinities and energy scores of SBFI26, SBFI50, and SBFI60 for FABP3, FABP5, and FABP7. Linear regression revealed an r^2 value of 0.744. The binding affinities and energy scores are derived from Table 1 and Table 2.

Table 1. Single-point energy calculations of inhibitors docked to FABPs.

Compound	FABP3	FABP5	FABP7
	(kcal/mol)	(kcal/mol)	(kcal/mol)
SBFI26	−35.85	−49.45	−58.44
SBFI50	−43.64	−36.20	−50.88
SBFI60	−37.30	−44.97	−58.95

GW6471 (Fig. 2E). In contrast, antagonism of CB_2 receptors with SR144528 or opioid receptors with naloxone failed to reverse the antinociceptive effects of SBFI26. As expected, administration of the antagonists in the absence of SBFI26 did not alter nociceptive responses.

FABP Inhibition Elevates Brain AEA Levels *in vivo*

The data presented thus far suggest that FABP inhibitors produce analgesia by potentiating endocannabinoid/NAE signaling. To examine this directly, we first determined the plasma and brain levels of SBFI26. Following i.p. injection, plasma and brain levels of SBFI26 peaked within one hour and gradually decreased over time (Fig. 3A). The compound displayed a plasma and brain half-life of approximately 3 hrs with levels returning to baseline by 24 hrs. As expected, the brain levels were lower than the plasma levels.

The brain levels of PEA, OEA, AEA, and 2-AG were examined following SBFI26 administration. Injection of SBFI26 significantly elevated AEA levels while the levels of PEA, OEA, and 2-AG were unaffected (Fig. 3B). SBFI26 did not inhibit AEA hydrolysis (Fig. 3C), excluding the possibility that it elevates AEA levels by inhibiting FAAH. Similar results were found with the other FABP inhibitors. Furthermore, we have previously demonstrated that SBFI26 does not activate CB_1 [31], indicating that its antinociceptive effects do not stem from direct activation of CB_1. This is further supported by the inability of SBFI26 to reduce locomotor activity or rectal temperature (Figs. 3D and 3E), effects that are observed following administration of CB_1 agonists [41,42]. Collectively, these data are the first to demonstrate that inhibition of FABPs elevates brain AEA levels to produce analgesia.

FABP Inhibitors Reduce Thermal Hyperalgesia Associated With Neuropathic Pain

To date, the antinociceptive effects of FABP inhibitors have been investigated in models of inflammatory pain. To ascertain whether FABP inhibitors reduce nociception associated with neuropathic pain, SBFI26 was administered to rats subjected to chronic constriction injury (CCI) of the sciatic nerve, a model of neuropathic pain. As expected, CCI rats developed thermal hyperalgesia and mechanical allodynia (Fig. 4A and B). Treatment with SBFI26 completely reversed thermal hyperalgesia at 1 hr post-administration with the effects persisting for up to 4 hrs (Fig. 4A). In contrast, SBFI50, which exhibits lower affinity for FABP5, was without effect (data not shown). Neither compound altered mechanical thresholds (Fig. 4B and data not shown).

Discussion

Chronic pain affects approximately fifteen percent of the population [43,44]. The endocannabinoid/NAE system has emerged as a promising target for the development of pain medications and cannabinoid receptor agonists have shown therapeutic efficacy in patients suffering from peripheral neuropathies [45–47]. However, cannabinoid receptor agonists suffer from untoward psychotropic effects [45,48], highlighting the need to develop novel non-narcotic analgesics that lack the side-effects and abuse potential of cannabinoid receptor agonists and other clinically used analgesics.

Our group has recently identified FABPs as intracellular endocannabinoid/NAE binding proteins [8,9]. Furthermore, we have demonstrated that pharmacological inhibition of FABPs produces antinociceptive effects that are mediated by cannabinoid receptors [31], suggesting that FABP inhibitors may reduce nociception by potentiating endocannabinoid signaling. To date, a direct demonstration that FABPs regulate endocannabinoid levels *in vivo* has not been reported. In addition, the development of FABP inhibitors as antinociceptive and anti-inflammatory agents requires demonstration of their broad efficacy in diverse models of pain. Here, we sought to begin addressing both of these outstanding questions.

In the current study, we show that inhibition of FABPs reduces nociception in models of inflammatory, visceral, and neuropathic pain. Of the inhibitors tested, SBFI26 was the most efficacious, followed by SBFI50 and SBFI60, with SBFI62 completely lacking efficacy. These results mirrored the experimental binding affinities

Table 2. Binding affinities of SBFI26, SBFI50, SBFI60, and SBFI62 to FABPs.

Compound	FABP3	FABP5	FABP7
	K_i (μM)	K_i (μM)	K_i (μM)
SBFI26	3.9±0.7	0.9±0.1	0.4±0.0
SBFI50	3.5±0.3	1.3±0.2	0.6±0.1
SBFI60	>10	1.6±0.0	0.3 ±0.0
SBFI62	2.6±1.1	3.3±0.7	6.1±0.5

The K_i values represent averages ± S.E. of three independent experiments.

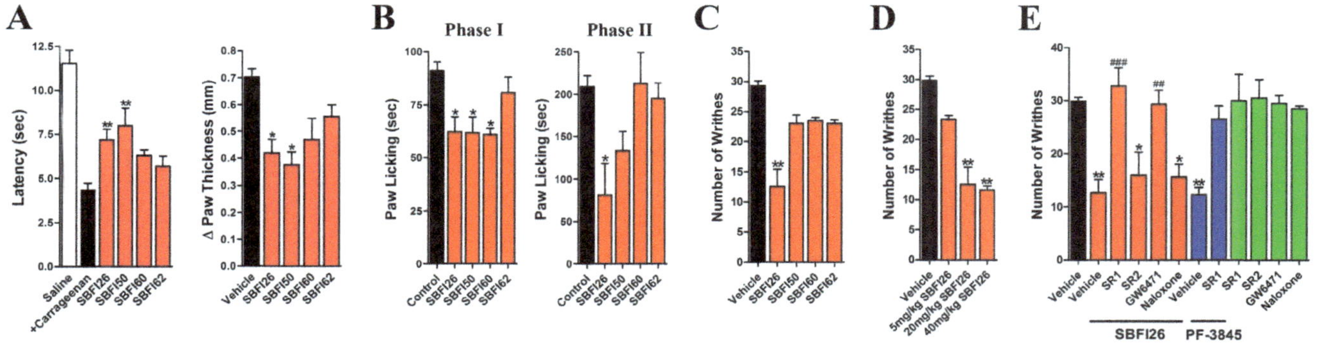

Figure 2. FABP inhibitors reduce nociception in models of inflammatory and visceral pain. (A) Effects of SBFI26, SBFI50, SBFI60, and SBFI62 (20 mg/kg, i.p.) upon carrageenan-induced thermal hyperalgesia (left panel) and paw edema (right panel) in mice. *, $p<0.05$; **, $p<0.01$ versus carrageenan injected animals (black bar) ($n=6$). (B) Effect of FABP inhibitors (20 mg/kg, i.p.) upon the first (left panel) and second phases (right panel) of formalin-induced nociception in mice. *, $p<0.05$ versus vehicle control ($n=6$). (C) SBFI26 reduces acetic acid-induced writhing in mice. **, $p<0.01$ ($n=6$). (D) Dose-response of SBFI26-mediated inhibition of acetic acid writhing in mice. **, $p<0.01$ ($n=6$). (E) The antinociceptive effects of SBFI26 are reversed by the cannabinoid receptor 1 antagonist rimonabant (SR1, 3 mg/kg) and the peroxisome proliferator-activated receptor alpha antagonist GW6471 (4 mg/kg). In contrast, the cannabinoid receptor 2 antagonist SR144518 (SR2, 3 mg/kg) and the opioid antagonist naloxone (2 mg/kg) were without effect. Rimonabant also reversed the antinociceptive effects of the FAAH inhibitor PF-3845 (blue bars). When administered alone, the antagonists did not modulate nociception (green bars). *, $p<0.05$; **, $p<0.01$ versus vehicle control. ##, $p<0.01$; ###, $p<0.001$ versus SBFI26 treated mice ($n=6$–9).

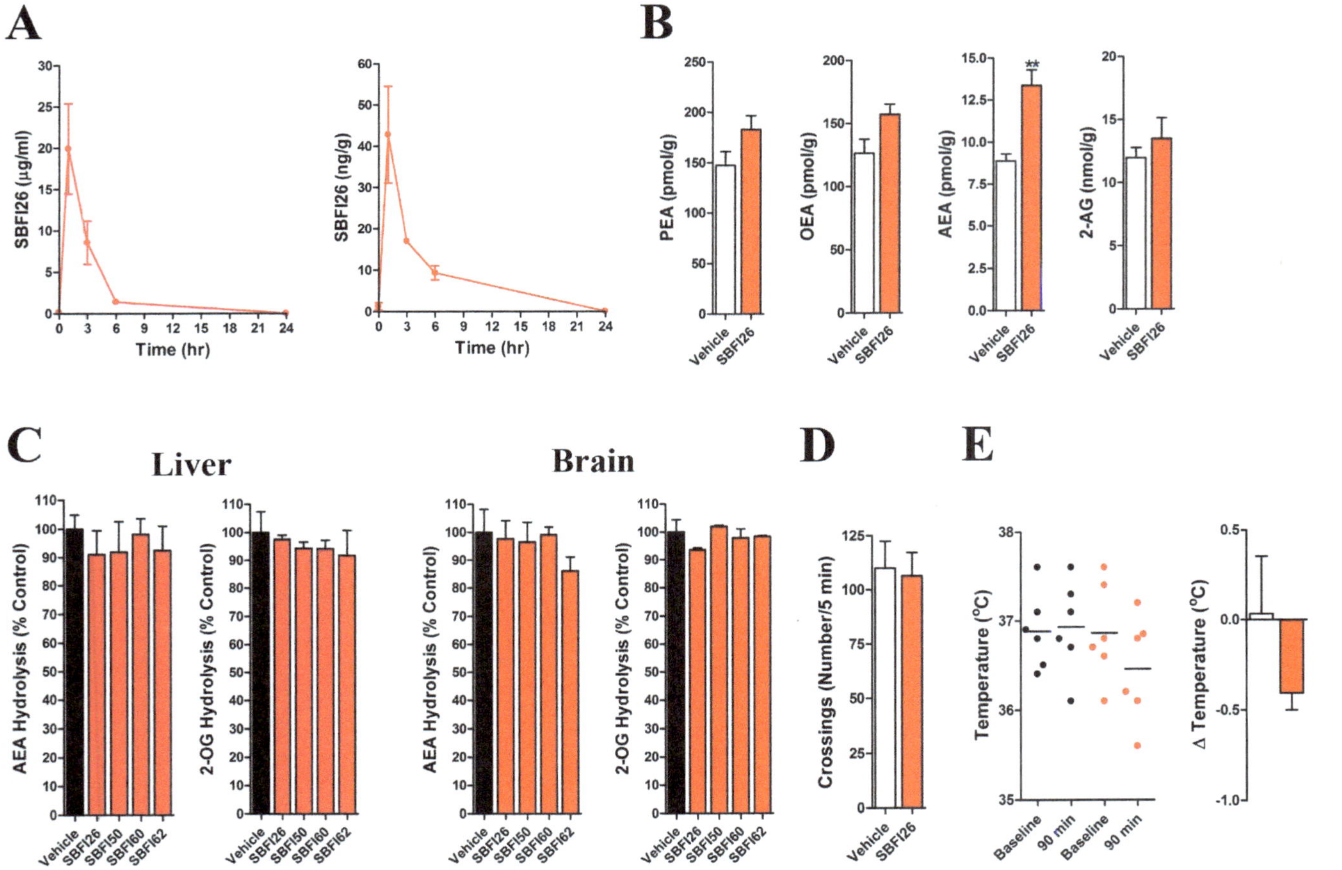

Figure 3. SBFI26 pharmacokinetics and its effect upon brain endocannabinoid levels. (A) Time course of SBFI26 levels in mouse plasma (left panel) and brain (right panel) following a single injection (20 mg/kg, i.p.) ($n=5$). (B) SBFI26 (20 mg/kg, i.p.) elevates brain levels of the AEA. Tissues were harvested 90 min after SBFI26 administration. **, $p<0.01$ ($n=6$). (C) Effect of FABP inhibitors (20 mg/kg, i.p.) upon AEA and 2-OG hydrolysis by mouse brain and liver homogenates following a single injection ($n=3$). (D) SBFI26 (20 mg/kg, i.p.) does not alter locomotor activity in mice. Locomotor activity was measured 90 min after SBFI26 administration ($n=6$). (E) SBFI26 (20 mg/kg, i.p.) does not reduce rectal temperature in mice. Left graph: scatterplot of rectal temperatures at baseline and 90 min following injection of vehicle (black circles) or SBFI26 (red circles). Right graph: change in rectal temperature between baseline and 90 min following administration of vehicle (white bar) or SBFI26 (red bar). Statistical analysis was performed by paired t-test ($p=0.205$) ($n=6$).

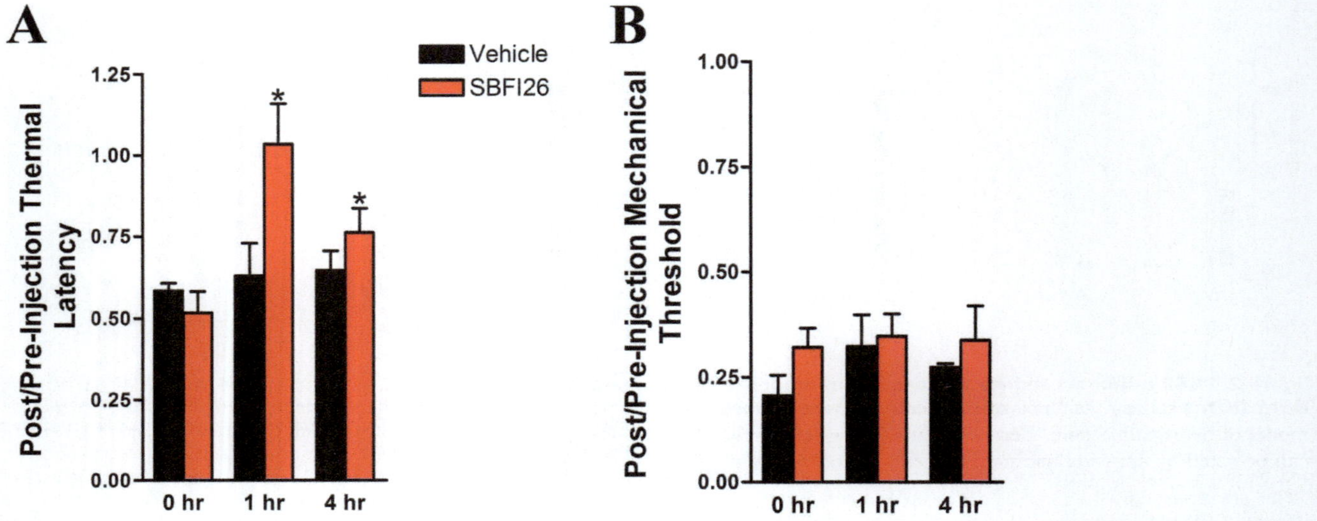

Figure 4. SBFI26 blocks thermal hyperalgesia in a rat model of neuropathic pain. (A) Thermal latencies and (B) mechanical thresholds in rats subjected to CCI were measured following injection of 20 mg/kg SBFI26. SBFI26 was injected at the 0 hr time point and evoked behaviors were measured at 1 and 4 hrs post-administration. The results are expressed as fraction of the pre-injury baseline measurement per animal (mean +/− SEM). Pre-injury thermal latency was 23.5 +/− 0.7 s and mechanical threshold was 29.9 +/− 0.6 g (mean +/− SEM). Results were analyzed by repeated measures ANOVA followed by Tukey's post-hoc analysis. *, $p<0.05$ versus 0 hr time point (n = 6).

of these compounds for FABP5 (Table 2), suggesting that high affinity binding to this protein may underlie the antinociceptive effects of FABP inhibitors. Indeed, SBFI50 and SBFI60, which exhibit lower affinity for FABP5 compared to SBFI26, were ineffective in the acetic acid test and similarly SBFI50 did not alter nociception in the CCI model. Furthermore, SBFI26, SBFI50, and SBFI60 bind to FABP7 with high affinity yet display markedly different *in vivo* efficacies, indicating that inhibition of FABP7 is unlikely to mediate the antinociceptive effects of these compounds. Future experiments employing mice lacking subsets of FABPs will be required to substantiate this hypothesis.

We have recently shown that AEA interacts with and is transported by FABPs to FAAH for catabolism [8,9]. Indeed, knockdown of FABP5 in cultured cells reduced AEA uptake and hydrolysis [9]. Our current results are in agreement with these studies and constitute the first direct observation that FABP inhibition elevates brain AEA levels *in vivo*. Given that FABPs exhibit a more restricted expression profile compared to the global expression of FAAH in the brain [49], our data suggest that FABPs may be major regulators of the AEA tone in a subset of brain regions.

NAEs activate diverse receptor systems, including cannabinoid and PPARα receptors [12,13]. In addition to AEA, FABPs bind to other NAEs [9], suggesting that the antinociceptive effects observed in FABP inhibitor treated mice may be mediated by

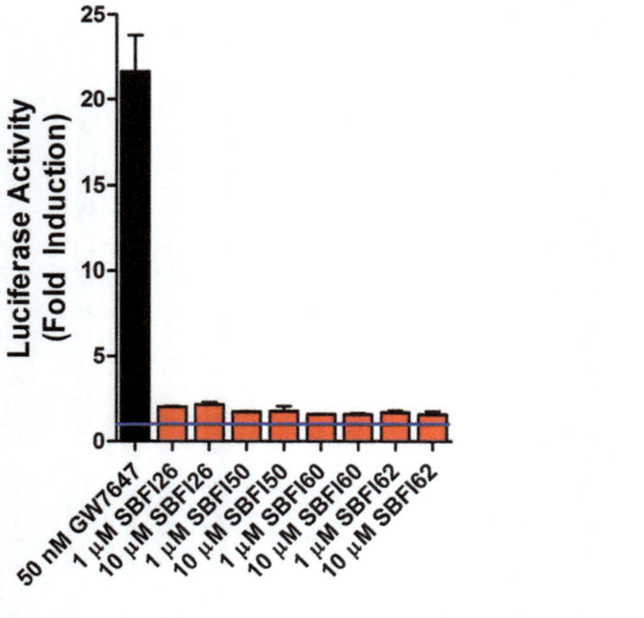

Figure 5. Activation of PPARα by FABP inhibitors. HeLa cells transfected with a PPARα reporter were incubated with the indicated compounds for 6 hours and luciferase and β-galactosidase activities were subsequently measured. Luciferase activity was normalized to β-galactosidase. The blue line represents baseline PPARα activation in the absence of agonists (n = 3).

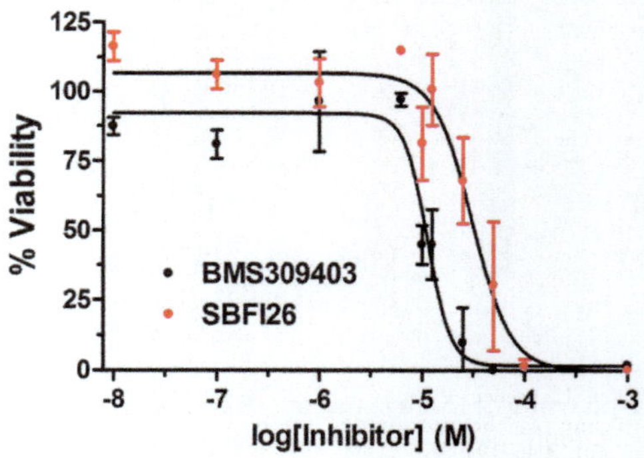

Figure 6. Cytotoxicity of SBFI26 and BMS309403 in HeLa cells. Cells were incubated with the indicated compounds and viability was assessed 24 hrs later. SBFI26 and BMS309403 reduced cell viability with IC_{50} values of 31.1±4.1 μM and 11.3±0.9 μM, respectively (n = 3).

NAEs that engage cannabinoid and/or PPARα receptors. Indeed, our findings demonstrate the involvement of CB_1 and PPARα receptors. It is noteworthy that inhibition of FABPs did not elevate PEA levels in mouse brains. Therefore, it is possible that the PPARα-mediated antinociceptive effects may stem from elevated PEA levels in peripheral nerves [29] or possibly in subsets of brain regions that regulate nociception, such that local changes in PEA levels may have eluded our analysis. Alternatively, FABPs may regulate the signaling of a lipid distinct from PEA that engages PPARα receptors. Lastly, it is unlikely that SBFI26 exerts its antinociceptive effects by directly activating PPARα. Indeed, while all four FABP inhibitors served as weak agonists at PPARα (Fig. 5), only SBFI26 exerted significant antinociceptive effects, which mirrors its higher affinity for FABP5.

Our findings also reveal that FABP inhibition modulates thermal hyperalgesia but not mechanical allodynia in the CCI model of neuropathic pain. Because heat and mechanical stimuli can be gated by non-overlapping peripheral sensory neurons [50–52], the selective modulation of heat sensitivity by FABPs may result from their expression in heat sensitive fibers and possibly their exclusion from mechanically-sensitive fibers. Alternatively, it is possible that greater CNS penetration of FABP inhibitors is required to modulate mechanical allodynia as reported for FAAH inhibitors [28].

In conclusion, our findings demonstrate that FABP inhibitors suppress nociception in multiple pain models, effects that are mediated by both CB_1 and PPARα receptors. Future medicinal chemistry efforts will be aimed at enhancing the potency, selectivity, and CNS penetration of FABP inhibitors. Because SBFI26 exhibits lower cytotoxicity compared to the previously described FABP inhibitor BMS309403 (Fig. 6) [53], inhibitors built upon this chemical scaffold may be better tolerated *in vivo*. Importantly, the compounds described herein weakly interact with FABP3, which may be advantageous as previous work has shown that mice lacking FABP3 develop age-dependent cardiac hypertrophy [39].

Acknowledgments

We would like to thank Robert Rieger at the Stony Brook Proteomics Center for help with mass spectrometry and Drs. Peter Glass and Helene Benveniste and the department of Anesthesiology for continued support. We would also like to thank Dr. Friedhelm Schroeder for advice regarding the NBD-stearate binding assay.

Author Contributions

Conceived and designed the experiments: MK MJR. Performed the experiments: MK MJR BPR WG MWE STG. Analyzed the data: MK MJR RCR DGD IO. Contributed reagents/materials/analysis tools: YHGT WTB LW. Wrote the paper: MK MJR BPR RCR DGD IO.

References

1. Furuhashi M, Hotamisligil GS (2008) Fatty acid-binding proteins: role in metabolic diseases and potential as drug targets. Nat Rev Drug Discov 7: 489–503.
2. De Leon M, Welcher AA, Nahin RH, Liu Y, Ruda MA, et al. (1996) Fatty acid binding protein is induced in neurons of the dorsal root ganglia after peripheral nerve injury. J Neurosci Res 44: 283–292.
3. Boneva NB, Mori Y, Kaplamadzhiev DB, Kikuchi H, Zhu H, et al. (2010) Differential expression of FABP 3, 5, 7 in infantile and adult monkey cerebellum. Neurosci Res 68: 94–102.
4. Boneva NB, Kaplamadzhiev DB, Sahara S, Kikuchi H, Pyko IV, et al. (2011) Expression of fatty acid-binding proteins in adult hippocampal neurogenic niche of postischemic monkeys. Hippocampus 21: 162–171.
5. Yamamoto T, Yamamoto A, Watanabe M, Matsuo T, Yamazaki N, et al. (2009) Classification of FABP isoforms and tissues based on quantitative evaluation of transcript levels of these isoforms in various rat tissues. Biotechnol Lett 31: 1695–1701.
6. Hawrylycz MJ, Lein ES, Guillozet-Bongaarts AL, Shen EH, Ng L, et al. (2012) An anatomically comprehensive atlas of the adult human brain transcriptome. Nature 489: 391–399.
7. Schug TT, Berry DC, Shaw NS, Travis SN, Noy N (2007) Opposing effects of retinoic acid on cell growth result from alternate activation of two different nuclear receptors. Cell 129: 723–733.
8. Kaczocha M, Glaser ST, Deutsch DG (2009) Identification of intracellular carriers for the endocannabinoid anandamide. Proc Natl Acad Sci U S A 106: 6375–6380.
9. Kaczocha M, Vivieca S, Sun J, Glaser ST, Deutsch DG (2012) Fatty acid-binding proteins transport N-acylethanolamines to nuclear receptors and are targets of endocannabinoid transport inhibitors. J Biol Chem 287: 3415–3424.
10. Hanhoff T, Lucke C, Spener F (2002) Insights into binding of fatty acids by fatty acid binding proteins. Mol Cell Biochem 239: 45–54.
11. LoVerme J, Russo R, La Rana G, Fu J, Farthing J, et al. (2006) Rapid broad-spectrum analgesia through activation of peroxisome proliferator-activated receptor-alpha. J Pharmacol Exp Ther 319: 1051–1061.
12. Lo Verme J, Fu J, Astarita G, La Rana G, Russo R, et al. (2005) The nuclear receptor peroxisome proliferator-activated receptor-alpha mediates the anti-inflammatory actions of palmitoylethanolamide. Mol Pharmacol 67: 15–19.
13. Devane WA, Hanus L, Breuer A, Pertwee RG, Stevenson LA, et al. (1992) Isolation and structure of a brain constituent that binds to the cannabinoid receptor. Science 258: 1946–1949.
14. Shioda N, Yamamoto Y, Watanabe M, Binas B, Owada Y, et al. (2010) Heart-type fatty acid binding protein regulates dopamine D2 receptor function in mouse brain. J Neurosci 30: 3146–3155.
15. Gerstner JR, Vanderheyden WM, Shaw PJ, Landry CF, Yin JC (2011) Fatty-acid binding proteins modulate sleep and enhance long-term memory consolidation in Drosophila. PLoS One 6: e15890.
16. Furuhashi M, Fucho R, Gorgun CZ, Tuncman G, Cao H, et al. (2008) Adipocyte/macrophage fatty acid-binding proteins contribute to metabolic deterioration through actions in both macrophages and adipocytes in mice. J Clin Invest 118: 2640–2650.
17. Cao H, Gerhold K, Mayers JR, Wiest MM, Watkins SM, et al. (2008) Identification of a lipokine, a lipid hormone linking adipose tissue to systemic metabolism. Cell 134: 933–944.
18. Hotamisligil GS, Johnson RS, Distel RJ, Ellis R, Papaioannou VE, et al. (1996) Uncoupling of obesity from insulin resistance through a targeted mutation in aP2, the adipocyte fatty acid binding protein. Science 274: 1377–1379.
19. Liu JW, Almaguel FG, Bu L, De Leon DD, De Leon M (2008) Expression of E-FABP in PC12 cells increases neurite extension during differentiation: involvement of n-3 and n-6 fatty acids. J Neurochem 106: 2015–2029.
20. Reynolds JM, Liu Q, Brittingham KC, Liu Y, Gruenthal M, et al. (2007) Deficiency of fatty acid-binding proteins in mice confers protection from development of experimental autoimmune encephalomyelitis. J Immunol 179: 313–321.
21. Furuhashi M, Tuncman G, Gorgun CZ, Makowski L, Atsumi G, et al. (2007) Treatment of diabetes and atherosclerosis by inhibiting fatty-acid-binding protein aP2. Nature 447: 959–965.
22. Maeda K, Cao H, Kono K, Gorgun CZ, Furuhashi M, et al. (2005) Adipocyte/macrophage fatty acid binding proteins control integrated metabolic responses in obesity and diabetes. Cell Metab 1: 107–119.
23. Erbay E, Babaev VR, Mayers JR, Makowski L, Charles KN, et al. (2009) Reducing endoplasmic reticulum stress through a macrophage lipid chaperone alleviates atherosclerosis. Nat Med 15: 1383–1391.
24. Hui X, Li H, Zhou Z, Lam KS, Xiao Y, et al. (2010) Adipocyte fatty acid-binding protein modulates inflammatory responses in macrophages through a positive feedback loop involving c-Jun NH2-terminal kinases and activator protein-1. J Biol Chem 285: 10273–10280.
25. Babaev VR, Runner RP, Fan D, Ding L, Zhang Y, et al. (2011) Macrophage Mal1 Deficiency Suppresses Atherosclerosis in Low-Density Lipoprotein Receptor-Null Mice by Activating Peroxisome Proliferator-Activated Receptor-{gamma}-Regulated Genes. Arterioscler Thromb Vasc Biol 31: 1283–1290.
26. Cravatt BF, Demarest K, Patricelli MP, Bracey MH, Giang DK, et al. (2001) Supersensitivity to anandamide and enhanced endogenous cannabinoid signaling in mice lacking fatty acid amide hydrolase. Proc Natl Acad Sci U S A 98: 9371–9376.
27. Lichtman AH, Shelton CC, Advani T, Cravatt BF (2004) Mice lacking fatty acid amide hydrolase exhibit a cannabinoid receptor-mediated phenotypic hypoalgesia. Pain 109: 319–327.
28. Booker L, Kinsey SG, Abdullah RA, Blankman JL, Long JZ, et al. (2012) The fatty acid amide hydrolase (FAAH) inhibitor PF-3845 acts in the nervous system to reverse LPS-induced tactile allodynia in mice. Br J Pharmacol 165: 2485–2496.

29. Clapper JR, Moreno-Sanz G, Russo R, Guijarro A, Vacondio F, et al. (2010) Anandamide suppresses pain initiation through a peripheral endocannabinoid mechanism. Nat Neurosci 13: 1265–1270.
30. Long JZ, Li W, Booker L, Burston JJ, Kinsey SG, et al. (2009) Selective blockade of 2-arachidonoylglycerol hydrolysis produces cannabinoid behavioral effects. Nat Chem Biol 5: 37–44.
31. Berger WT, Ralph BP, Kaczocha M, Sun J, Balius TE, et al. (2012) Targeting Fatty Acid Binding Protein (FABP) Anandamide Transporters - A Novel Strategy for Development of Anti-Inflammatory and Anti-Nociceptive Drugs. PLoS One 7: e50968.
32. Mukherjee S, Balius TE, Rizzo RC (2010) Docking validation resources: protein family and ligand flexibility experiments. J Chem Inf Model 50: 1986–2000.
33. Pettersen EF, Goddard TD, Huang CC, Couch GS, Greenblatt DM, et al. (2004) UCSF Chimera—a visualization system for exploratory research and analysis. J Comput Chem 25: 1605–1612.
34. Balius TE, Allen WJ, Mukherjee S, Rizzo RC (2013) Grid-based molecular footprint comparison method for docking and de novo design: application to HIVgp41. J Comput Chem 34: 1226–1240.
35. Dinh TP, Kathuria S, Piomelli D (2004) RNA interference suggests a primary role for monoacylglycerol lipase in the degradation of the endocannabinoid 2-arachidonoylglycerol. Mol Pharmacol 66: 1260–1264.
36. Hargreaves K, Dubner R, Brown F, Flores C, Joris J (1988) A new and sensitive method for measuring thermal nociception in cutaneous hyperalgesia. Pain 32: 77–88.
37. Bennett GJ, Xie YK (1988) A peripheral mononeuropathy in rat that produces disorders of pain sensation like those seen in man. Pain 33: 87–107.
38. Owada Y, Yoshimoto T, Kondo H (1996) Spatio-temporally differential expression of genes for three members of fatty acid binding proteins in developing and mature rat brains. J Chem Neuroanat 12: 113–122.
39. Binas B, Danneberg H, McWhir J, Mullins L, Clark AJ (1999) Requirement for the heart-type fatty acid binding protein in cardiac fatty acid utilization. FASEB J 13: 805–812.
40. Ahn K, Johnson DS, Mileni M, Beidler D, Long JZ, et al. (2009) Discovery and characterization of a highly selective FAAH inhibitor that reduces inflammatory pain. Chem Biol 16: 411–420.
41. Kinsey SG, Mahadevan A, Zhao B, Sun H, Naidu PS, et al. (2011) The CB2 cannabinoid receptor-selective agonist O-3223 reduces pain and inflammation without apparent cannabinoid behavioral effects. Neuropharmacology 60: 244–251.
42. Smith PB, Compton DR, Welch SP, Razdan RK, Mechoulam R, et al. (1994) The pharmacological activity of anandamide, a putative endogenous cannabinoid, in mice. J Pharmacol Exp Ther 270: 219–227.
43. Gaskin DJ, Richard P (2012) The economic costs of pain in the United States. J Pain 13: 715–724.
44. Turk DC (2002) Clinical effectiveness and cost-effectiveness of treatments for patients with chronic pain. Clin J Pain 18: 355–365.
45. Bestard JA, Toth CC (2010) An Open-Label Comparison of Nabilone and Gabapentin as Adjuvant Therapy or Monotherapy in the Management of Neuropathic Pain in Patients with Peripheral Neuropathy. Pain Pract.
46. Flachenecker P (2013) A new multiple sclerosis spasticity treatment option: effect in everyday clinical practice and cost-effectiveness in Germany. Expert Rev Neurother 13: 15–19.
47. Notcutt W, Langford R, Davies P, Ratcliffe S, Potts R (2012) A placebo-controlled, parallel-group, randomized withdrawal study of subjects with symptoms of spasticity due to multiple sclerosis who are receiving long-term Sativex(R) (nabiximols). Mult Scler 18: 219–228.
48. Cravatt BF, Lichtman AH (2004) The endogenous cannabinoid system and its role in nociceptive behavior. J Neurobiol 61: 149–160.
49. Egertova M, Cravatt BF, Elphick MR (2003) Comparative analysis of fatty acid amide hydrolase and cb(1) cannabinoid receptor expression in the mouse brain: evidence of a widespread role for fatty acid amide hydrolase in regulation of endocannabinoid signaling. Neuroscience 119: 481–496.
50. Cavanaugh DJ, Lee H, Lo L, Shields SD, Zylka MJ, et al. (2009) Distinct subsets of unmyelinated primary sensory fibers mediate behavioral responses to noxious thermal and mechanical stimuli. Proc Natl Acad Sci U S A 106: 9075–9080.
51. Mishra SK, Tisel SM, Orestes P, Bhangoo SK, Hoon MA (2011) TRPV1-lineage neurons are required for thermal sensation. EMBO J 30: 582–593.
52. Abrahamsen B, Zhao J, Asante CO, Cendan CM, Marsh S, et al. (2008) The cell and molecular basis of mechanical, cold, and inflammatory pain. Science 321: 702–705.
53. Sulsky R, Magnin DR, Huang Y, Simpkins L, Taunk P, et al. (2007) Potent and selective biphenyl azole inhibitors of adipocyte fatty acid binding protein (aFABP). Bioorg Med Chem Lett 17: 3511–3515.

3

Multi-Indication Carbamazepine and the Risk of Severe Cutaneous Adverse Drug Reactions in Korean Elderly Patients: A Korean Health Insurance Data-Based Study

Ji Young Kim[1], Joongyub Lee[2], Young-Jin Ko[1], Ju-Young Shin[3], Sun-Young Jung[3], Nam-Kyong Choi[2], Byung-Joo Park[1,3]*

1 Department of Preventive Medicine, Seoul National University College of Medicine, Seoul, Republic of Korea, **2** Medical Research Collaborating Center, Seoul National University Hospital, Seoul, Republic of Korea, **3** Korea Institute of Drug Safety and Risk Management, Seoul, Republic of Korea

Abstract

Objective: To evaluate the risk of severe cutaneous adverse drug reactions (SCAR) after exposure to multi-indication antiepileptic drugs for in Korean elderly patients.

Methods: We used a nationwide database from the Korean Health Insurance Review and Assessment Service claims constructed for the monitoring of drug utilization among the entire Korean elderly population from January 2005 to June 2006. We identified cases of SCARs among inpatients aged ≥65 years and those newly diagnosed with erythema multiforme according to the International Classification of Diseases, 10th revision code (L51). Each case was matched to four controls for gender, age, and the first hospitalization date as the index date. The use of carbamazepine, gabapentin, lamotrigine, topiramate, phenobarbital, phenytoin, and valproate during a 60-day period before the index date was compared. A conditional logistic regression analysis was performed to calculate the odds ratios (OR) and 95% confidence intervals (CI) of SCARs for antiepileptic drug.

Results: We identified 286 cases of SCAR and 1,144 matched controls. Among the 25 patients who were prescribed antiepileptic drugs within 60 days of the index date. There were 11 cases (3.8%) of severe ocular manifestations, and most elderly patients were first-time or short-term users of antiepileptic drugs. Among the 10 cases of carbamazepine use, only 2 cases were prescribed carbamazepine for seizure. All antiepileptic drugs were associated with an increased SCAR risk (adjusted OR = 3.42, 95% CI: 1.75–6.63). The SCAR risk was highest in patients treated with carbamazepine (adjusted OR = 10.39, 95% CI: 2.64–40.86, for multi-indication; adjusted OR = 6.84, 95% CI: 1.55–30.10, for neuropathic pain).

Conclusion: Carbamazepine use was associated with a nearly 10-fold increase in severe cutaneous drug reactions in Korean elderly patients. This association was consistently high with SCAR patients who received carbamazepine for neuropathic pain.

Editor: Alfonso Carvajal, Universidad de Valladolid, Spain

Funding: This study was supported by a grant from the Korean Food and Drug Administration (07072KFDA224). The funders had no role in study design, data collection and analysis, decision to publish, or preparation of the manuscript.

Competing Interests: The authors have declared that no competing interests exist.

* E-mail: bjpark@snu.ac.kr

Introduction

Antiepileptic drugs including carbamazepine, valproate, phenytoin, and phenobarbital consistently increase the risk of severe cutaneous adverse drug reactions (SCARs) such as Stevens-Johnson syndrome (SJS) and toxic epidermal necrolysis (TEN) [1–3]. Nevertheless, the use of antiepileptic drugs has steadily increased in elderly patients. Antiepileptic drugs are prescribed for the treatment of diverse conditions including migraines, mood disorders, neuropathic pain, and epilepsy [4–6]. The use of antiepileptic drugs peaked in those aged 80–84 years in Australia [4] and according to the Norwegian Prescription Database constructed between 2004 and 2007, 24.5% of antiepileptic drugs users were elderly people (aged 60–102 years) [5]. Neuropathic pain such as post-herpes neuralgia, diabetic neuropathy, and central post-stroke pain, as well as post-stroke seizure and epilepsy are the most common reasons for antiepileptic drug use in the elderly [7,8]. Moreover, the clearance rate of most antiepileptic drugs in the elderly has decreased by approximately 20–40% [9].

Elderly patients are more vulnerable to adverse drug reactions than younger patients, because of multi-morbidity and polypharmacy [10,11]. These factors are important cause of hospital admissions in the elderly [12,13]. One study found that inpatients with adverse drug reactions (ADRs) were significantly older (median age, 76 years) than patients without ADRs (median age, 66 years) [13]. Most of the cutaneous ADRs are not life threatening, but they can be a major cause of poor quality of life among the elderly [14]. SJS and TEN have a high mortality rate of 20%–25%, and long-lasting sequelae including corneal

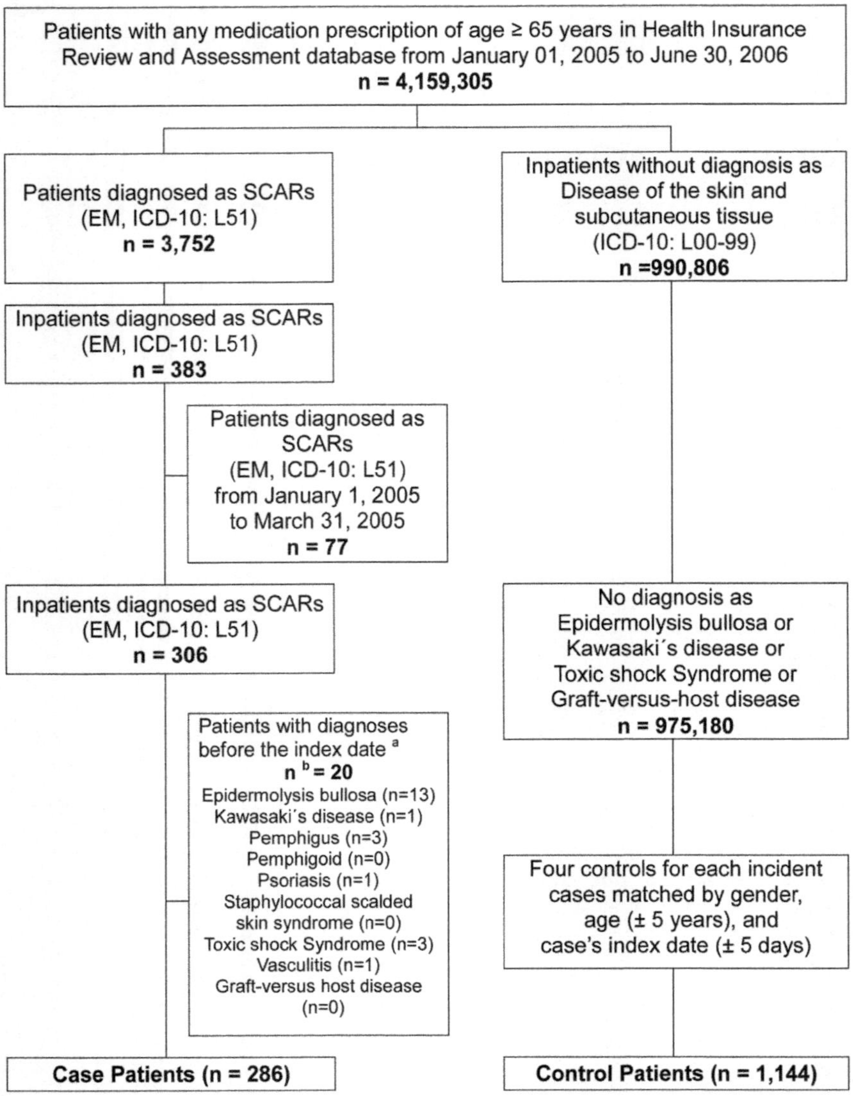

Figure 1. Sampling procedures of cases and controls. Abbreviations; EM, Erythema multiforme; SCARs, Severe cutaneous adverse drug reactions [a] Index date: The first SCAR (EM, ICD-10: L51) hospitalization date for the cases. [b] The sum of the numbers for the three exclusion criteria is greater than the total number because some patients met more than one exclusion criterion.

ulcerations represent a considerable disease burden [15]. Additionally, the mortality in SJS and TEN patients increased with age [16]. Recently, a 1-year follow-up study of patients with SCARs reported that high in-hospital mortality and after-discharge deaths were associated with older age [17].

There are few recent data on the epidemiology of SCARs in the elderly. Previous studies on SCAR were conducted across all age groups in the West, but did not specifically focus on the elderly. A recent SCAR study using the National Health Insurance database in Taiwan focused on bipolar disorders in middle-aged patients (mean age, 41 years) [18].

To our knowledge, there are no previous large-scale epidemiological studies of antiepileptic drug-related SCARs on the Korean elderly. In 2007, a nationwide database was constructed for monitoring drug utilization among the elderly in Korea. The aim of this study was to evaluate the risk of SCARs after exposure to multi-indication antiepileptic drugs in Korean patients aged ≥65 years. We conducted a case-control study based on the Korean Health Insurance Review and Assessment Service (HIRA) database constructed from January 1, 2005, to June 30, 2006.

Materials and Methods

Data Source

We used the Korean HIRA database of elderly patients aged ≥65 years, which was constructed between January 1, 2005, and June 30, 2006. The database contained information on 4,159,305 elderly patients aged ≥65 years and 100,838,744 prescriptions. The HIRA database contained information on the patients' de-identified number, age, gender, institutional region, diagnosis as per the International Classification of Diseases 10th Revision code (ICD-10 code), prescribed drug names, formulas, doses, prescription duration, and expenses [19]. The Korean National Health Insurance (KNHI) program was initiated in 1977 and achieved

Table 1. Characteristics of cases and controls (N = 1,430).

	Cases (n = 286)	Controls (n = 1,144)	*P*-value
Age (years, mean ± SD)	73.6±6.6	73.6±6.6	1.000
65–69	98 (34.3)	392 (34.3)	
70–74	74 (25.9)	296 (25.8)	
75–79	64 (22.4)	256 (22.4)	
80+	50 (17.5)	200 (17.5)	
Gender			1.000
Male	121 (43.3)	484 (43.3)	
Female	165 (57.7)	660 (57.7)	
Antiepileptic drugs			<0.001
Yes [a]	62 (21.7)	105 (9.2)	
Mono therapy	45 (15.7)	90 (7.9)	
Combination therapy	17 (5.9)	15 (1.3)	
No	286 (78.3)	934 (90.8)	
Charlson Comorbidity Index (mean ± SD)	2.0±1.5	1.4±1.3	<0.001
0	44 (15.4)	336 (29.4)	<0.001
1	80 (28.0)	357 (31.2)	
2	69 (24.1)	261 (22.8)	
3	45 (15.7)	122 (10.7)	
4 +	48 (16.8)	68 (5.9)	
Comorbidity [b]			
Cancer	31 (10.8)	105 (9.2)	0.392
Cerebrovascular disease	80 (28.0)	151 (13.2)	<0.001
Chronic pulmonary disease	92 (32.2)	323 (28.2)	0.190
Connective tissue/Rheumatic disease	29 (10.1)	55 (4.8)	0.001
Dementia	18 (6.3)	42 (3.7)	0.048
DM without complications	56 (19.6)	123 (10.8)	<0.001
DM with complications	41 (14.3)	104 (9.1)	0.009
Herpes viral infection	7 (2.5)	4 (0.4)	<.0001
Influenza	3 (1.1)	9 (0.8)	0.574
Mild liver disease	38 (13.3)	113 (9.9)	0.093
Myocardial infarction	11 (3.9)	23 (2.0)	0.068
Paraplegia or Hemiplegia	11 (3.9)	22 (1.9)	0.053
Peptic ulcer disease	78 (27.3)	274 (24.0)	0.244
Peripheral vascular disease	19 (6.6)	79 (6.9)	0.875
Renal disease	20 (6.7)	17 (1.5)	<0.001
AIDS/HIV infection	0 (0.0)	0 (0.0)	1.000
Others [c]	0 (0.0)	0 (0.0)	1.000
Major indications for antiepileptic drugs			
Bipolar disorder	1 (0.4)	2 (0.2)	0.563
Diseases of spinal cord	4 (1.4)	6 (0.5)	0.113
Neuropathy	42 (14.7)	122 (10.7)	0.056
Seizure	35 (12.2)	27 (2.4)	<0.001
Trigeminal neuralgia	13 (4.6)	31 (2.7)	0.108

Abbreviations; AIDS/HIV, acquired immune deficiency syndrome/human immunodeficiency virus; DM, diabetes mellitus; SD, standard deviation
Values are presented as number (%).
[a]Use of all antiepileptic drugs before the index day.
[b]Patients with more than one underlying disease.
[c]Other diseases, including histoplasmosis, mycoplasma pneumonia, and mumps.

Table 2. Estimates of SCAR risk from antiepileptic drugs within 60 days of index date (N = 1,345).

Antiepileptic drugs	Cases (n = 269)	Controls (n = 1,076)	cOR (95% CI)	aOR [b] (95% CI)
All †	25 (9.3)	30 (2.8)	3.72 (2.44–8.76)	3.40 (1.76–6.58)
Carbamazepine†	10 (3.7)	4 (0.4)	12.59[a] (3.22–71.52)	10.69 (2.75–41.57)
Gabapentin	7 (2.6)	22 (2.0)	1.29[a] (0.46–3.19)	1.13 (0.41–3.17)
Lamotrigine	1 (0.4)	0 (0.0)	4.00[a] (0.21–∞)	-
Topiramate	0 (0.0)	1 (0.1)	4.00[a] (0.00–76.00)	-
Phenobarbital	2 (0.3)	3 (0.7)	2.67[a] (0.22–23.27)	1.79 (0.21–15.49)
Phenytoin	4 (1.5)	0 (0.0)	21.14[a] (3.59–∞)	-
Valproate	1 (0.4)	1 (0.1)	4.00[a] (0.05–313.99)	8.89 (0.42–189.92)

Abbreviations; aOR, adjusted odds ratios; cOR, crude odds ratios; SCARs, severe cutaneous adverse drug reactions; 95% CI, 95% confidence interval
Values are presented as number (%).
[a]Odds ratios calculated by exact conditional logistic regression.
[b]Odds ratios adjusted for cerebrovascular disease, connective tissue/rheumatic disease, diabetes mellitus, herpes viral infection, seizure, renal disease, Charlson comorbidity index scores, previously highly suspected drugs (allopurinol, aminopenicillins, cephalosporins, imidazoles, macrolides, sulfonamides, tetracyclines and quinolones).
†P-value <0.001

universal coverage for the entire Korean population of approximately 50 million individuals by 1989 [20]. The HIRA provided de-identified patient claim data for the purpose of public health research. In the HIRA database, the positive predictive value (PPV) for the diagnosis of inpatients was 81.8% [21].

Ethics Statement

This study was approved by the Institutional Review Board of Seoul National University College of Medicine/Seoul National University Hospital (E-1305-036-487).

Definition of Case and Control Patients

Cases were defined as inpatients aged ≥65 years who newly diagnosed with erythema multiforme (ICD-10 code: L51) between April 1, 2005, and June 30, 2006 [18,22–24]. The first hospitalization due to erythema multiforme was defined as the index date for the case. To identify incident cases of SCAR, we excluded patients with pre-existing erythema multiforme during the preceding 3 months, from January 1, 2005, to March 31, 2005. Among them, patients diagnosed prior to the index date with epidermolysis bullosa (Q81), Kawasaki's disease (Q81), pemphigus (L10), pemphigoid (L12), psoriasis (L40), staphylococcal scalded skin syndrome (L00), toxic shock syndrome (A48.3), vasculitis (L95), or graft-versus-host disease (T86.0), according to the exclusion criteria of the European Registry of Severe Cutaneous Adverse Reactions (RegiSCAR) study, were also excluded in order to increase the validity of SCAR diagnosis [17,25]. Potential controls were selected among inpatients with no diagnosis of skin and subcutaneous tissue disease (L00–L99) during the study periods. The exclusion criteria in controls were also based on the same as the criteria used in the cases. The index date of control patients were defined as the date of hospital admission for treatment. For each incident case, four controls were matched by gender, age (±5 years), and index date (±5 days).

Exposure Assessment

Patients who were prescribed at least one antiepileptic drug before the index date were defined as the antiepileptic drugs prescription group. Seven antiepileptic drugs – carbamazepine, gabapentin, lamotrigine, topiramate, phenobarbital, phenytoin, and valproate – were selected as the exposure agents. Patients who were simultaneously prescribed different antiepileptic drugs during the research period were classified into the combination-therapy group, and those who were prescribed only one medication were classified into the mono-therapy group. The exposure period was defined as the prescription of antiepileptic drugs within 60 days before the index date. Previous studies reported that the risk of SCARs increases within 8 weeks following the first use of such drugs [3,18,26]. To estimate the time delay between the beginning of antiepileptic drug use and the occurrence of SCARs, the latent

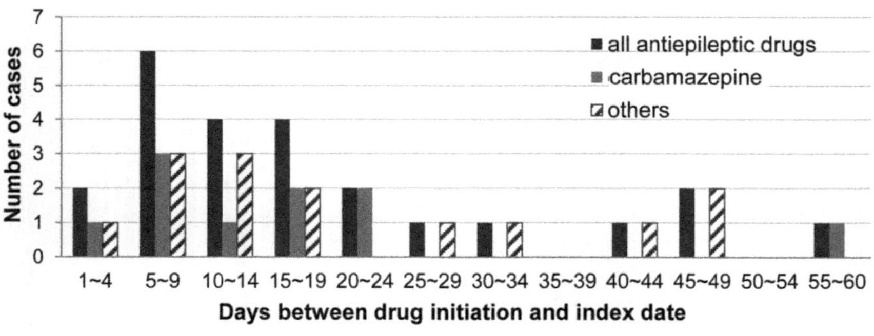

Figure 2. Distribution of latent periods for antiepileptic drugs.

Table 3. Duration of prescription and latent period before onset of SCARs in 25 cases. [a]

		Prescription duration (days)		Latent period (days)	
Antiepileptic drugs	**n**	**Mean ± SD**	**Median (Range)**	**Mean ± SD**	**Median (Range)**
All	25	19.3±14.0	15.0 (3–41)	19.1±15.2	16.0 (3–56)
Carbamazepine	10	20.5±14.3	17.0 (3–41)	17.3±15.4	15.0 (3–56)
Gabapentin	7	11.6±11.4	7.0 (3–31)	23.3±19.3	17.0 (4–49)
Phenobarbital	2	16.0±18.4	16.0 (3–29)	14.0±2.8	14.0 (12–16)
Lamotrigine	1	40.0		17.0	
Phenytoin	4	29.0±10.5	31.5 (15–38)	22.3±16.5	21.0 (5–42)
Valproate	1	8.0		8.0	

Abbreviations; SCARs, severe cutaneous adverse drug reactions; SD, standard deviation
[a]Cases with prescribed antiepileptic drugs within 60 days of index date.

period was defined as the duration between the date of the antiepileptic drug prescription and the index date. To evaluate the effect of short- or long-term use, the prescription duration was defined as the total period for which antiepileptic drugs were prescribed before the index date.

Confounding Factors

Information on confounding factors was collected using ICD-10 codes for diagnoses and drug prescriptions in the HIRA database. Cancer (C00-C97), connective tissue/rheumatic diseases (M05, M06, M32-M 34, M31.5, M35.1, M35.3, M36.0), herpes virus infection (B00), Human immunodeficiency virus (HIV) infection (B20–B24), influenza (J11), histoplasmosis (B39), and mycoplasma pneumonia (J15.7), which are non-medication risk factors for SJS or TEN, were included [3,26]. To adjust for the severity of accompanying diseases, Charlson Comorbidity Index scores were calculated [27]. In addition, bipolar disorder (F31), diseases of the spinal cord (G95), neuropathy (G56–G64, G99), trigeminal neuralgia (G50, G53), seizures (G40, G41, R56), cerebrovascular diseases (G45, G46, I60–I69, H34.0), diabetes mellitus (E10–E14), and renal diseases (N18, N19, N05.2–N05.7, N03.2–N03.7, Z49.0–Z49.2) were included as underlying diseases before the index date. Other concomitant medications such as acetate derivative non-steroidal anti-inflammatory drugs (NSAIDs), allopurinol, aminopenicillins, cephalosporin, imidazole, macrolide, oxicam NSAIDs, quinolones, sulfonamide, and tetracyclines, which are related to the risk of SCARs, were considered as confounding factors [28].

Statistical Analysis

The general characteristics of patients, including age, gender, prescription of antiepileptic drugs, comorbidities, and Charlson Comorbidity Index scores, were analyzed. Categorical variables are presented as numbers and percentages and continuous variables are presented as means and standard deviations (SD). For the continuous variables, we used the Wilcoxon signed-ranks test to compare means. Comorbidities of cases and controls were compared using the McNemar test. For each incident case, four controls were matched by gender, age (±5 years) and index date (±5 days) using the Greedy method. Because controls were matched individually, conditional logistic regression was used to assess the risk of SCARs after use of antiepileptic drugs. If exposure rate of the antiepileptic drug in the controls is assumed to be 2% and the odds ratios (OR), 3.0 based on results of previous studies, then on taking into account the 1:4 matched case-control study design, the appropriate number of study subjects was calculated to be 284 in the case group, which would yield a 80% statistical power and 5% significance. Univariate and multivariate conditional logistic regression analyses were performed to calculate the ORs and 95% confidence intervals (CI) of SCARs for each antiepileptic drug. For some antiepileptic drugs taken by few or no patients, we used the exact method for estimating ORs. Among comorbidities and co-medications previously established as risk

Table 4. Estimates of SCAR risk from carbamazepine.

	Cases	Controls	cOR (95% CI)	aOR [b] (95% CI)
Sensitivity analysis	**n = 269**	**n = 1,076**		
Latent periods less than 30 days[†]	9 (3.4)	3 (0.3)	12.00[a] (2.30–68.91)	9.91 (2.48–39.62)
Indications for neuropathic pain[†]	6 (2.2)	3 (0.3)	8.00[a] (1.71–49.44)	6.84 (1.55–30.10)
Subgroup analysis	**n = 134**	**n = 536**		
Diagnosis with SJS or TEN [†]	5 (3.7)	3 (0.6)	8.93[a] (1.43–95.07)	10.22 (1.64–3.60)

Abbreviations; aOR, adjusted odds ratios; cOR, crude odds ratios; SCARs, severe cutaneous adverse drug reactions; SJS, Stevens-Johnson syndrome; TEN, Toxic epidermal necrolysis; 95% CI, 95% confidence interval
[a]Odds ratios calculated by exact conditional logistic regression.
[b]Odds ratios adjusted for cerebrovascular disease, connective tissue/rheumatic disease, diabetes mellitus, seizure, renal disease, Charlson comorbidity index scores, previously highly suspected drugs (allopurinol, aminopenicillins, cephalosporins, imidazoles, oxicams NSAIDs, sulfonamides, tetracyclines and quinolones).
[†]*P*-value <0.001.

Table 5. Clinical features of 10 cases who prescribed carbamazepine within 60 days of SCARs.

No	Age/gender	Underlying diseases	Indications for CBZ	No of CBZ Prescription	Dose (mg/day)	Duration (days)	Co-medication	Latent period (days)	Acute complications
1	82/Female	HTN, OA	CVD, Trigeminal neuralgia	2	400	8	acetate NSAIDs, aminopenicillins, cephalosporins	3	ND
2	73/Female	HTN	CVD, Trigeminal neuralgia	2	200	38	acetate NSAIDs, oxicams NSAIDs	7	Pneumonia
3	73/Female	Dementia, UTI	ND	2	600	41	aminopenicillins, cephalosporins, sulfonamides	18	ND
4	69/Female	Asthma, HTN, Dementia, MDD, Chronic bronchitis	ND	1	400	11	None	56	Nephritis
5	68/Male	Asthma, COPD	Trigeminal neuralgia	3	400	34	cephalosporins, macrolides	6	ND
6	68/Female	Lumbar disc rupture	CVD, Seizure, Neuropathy	2	400	30	acetate NSAIDs, cephalosporins	23	ND
7	67/Female	Lung cancer, PU	Seizure	1	200	10	acetate NSAIDs, cephalosporins, macrolides	13	Bronchitis
8	67/Female	MDD, OA, Cervical disc disorder	Post-herpetic neuralgia	1	200	23	acetate NSAIDs, aminopenicillins, oxicams NSAIDs	23	ND
9	66/Male	Mild liver disease	Neuropathy	1	200	7	acetate NSAIDs, aminopenicillins, quinolones	7	ND
10	66/Female	Rheumatic disease, DM, PU	Neuropathy	1	200	3	cephalosporins, imidazoles, quinolones	17	Bronchitis

Abbreviations; CBZ, carbamazepine; COPD, chronic obstructive pulmonary diseases; CVD, cerebrovascular disease; DM, diabetes mellitus; HTN, hypertension; MDD, major depressive disorder; ND, not determined; OA, osteoarthritis; PU, peptic ulcer diseases;UTI,urinary tract infection.

factors, variables with p-values <0.2 in the univariate analysis were selected as potential confounders for the final multivariate model. Subgroup analyses were performed only for SJS (L51.1) or TEN (L51.2) with the four-digit ICD-10 codes to assess the validated patients with SCAR. Latent periods and prescription durations were calculated using both medians (range) and means (SD). All p-values of <0.05 were considered statistically significant, and all tests were two-tailed. All data were analyzed using SAS 9.3 (SAS Institute Inc., Cary, NC, USA).

Results

A flowchart of the inclusion and exclusion criteria is shown in Figure 1. Our study identified 286 cases and 1,144 matched controls. Table 1 shows the demographic characteristics and use of antiepileptic drugs for both groups before the onset of SCARs. There were 286 cases (121 men and 165 women), with a mean age ± SD of 73.6±6.6 years. Sixty-two (21.7%) cases and 105 (9.2%) controls received at least one antiepileptic drug before the index date. The proportion of antiepileptic drug prescriptions in the cases was significantly higher than that in the controls. The mean Charlson Comorbidity Index score was 2.0 ± 1.5 for cases and 1.4±1.3 for controls, and this difference was statistically significant. Underlying diseases such as cerebrovascular diseases, diabetes mellitus, seizures, and renal diseases were frequent among the cases ($p<0.001$). Similarly, the proportion of patients with connective tissue/rheumatic diseases and herpes virus infection was higher among the cases than the controls. Recent herpes viral infection within 3 months before the index date was reported in only 7 cases and 4 controls. No patients had HIV infection, histoplasmosis, mycoplasma pneumonia, or mumps. There were no statistically significant differences between the two groups in terms of the incidence of other diseases. Eleven (3.8%) cases were diagnosed with severe ocular complications: 2 with corneal ulcer, 2 with corneal ulcers and entropion, 2 with corneal scars and opacities, 2 with entropion, and 3 with visual impairment (table not shown).

Table 2 shows the risk estimates of SCARs associated with antiepileptic drugs, calculated by multiple conditional logistic regression analysis. We excluded the antiepileptic drug combination-therapy group, and the final analysis was based on 269 cases matched with 1,076 controls with prescriptions within 60 days of the index date. All antiepileptic drugs showed an increased risk of SCARs (adjusted OR = 3.42; 95% CI: 1.75–6.63). Among the antiepileptic drugs, carbamazepine was associated with the highest risk of SCARs (adjusted OR = 10.39; 95% CI: 2.64–40.86). For gabapentin, phenobarbital, and valproate, the adjusted ORs were 1.10, 2.10, and 8.89, respectively, but no significant association was observed. The risk estimate was consistent when analysis was restricted to patients without recent herpes viral infection. The adjusted OR was 3.69 (95% CI: 1.89–7.23) for all antiepileptic drugs (table not shown).

Figure 2 shows the distribution of the latent period in the 25 cases exposed to antiepileptic drugs within 60 days before the index date. Nineteen cases (76%) initiated their treatment less than 30 days before the index date. The median duration of latency (range) for all antiepileptic drugs was 16.0 (range, 3–56) days. The mean duration of prescription for all antiepileptic drugs was 19.3±14.0 days (Table 3). All 25 cases were short-term users (less than 60 days of antiepileptic drugs treatment), and 12 cases (48%) were new users with the first prescription of antiepileptic drugs given during the study period (table not shown).

A subgroup analysis was conducted for 134 cases with SJS or TEN selected using the four-digit ICD-10 codes. Among the 134 cases, 80.6% (n = 108) were classified as having SJS, 17.2% (n = 23) as having TEN, and 2.2% (n = 3) as having both SJS/TEN. The adjusted OR was 10.22 (95% CI: 1.64–63.60) for carbamazepine. The SCAR risk was consistently high in patients treated with carbamazepine for neuropathic pain (adjusted OR = 6.84, 95% CI: 1.55–30.10) (Table 4). Among the 10 cases of carbamazepine use, 8 patients were women; additionally, only 2 of the 10 cases were prescribed carbamazepine for seizure (Table 5).

Discussion

In elderly Korean patients, the use of antiepileptic drugs increased the risk of SCARs about three-fold as compared to patients who had not used antiepileptic drugs, and the use of carbamazepine was associated with the greatest increase in the risk of SCARs (adjusted OR = 10.69, 95% CI: 2.75–41.57). Among individual antiepileptic drugs, gabapentin, phenobarbital, and valproate increased the risk of SCARs, but this increase was not statistically significant.

The increased risk of SCARs associated with the use of antiepileptic drugs in the general population has been a consistent finding in several studies [18,26,28,29]. In 2008, one study using the database from Taiwan National Health Insurance showed that the use of carbamazepine and valproate as mood stabilizers increased the risk of SCARs (carbamazepine: adjusted OR = 3.10, 95% CI: 1.51–6.35; valproate: adjusted OR = 5.17, 95% CI: 1.26–5.92). In Taiwan, Gau et al. investigated patients with bipolar disorder only, and the mean age of the subjects was 41 years [18]. Therefore, we cannot make a direct comparison between the results of the study by Gau et al. and our results which focused on elderly patients. In France, the incidence of TEN was 2.7-fold higher among patients aged above 65 years than in those aged below 65 years. This study was performed 20 years ago with a relatively small sample size of only 77 patients [30]. In the pooled analysis of children aged <15 years, Levi et al. found that the crude OR was 91 (95% CI: 14–∞) for all antiepileptic drugs as a group and 15 (95% CI: 1.8–∞) for carbamazepine. However, Levi at al. reported 24 cases and only one control exposed to antiepileptic drugs (total, 80 cases and 216 controls), and therefore, they did not conduct multivariate analysis after adjusting for confounders [29]. According to the SCAR and EuroSCAR studies conducted in European countries, the multivariate relative risk (mRR) of carbamazepine was 12 (95% CI 3.5–38) [26] and 72 (95% CI: 23–225) [28], respectively.

Herpes infection has previously been reported to increase the risk of SCAR in the general population [31,32]. Our results show significant differences between cases and controls with recent herpes infection. Therefore, we conducted analysis after exclusion of patients with recent herpes infection and the risk of SCAR consistently increased. However, in children, recent herpes infection had no significant association with SCARs [29].

Our results did not find an association between SCARs and lamotrigine, topiramate, phenobarbital, phenytoin, and valproate in the elderly. Because of the small number of patients by each antiepileptic drug, our study did not have enough statistical power to identify certain SCAR risks. However, in the general population, these antiepileptic drugs have frequently been reported to increase the risk of SJS or TEN [1–3]. Our study did not show a significantly increased SCARs risk with the use of gabapentin. Gabapentin is usually considered a safe medication for patients with a genetic risk factor of carbamazepine-induced SJS [22] and only a few studies have reported an association between SJS or TEN risk and gabapentin use [33–35]. However, in 2011, the US FDA cautioned that potentially serious, multi-organ hypersensitivity, known as drug reaction with eosinophilia and systemic symptoms, has been reported following gabapentin use.

Patients with SJS or TEN frequently had ocular manifestations ranging from conjunctivitis to corneal ulceration [1], which significantly impaired their overall quality of life [36]. Yip et al. reported that 81 (69%) patients with SJS or TEN had ocular complications and 4% had severe ocular involvement during a median follow-up period of 2 months [37]. In our study, only 11 (3.8%) cases diagnosed with severe ocular complications.

Among 25 cases in our study, 13 (52%) patients were prescribed antiepileptic drugs for the first time during the study period. This finding is consistent with previous reports showing an increased risk of antiepileptic drug-induced SCARs, which was mostly observed in short-term or recent-start drug users in the general population [3,28]. In our study, the mean prescription duration for carbamazepine use was 20.5±14.3 days, which was similar to that for carbamazepine (27.4±14.3 days) in Taiwan [18]. Recently in Korea, Kim et al. reported that the mean treatment duration of carbamazepine was 25.9±15.1 days in 24 carbamazepine-induced SCAR patients [38]. The latent period in our study was defined as the time from the intake of antiepileptic drugs to the first hospitalization due to SCARs, and thus, the mean latent period was 19.1 days for all antiepileptic drug users and 17.3 days for carbamazepine users. The latent period in elderly patients with SCARs was not prolonged as compared to the results of studies in the general population. In the EuroSCAR study, the distribution of the latent period for carbamazepine was similar, ranging from 4 days to 28 days [28]. Yang et al. reported that among 154 SCARs patients, the latent period was 12.32±5.07 days for carbamazepine users and ≤27 days for antiepileptic drug users (lamotrigine, oxcarbazepine, phenobarbital, and phenytoin) [1]. In a recent study based on the EuroSCAR and RegiSCAR databases, Lee et al. showed that prior exposure to corticosteroids prolonged the period of latency before the onset of SJS and TEN [19]. In our analysis, there were only two cases of antecedent corticosteroid users (gabapentin exposure) as per the criteria of Lee et al., and therefore, the result of the latent period was minimally affected. In reality, a mean lag time of 3–3.9 days exists between the date of skin lesion occurrence and the date of hospitalization in children [29]. Therefore, it is reasonable to assume that skin reactions occur 3–4 days before the latent period, and this period can be important for prognosis improvement.

In the present study, a patient admitted to hospital and diagnosed with SJS or TEN with the four-digit ICD-10 codes was considered more valid and severe case, because recording of diagnosis with the four-digit ICD-10 code was not compulsory in Korean clinics during the study period. We applied subgroup analysis for 134 cases with SJS or TEN selected using the four-digit ICD-10 codes, and the results were as follows: for carbamazepine, adjusted OR = 10.22 (95% CI: 1.64–63.60). This result was similar to the result of the initial analysis. Among the 10 cases of carbamazepine use, only 2 patients were prescribed carbamazepine for seizure. Treating pain of neurologic origin was the most common indication of carbamazepine in our study. In Taiwan, peripheral neuropathy was the most frequent underlying disease in antiepileptic drugs-induced SCAR patients [1]. When sensitivity analysis was conducted after selecting cases of carbamazepine use for neuropathic pain, the adjusted OR was 6.84 (95% CI 1.55–30.10). As therapeutic indications have extended, antiepileptic drugs have been used more frequently in pain management [39]. In addition to its use in epilepsy, carbamazepine is also effective in many patients with chronic neuropathic pain [40]. However, carbamazepine is the most common causative agent for SJS or TEN in Southeast Asia, accounting for 26% of cases in Taiwan and 35.7% in Malaysia [41]. Our finding showed that patients who received carbamazepine for pain were consistently associated with risk of SCAR. Physicians should consider medications other than carbamazepine, especially when initiating therapy for pain in elderly patients.

The present study has several limitations. First, lifestyle factors of individual patients, such as smoking, alcohol drinking, family history, and past medical history before the study period were not available. However, the severity of comorbidities was adjusted in the analysis using the Charlson Comorbidity Index score. Moreover, other lifestyle factors are less affected because most SCARs are caused by medication or medical conditions. Second, we used a case-control design in our study. To avoid misclassification bias, the controls were selected from patients who were not hospitalized previously for skin diseases. Lastly, hospital inpatients were selected as controls for each case. Hospital-based controls are unlikely to be representative of the general population and may result in a selection bias because of different hospital admission rates. We compared the admission diagnosis and rate of our study subjects and that of the general population during the study period. The distributions of the admission diagnosis and rate for the controls were consistent with that of the national annual report on elderly patients in Korea.

Conclusions

In conclusion, the use of carbamazepine increased the risk of severe cutaneous adverse drug reactions by almost 10-fold in Korean elderly patients aged ≥65 years. This association was consistently high with SCAR patients of carbamazepine use for neuropathic pain. When prescribing carbamazepine for the first time to elderly patients, prodromal symptoms that may occur before the skin lesions should be assessed, and special care should be taken to achieve earlier diagnosis and referral in order to improve prognosis.

Author Contributions

Conceived and designed the experiments: JYK SYJ BJP. Performed the experiments: JYK JL YJK. Analyzed the data: JYK YJK JYS. Contributed reagents/materials/analysis tools: NKC BJP. Wrote the paper: JYK JL.

References

1. Yang CY, Dao RL, Lee TJ, Lu CW, Yang CH, et al. (2011) Severe cutaneous adverse reactions to antiepileptic drugs in Asians. Neurology 77: 2025–2033.
2. Mockenhaupt M, Messenheimer J, Tennis P, Schlingmann J (2005) Risk of Stevens-Johnson syndrome and toxic epidermal necrolysis in new users of antiepileptics. Neurology 64: 1134–1138.
3. Rzany B, Correia O, Kelly JP, Naldi L, Auquier A, et al. (1999) Risk of Stevens-Johnson syndrome and toxic epidermal necrolysis during first weeks of antiepileptic therapy: a case-control study. Study Group of the International Case Control Study on Severe Cutaneous Adverse Reactions. Lancet 353: 2190–2194.
4. Hollingworth SA, Eadie MJ (2010) Antiepileptic drugs in Australia: 2002–2007. Pharmacoepidemiol Drug Saf 19: 82–89.
5. Johannessen Landmark C, Larsson PG, Rytter E, Johannessen SI (2009) Antiepileptic drugs in epilepsy and other disorders-a population-based study of prescriptions. Epilepsy Res 87: 31–39.
6. Tsiropoulos I, Gichangi A, Andersen M, Bjerrum L, Gaist D, et al. (2006) Trends in utilization of antiepileptic drugs in Denmark. Acta Neurol Scand 113: 405–411.
7. Sheorajpanday RV, De Deyn PP (2007) Epileptic fits and epilepsy in the elderly: general reflections, specific issues and therapeutic implications. Clin Neurol Neurosurg 109: 727–743.

8. Ahmad M, Goucke CR (2002) Management strategies for the treatment of neuropathic pain in the elderly. Drugs Aging 19: 929–945.
9. Italiano D, Perucca E (2013) Clinical pharmacokinetics of new-generation antiepileptic drugs at the extremes of age: an update. Clin Pharmacokinet 52: 627–645.
10. Field TS, Gurwitz JH, Harrold LR, Rothschild J, DeBellis KR, et al. (2004) Risk factors for adverse drug events among older adults in the ambulatory setting. J Am Geriatr Soc 52: 1349–1354.
11. Green JL, Hawley JN, Rask KJ (2007) Is the number of prescribing physicians an independent risk factor for adverse drug events in an elderly outpatient population? Am J Geriatr Pharmacother 5: 31–39.
12. Shamliyan T (2010) Adverse drug effects in hospitalized elderly: data from the healthcare cost and utilization project. Clin Pharmacol 2: 41–63.
13. Pirmohamed M, James S, Meakin S, Green C, Scott AK, et al. (2004) Adverse drug reactions as cause of admission to hospital: prospective analysis of 18 820 patients. BMJ 329: 15–19.
14. Carneiro SC, Azevedo-e-Silva MC, Ramos-e-Silva M (2011) Drug eruptions in the elderly. Clin Dermatol 29: 43–48.
15. Rzany B, Mockenhaupt M, Baur S, Schroder W, Stocker U, et al. (1996) Epidemiology of erythema exsudativum multiforme majus, Stevens-Johnson syndrome, and toxic epidermal necrolysis in Germany (1990–1992): structure and results of a population-based registry. J Clin Epidemiol 49: 769–773.
16. Bastuji-Garin S, Fouchard N, Bertocchi M, Roujeau JC, Revuz J, et al. (2000) SCORTEN: a severity-of-illness score for toxic epidermal necrolysis. J Invest Dermatol 115: 149–153.
17. Sekula P, Dunant A, Mockenhaupt M, Naldi L, Bouwes Bavinck JN, et al. (2013) Comprehensive survival analysis of a cohort of patients with Stevens-Johnson syndrome and toxic epidermal necrolysis. J Invest Dermatol 133: 1197–1204.
18. Gau SS, Chao PF, Lin YJ, Chang CJ, Gau CS (2008) The association between carbamazepine and valproate and adverse cutaneous drug reactions in patients with bipolar disorder: a nested matched case-control study. J Clin Psychopharmacol 28: 509–517.
19. Lee J, Youn K, Choi NK, Lee JH, Kang D, et al. (2013) A population-based case-control study: proton pump inhibition and risk of hip fracture by use of bisphosphonate. J Gastroenterol 48: 1016–1022.
20. Choi NK, Chang Y, Jung SY, Choi YK, Lee J, et al. (2011) A population-based case-crossover study of polyethylene glycol use and acute renal failure risk in the elderly. World J Gastroenterol 17: 651–656.
21. Park BJ, Sung JH, Park KD (2003) Report of the evaluation for validity of discharged diagnoses in Korean Health Insurance database [in Korean]. Seoul: Seoul National University.
22. Chen P, Lin JJ, Lu CS, Ong CT, Hsieh PF, et al. (2011) Carbamazepine-induced toxic effects and HLA-B*1502 screening in Taiwan. N Engl J Med 364: 1126–1133.
23. Lin MS, Dai YS, Pwu RF, Chen YH, Chang NC (2005) Risk estimates for drugs suspected of being associated with Stevens-Johnson syndrome and toxic epidermal necrolysis: a case-control study. Intern Med J 35: 188–190.
24. Strom BL, Carson JL, Halpern AC, Schinnar R, Snyder ES, et al. (1991) A population-based study of Stevens-Johnson syndrome. Incidence and antecedent drug exposures. Arch Dermatol 127: 831–838.
25. Genin E, Schumacher M, Roujeau JC, Naldi L, Liss Y, et al. (2011) Genome-wide association study of Stevens-Johnson Syndrome and Toxic Epidermal Necrolysis in Europe. Orphanet J Rare Dis 6: 52.
26. Roujeau JC, Kelly JP, Naldi L, Rzany B, Stern RS, et al. (1995) Medication use and the risk of Stevens-Johnson syndrome or toxic epidermal necrolysis. N Engl J Med 333: 1600–1607.
27. Quan H, Sundararajan V, Halfon P, Fong A, Burnand B, et al. (2005) Coding algorithms for defining comorbidities in ICD-9-CM and ICD-10 administrative data. Medical Care 43: 1130–1139.
28. Mockenhaupt M, Viboud C, Dunant A, Naldi L, Halevy S, et al. (2008) Stevens-Johnson syndrome and toxic epidermal necrolysis: assessment of medication risks with emphasis on recently marketed drugs. The EuroSCAR-study. J Invest Dermatol 128: 35–44.
29. Levi N, Bastuji-Garin S, Mockenhaupt M, Roujeau JC, Flahault A, et al. (2009) Medications as risk factors of Stevens-Johnson syndrome and toxic epidermal necrolysis in children: a pooled analysis. Pediatrics 123: e297–304.
30. Bastuji-Garin S, Zahedi M, Guillaume JC, Roujeau JC (1993) Toxic epidermal necrolysis (Lyell syndrome) in 77 elderly patients. Age Ageing 22: 450–456.
31. Golden HE (1993) Stevens-Johnson syndrome associated with herpes simplex virus. Arch Intern Med 153: 1396.
32. Rzany B, Hering O, Mockenhaupt M, Schroder W, Goerttler E, et al. (1996) Histopathological and epidemiological characteristics of patients with erythema exudativum multiforme major, Stevens-Johnson syndrome and toxic epidermal necrolysis. Br J Dermatol 135: 6–11.
33. Gonzalez-Sicilia L, Cano A, Serrano M, Hernandez J (1998) Stevens-Johnson syndrome associated with gabapentin. Am J Med 105: 455.
34. DeToledo JC, Minagar A, Lowe MR, Ramsay RE (1999) Skin eruption with gabapentin in a patient with repeated AED-induced Stevens-Johnson's syndrome. Ther Drug Monit 21: 137–138.
35. Ma JE, Kim HS, Park DJ, Kim HC, Lee JD, et al. (2007) A Case of Stevens-Johnson Syndrome Induced by Gabapentin [in Korean]. Korean J Asthma Allergy Clin Immunol 27: 283–286.
36. Paquet P, Pierard GE (2010) New insights in toxic epidermal necrolysis (Lyell's syndrome): clinical considerations, pathobiology and targeted treatments revisited. Drug Saf 33: 189–212.
37. Yip LW, Thong BY, Lim J, Tan AW, Wong HB, et al. (2007) Ocular manifestations and complications of Stevens-Johnson syndrome and toxic epidermal necrolysis: an Asian series. Allergy 62: 527–531.
38. Kim SH, Lee KW, Song WJ, Jee YK, Lee SM, et al. (2011) Carbamazepine-induced severe cutaneous adverse reactions and HLA genotypes in Koreans. Epilepsy Res 97: 190–197.
39. Hall GC, Carroll D, McQuay HJ (2008) Primary care incidence and treatment of four neuropathic pain conditions: a descriptive study, 2002–2005. BMC Fam Pract 9: 26.
40. Wiffen PJ, Derry S, Moore RA, McQuay HJ (2011) Carbamazepine for acute and chronic pain in adults. Cochrane Database Syst Rev: CD005451.
41. Chung WH, Hung SI, Chen YT (2010) Genetic predisposition of life-threatening antiepileptic-induced skin reactions. Expert Opin Drug Saf 9: 15–21.

4

Glucocorticoid-Mediated Enhancement of Glutamatergic Transmission May Outweigh Anti-Inflammatory Effects under Conditions of Neuropathic Pain

Glenn-Marie Le Coz, Fernand Anton, Ulrike Hanesch*

Laboratory of Neurophysiology & Psychobiology, University of Luxembourg, Luxembourg, Luxembourg

Abstract

At the clinical level comorbidity between chronic pain and dysfunctional hypothalamus-pituitary-adrenal (HPA) axis is well established. We aimed to identify causal relationships in a model of neuropathic pain (chronic constriction injury, CCI) by studying the effects of glucocorticoid receptor agonist (dexamethasone) and antagonist (RU-486) administration on pain behavior and spinal biochemical mediators. Daily injections were performed in Sprague Dawley rats. Weight, plasma corticosterone levels and mechanical pain thresholds were assessed before and during 21 days post-CCI. At days four and 21 we investigated the mRNA expression of spinal mediators. In the dexamethasone-injected group, we observed a diminution of body weight and plasma corticosterone levels during the 21 days post surgery period and a more pronounced pain sensitivity until day 7 post-CCI. This enhanced pain sensitivity in the early period following nerve injury was accompanied by a transient increase of the glutamate receptors mGluR5 and NMDA at day 4. However, at this time point we did not observe any effect of the agonist/antagonist injections on the mRNA expression of pro-inflammatory cytokines. The RU-486-injected rats showed a slight mechanical hypoalgesia until 7 days post-CCI, but without any significant correlation with the expression of the measured markers. Our results indicate that glucocorticoid-related modulations of neuropathic pain processing may rather depend on a modification of glutamatergic transmission than on a change in pro-inflammatory cytokine expression.

Editor: Claudia Sommer, University of Würzburg, Germany

Funding: This work was supported by grant from the University of Luxembourg (F3R-INS-PUL-08MPMG and F3R-INS-PUL-11STPA). The funder had no role in study design, data collection and analysis, decision to publish, or preparation of the manuscript.

Competing Interests: The authors have declared that no competing interests exist.

* E-mail: ulrike.hanesch@uni.lu

Introduction

Comorbidities between chronic pain states and a dysfunctional hypothalamus-pituitary-adrenal (HPA) axis have repeatedly been described [1,2]. In this framework, research has mainly focused on relationships between adrenocortical reactivity and inflammatory pain states [3,4]. Recently, experimental studies have used pharmacological approaches to confirm that altered glucocorticoid processing may have a causal influence on pain sensitivity [5,6]. A reduced adrenocortical reactivity (relative hypocortisolism) that may e.g. be related to chronic exposure to stress may hence lead to an exacerbation of pain [7].

Under physiological conditions, the activation of the HPA axis leads to the production of glucocorticoids (GCs), steroid hormones that bind to two kinds of receptors, the mineralocorticoid receptors (MR) and the glucocorticoid receptors (GR) [8]. The GCs can act at the transcriptional level *via* the translocation of the complex GC-GR to the nucleus which will in turn lead to an enhancement or repression of the transcription of specific target genes [9,10]. The GCs are known to have an impact on neuropathic pain, especially through their GR receptor, which is upregulated after chronic constriction injury (CCI) [11,12]. Allodynia and hyperalgesia were prevented by a treatment with a GR antagonist, RU-486 while a GR agonist (dexamethasone) administration exacerbated the pain sensitivity in CCI rats [11].

In neuropathic pain models, an inflammatory component is involved, especially in CCI [13,14]. Potential effects of pro-inflammatory cytokines should hence be taken into account. Due to the activation of glial cells during central and peripheral sensitization, a release of pro-inflammatory cytokines having a major impact on neuronal activation, on glial cell activity and on the secretion of other factors from these cells has been observed. TNFα is known to be implicated in the initiation and maintenance of central sensitization [15] and to enhance neuronal sensitivity to thermal and mechanical stimulation [16]. Il-1β is well known to increase calcium conductance to the intracellular milieu through the NMDA receptor in nociceptive spinal cord neurons [17]. The GCs have powerful anti-inflammatory effects that could e.g. reduce the pain response *via* an inhibition of the release of the mentioned pro-inflammatory cytokines [18].

Additional biochemical pathways depending on glucocorticoids and significantly altering nociceptive processing have mainly been described in neuropathic pain models. The activation of GR can impact on the glutamatergic system through an upregulation of NMDA receptors and a downregulation of the excitatory amino-acid transporter EAAT3 [11,19,20]. In contrast to the inhibition of cytokine release and concomitant reduction of pain sensitivity, GR activation may hence also lead to an enhancement of glutamatergic transmission resulting in exacerbated nociceptive processing. In this case, the glucocorticoids play an important active role in central sensitization, participating in the initiation of neuropathic pain and facilitating the accumulation of extracellular glutamate [21]. In a normal configuration, glutamate is removed from the synaptic cleft by transporters located on neurons (EAAT3) and on glial cells (EAAT2). Besides the involvement of the ionotropic NMDA receptor, the metabotropic receptor mGluR5 has also been demonstrated to be implicated in the central sensitization induced by a CCI model of neuropathic pain [22].

The goal of the present pharmacological study was to investigate the impact of GC on spinal markers of nociceptive processing in a model of neuropathic pain. To mimic states of hyper- and hypo-cortisolism, we used daily administrations of GR agonists (dexamethasone) and antagonists (RU-486) in rats with chronic constriction injury.

We measured metabolic parameters, such as the weight and the plasma corticosterone levels, as well as the repercussion of these treatments on mechanical pain thresholds. Concerning potentially involved biochemical cascades, we investigated markers of the two opposite pathways described above. More specifically, we studied the mRNA expression of the pro-inflammatory cytokines TNFα and IL-1β, of ionotropic (NMDA, through its subunits NR1 and NR2a) and metabotropic (mGluR5) glutamate receptors as well as of the glial and neuronal glutamate transporters EAAT2 and EAAT3.

Materials and Methods

Animals

Experiments were performed in 50 adult 50–60 days old male Sprague Dawley rats weighing 207–382 g. Male rats were used to avoid effects of estrogens on glucocorticoid release. The animals (Harlan Laboratories, Netherlands) were housed three per cage in a temperature-controlled room (20–22°C) under a 12 h day-night cycle. Food and water were provided *ad libitum*. The body weight was regularly controlled. Starting two weeks before initiation of the experiments, the animals were handled daily and habituated to the behavioral testing room and devices. The Animal Care and Use Committee of the University of Luxembourg approved all animal procedures.

CCI surgery

For chronic constriction injury (CCI) surgery, all rats were anesthetized with isoflurane using an anesthesia unit (Univentor 400, Zejtun, Malta). The right sciatic nerve was exposed and three natural chromic gut 4–0 (Stoelting Europe, Dublin, Ireland) loose ligatures were placed around the nerve. The distance between two ligatures was 1 mm. The muscle layer was closed with 4–0 silk sutures and the skin layer was closed with surgical skin staples.

Experimental protocol

The rats were divided into three groups receiving daily injections of either dexamethasone (DEX, n = 16), or RU-486 (RU, n = 17) or vehicle (CON, n = 17) from two days before the surgery until the end of the experiment. Ten animals per group were sacrificed already 4 days after the CCI surgery to measure early changes in the expression level of spinal mediators. The remaining rats (DEX: n = 6, RU: n = 7, CON: n = 7) underwent a long term experiment. They were sacrificed at day 21 post surgery and their spinal cord was also examined for spinal mediator mRNA.

The course of the experiments was as follows: mechanical pain thresholds were assessed on three consecutive days (d-5, d-4 and d-3) to reveal baseline values (BS). The daily pharmacological treatment started at d-2 and on this day and the two following ones (d-2, d-1, d0) mechanical thresholds were also measured (baseline with injections, BSi) to test for drug effects. At d0 CCI surgery was performed and pain sensitivity measurements were done on days 4, and for the long term groups additional on days 7, 10, 14, and 21. Blood sampling was carried out on d-2 (BS), d0 (BSi) and on days 1, 4, and 7, 14 and 21 following CCI surgery. Animals were sacrificed after the experiments on day 4 or 21 and the spinal cord was removed and processed for qPCR. Weight, corticosterone levels and behavioral data of the animals sacrificed at day 4 were in the same range as those measured in the long term group. For this reason only the data covering the 21 days of experiment are presented.

Von Frey monofilament test

The Von Frey test was used to measure mechanical allodynia/hyperalgesia. Rats were placed in Plexiglas® cages with wire mesh bottoms and given 10 min to acclimate. Each monofilament (OptiHair, MarstockNervTest, Germany) was placed perpendicularly onto the midplantar region of the hind paw and pressure was increased until the point of deflection of the filament was reached. Pain thresholds were determined by the ascending and descending method of limits with forces ranging from 8 to 256 mN in 11 logarithmic steps [23]. Each test was repeated three times and the mean was calculated for each paw.

We set the values of the left unaffected side (control) to 100% and expressed the threshold of the right injured paw as a percentage of the left one.

Blood sampling and measurement of corticosterone levels

Blood sampling was performed in awake animals between 9 h and 9 h30, half an hour before the injections. To minimize stress reactions, rats were loosely held in a towel and then a small incision at about 15 mm from the end of the tail was performed using a scalpel. 300 μl of blood was collected with a capillary tube coated with EDTA (Microvette CB300, Sarstedt, Essen, Belgium). The samples were immediately placed on ice, then centrifuged for 10 min at 4°C and the plasma was removed and stored at −20°C.

Serum corticosterone levels were measured using an ELISA (Enzyme-Linked Immunosorbent Assay) kit (Assay Designs, USA). Analysis was done according to the manufacturer's protocol. Data were acquired via a plate reader (Sunrise Magellan, Austria) using an adequate software package (Magellan software, v6.4 standard, Austria).

Injections of dexamethasone, RU-486, or vehicle

The first day of injection (d-2) preceded the surgery by two days and the injections were repeated daily until the end of experimentation at d4 or d21. The groups received daily intraperitoneal injections of either dexamethasone, a GR agonist (dexamethasone 21-phosphate disodium salt, Sigma Aldrich, Germany), at a dose of 0.5 mg/kg/d dissolved in sterile saline 0.9%, or RU-486, a GR antagonist (mifepristone, Sigma Aldrich, Germany), at a dose of 4 mg/kg/d liquefied in olive oil containing 1% ethanol. The control group was treated either with olive oil containing 1% ethanol (8 animals) or saline 0.9% (9 animals). Since these two control groups did not differ in their results, we pooled the data. The daily injected volume was 0.2 ml. Injections were always performed at the same hour (10 am), 30 min before starting the behavioral tests.

Sample and RNA collection

At day 4 or 21 post surgery, rats were deeply anesthetized with isoflurane and decapitated. Levels L4/L5 of the spinal cord were removed and the total RNA was extracted with the Invitrap Spin Tissue RNA Microkit (Invitek, Germany). The RNA concentration was determined by measuring the absorbance at 260 nm, using a Nanodrop ND-2000 spectrophotometer (Thermo Fisher Scientific, Wilmington, U.S.A.).

Reverse transcription and Real-Time qPCR

Total RNA (500 ng) was reverse transcribed into cDNA using the ImProm-II Reverse Transcription System (Promega Corporation, Madison, USA). Real-Time PCR reactions were performed from 10 ng of cDNA with a CFX-96 thermocycler (Bio-Rad Laboratories, Nazareth, Belgium) using SYBR green Supermix PerfeCTa (95053–02K, Quanta Biosciences, Gaithersburg, MD, USA) and primers for the reference gene, β-actin, and the genes of interest presented in Table 1.

The steps consisted of one cycle of 3 min at 95°C and 40 cycles of amplification (10 sec at 95°C, 30 sec at 61°C). All samples were run in triplicate. Relative expression was estimated using the ΔΔCt- method [24] with β-actin as the reference. Threshold cycle values (CT) were used to compute the amount of target gene mRNA in relation to the reference gene mRNA (β-actin). ΔCT represents the difference between the number of cycles that were necessary to detect the PCR products of the target and the reference genes. The ΔΔCT indicates the difference between the ΔCT of the pharmacologically treated groups and the ΔCT of the vehicle treated (CON) animals. The data were expressed as $2^{-\Delta\Delta CT}$ and the mean of the right injured as well as of the left not affected side was computed for each group. Since we did not notice any significant differences in the relative expression levels, we only present the data for the right affected side of the spinal cord.

Statistical analysis

Statistical analyses for mechanical thresholds and qPCR were carried out using an analysis of variance (ANOVA) followed by a Scheffé *post hoc* test to identify differences between groups. Regarding the weight and corticosterone levels a Dunnett T3 *post hoc* test was used. $P<0.05$ was defined as the level of statistical significance. Statistical tests were performed with IBM SPSS Statistics version 19 (IBM corporation, Somers, NY, USA).

Results

Effect of GR-antagonist/agonist administration and CCI surgery on metabolism

The weight of the rats was followed up from 7 days before to 21 days post-CCI at different time intervals (Fig. 1). At the start of the experiment, at d-7, the mean weight was identical in all three groups (DEX: 289.83±18.25 g, RU: 297.33±20.18 g, CON: 291±18.15 g). A normal increase in weight was then observed at d-5 (DEX: 309.75±14.60 g, RU: 319.17±16.20 g, CON: 313.17±14.24 g).

With the start of the drug injections the animal weight in the DEX group decreased constantly, regardless of the CCI surgery, until the end of the experiment at d21 (248.27±10.33 g). In contrast, the rats in the RU group gained weight until d21 (355.75±11.05 g) in a time course comparable to the one seen for CON (d21: 361.83±10.03 g). In the two latter groups the nerve constriction on d0 only slightly slowed down the increase in weight.

Statistical analysis revealed a significant difference between the mean weight of DEX animals and CON from d4 ($p<0.05$) to d21 ($p<0.001$) and between DEX and RU rats from d7 ($p<0.01$) until the end of the experiment at d21 ($p<0.001$).

Table 1. Sequences of primers used in this study.

Name	Accession	Sequence
β-actin	NM_031144	5′ GCT GAG AGG GAA ATC GTG CGT GAC 3′
		5′ GGA GGA AGA GGA TGC GGC AGT GG 3′
EAAT2	NM_017215	5′ ATG CTC CTC ATT CTC ACA G 3′
	NM_001035233	5′ CTA CAT TGA CCG AAG TTC TC 3′
EAAT3	NM_013032.3	5′ TCA TAG TCG GGA AGA AC 3′
		5′ AGC GGA ATG TAA CTG GAA GG 3′
IL-1β	NM_031512	5′ GTT GAA TCT ATA CCT GTC CTG TG 3′
		5′ TGG TCT TGA CTT CTA TCT TGT TG 3′
TNFα	NM_012675	5′ GCT CTT CTG TCT ACT GAA CTT C 3′
		5′ GAT CTG AGT GTG AGG GTC TG 3′
mGluR5	NM_017012.1	5′ ACA ACC TCT ACA GTG GTA CG 3′
		5′ GGC CCA AGT CAC AGA TTT TC 3′
NR1	NM_001270607	5′ GGT TGC GTG GGC AAC ACC AA 3′
		5′ CCG TCC GCA TAC TTA GAA GA 3′
NR2a	NM_012573.3	5′ CAG ATA ACA ATA AGA ACC ACA AG 3′
		5′ AAC ATC GCT ACA GTC CTT 3′

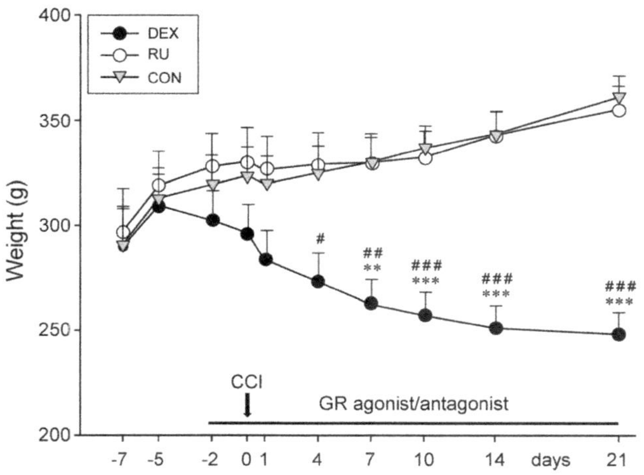

Figure 1. Animal weight changes following GR-agonist/antagonist treatment and CCI. Influence of daily injections of the GR agonist dexamethasone (DEX), the GR antagonist RU-486 (RU), or vehicle (CON) in combination with chronic constriction injury (CCI) on the rat weight. Administration of the GR agonist resulted in a constant loss of weight, unaffected by CCI surgery. GR antagonist or vehicle treated animals exhibited a normal gain of weight, only slightly slowed down by the CCI surgery. Data are shown as mean ± s.e.m. **$p<0.01$, ***$p<0.001$ indicate significant differences between DEX and RU and #$p<0.05$, ##$p<0.01$, ###$p<0.001$ represent significant differences between DEX and CON.

Alterations of plasma corticosterone concentrations in response to GR-antagonist/agonist injections and CCI surgery

The three groups of rats displayed comparable plasma corticosterone levels at d-5 before the administration of the GR-agonist or -antagonist (DEX: 219±41 ng/ml, RU: 209±28 ng/ml, CON: 173±21 ng/ml) (Fig. 2).

Injections of vehicle (CON group) did not alter the blood corticosterone levels *per se* (d-1: 159±22 ng/ml). The nerve injury on d0 however resulted in an increase of the corticosterone concentration from d1 (205±29 ng/ml) to the end of the experiment (d21: 273±55 ng/ml). In the DEX group the concentration of circulating corticosterone decreased following the administration of dexamethasone and persisted at this low level throughout the course of the experiment despite the CCI surgery. Compared to the CON animals the DEX group exhibited significantly lower corticosterone levels at d1 ($p<0.05$) and d14 ($p<0.01$) but not at d7 and d21.

In contrast, injections of the GR-antagonist RU-486 did not lead to alterations in blood corticosterone levels in the pre-surgery period (d-1: 216±19 ng/ml). However, the nerve constriction on d0 led to an increase in the concentration of circulating corticosterone measured on d1 (302±36 ng/ml). Throughout the course of neuropathy the levels remained enhanced. In comparison with the control group no significant differences were seen.

Comparing the DEX and RU groups statistically significant differences were observed at all time points after CCI surgery except at d14 (d1: $p<0.01$; d4: $p<0.01$; d7: $p<0.05$; d14: $p=0.129$; d21: $p<0.05$), confirming a strong effect of dexamethasone on the plasma corticosterone levels.

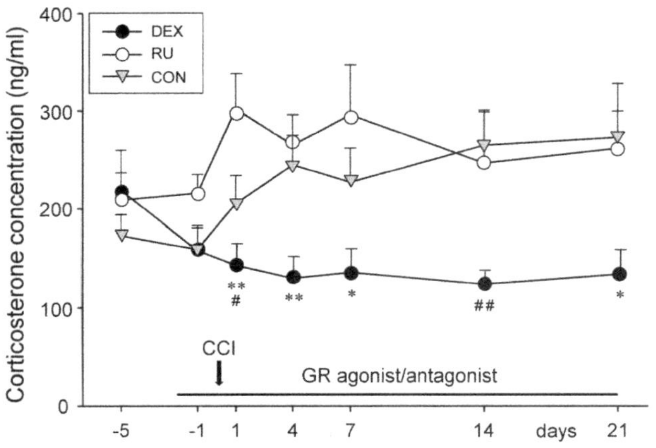

Figure 2. Changes in blood corticosterone concentration throughout drug administration and CCI periods. Despite CCI surgery, daily administration of the GR agonist dexamethasone (DEX) led to a slight decrease of plasma corticosterone levels, persisting throughout the experiment. Injections of the GR antagonist RU-486 (RU) or vehicle (CON) *per se* had no effect on the concentration of circulating corticosterone. The chronic constriction injury (CCI) however triggered a persistent increase in plasma corticosterone levels. Data are presented as mean ± s.e.m. *$p<0.05$, **$p<0.01$ indicate significant differences between DEX and RU and #$p<0.05$, ##$p<0.01$ between DEX and CON.

Effect of systemic GR-antagonist/agonist treatment on nerve injury-related mechanical allodynia/hyperalgesia

On the three consecutive days (d-5 to d-3) preceding any manipulation, rats were tested for baseline mechanical paw withdrawal (BS). The pain thresholds were expressed in percentages of the right injured paw compared to the left paw that served as control (Fig. 3). As expected, no difference between the three groups could be observed (DEX: 98.5±4.92%, RU: 102.5±3.79%, CON: 100.7±1.66%). Thereafter, animals were injected daily and pain thresholds were again assessed during the three following days (d-2 to d0) to obtain a baseline under conditions of drug application (BSi = baseline with injections). We did not observe any significant differences between the groups neither under BSi conditions (DEX: 102.6±2.57%, RU: 100±1.26%, CON: 99.3±4.24%), nor under BS control conditions.

Four days after CCI we noticed, as expected, a pronounced nerve injury-related increase in pain sensitivity for all three groups. However, the degree of increase differed between groups. Whereas the RU animals appeared less sensitive (48.4±12.59%) to noxious mechanical stimulation than CON (31.7±6.43%), the DEX rats exhibited a higher pain sensitivity (12.4±2.04%). This differential pain sensitivity of the groups was still seen 7 days after surgery (RU: 52.20±9.80%, CON: 29.4±3.58%, DEX: 13.2±2.64%). At d10 and 14, the pain thresholds of RU (16.4±1.95%) and CON (15±1.13%) further decreased, reaching the same level as DEX (11.3±0.46%). Only at d21, the mechanical pain sensitivity slightly decreased in all three groups (DEX: 39.5±9.54%, RU: 40.8±5.83%, CON: 22.5±1.75%).

Intergroup comparisons revealed that rats receiving systemic RU 486 treatment were less sensitive to noxious mechanical stimulation for up to 7 days after CCI surgery than rats with dexamethasone administration (d4: $p<0.05$; d7: $p<0.01$).

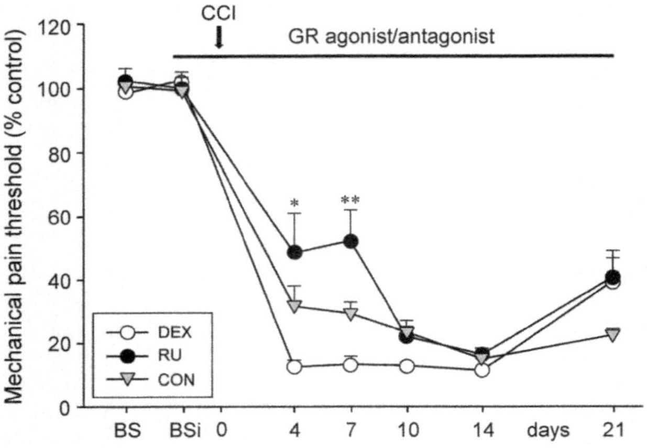

Figure 3. Influence of GR-agonist/antagonist treatment and CCI on mechanical pain thresholds. Treatment of the animals with either GR agonist dexamethasone (DEX), GR antagonist RU-486 (RU), or vehicle (CON) did not change the mechanical sensitivity *per se*. Chronic constriction injury (CCI) resulted in an increase of pain sensitivity in all three groups. Dexamethasone receiving rats were more sensitive to mechanical stimulation than RU-486 injected rats up to seven days post surgery. Data of the right affected paw are presented as percentage of the left control paw (mean ± s.e.m.). Asterisks indicate a significant difference between the DEX and RU group for the individual time point (* $p<0.05$, ** $p<0.01$).

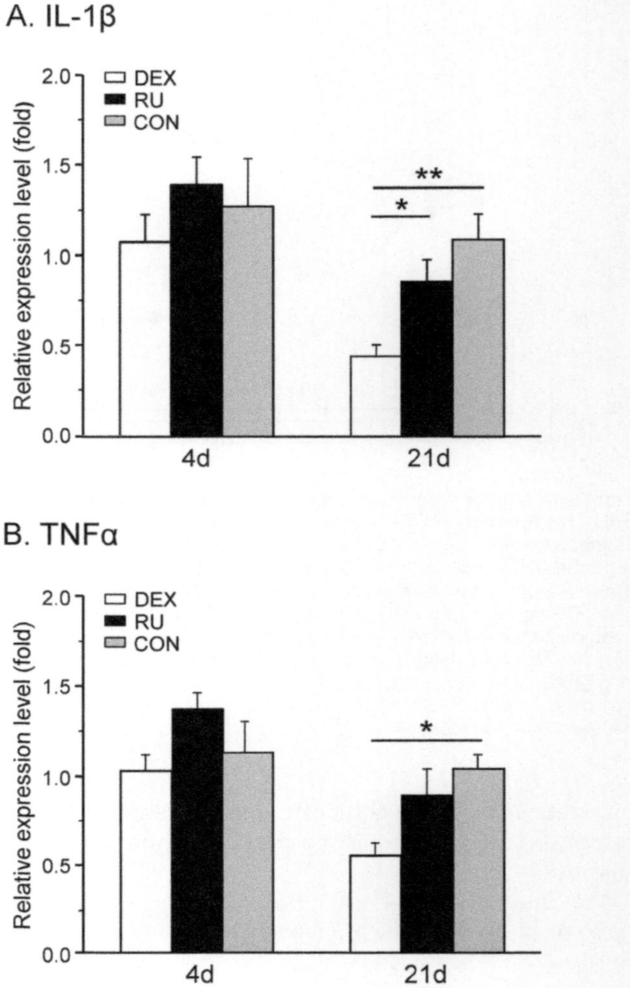

Figure 4. Spinal cytokine mRNA expression following CCI in dexamethasone and RU-486 treated rats. The relative mRNA expression levels of (**A**) IL-1β and (**B**) TNFα in the right spinal cord segment L4/L5 were measured at days four and 21 after CCI surgery in three groups of rats receiving either daily dexamethasone (DEX), RU-486 (RU), or vehicle (CON) injections. Early after injury activation or inhibition of GR did not alter the relative expression levels of both cytokines. In the later phase, the mRNA of IL-1β was downregulated by dexamethasone and RU-486 treatment, whereas TNFα mRNA levels were reduced only by GR activation. Data are expressed as mean ± s.e.m. *$p<0.05$, **$p<0.01$, ***$p<0.001$.

Alteration of cytokine expression following dexamethasone or RU-486 treatment

IL-1β and TNFα are cytokines known to be implicated in neuropathic pain mechanisms. Four days after surgery the IL-1β mRNA expression did not display any difference in the three groups (DEX: 1.36±0.21, RU: 1.17±0.14 and CON: 1.32±0.35) (Fig. 4A). At d21 post-CCI the expression of this cytokine was reduced in the DEX group (0.41±0.06) but not significantly changed in rats treated with RU-486 (0.79±0.11) in comparison with the control group (1.00±0.13). Statistical analysis revealed a significant difference at day 21 between DEX and CON ($p<0.01$) and also between DEX and RU ($p<0.05$).

We could observe the same temporal regulation profile for TNFα. At d4, no significant up- or downregulation of the mRNA expression of this cytokine was observed in the treated groups (DEX: 0.83±0.10, RU: 1.53±0.19 and CON: 1.05±0.11). 21 days post surgery the mRNA expression was downregulated in the DEX group (0.54±0.07) but not in the RU rats (0.87±0.15) (Fig. 4B). At this time point we observed a significant difference between the DEX group and CON ($p<0.05$).

These data confirm a (late) regulatory effect of dexamethasone but not of RU-486 on the mRNA expression of the two studied pro-inflammatory cytokines.

Impact of GR-agonist/antagonist administration on components of the glutamatergic system

Expression of excitatory amino-acid transporters. Excitatory amino-acid transporters (EAATs) also known as glutamate transporters are essential to homeostasis, permitting the uptake of the neurotransmitter from the synaptic cleft to regulate its effects. In the present study, we focused on two of the five subtypes, one, which is located in the membrane of glial cells (EAAT2) and the other which can be found in the membrane of neurons (EAAT3, also known as EAAC1).

The mRNA expression of the glial transporter EAAT2 showed no significant change in the RU group four days (1.94±0.10) and 21 days (0.79±0.11) after surgery (Fig. 5A). Likewise, the administration of the GR-agonist had no statistic effect on the expression of EAAT2, neither under short term (1.45±0.3) nor under long term (1.00±0.12) neuropathic conditions.

Regarding the neuronal transporter EAAT3, no significant alteration in the mRNA expression was found in the DEX group in the early period (1.76±0.29) as well as three weeks following nerve constriction (0.93±0.15). Systemic treatment with RU-486 induced a significant increase in the expression of EAAT3 after four days (2.53±0.22; $p<0.01$ compared to CON) and came back to control levels at 21 days (0.96±0.11) (Fig. 5B).

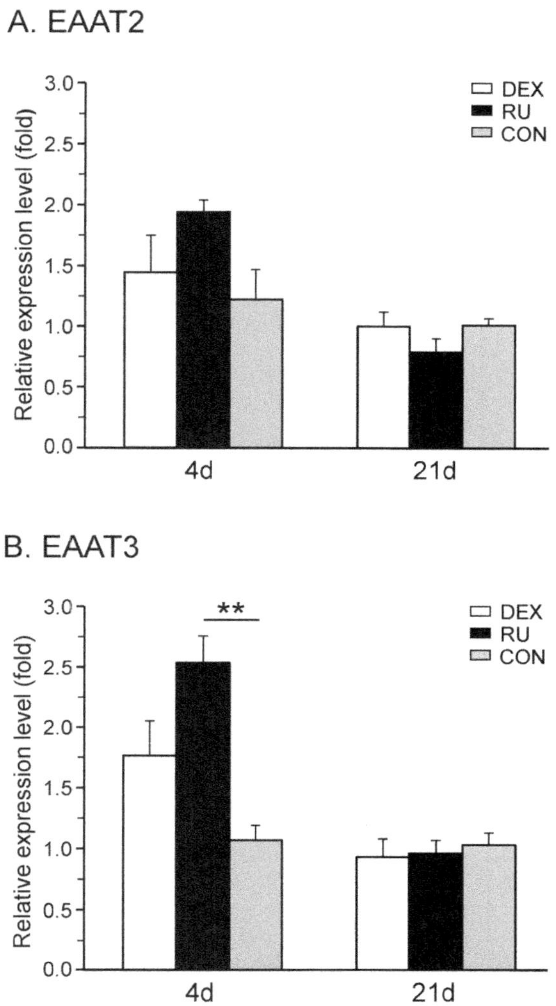

Figure 5. CCI-mediated mRNA expression of spinal EAATs under GR-agonist/antagonist treatment. The relative mRNA expression levels of (**A**) the glial glutamate transporter EAAT2 and (**B**) the neuronal glutamate transporter EAAT3 were measured in the right spinal cord segment L4/L5 at days four and 21 after CCI surgery in three groups of rats receiving daily injections of either GR agonist dexamethasone (DEX), GR antagonist RU-486 (RU), or vehicle (CON). Neither activation nor inhibition of GR significantly influenced the relative expression levels of EAAT2 at both time points (**A**). EAAT3 mRNA was upregulated in the acute phase of neuropathy by RU-486 administration but not by dexamethasone. At later stages, modulation of GR activity did not result in any effect on EAAT3 transcription (**B**). Data are expressed as mean±s.e.m.

Taken together, the systemic administration of the GR-antagonist resulted in a significant increase in mRNA levels of merely the neuronal glutamate transporter EAAT3. In contrast, dexamethasone displayed no significant influence on the regulation of the excitatory amino-acid transporters, neither in the early development nor in later phases of neuropathy.

Expression of glutamate receptors. The metabotropic glutamate receptor mGluR5 as well as the ionotropic NMDA receptor are claimed to be involved in neuropathic pain syndromes. For the latter, seven subunits have been described. Here, we focused on the two commonly expressed NR1 and NR2a subunits.

Regarding the mRNA expression of the metabotropic receptor mGluR5, a transient and significant increase was only seen early after nerve injury in the DEX (2.88 ± 0.14; $p<0.001$) as well as the RU group (2.37 ± 0.12; $p<0.001$) as compared to CON (1.18 ± 0.25). At d21 the mRNA expression of mGluR5 came back to control levels in both treatment groups (DEX: 1.17 ± 0.09; RU: 1.02 ± 0.10; CON: 1.09 ± 0.21) (Fig. 6A).

For the NR1 mRNA expression, a significant increase was noticed in the DEX group at d4 (1.73 ± 0.16) compared to CON (1.00 ± 0.16; $p<0.05$). The level returned to baseline at d21 post surgery (DEX: 1.17 ± 0.09, CON: 1.06 ± 0.15) (Fig. 6B). Administration of the GR-antagonist RU-486 had no significant influence on the NR1 regulation at d4 (1.44 ± 0.09) and d21 (1.02 ± 0.10).

Neither activation nor inhibition of the GR led to any significant modification of the NR2a mRNA expression early after nerve constriction (RU: 1.61 ± 0.07; DEX: 1.32 ± 0.19; CON: 1.15 ± 0.19) (Fig. 6C). However, in the later phase of neuropathy, the RU group displayed a significant decrease of the relative expression level (0.58 ± 0.0; $p<0.05$) whereas the level measured in the DEX group (0.78 ± 0.06) was not statistically different from control (1.08 ± 0.19).

Summarizing the effects of pharmacological GR-manipulation on the expression of glutamate receptors, we observed an early GR-activation mediated upregulation of metabotropic and ionotropic receptors and a late downregulation of one subunit of the NMDA receptor related to GR-antagonist application.

Discussion

In the present work, we aimed to determine the role of GCs in the onset and maintenance of mechanical allodynia/hyperalgesia in a CCI model of neuropathic pain. Our observations included: **1**. A decrease in body weight for the DEX group throughout the 21 days following CCI surgery; **2**. A higher sensitivity to painful mechanical stimulation of the DEX group until day 7 post surgery; **3**. A lack of effects of dexamethasone or RU-486 injections on early pro-inflammatory cytokine mRNA expression; **4**. No significant differences in EAAT2 mRNA expression at days 4 and 21 after the CCI surgery but a RU-486-related increase at day 4 for EAAT3; **5**. A pronounced transient increase in NMDA receptor subunit NR1 and in mGluR5 mRNA expression in the DEX group at 4 days post surgery; **6**. A decrease in the NMDA receptor subunit NR2a mRNA expression only 21 days post CCI in the RU group.

Metabolic effects of GR-agonist or -antagonist administration

In the DEX group consistent decrease in body weight was observed from the starting day of the injections until the end of the experiment. Since glucocorticoids are known to imply the mobilization of fatty acids [8], our findings may be related to dexamethasone mimicking the effects of endogenous GCs and provoking a utilization of the mentioned fatty acids and the concomitant loss of weight. In the present study, plasma corticosterone levels reflecting HPA axis activity under physiological conditions have been modified by the dexamethasone or RU-486 injections. In the first days of the observation, i.e. in the absence of any manipulation, no differences were observed between the three groups. After starting the drug injections, the plasma corticosterone levels of the DEX group decreased and then stayed at a stable level from day one to the end of the experiment. This is consistent with the fact that dexamethasone mimics endogenous GC effects leading to an activation of the negative

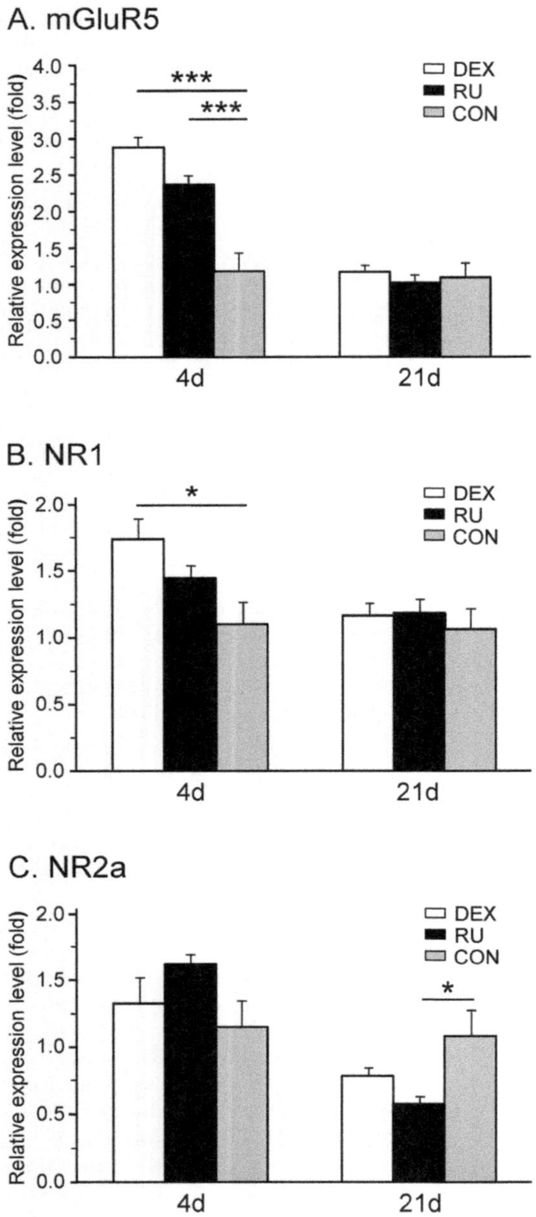

Figure 6. mRNA expression of spinal ionotropic and metabotropic glutamate receptors following GR-agonist/antagonist administration and CCI. The relative mRNA expression levels of (**A**) the metabotropic receptor mGluR5, (**B**) the subunit NR1 and (**C**) the subunit NR2a of the ionotropic NMDA receptor were measured in the right spinal cord segment L4/L5 at days four and 21 after CCI surgery in three groups of rats receiving daily injections of either dexamethasone (DEX), RU-486 (RU), or vehicle (CON). Early after CCI the mGluR5 mRNA was significantly upregulated by GR activation and inhibition, whereas the NR1 subunit was significantly upregulated only in the DEX group. For both receptors no change from control was seen in the late phase of neuropathy. On the other hand, the NR2a mRNA was not altered in acute conditions but downregulated at 21 days in the RU group treated with the GR antagonist. Data are expressed as mean ± s.e.m. *$p<0.05$.

feedback control of the HPA axis. For the other two groups, the increase observed at day one was probably mainly due to the surgery performed at day zero. At this time point, the dexamethasone administration probably masked these surgery-related variations in the DEX group via the described activation of the negative feedback loop. The corticosterone concentration in the RU and CON groups stayed at a higher and relatively constant level throughout the experiment. This is consistent with data from Soro and colleagues [25] who failed to observe an effect of RU-486 on the corticosterone level of Sprague Dawley rats.

Development and maintenance of mechanical allodynia/hyperalgesia

The measurement of mechanical allodynia/hyperalgesia during three days without interventions and the three days with drug injections did not reveal any differences between the groups. In the absence of any injury, the administration of GR agonists or antagonists did hence not have any effect on the mechanical pain thresholds. However, 4 to 7 days after the CCI surgery, the RU group was significantly less sensitive than the DEX group. This observation is in accordance with a recent study of Ou and colleagues [26] highlighting a protective effect of another GR antagonist, M8046, in CCI-induced neuropathic pain. The pain thresholds of the CON rats were located between those of the pharmacologically treated groups during the same period. Our observations are consistent with studies showing that intrathecal injections of dexamethasone increase pain-like behaviors in a spared nerve injury (SNI) model [19] and CCI model of neuropathic pain and that GR antagonists like RU-486 attenuate them [20]. These effects are opposite to the well-known anti-inflammatory and hypoalgesic effects of GR activation and may suggest that other pathways involving the glutamatergic system known to have a role in neuropathic pain (for review see [27]) should be more implied in the onset of mechanical allodynia than the local inflammation. No significant differences in pain sensitivity between the groups were detected in the later period following CCI surgery. This could be due to adaptive biochemical processes and to the implication of other mediators coming into play following pronounced ongoing pharmacological activation or inactivation of GRs. It should be noted here that effects related to pharmacological manipulation of the HPA axis have been described to display complex and even paradoxical patterns, depending on factors like dose, site and mode of application and on duration of the treatment [28]. In this context, Kingery and co-workers [29] have e.g. observed that once-daily injections of methylprednisolone had no antihyperalgesic effect in a rat sciatic nerve transection model while continuous infusion reversed heat and mechanical hyperalgesia. More specifically turning to glucocorticoid receptor antagonists, Takasaki and colleagues [12] described that intrathecal and intraperitoneal injections of RU-486 produced antinociceptive effects in a mouse model of neuropathic pain while intracerebroventricular injections had no effect. The authors however only provided short term observations. We are not aware of any data on long term effects in this context. The measurement of the mRNA expression of the mentioned cytokines as well as glutamate transporters and transmitters at d21 was partly aimed at considering the time dependent involvement of implied mediators.

Taken together, our behavioral results seem to emphasize a more important role of GR modulation in the onset of mechanical allodynia/hyperalgesia rather than in the longer term maintenance.

Involvement of pro-inflammatory cytokines

As mentioned in the final paragraph of the methods section, we did not observe significant side differences in the expression levels of cytokine mRNAs. The same was true for the other examined biochemical markers. This at first astonishing finding is reminiscent of the implication of spinal glia and pro-inflammatory cytokines in mirror-image neuropathic pain [30]. Bilateral labelling of activated microglia in the spinal cord dorsal horn following a unilateral spared nerve injury has e.g. been described in rats [31]. The fact that we did not observe altered pain behavior induced by stimulation of the contralateral (control) paw in spite of the quite symmetrical biochemical expression of mRNA levels may be related to a time dependent dissociation between pain behavior and the measured biochemical parameters. In this sense, Huiging Li and colleagues [32], using a spared nerve injury model in rats, have e.g. observed elevated pro-inflammatory cytokine levels with effects of steroid treatment gradually becoming less apparent while the effects of the same drug on mechanical sensitivity remained evident on day 7 post surgery. In our hands, there may also have been a more pronounced ipsilateral expression of spinal mediators in the initial phase preceding day 4 after CCI which gradually decayed and converged with the respective values of the untreated side.

Pro-inflammatory cytokines such as IL-1β and TNFα play an important role in inflammatory reactions and may also be involved in neuropathic pain [9,33] and in the initiation and maintenance of central sensitization [34].

We only observed a pronounced decrease in IL-1β mRNA expression at day 21 post CCI surgery for the DEX group, as compared to the two other groups. This is consistent with studies from cell cultures exhibiting an important diminution in IL-1β mRNA expression after corticosteroid administration [9,35]. Surprisingly, we did not observe any DEX-related effects on the mRNA expression of this cytokine at day 4. This negative finding could reflect that IL-1β may not be involved in the onset of mechanical allodynia following CCI. We did not have the possibility to include measurements of protein levels in the present study. These data could be important for the consideration of potential posttranscriptional regulation-related effects which may play a critical role in the regulation of pro-inflammatory cytokine expression by mitogen activated protein kinase signal transduction pathways as well as by anti-inflammatory agents and mediators (for review see [36]). These may in turn depend on a host of factors that have recently been discussed in detail by Ji and colleagues [37]. The absence of dexamethasone effects at day 4 post CCI is however in line with the enhanced sensitivity to mechanical allodynia/hyperalgesia that may be linked to pro-inflammatory cytokine-mediated effects.

The TNFα mRNA expression was likewise downregulated in the DEX group at day 21. This is also in line with other studies showing a decrease of TNFα expression after administration of dexamethasone [38,39] and an inhibition of TNFα translation by GCs [40]. The absence of a significant decrease after 4 days is coherent with delayed modifications regarding this pro-inflammatory cytokine. In agreement with our results, an inhibition of spinal TNFα receptor expression following administration of the synthetic GC methylprednisolone has also been shown, an effect that may be reversed by the administration of RU-486 [41].

Taken together, our results are in accordance with the anti-inflammatory effects of GR activation in a later phase. TNFα and IL-1β are known to activate glia cells [42]. Effects of GR activation or inactivation on this type of cells thus remain to be considered in the present context. On the other hand, the fact that the DEX group was more sensitive to mechanical allodynia/hyperalgesia in the early phase after surgery may point to the dominance of GR-mediated enhancement of glutamatergic processing as will be discussed below.

Role of glutamate transporters

Dexamethasone has been shown to have an inhibitory effect on the downregulation of glutamate transporters such as EAAT1 (=GLAST), EAAT2 (=GLT1) and EAAT3 (=EAAC1) after chronic morphine administration [43]. Along this line Kalariti and colleagues [44] have demonstrated an increase in EAAT1 protein but not mRNA expression *in vitro* following dexamethasone administration. GR-activation has also been reported to diminish EAAT3 expression under conditions of nerve injury, effects reversed by administration of RU 486 [19]. The decreased glutamate transporter expression leads to an increase of extracellular glutamate resulting in amplified synaptic transmission [11,19,20].

In the present study we did not observe any significant change of EAAT3 mRNA expression in the dexamethasone treated group at day 4, whereas, at the same time point, the RU group exhibited an important increase. The EAAT2 mRNA expression was not affected, neither by dexamethasone nor by RU-486.

Although pointing towards the same direction, these results are not fully consistent with the studies mentioned above. These discrepancies may be related to the different models used to induce neuropathic pain as well as to the doses of the respective drugs that have been administered. The RU-486 injection-related increase is however in accordance with the literature. It may participate in the enhancement of glutamate uptake from the synaptic cleft leading to a reduction of glutamatergic transmission and of pain sensitivity as observed in the RU group at days 4 and 7.

Impact on glutamate receptors

Glutamate receptors have also been shown to be involved in GC-mediated effects in a context of neuropathic pain. In this framework, the role of the metabotropic receptor mGluR5 has been investigated under conditions of GR agonist and antagonist treatment. Kalariti and colleagues [44] demonstrated *in vitro* that dexamethasone administration increased mGluR5 mRNA and protein expression. This result is consistent with our observation at day 4, where a large increase of mGluR5 mRNA expression was seen in the DEX group. However, these differences had vanished at day 21, when the groups also displayed similar mechanical pain thresholds. These findings seem to support the assumption that mGluR5 could be more implicated in the onset rather than in the maintenance of the hypersensitivity observed in the DEX group.

Glucocorticoid-mediated effects on NMDA receptor regulation have also been studied quite extensively. It has e.g. been shown that GR activation leads to an upregulation of the NMDA receptor expression in the hippocampus and that enhanced GCs levels lead to an increase in glutamatergic transmission [21]. In addition, after a peripheral nerve injury, a time-dependent and region-specific upregulation of two subunits of the NMDA receptor has been observed [11]. More precisely, NR1 and NR2 mRNA expression have been shown to be increased in the ipsilateral spinal dorsal horn in a CCI model. Furthermore, these subunit expressions decrease under conditions of RU-486 administration. These data are in agreement with our results showing a dexamethasone-related enhancement of mRNA expression of NR1 four days after surgery in the ipsilateral spinal cord. This increased expression is accompanied by pain hypersensitivity exhibited by the DEX group rats at this early time point. Moreover, we can confirm an antagonist-related downregulation of the NR2 subunit in later phases of experimentally induced CCI.

In our hands the NMDA receptor subunit NR1 played a role in the onset rather than in the maintenance of mechanical allodynia/hyperalgesia whereas the NR2a subunit could subsequently have taken over a more dominant role.

Limitations of the study

A limitation of the study is that we only present mRNA expression data for the spinal mediators. Regulations on a post-transcriptional level, e.g. via micro-RNAs could play an important role. Therefore, measurement of protein expression via western blotting should be included in further experiments. It should however be noted that the reliability of this kind of protein quantification (by using house keeping genes) is currently also under debate.

Conclusion

The present study demonstrated that at an early time point post-CCI, the activation of GR leads to an enhancement of mRNA expression of glutamate receptors accompanied by an increase in mechanical pain sensitivity.

Under these conditions, GR activation may hence lead to an intensification of glutamatergic transmission that may outweigh putative anti-inflammatory effects. Further investigations aimed at confirming this assumption and at elucidating the underlying mechanisms will have to include the assessment of protein levels. The involvement of altered descending pain control pathways will also have to be considered.

Acknowledgments

The authors thank Jessica Tapp for her technical assistance.

Author Contributions

Conceived and designed the experiments: FA UH. Performed the experiments: G-MLC. Wrote the paper: G-MLC FA UH. Analyzed and interpreted the data: G-MLC UH.

References

1. Davis MC, Zautra AJ, Reich JW (2001) Vulnerability to stress among women in chronic pain from fibromyalgia and osteoarthritis. Ann Behav Med 23: 215–26.
2. Aloisi AM, Buonocore M, Merlo L, Galandra C, Sotgiu A, et al. (2011) Chronic pain therapy and hypothalamic-pituitary-adrenal axis impairment. Psychoneuroendocrino 36: 1032–1039.
3. Kanczkowski W, Alexaki VI, Tran N, Großklaus S, Zacharowski K, et al. (2013) Hypothalamo-pituitary and immune-dependent adrenal regulation during systemic inflammation. P Natl Acad Sci USA 110: 14801–14806.
4. Straub RH, Bijlsma JW, Masi A, Cutolo M (2013) Role of neuroendocrine and neuroimmune mechanisms in chronic inflammatory rheumatic diseases -The 10-year update. Semin Arthritis Rheum in press. doi:10.1016/j.semarthrit.2013.04.008.
5. Kuehl LK, Michaux GP, Richter S, Schächinger H, Anton F (2010) Increased basal mechanical pain sensitivity but decreased perceptual wind-up in a human model of relative hypocortisolism. Pain 149: 539–46.
6. Michaux GP, Magerl W, Anton F, Treede RD (2012) Experimental characterization of the effects of acute stresslike doses of hydrocortisone in human neurogenic hyperalgesia models. Pain 153: 420–428.
7. Chrousos GP (2000) Stress, chronic inflammation, and emotional and physical well-being: Concurrent effects and chronic sequelae. J Allergy Clin Immunol 106: S275–291.
8. Newton R (2000) Molecular mechanisms of glucocorticoid action: what is important? Thorax 55: 603–613.
9. Lee SW, Tsou AP, Chan H, Thomas J, Petrie K, et al. (1988) Glucocorticoids selectively inhibit the transcription of the interleukin 1 beta gene and decrease the stability of interleukin 1 beta mRNA. Proc Natl Acad Sci USA 85: 1204–1208.
10. Liberman AC, Druker J, Perone MJ, Arzt E (2007) Glucocorticoids in the regulation of transcription factors that control cytokine synthesis. Cytokine Growth F R 18: 45–56.
11. Wang S, Lim G, Zeng Q, Sung B, Yang L, et al. (2005) Central glucocorticoid receptors modulate the expression and function of spinal NMDA receptors after peripheral nerve injury. J Neurosci 25: 488–495.
12. Takasaki I, Kurihara T, Saegusa H, Zong S, Tanabe T (2005) Effects of glucocorticoid receptor antagonists on allodynia and hyperalgesia in mouse model of neuropathic pain. Eur J Pharmacol 524: 80–83.
13. Bennett GJ, Xie YK (1988) A peripheral mononeuropathy in rat that produces disorders of pain sensation like those seen in man. Pain 33: 87–107.
14. Gómez-Nicola D, Valle-Argos B, Suardíaz M, Taylor JS, Nieto-Sampedro M (2008) Role of IL-15 in spinal cord and sciatic nerve after chronic constriction injury: regulation of macrophage and T-cell inflitration. J Neurochem 107: 1741–1752.
15. Oprée A, Kress M (2000) Involvement of the proinflammatory cytokines tumor necrosis factor-alpha, IL-1 beta, and IL-6 but not IL-8 in the development of heat hyperalgesia: effects on heat-evoked calcitonin gene-related peptide release from rat skin. J Neurosci 20: 6289–6293.
16. Junger H, Sorkin LS (2000) Nociceptive and inflammatory effects of subcutaneous TNFalpha. Pain 85: 145–151.
17. Milligan ED, Watkins LR (2009) Pathological and protective roles of glia in chronic pain. Nat Rev Neurosci 10: 23–36.
18. Coutinho AE, Chapman KE (2011) The anti-inflammatory and immunosuppressive effects of glucocorticoids, recent developments and mechanistic insights. Mol Cell Endocrinol 335: 2–13.
19. Alexander JK, DeVries AC, Kigerl KA, Dahlman JM, Popovich PG (2009) Stress exacerbates neuropathic pain via glucocorticoid and NMDA receptor activation. Brain Behav Immun 23: 851–860.
20. Wang S, Lim G, Zeng Q, Sung B, Ai Y, et al. (2004) Expression of central glucocorticoid receptors after peripheral nerve injury contributes to neuropathic pain behaviors in rats. J Neurosci 24: 8595–8605.
21. Lu J, Goula D, Sousa N, Almeida OF (2003) Ionotropic and metabotropic glutamate receptor mediation of glucocorticoid-induced apoptosis in hippocampal cells and the neuroprotective role of synaptic N-methyl-d-aspartate receptors. Neuroscience 121: 123–131.
22. Urban MO, Hama AT, Bradbury M, Anderson J, Varney MA, et al. (2003) Role of metabotropic glutamate receptor subtype 5 (mGluR5) in the maintenance of cold hypersensitivity following a peripheral mononeuropathy in the rat. Neuropharmacology 44: 983–993.
23. Chaplan SR, Bach FW, Pogrel JW, Chung JM, Yaksh TL (1994) Quantitative assessment of tactile allodynia in the rat paw. J Neurosci Methods 53: 55–63.
24. Pfaffl M (2001) A new mathematical model for relative quantification in real-time RT-PCR. Nucleic Acids Res 29: 2002–2007.
25. Soro A, Panarelli M, Holloway CD, Fraser R, Keuron CJ (1995) Effects of the glucocorticoid antagonist RU 486 in spontaneously hypertensive and Sprague Dawley rats. J Endocrinol Invest 18: 833–839.
26. Ou GK, Wang RX, Li JJ, Cao H, Lian QQ, et al. (2013) Effect of M8046 on expression of COX-2/PGE2 in spinal cord and DRG in rats with neuropathic pain. Zhongguo Zhong Yao Za Zhi 29: 97–100.
27. Osikowicz M, Mika J, Przewlocka B (2013) The glutamatergic system as a target for neuropathic pain relief. Exp Physiol 98: 372–384.
28. McEwen BS, Kalia M (2010) The role of corticosteroids and stress in chronic pain conditions. Metabolism 59 (Suppl 1): S9–S15.
29. Kingery WS, Agashe GS, Sawamura S, Davies F, Clark JD, et al. (2001) Glucocorticoid inhibition of neuropathic hyperalgesia and spinal Fos expression. Anesth Analg 92: 476–482.
30. Milligan ED, Twining C, Chacur M, Biedenkapp J, O'Connor K, et al. (2003) Spinal glia and proinflammatory cytokines mediate mirror-image neuropathic pain in rats. J Neurosci 23: 1026–1040.
31. Wen YR, Suter MR, Kawasaki Y, Huang J, Pertin M, et al. (2007) Nerve conduction blockade in the sciatic nerve prevents but does not reverse the activation of p38 mitogen-activated protein kinase in spinal microglia in the rat spared nerve injury model. Anesthesiology 107: 312–321.
32. Li H, Xie W, Strong JA, Zhang J-M (2007) Systemic anti-inflammatory corticosteroid reduces mechanical pain behaviour, sympathetic sprouting, and elevation of pro-inflammatory cytokines in a rat model of neuropathic pain. Anesthesiology 107: 489–477.
33. Leung L, Cahill C (2010) TNF-α and neuropathic pain - a review. J Neuroinflamm 7: 27–39.
34. McMahon SB, Cafferty WB, Marchand F (2005) Immune and glial cell factors as pain mediators and modulators. Exp Neurol 192: 444–462.
35. Snyder DS, Unanue ER (1982) Corticosteroids inhibit murine macrophage Ia expression and interleukin 1 production. J Immunol 129: 1803–1805.
36. Clark A (2000) Post-transcriptional regulation of pro-inflammatory gene expression. Arthritis Res 2: 172–174.
37. Ji R-R, Berta T, Nedergaard M (2013) Glia and pain: is chronic pain a gliopathy? Pain 154 (Suppl 1): S10–S28.
38. Abraham SM, Lawrence T, Kleiman A, Warden P, Medghalchi M, et al. (2006) Antiinflammatory effects of dexamethasone are partly dependent on induction of dual specificity phosphatase 1. J Exp Med 203: 1883–1889.
39. Dawson J, Rordorf-Adam C, Geiger T, Towbin H, Kunz S, et al. (1993) Interleukin-1 (IL-1) production in a mouse tissue chamber model of inflammation. II. Identification of (tissue) macrophages as the IL-1 producing cells and the effect of anti-inflammatory drugs. Agents Actions 38: 255–264.
40. Swantek JL, Cobb MH, Geppert TD (1997) Jun N-terminal kinase/stress-activated protein kinase (JNK/SAPK) is required for lipopolysaccharide stimulation of tumor necrosis factor alpha (TNF-alpha) translation: glucocorticoids inhibit TNF-alpha translation by blocking JNK/SAPK. Mol Cell Biol 17: 6274–6282.

41. Yan P, Liu N, Kim GM, Xu J, Li Q, et al. (2003) Expression of the type 1 and type 2 receptors for tumor necrosis factor after traumatic spinal cord injury in adult rats. Exp Neurol 183: 286–297.

42. Aschner M (1998) Astrocytes as mediators of immune and inflammatory responses in the CNS. Neurotoxicology 19: 269–281.

43. Wen ZH, Wu GJ, Chang YC, Wang JJ, Wong CS (2005) Dexamethasone modulates the development of morphine tolerance and expression of glutamate transporters in rats. Neuroscience 133: 807–817.

44. Kalariti N, Lembessis P, Papageorgiou E, Pissimissis N, Koutsilieris M (2007) Regulation of the mGluR5, EAAT1 and GS expression by glucocorticoids in MG-63 osteoblast-like osteosarcoma cells. J Musculoskelet Neuronal Interact 7: 113–118.

5

Gene Therapy for Neuropathic Pain by Silencing of TNF-α Expression with Lentiviral Vectors Targeting the Dorsal Root Ganglion in Mice

Nobuhiro Ogawa[1], Hiromichi Kawai[1], Tomoya Terashima[1]*, Hideto Kojima[2], Kazuhiro Oka[3], Lawrence Chan[3], Hiroshi Maegawa[1]

1 Department of Medicine, Molecular Genetics in Medicine, Shiga University of Medical Science, Otsu, Shiga, Japan, **2** Department of Molecular Genetics in Medicine, Shiga University of Medical Science, Otsu, Shiga, Japan, **3** Departments of Medicine and Molecular and Cellular Biology, Baylor College of Medicine, Houston, Texas, United States of America

Abstract

Neuropathic pain can be a debilitating condition. Many types of drugs that have been used to treat neuropathic pain have only limited efficacy. Recent studies indicate that pro-inflammatory mediators including tumor necrosis factor α (TNF-α) are involved in the pathogenesis of neuropathic pain. In the present study, we engineered a gene therapy strategy to relieve neuropathic pain by silencing TNF-α expression in the dorsal root ganglion (DRG) using lentiviral vectors expressing TNF short hairpin RNA1-4 (LV-TNF-shRNA1-4) in mice. First, based on its efficacy in silencing TNF-α *in vitro*, we selected shRNA3 to construct LV-TNF-shRNA3 for *in vivo* study. We used L5 spinal nerve transection (SNT) mice as a neuropathic pain model. These animals were found to display up-regulated mRNA expression of activating transcription factor 3 (ATF3) and neuropeptide Y (NPY), injury markers, and interleukin (IL)-6, an inflammatory cytokine in the ipsilateral L5 DRG. Injection of LV-TNF-shRNA3 onto the proximal transected site suppressed significantly the mRNA levels of ATF3, NPY and IL-6, reduced mechanical allodynia and neuronal cell death of DRG neurons. These results suggest that lentiviral-mediated silencing of TNF-α in DRG relieves neuropathic pain and reduces neuronal cell death, and may constitute a novel therapeutic option for neuropathic pain.

Editor: Simone Di Giovanni, Hertie Institute for Clinical Brain Research, University of Tuebingen, Germany

Funding: This work was supported by a Grant-in-Aid (#23590378 to H. Kojima) for Scientific Research from the Ministry of Education, Culture, Sports, Science and Technology, Japan, and grants from the US National Institutes of Health (R01-HL051586 (to L. Chan), and the President's Discretionary Fund from Shiga University of Medical Science (no. 1515503L and no. 1515503F to H. Kojima). The funders had no role in study design, data collection and analysis, decision to publish, or preparation of the manuscript.

Competing Interests: The authors have declared that no competing interests exist.

* E-mail: tom@belle.shiga-med.ac.jp

Introduction

Neuropathic pain is defined as pain caused by a lesion or disease in the somatosensory nervous system [1]. Its severity varies but is often so debilitating that it has been called "the most terrible of all tortures, which a nerve wound may inflict" [2]. Neuropathic pain is characterized by sensory abnormalities that range from unpleasant abnormal sensations (dysesthesia), to an increased response to painful stimuli (hyperalgesia), and to pain in response to a stimulus that does not normally provoke pain (allodynia) [3]. These three kinds of pain are the most difficult types of chronic pain to treat, and are often associated with autoimmune diseases such as rheumatoid arthritis or Sjögren's syndrome, metabolic diseases such as diabetes mellitus, side effects of drugs for cancer or HIV chemotherapy, toxin exposure, infection and trauma [4–7]. Neuropathic pain impairs a patient's daily activities and quality of life. Currently available treatments for neuropathic pain include sodium channel blockers, anti-depressants and anti-epileptic drugs, but they are grossly inadequate; novel treatment methods with better efficacy are much needed.

A number of animal models have been developed that can be used to study the mechanism of neuropathic pain and to examine the efficacy of new therapies [8]. For example, L5 spinal nerve injury mouse models are widely used, so is the modified spinal nerve ligation model [9], in which severe mechanical allodynia and hyperesthesia occur without motor deficit. Another model, the spinal nerve transection (SNT) mice [10] requires skillful surgery; these mice display a stable type of neuropathic pain and is especially suitable for pain studies and behavioral tests.

Recently, peripheral nerve and spinal nerve injury models have also been used for research into the pathogenesis of neuropathic pain. Studies in these models revealed that pro-inflammatory mediators, such as tumor necrosis factor α (TNF-α), interleukin (IL)-1β and IL-6, are up-regulated in the dorsal root ganglion (DRG) and may be important mediators of neuropathic pain in rodents [7,11–15]. Of note, TNF-α signaling was shown to stimulate sensory neuronal excitability [16] and produce neuropathic pain [17,18]. TNF-α and caspase-related signaling pathways also result in cell death and neuropathic pain [19], establishing TNF-α expression in the DRG as a key mediator of neuropathic pain. In addition, we previously reported that TNF-α was involved in the pathogenesis of diabetic neuropathy in mice and that inactivation or inhibition of TNF-α ameliorated diabetic neuropathy and reduced hyperalgesia [20,21]. In nondiabetic injury neuropathic pain models, the inhibition of TNF-α also reduced neuropathic pain-related behavior [13,22–24]. Furthermore, in human studies, TNF-α was found to be up-regulated in sensory nerve and DRG, and contributed to neuropathic pain in sensory neuronopathy, inflammatory diseases or nerve injury [7,25–27]. We therefore hypothesized that TNF-α may be a suitable therapeutic target for the treatment of neuropathic pain and neuropathy. Indeed, human studies have suggested that anti-TNF-α drugs ameliorate neuropathic pain and neuropathy in Sjögren's syndrome [25], sciatica and disc-herniation [28–30]. However, the need for these drugs to be delivered systemically led to serious side effects such as infection, interstitial pneumonia and liver failure because generalized TNF-α inhibition suppresses the normal immune system. Thus, to avoid inducing systemic side effects, we selected the local administration of gene delivery vectors to target the TNF-α at the site of injection.

Here, we present a gene therapy strategy that relieves SNT-induced neuropathic pain by silencing TNF-α expression in DRG using RNA interference technology with lentiviral vectors. This strategy was effective in suppressing neuropathic pain and protecting DRG neurons from cell death. These results constitute a proof of principle that the therapeutic strategy can potentially be used to treat neuropathic pain and sensory neuronopathy in people.

Materials and Methods

Ethics statement

All animal protocols were approved by the Institutional Animal Care and Use Committee of Shiga University of Medical Science (Approved Number: 2012-8-5). All procedures were performed in accordance with the guidelines of the Research Center for Animal Life Science of Shiga University of Medical Science.

Construction of mouse TNF-α over-expression or silencing plasmids for lentiviral vectors

The full-length mouse TNF-α cDNA was inserted into pLL3.7 plasmid including elongation factor 1 (EF-1) promoter and DsRed as a reporter gene (TNF-α over-expression plasmid: LV-TNF-DsRed). Four short hairpin RNAs (shRNA) were individually inserted into pLL3.7 plasmid including U6 promoter and enhanced green fluorescent protein (GFP), as a reporter gene, driven by cytomegalovirus (CMV) promoter (TNF-α silencing plasmid: LV-TNF-shRNA1-4). The full-length TNF-α coding sequence (NM_013693) was isolated from RAW cells with lipopolysaccharide stimulation. shRNA sequences against mouse TNF-α were designed using a web site from The RNAi Consortium (TRC) algorithm (Available: http://www.broadinstitute.org/rnai/trc. Accessed on 2014 Feb 20.).

Production of mouse TNF-α over-expressing or silencing lentiviral vectors

To produce recombinant lentiviral particles, psPAX2 (a packaging plasmid), pMD2.G (an envelope plasmid, which has the vesiculo-stomatitis virus G-protein), a gift of Dr. Didier Trono (École Polytechnique Fédérale de Lausanne, Switzerland), and TNF-α over-expression plasmid (or silencing plasmid) were co-transfected into 293T cells using the calcium phosphate method as described previously [31]. After 6 h incubation, the culture medium was exchanged. Culture medium containing lentiviral particles was collected after 48 h incubation, and was filtered through a 0.45 μm pore size cellulose acetate filter. Lentiviral vectors were concentrated using Lenti-X Concentrator (Takara Bio Inc., Otsu, Japan), and were stocked at a concentration of 1.8×10^8 infectious units (IFU)/ml at −80°C after the determination of IFU using 293T cells. Finally, we produced LV-TNF-DsRed (mouse TNF-α and DsRed expression vector), LV-GFP (control vector expressing GFP without shRNA sequence) and LV-TNF-shRNA1-4 (TNF-α silencing vector with GFP expression).

Co-infection test of mouse TNF-α over-expressing and silencing lentiviral vectors

One day before infection, 293T cells were split to 6 well-culture dishes at a density of 1.0×10^5 cells per well. The confluency of 293T cells was approximately 70% at the time of infection. At 6 h after infection of LV-TNF-DsRed (3.6×10^5 IFU), 3.6×10^5 IFU LV-GFP or LV-TNF-shRNA1-4 was separately added into each well of LV-TNF-DsRed-infected 293T cells. At 72 h later, DsRed and GFP expression were observed under fluorescence microscopy and TNF-α mRNA expression was determined by quantitative RT-PCR analysis.

Animals

Male 9–10 week-old C57BL6 (Japan CLEA, Osaka, Japan) mice weighing 19.0–22.0 g were used in this study. The mice were housed in separated cages and the room kept under 12:12 light-dark cycle with free access to food and water.

Surgical procedures

The neuropathic pain model by L5 spinal nerve transection (SNT) was generated by the method described previously (**Figure 1A**) [9,10]. Briefly, mice were anesthetized by intraperitoneal administration of sodium pentobarbital (5 mg/kg). After the midline incision of mouse back skin, the bilateral L5 transverse processes of the lumbar spine were clearly removed. Bilateral L5 spinal nerves were exposed on the visual field. Only the left nerve was pinched and transected. Immediately after transection, 1 μl (1.8×10^5 IFU/μl) of lentiviral vector was injected onto proximal transected site of left L5 spinal nerve using a Hamilton syringe (8001 1701LT, Hamilton company, Nevada, USA) with a 30G needle. The right spinal nerve, as a control side, was clearly exposed without transection or administration of lentiviral vector.

Behavioral test

Mechanical allodynia was assessed prior to injury (day -2) and at 1, 3, 5, 7, 10 and 14 days after SNT, using a dynamic planter aesthesiometer (Ugo Basil, Varese, Italy) as described previously [32]. Paw withdrawal in response to mechanical stimuli was measured. Briefly, each mouse was placed in a polypropylene box with a metallic mesh floor and allowed to acclimatize to the testing environment for at least 1 h. A stimulating filament probe was positioned under the hind paw, which was gradually applied until mice withdrew their paw. The pressure was increased at approximately 10 g/mm^2/sec. The test was performed on both the intact right or neuropathic left hind paw. The withdrawal threshold was determined by mean of three trials.

Reverse transcription-PCR and quantitative RT-PCR analysis

Animal tissues were removed under deep anesthesia and immediately frozen in liquid nitrogen. Total RNA was extracted from cultured cells and frozen tissues using RNeasy mini kit (Qiagen, Valencia, CA) with DNase I (Rnase-free DNase set, Qiagen) treatment. Reverse transcription was performed from 100 ng of total RNA in each tube using Prime Script perfect Real time (Takara Bio Inc.).

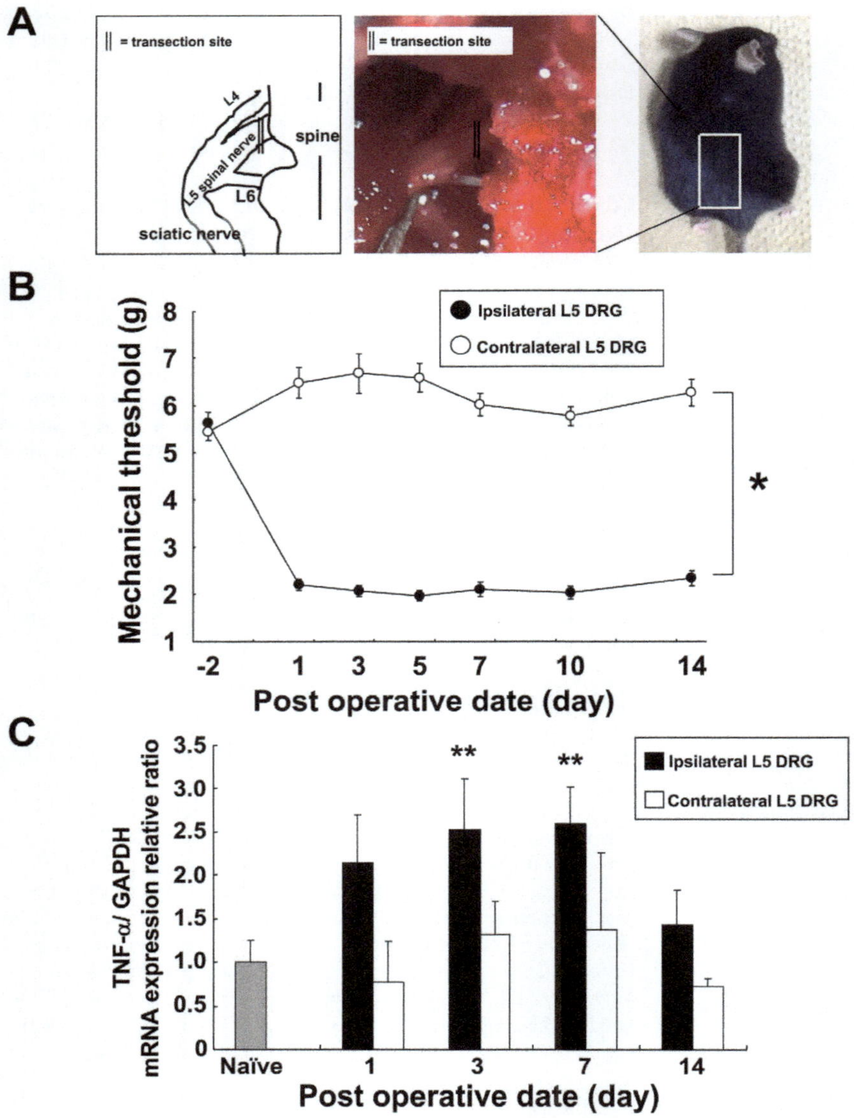

Figure 1. L5 spinal nerve transection as a neuropathic pain model. (**A**) Schematic presentation of left L5 spinal nerve transection (SNT) surgical procedure. Left and middle panels show the anatomical enlargement scene of the same field as the square of the mouse back in the right panel. The left panel shows a schematic view of the middle panel picture. The double lines show the L5 spinal nerve transection site in the left and middle panels. (**B**) The threshold of mechanical allodynia in the neuropathic model mice induced by SNT for 14 days. Black circles indicate ipsilateral and white circles indicate contralateral responses for mechanical stimuli. The threshold values were measured for five mice at each time point. Data show means ± S.E. **p*<0.01. (**C**) TNF-α mRNA expression in bilateral L5 DRG of neuropathic pain model mice for 14 days after SNT. The data are normalized to GAPDH and presented as the relative ratio to naïve DRG (no SNT mice) (n = 3–5 per each time course group). Gray bar is naïve DRG group, black bars are ipsilateral L5 DRG group, and open bars are contralateral L5 DRG group. Bars show means ± S.E. ***p*<0.05, compared with naïve.

RT-PCR was performed with the following primers: 5′-CACGTCGTAGCAAACCACCAAGTGG-3′ and 5′-GATAGCAAATCGGCTGACGGTGTGG-3′ for mouse TNF-α, 5′-AGGACGACGGCAACTACAAGAC-3′ and 5′-GAAGTTCACCTTGATGCCGTTC-3′ for GFP, 5′-AAATCCCATCACCATCTTCCA-3′ and 5′-AATGAGCCCCAGCCTTCTC-3′ for human GAPDH (for 293T cell), 5′-AACGACCCCTTCATTGAC-3′ and 5′-TCCACGACATACTCAGCAC-3′ for mouse GAPDH (for mouse tissues). For RT-PCR by TaqMan method, the following primers were used: Mn_99999915_g1 (Invitrogen, Carlsbad, USA) for mouse GAPDH and 5′-CATCTTCTCAAAATTCGAGTGACAA-3′, 5′-TCGGAGTAGACAAGGTAGAACCC-3′ and 5′-FAM-GCACGTCGTAGCAAACCACCACCAAGTGGA-TAMRA-3′ (probe) for mouse TNF-α. The PCR reaction consisted of denaturation at 94°C for 30 seconds, annealing at 60°C for 30 seconds, extension at 72°C for 30 seconds. The PCR products were analyzed with FAS-IV (Japan Genetics, Tokyo, Japan).

For quantification of each gene, real time PCR assay was performed using a LightCycler 480 (Roche Diagnostics, Manheim, Germany) with SYBR Green method (for activating transcription factor 3 (ATF3), calcitonin gene related peptide (CGRP), IL-6, neuropeptide Y (NPY), human GAPDH, mouse GAPDH and mouse TNF-α) and TaqMan method (for mouse GAPDH and mouse TNF-α). The PCR parameters were one cycle of 95°C for three min, followed by 50 cycles of denaturation at 95°C for 30 sec, annealing at 60°C for 30 sec and extension at 72°C for 30 sec. The emitted fluorescence for each reaction was measured three times during the annealing extension phase, and amplification plots were analyzed using LightCycler 480 software, version 1.5 (Roche Diagnostics Manheim, Germany). Potential genomic DNA contamination was controlled by the use of intron-encompassing primers and DNase digestion. GAPDH and MAPK6 have been reported to be the most stable reference genes for use in normalizing transcript level of interest genes although the expression of other many house-keeping genes reduced on the early phase in DRG after nerve injury [33]. Therefore, the normalization and relative expression analysis of target genes were performed using the $2^{-\Delta\Delta Ct}$ method with GAPDH as a control, which expression levels were confirmed not to be changed among day -2, 3, 7 and 14.

Immunohistochemistry

Animals were anesthetized by intraperitoneal administration of sodium pentobarbital (50 mg/kg) and intracardially perfused with 30 ml of PBS followed by a fixative containing 4% paraformaldehyde in 0.1 M PB. After perfusion fixation, animal tissues were kept in the same fixative at 4°C for 18 h and permeated with 15% (w/v) sucrose buffer with agitation. Each tissue was embedded in Tissue-Tek O.C.T compound (Sakura, Tokyo, Japan), frozen with liquid nitrogen and cut on a cryostat at 8 μm sections collected on MAS (Matsunami aggressive silane)-coated glass slides. Sections were blocked with 3% normal goat serum in PBS at room temperature for 15 min and processed for immunohistochemistry. The following antibodies were used: anti-TNF-α (1:100, Abcam, Cambridge, United Kingdom), anti-GFP (1:100, Medical & Biological Laboratories, Nagoya, Japan), anti-cleaved caspase3 (1:100, Cell Signaling Technology Japan, Tokyo, Japan), and AlexaFluor 488, 594 and 633 (1:1000, Abcam) as primary and secondary antibodies. For marker stains, we used 4′,6-diamidino-2-phenylindole (DAPI) for nuclei and fluorescent Nissl (NeuroTrace 435/455 or 530/615, Molecular Probes, Eugene, Oregon, USA) for neurons. Fluorescence images were captured and analyzed using Nikon C1si and the software, EZ-C1 version 3.90 (Nikon, Tokyo Japan).

DRG neuron cell count

To evaluate the neuronal cell survival in ipsilateral L5 DRG after SNT, we perfused mice transcardially with 4% paraformaldehyde in 0.1 M PBS, and isolated DRG tissues and embedded them in paraffin. L5 DRG paraffin blocks were sectioned at 10 μm thickness and stained with 0.1% Cresyl violet (Nissl stain, Muto Pure Chemicals Co. Ltd, Tokyo, Japan). After Nissl staining (Cresyl violet), all visible neurons in each left L5 DRG were counted in consecutive sections (20 μm intervals). For the evaluation of apoptosis after SNT with or without gene therapy, we counted the number of cleaved caspase3 positive neurons. Approximately 300 neurons were analyzed in consecutive sections (30 μm intervals) for each left L5 DRG.

Transduction efficacy and treatment effects of gene therapy by lentiviral vector *in vivo* were evaluated by counting the number of GFP or TNF-α positive neurons with the neuronal marker stain of fluorescent Nissl (NeuroTrace 435/455 for GFP or NeuroTrace 530/615 for TNF-α) in DRG after SNT with or without gene therapy. We analyzed approximately 300 neurons in consecutive sections (30 μm intervals) for each L5 DRG.

Statistical analysis

Statistical analysis was performed with SPSS 17.0 software (SPSS Inc., Chicago, USA). All data are shown as mean ± standard error of the mean (S.E.). The one-way ANOVA followed by Tukey's test was used to calculate statistical significance for multiple data sets. For behavioral test, two-way ANOVA was used. Data were considered significant difference at $p<0.05$.

Results

TNF-α expression and behavior testing in a spinal nerve transection (SNT) mouse model of neuropathic pain

We induced neuropathic pain in mice by SNT on the left side of the L5 spinal nerve at a location close to the spine (ipsilateral side, **Figure 1A**). The right L5 spinal nerve was not transected (contralateral side). SNT induced severe mechanical allodynia and hyperesthesia in the ipsilateral hind paw. We measured the hind paw withdrawal threshold against the mechanical stimuli (mechanical threshold) for the ipsilateral and contralateral paws for 14 days after SNT and found that the threshold was markedly decreased the day after SNT and remained at the same low level for 14 days (**Figure 1B**). We quantified TNF-α mRNA expression in L5 DRG by RT-PCR on day 1, 3, 7 and 14 after left SNT-induced neuropathic pain (**Figure 1C**) and found that SNT led to elevation of TNF-α mRNA expression in the DRG on the ipsilateral side, which was approximately 2.5-fold higher than the level in the naïve L5 DRG on day 3 and 7 after SNT, and returned towards baseline levels on day 14 after SNT (**Figure 1C**).

Design and evaluation of shRNA sequences against TNF-α expression in cultured cells

To develop an shRNA gene therapy against TNF-α in the SNT model, we designed 4 candidate shRNA sequences against TNF-α based on scoring algorithms presented by The RNAi Consortium (TRC, available: http://www.broadinstitute.org/rnai/trc. Accessed on 2014 Feb 20.) (Target sites of these four shRNA against mouse TNF-α are shown in **Figure 2A**). We cloned the individual shRNA sequences (shRNA1-4 in **Figure 2A**) into a pLL3.7 plasmid to produce lentiviral vectors designated LV-TNF-shRNA1-4 (**Figure 2B**). In these vectors, the shRNA sequence was driven by the U6 promoter and the GFP was driven by the CMV promoter (**Figure 2B**).

We created TNF-α-expressing 293T cells by infecting them with lentiviral vector over-expressing TNF-α and DsRed driven by EF-1 promoter (LV-TNF-DsRed in **Figure 2B**). We next tested the capacity of LV-TNF-shRNA1-4 to silence TNF-α expression by infecting these cells with LV-TNF-shRNA1-4 or LV-GFP (control GFP vector with no shRNA sequence). Seventy-two hours later, we observed these cells under the fluorescence microscope. We found that in the LV-TNF-shRNA1-4 and LV-GFP groups, the GFP signals were similar in 293T cells (lower panels in **Figure 2C**) confirming approximately similar level of infection of the 4 silencing vectors. In cells that were infected with silencing vectors (LV-TNF-shRNA1-4), the DsRed signal was markedly attenuated in all 4 groups compared with the LV-GFP group or single infection LV-TNF-DsRed ('none' group) (upper panels in **Figure 2C**). Next, we quantified TNF-α mRNA expression by RT-PCR and found that the level of TNF-α mRNA was significantly reduced in the 4 LV-TNF-shRNA groups compared with LV-GFP control group ($n=5$, $p<0.01$, the relative percent lowering in mRNA level were as follows: 47.8% by LV-TNF-shRNA1, 75.1% by LV-TNF-shRNA2, 89.1% by LV-TNF-shRNA3, and 84.7% by LV-TNF-shRNA4; **Figure 2D**). Thus, of the 4 vectors that we analyzed, we found LV-TNF-shRNA3 to

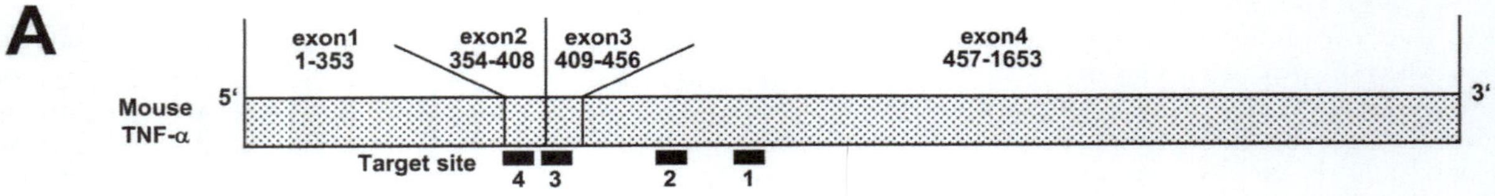

(target site)	sense	hairpin	antisense
shRNA1 (651-671)	TGGCTATCTCATACCAGGAGAAA	CTCGAG	TTTCTCCTGGTATGAGATAGCTTTTTTC
shRNA2 (560-580)	TGCGATGGGTTGTACCTTGTCTA	CTCGAG	TAGACAAGGTACAACCCATCGTTTTTTC
shRNA3 (403-423)	TGCCTCCCTCTCATCAGTTCTAT	CTCGAG	ATAGAACTGATGAGAGGGAGGTTTTTTC
shRNA4 (368-388)	TGCACTCAGATCATCTTCTCAAA	CTCGAG	TTTGAGAAGATGATCTGAGTGTTTTTTC

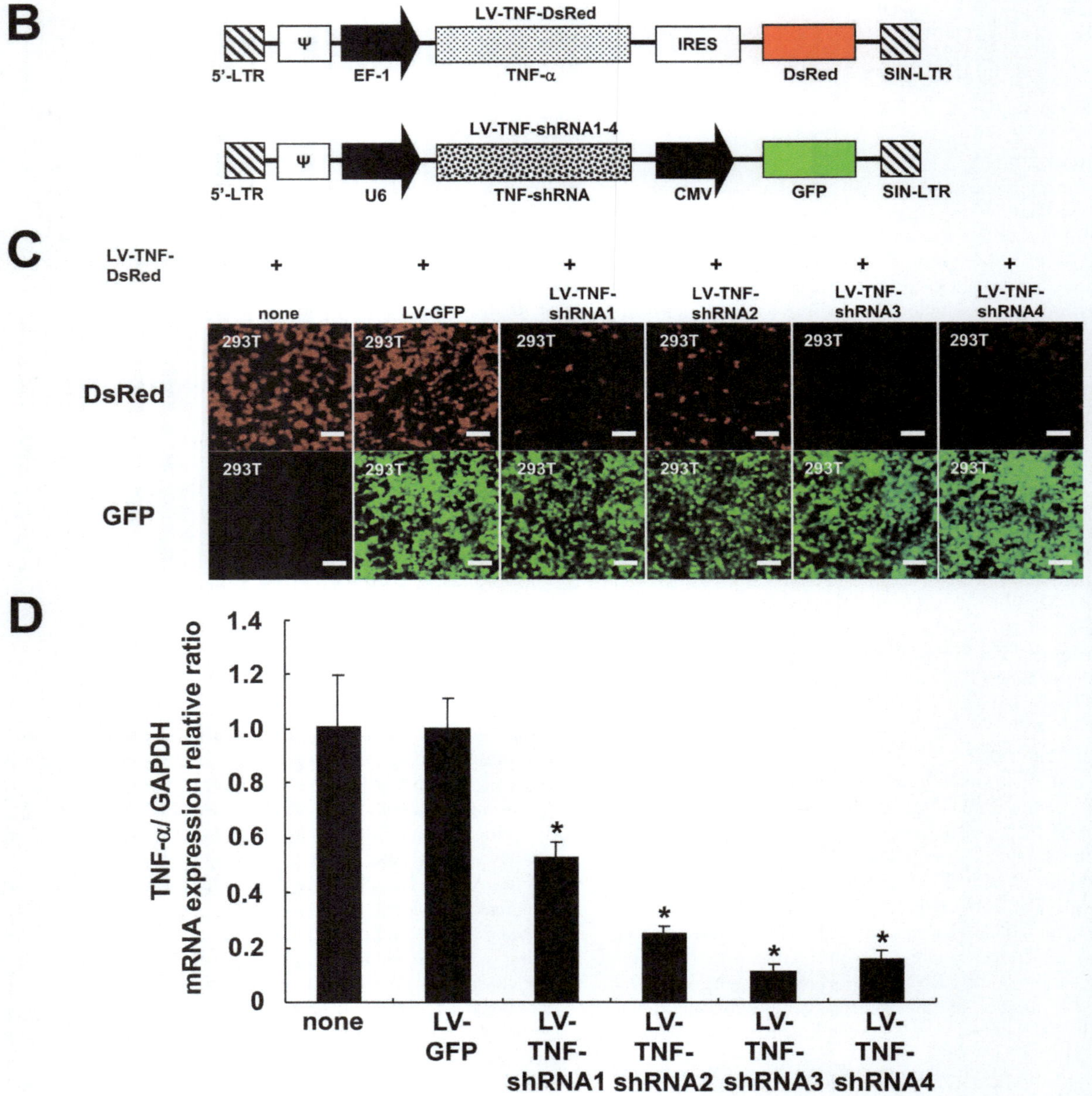

Figure 2. Construction of mouse TNF-α over-expression and shRNA lentiviral vectors and silencing efficacy of LV-TNF-shRNAs. (**A**) Four candidate shRNA sequences against TNF-α (shRNA1 to shRNA4) and schematic presentation of target site of these shRNAs on mouse TNF-α sequence. The black bars and the number 1 to 4 under the scheme of mouse TNF-α cDNA indicate the location of mouse TNF-α cDNA targeted by shRNA1-4. The numbers in the parentheses beside shRNA1-4 mean the location of target site against the mouse TNF-α cDNA. (**B**) Schematic presentation of LV-TNF-DsRed (TNF-α over-expression vector, upper) and LV-TNF-shRNA1-4 (TNF-α silencing vector, lower). LTR: long terminal repeat,

Ψ: packaging signal, EF-1: elongation factor 1 promoter, IRES: internal ribosome entry sites, SIN-LTR: self inactivating-LTR, CMV: cytomegalovirus promoter. (**C**) Fluorescence in 293T cells at 72 h after co-infection with two lentiviral vectors, LV-TNF-DsRed and LV-TNF-shRNA1-4, LV-GFP (GFP control vector with no TNF-shRNA sequence) or none. Upper panels show TNF-α expression (red), lower panels show each transduction of LV-TNF-shRNA1-4 therapeutic vectors or LV-GFP (green). Scale bar = 50 μm. (**D**) TNF-α mRNA expression in 293T cells at 72 h after infection of LV-TNF-DsRed with LV-TNF-shRNA1-4, LV-GFP, or none (n = 5 per group). The data were normalized by GAPDH. Bars indicate means ± S.E. *$p<0.01$ compared with LV-GFP group.

be the most efficacious in silencing TNF-α expression in 293T cells. We therefore tested the efficacy of using LV-TNF-shRNA3 therapy on neuropathic pain in the SNT mouse model.

Evaluation of transduction efficiency with LV-TNF-shRNA3 injection onto left L5 spinal nerve

We determined the efficiency of gene delivery after the treatment by histological analysis and mRNA expression of GFP (reporter gene) in bilateral DRG tissues after infection of LV-TNF-shRNA3 targeting the transected left L5 spinal nerve. Infection-induced GFP mRNA expression in ipsilateral L5 DRG was confirmed between day 3 to day 14 after local injection onto the left L5 spinal nerve (**Figure 3A**). mRNA expression was also observed in the contralateral L5 DRG, but the expression levels were much lower compared with the ipsilateral side. GFP mRNA expression in ipsilateral L5 DRG gradually increased from day 3 to day 14, which was also observed in the contralateral side although the expression was significantly lower (complete set of data from all treated mice, corrected to GAPDH expression, **Figure 3A**). In addition, GFP protein signals were detected mainly in neurons of L5 ipsilateral DRG sections, which population gradually increased and reached 43.2%±6.1% on day 14 (**Figure 3B, C**). In L5 contralateral DRG, GFP protein signals were observed at 1 level significantly lower than in the ipsilateral DRG, reaching 18.9%±3.0% of the neurons on day 14 (**Figure 3B, C**). Therefore, administration of LV-TNF-shRNA3 induced high level of transgene expression in DRG tissues by local injection onto the spinal nerve.

LV-TNF-RNA3 suppressed TNF-α expression in ipsilateral L5 DRG after SNT

We quantified the relative degree of TNF-α silencing after LV-TNF-shRNA3 gene therapy by quantitative RT-PCR of TNF-α mRNA and immunohistochemistry of TNF-α protein in L5 DRG tissues. In SNT with LV-GFP group (control group), TNF-α mRNA expression increased approximately 4-fold compared with pretreatment expression levels in ipsilateral L5 DRG from day 3 to day 14 (left panel in **Figure 4A**). The increased TNF-α mRNA expression by SNT was markedly suppressed down to baseline levels in ipsilateral L5 DRG treated with LV-TNF-shRNA3 (therapy group) for 14 days (left panel in **Figure 4A**). In the contralateral L5 DRG, there was no significant change in TNF-α mRNA levels in the untreated LV-GFP groups (control group). The LV-TNF-shRNA3 group also did not show any change (right panel in **Figure 4A**). Immunohistochemistry in ipsilateral L5 DRG revealed markedly increased immunoreactive TNF-α in the cytosol of neurons after ipsilateral SNT in the LV-GFP group compared with naïve (control group) from day 3 to day 14 (**Figure 4B, C**). The immunostained TNF-α positive neurons (co-localized with Nissl stain) increased markedly in SNT with LV-GFP group compared with pretreatment DRG group (naïve) from day 3 to day 14 (the percentage of positive neuron were increased approximately 60% and peaked at day 7, **Figure 4B**). In gene therapy group with LV-TNF-shRNA3, the appearance of immunoreactive TNF-α-positive neurons induced in the vast majority of the DRG neurons by SNT was suppressed to baseline levels from day 3 to day 14 (**Figure 4B, C**). These results were consistent with the data on the level of TNF-α mRNA expression.

LV-TNF-RNA3 preserves DRG neurons from cell death caused by SNT

SNT induced cell death leading to reduced neuron number was reported to correlate with neuropathic pain [34]. We therefore used Nissl staining to quantify the number of surviving DRG neurons in ipsilateral L5 DRG in LV-GFP and LV-TNF-shRNA3 treatment groups on day 14 after SNT (**Figure 5A, B**). Neuronal cell numbers were significantly reduced by SNT in the ipsilateral L5 DRG in LV-GFP group (709.8±119.1 cells/DRG tissue) compared to naïve (2264±260.3 cells/DRG tissue) (**Figure 5A, B**). In contrast, DRG neuronal cell numbers were significantly preserved in the LV-TNF-shRNA3 treatment group (1501±154.8 cells/DRG tissue) compared with the LV-GFP group (**Figure 5A, B**).

We next used immunohistochemistry of cleaved caspase3 to quantify the number of apoptotic neurons in L5 ipsilateral DRG on day 14 after SNT and the therapeutic effects of TNF-α silencing. We detected a very low level of cleaved caspase3-immunoreactive DRG neurons under naïve basal conditions (3.35±1.00%, **Figure 6A, B**). However, the number of cleaved caspase3-positive neurons in ipsilateral L5 DRG 14 days after SNT increased significantly in the LV-GFP group (16.52±1.56%); this SNT-induced increase in number of apoptotic cells was significantly suppressed by LV-TNF-shRNA3 treatment (to 9.09±1.14%) (**Figure 6A, B**).

LV-TNF-shRNA3 reduces mRNA expression of neuropeptides, injury and inflammatory markers related to neuropathic pain

Many injury markers, cytokines and neuropeptides have been reported to be up-regulated in DRG neurons in mouse models of neuropathic pain. Thus, we measured the mRNA expression of the injury makers ATF3 and NPY, the inflammatory cytokine IL-6, and the neuropeptide CGRP in ipsilateral L5 DRG to evaluate the effect of TNF-α silencing. Both ATF3 and NPY mRNA levels increased markedly after SNT. The ATF3 mRNA peaked early at day 3, whereas NPY mRNA increased significantly at day 3 but peaked later at day 7 after SNT (**Figure 7A, B**). The peak ATF3 expression was significantly suppressed on day 3 and that of NPY was significantly suppressed on days 3 and 7 in the LV-TNF-RNA3 group compared with the LV-GFP group (**Figure 7A, B**). IL-6 mRNA expression was significantly elevated in L5 DRG by SNT in the LV-GFP group on day 3 (**Figure 7C**), and the level was significantly attenuated in the LV-TNF-shRNA3 group on day 3 (**Figure 7C**). We detected no significant change in the mRNA expression of CGRP, a neurotransmitter correlated with pain transmission (**Figure 7D**), and its level was not changed by LV-TNF-shRNA treatment (**Figure 7D**).

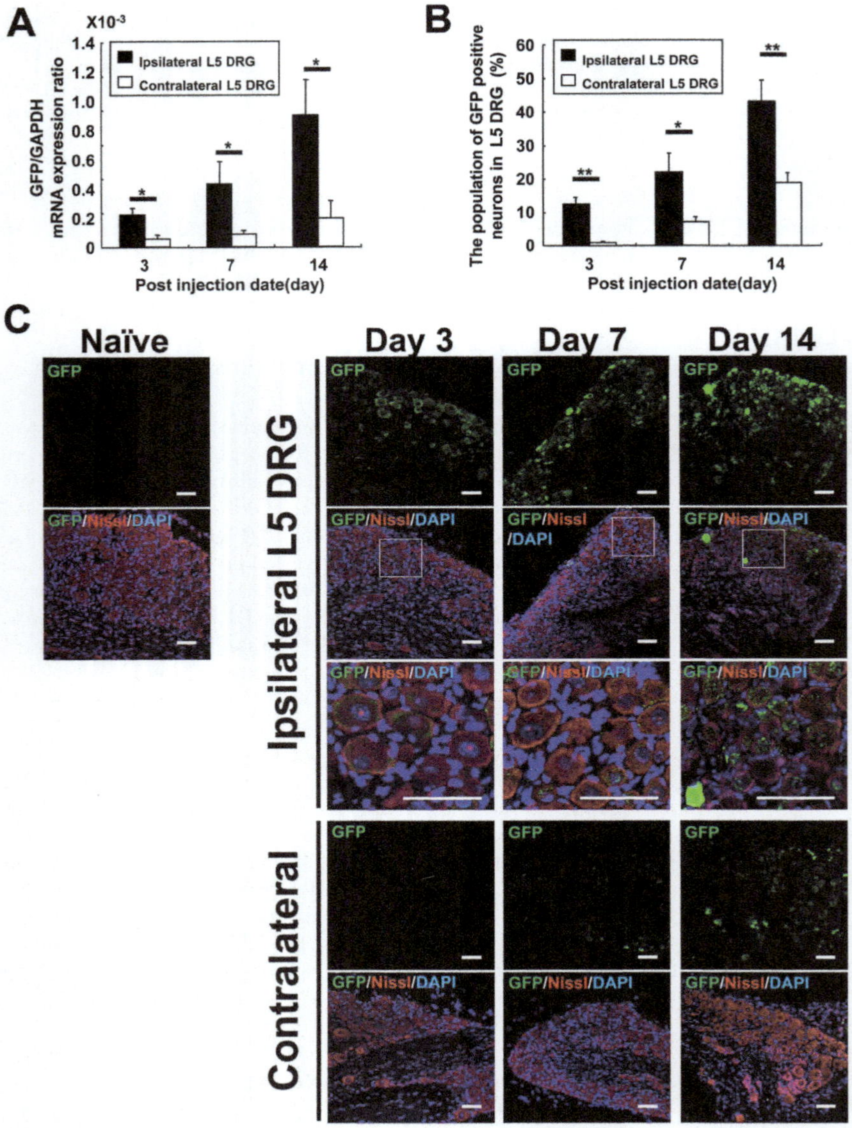

Figure 3. Transduction efficacy of LV-TNF-shRNA3 onto left L5 spinal nerve in L5 DRG tissues. (**A**) The quantification of GFP mRNA expression induced by LV-shRNA3 in bilateral L5 DRG on day 3, 7, 14 after SNT and injection of LV-TNF-shRNA3. The data were normalized to GAPDH. Black bars showed the results in ipsilateral L5 DRG (n = 5 per time point) and open bars showed the results in contralateral L5 DRG (n = 5 per time point). Bars indicate means ± S.E. *$p<0.05$. (**B**) The population of GFP positive neurons in L5 DRG on day 3, 7 and 14 after SNT and injection of LV-TNF-shRNA3. Black bars showed the results in ipsilateral L5 DRG (n = 5 per time point) and open bars showed the results in contralateral L5 DRG (n = 5 per time point). Bars indicate means ± S.E. *$p<0.05$, **$p<0.01$. (**C**) Immunohistochemical staining with anti-GFP antibodies (green), DAPI (blue) and Nissl (red) in the bilateral L5 DRG on day 3, 7 and 14 after SNT and injection of LV-TNF-shRNA3. Upper panels of each group showed immunostainigs of anti-GFP antibodies and 2nd lines' panels showed the merged images of GFP, Nissl and DAPI in each group. The square regions of 2nd lines' panels were enlarged in third lines' panels in ipsilateral L5 DRG group. Scale bar = 50 μm.

LV-TNF-shRNA3 gene therapy for neuropathic pain in the SNT mouse model

While we analyzed the various biochemical and immunohistochemical parameters induced by SNT, we also monitored the efficacy of LV-TNF-shRNA3 or LV-GFP (control vector) treatment by measuring the mechanical threshold every other day till day 7 and again on day 10 and 14 after treatment (**Figure 8**). The mechanical threshold in the ipsilateral hind paw was significantly impaired in both groups from day 1 to day 14, but the impairment was significantly attenuated throughout this period in the LV-TNF-shRNA3 group compared with the LV-GFP (control vector) group. Therefore, the LV-TNF-shRNA3 treatment led to an improvement in an objective behavior measurement in neuropathic pain in SNT mice.

Discussion

This study demonstrated that silencing of TNF-α expression with lentiviral vectors suppressed neuropathic pain induced by SNT. Lentiviral vectors targeted to DRG tissues decreased TNF-α expression in the affected (ipsilateral) DRG neurons. In addition, silencing of TNF-α expression in DRG resulted in the inhibition of

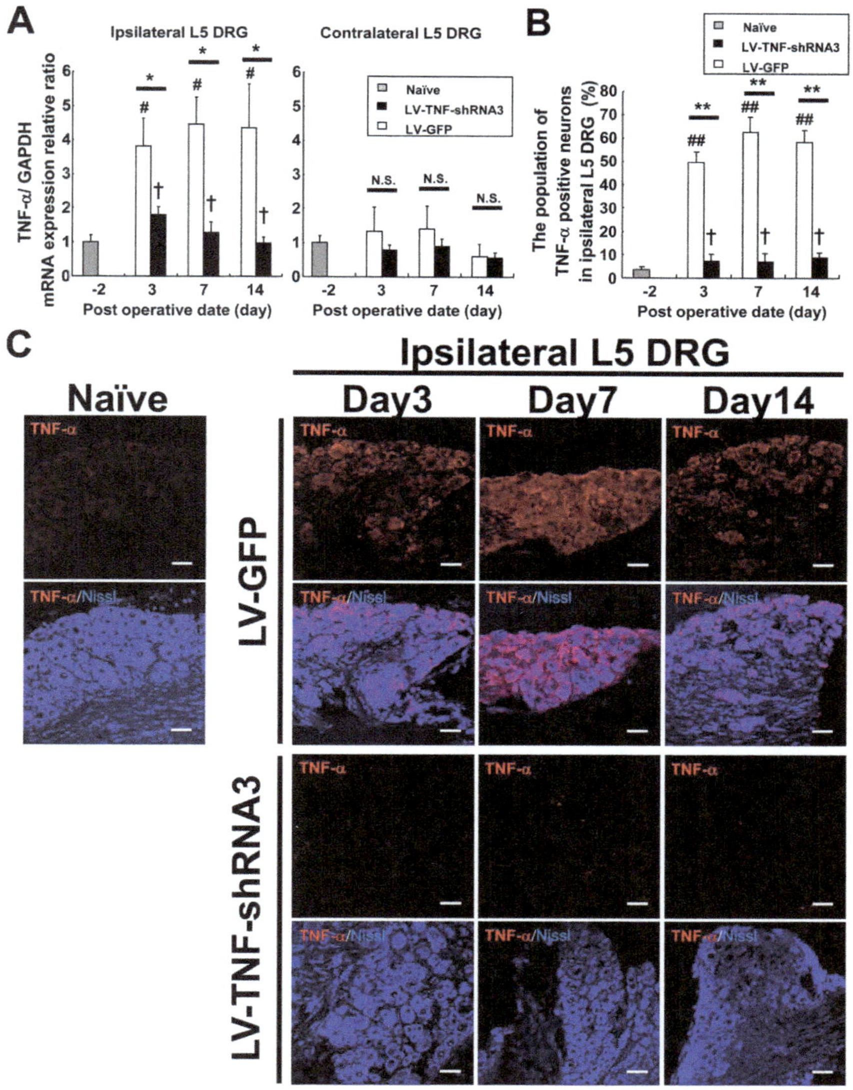

Figure 4. Suppression of TNF-α mRNA and protein expression in L5 DRG of SNT mice by LV-TNF-shRNA3. (**A**) TNF-α mRNA expression in bilateral L5 DRG from LV-GFP or LV-TNF-shRNA3 groups on day 3, 7, 14 after SNT and injection. Ipsilateral L5 DRG (left panel) and contralateral L5 DRG (right panel). The data are normalized to GAPDH and presented as a relative ratio to naïve DRG (on day −2). Gray bars showed the result in naïve DRG (on day −2, n = 6), white bars showed the results in LV-GFP group (n = 6–8 per time point) and black bars showed the results in LV-TNF-shRNA3 group (n = 6–8 per time point) Bars indicate means ± S.E. *$p<0.05$, #$p<0.05$ compared with naïve, ##$p<0.01$ compared with naïve, † the difference was not significant compared with naïve. N.S. means "not significant." (**B**) The population of TNF-α positive neurons in ipsilateral L5 DRG on day 3, 7 and 14 after SNT and injection of LV-GFP or LV-TNF-shRNA3. Gray bars showed the result in naïve DRG without SNT and injection (on day −2, n = 4), white bars showed the results in LV-GFP group (n = 4–5 per time point) and black bars showed the results in LV-TNF-shRNA3 group (n = 4–5 per time point) Bars indicate means ± S.E. ** $p<0.01$, ##$p<0.01$ compared with naïve, † the difference was not significant compared with naïve. (**C**) Immunohistochemical staining with anti-TNF-α antibodies (red) and Nissl (blue) in the ipsilateral L5 DRG on day 3, 7 and 14 after SNT and injection of LV-GFP or LV-TNF-shRNA3. Upper panels of each group showed immunostainigs of anti-TNF-α antibodies and lower panels showed the merged image of TNF-α and Nissl in each group. Scale bar = 50 μm

neuronal cell death and apoptosis caused by SNT. Furthermore, injury markers and inflammatory cytokines that were up-regulated by SNT were greatly attenuated by lentiviral gene therapy. Therefore, gene therapy-mediated TNF-α silencing may be an efficacious treatment strategy for protecting DRG neurons and ameliorate neuropathic pain induced by nerve injury.

Neuropathic pain and TNF-α

Neuropathic pain is caused by neuronal damage or dysfunction [1,35]. Recent studies suggest that a communication between the immune and the nervous systems may underlie neuropathic pain [11]. TNF-α is a pro-inflammatory cytokine commonly produced in response to different types of disease, inflammation and tissue damage. It is a short-lived inflammatory mediator that plays a central role in initiating inflammatory reactions of the innate immune system, including the induction of other cytokine production, activation and expression of adhesion molecules,

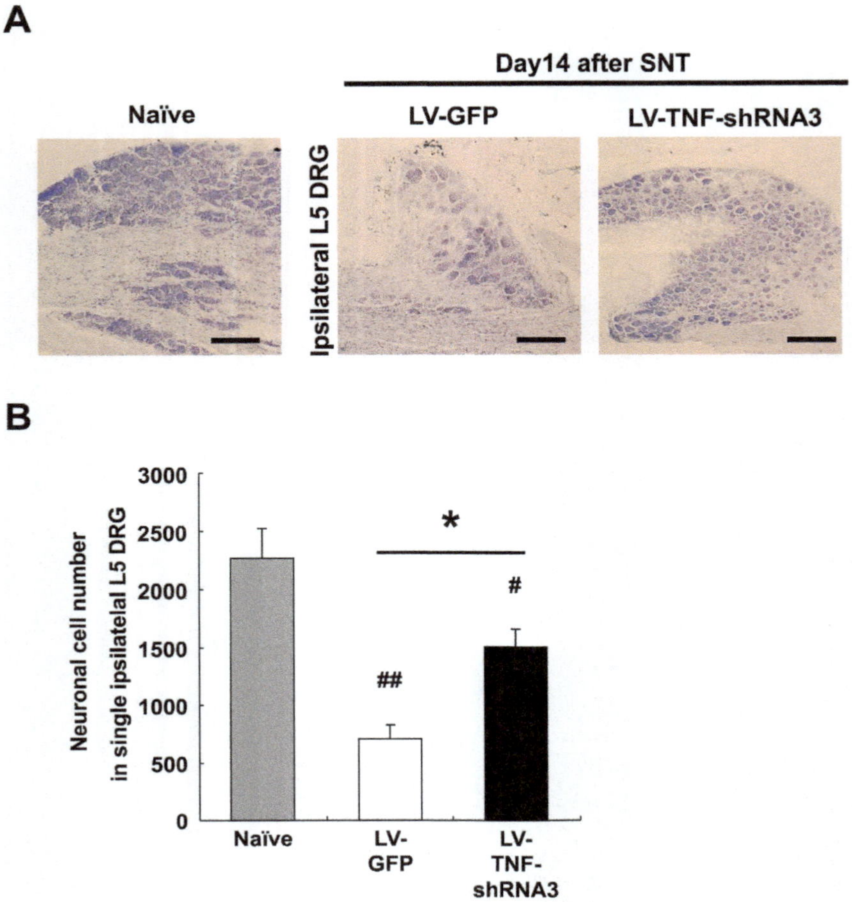

Figure 5. Evaluation of survival neurons in L5 DRG after SNT with LV-TNF-shRNA3. (**A**) Nissl stain of L5 ipsilateral L5 DRG on day 14 after SNT with LV-TNF-shRNA3 or LV-GFP. Scale bar = 50 μm. (**B**) Quantitative analysis of cell survival in L5 DRG neurons after SNT with LV-TNF-shRNA3 or LV-GFP (n = 5 per group). Gray bar - neuronal cell numbers including single ipsilateral L5 DRG in naïve DRG group; white bar - LV-GFP group; black bar - LV-TNF-shRNA3 group. Bars show means ± S.E. *$p<0.01$, $^{\#}p<0.05$ compared with naïve, $^{\#\#}p<0.01$ compared with naïve.

and stimulation of inflammatory cells in nerve injury [36]. Indeed, the direct application of TNF-α to the sciatic nerve and DRG leads to changes in the properties of neurons, such as ectopic firing in Aδ-, Aβ- and C-fibers [37,38], and induces thermal hyperalgesia and mechanical allodynia [18,39,40]. Furthermore, TNF-α enhances TTX-R Na^+ channels and increases membrane K^+ ion conductance by a non-voltage-gated mechanism in DRG neurons [41,42]. Therefore, TNF-α plays a pivotal role in multiple pathways involved in neuropathic pain and is clearly a treatment target for neuropathic pain. Here we found that silencing TNF-α in DRG partially suppressed mechanical allodynia though it did not produce a complete remission. Other cytokines, neurotrophic factors and chemokines such as IL-1β, nitric oxide, ATP, chemokine(C-C motif) ligand 2 and nerve growth factor, are involved in the pathogenesis of neuropathic pain, and they have direct actions as well as mediate crosstalks with TNF-α in nociceptive cascade in DRG neurons [43]. It is likely that the directed modulation of these molecules, in addition to TNF-α suppression, may be required for a more robust clinical remission of the neuropathic pain. Nonetheless, this study showed that gene therapy-mediated TNF-α-silencing is a useful strategy for the treatment of neuropathic pain.

Association between TNF-α and apoptosis or inflammation in spinal nerve injury

Spinal nerve injury leads to activated caspase3 and increased apoptosis [34] in DRG neurons [44,45]. TNF-α was known to be associated with apoptosis through the activation of caspase3 pathway [46]. In this study, TNF-α expression and caspase3 were elevated in DRG tissues 14 days after SNT, and we showed that TNF-α silencing in this setting suppressed caspase3 and increased the number of surviving DRG neurons. Therefore, silencing TNF-α not only suppresses neuropathic pain but also protects DRG neurons from apoptotic cell death after SNT, an effect that may have an impact on the functional maintenance and regeneration potential of sensory neurons.

IL-6 is up-regulated in DRG in response to peripheral nerve injury [47,48]. A recent study suggested that TNF-α induces the production of IL-6, which contributes to neuropathic pain in DRG [49] and spinal cord in a spinal nerve transection model [47–49]. ATF3 and NPY are widely used as injury markers of axotomy. These two molecules are also up-regulated in DRG neurons in nerve injury models [50,51], and are associated with phenotypic changes [52] in DRG neurons such as ion channel excitability and responses against neuropeptides [53,54]. Here, we showed that mRNA expression of ATF3, NPY and IL-6 is elevated in the early

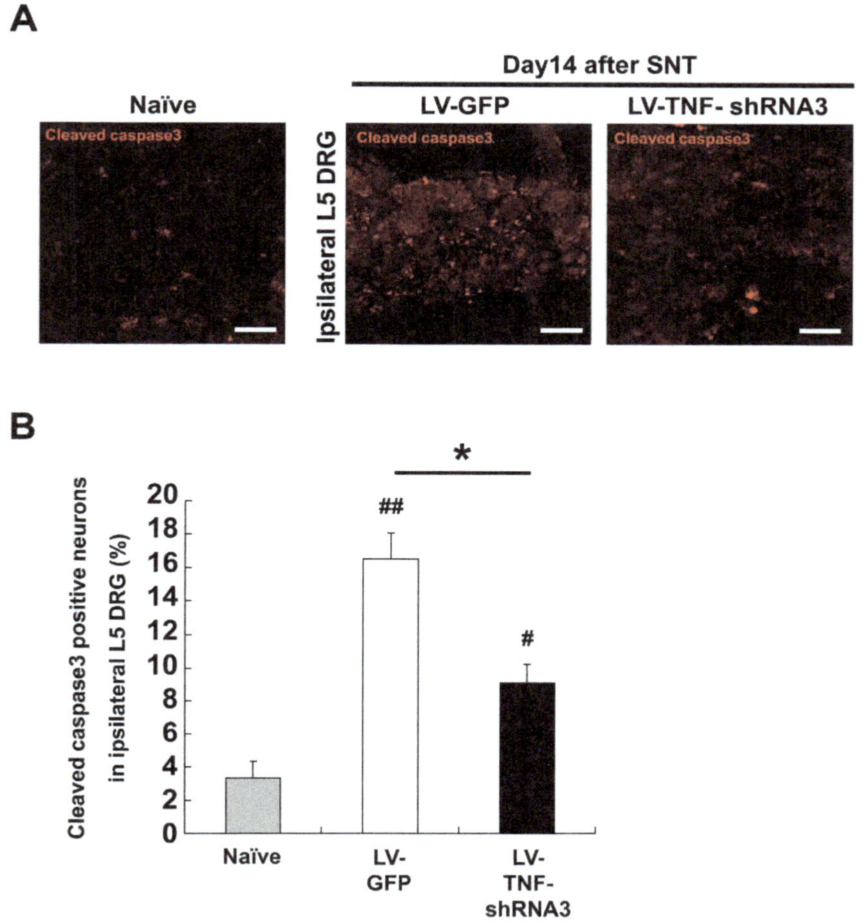

Figure 6. Immunohistochemical analysis of cleaved caspase3 in DRG tissues. Immunohistochemical staining of cleaved caspase3 (red) (**A**) and the quantitative analysis of cleaved caspase3 positive neurons (**B**) in ipsilateral L5 DRG after spinal nerve transection with LV-TNF-shRNA3 or LV-GFP on day 14 (n = 5 in each group). Bars show means ± S.E. *$p<0.01$, $^{\#}p<0.05$ compared with naïve, $^{\#\#}p<0.01$ compared with naïve. Scale bar = 50 μm.

phase after SNT but can be suppressed by TNF-α silencing, indicating that TNF-α is likely up-stream of the immune cascade during nerve injury. The multiple downstream effects of TNF-α silencing protect DRG neurons against inflammation induced by nerve injury by suppressing of ATF3, NPY and IL-6 expression, resulting in the reduction of apoptosis and suppression of neuropathic pain.

Benefits of lentiviral vector-mediated silencing of TNF-α

DRG-targeted gene delivery is a promising therapeutic option for the treatment of neuropathic pain. A number of viral gene vectors are available for gene delivery, including adenoviral (Ad) vectors, adeno-associated viral (AAV) vectors, and lentiviral vectors [55]. The selection of the appropriate viral vectors and route of delivery are important issues that must be considered.

In general, Ad vectors have high transduction efficiency in most cells with the coxsackie virus and adenovirus receptor (CAR) compared to AAV and lentiviral vectors after attachment to the target cells [56–58]. However, Ad vectors show relatively low affinity for mature neuronal cells with rare CAR [56,59]. In using AAV vectors for neural tissue transduction, several serotypes of AAV vectors are known to show tropism to neurons [55,60]. In lentiviral vectors, the tropism to the neurons is acquired by the specific envelop protein [55,61–63]. In this study, we used lentiviral vectors pseudotyped with vesiculo-stomatitis virus glycoprotein for gene therapy of neuropathic pain because this glycoprotein gives the letiviral vectors both the potential of tropism for neuronal cells and an ability to infect neuronal cells by axonal transport [63].

It is also important to consider the toxicity of various viral vectors. Ad vectors have been shown to induce a potent immune response against the capsid, double-stranded DNA genome, viral proteins expressed from the vector backbone, or incorporated transgenes, a limitation for *in vivo* gene therapy [64]. In contrast, AAV and lentiviral vectors generally elicit a relativelymild immune response as compared to Ad vectors [55,64]. Using lentiviral vectors might lead to a relatively mild immune response, when used *in vivo* in rodents [55,56,62].

For delivering transgenes by viral vectors to the DRG *in vivo*, it was reported mainly by three different approaches, intrathecally, direct injection into sciatic nerve or into the DRG itself [55,60–62,65,66]. A prior study using AAV vectors suggested that the direct injection of the vectors into the DRG or sciatic nerve could provide stronger gene expression in the DRG neurons than injection into subcutaneous tissue or subarachnoid space [65]. Moreover, direct injection of Ad vector and AAV vector into

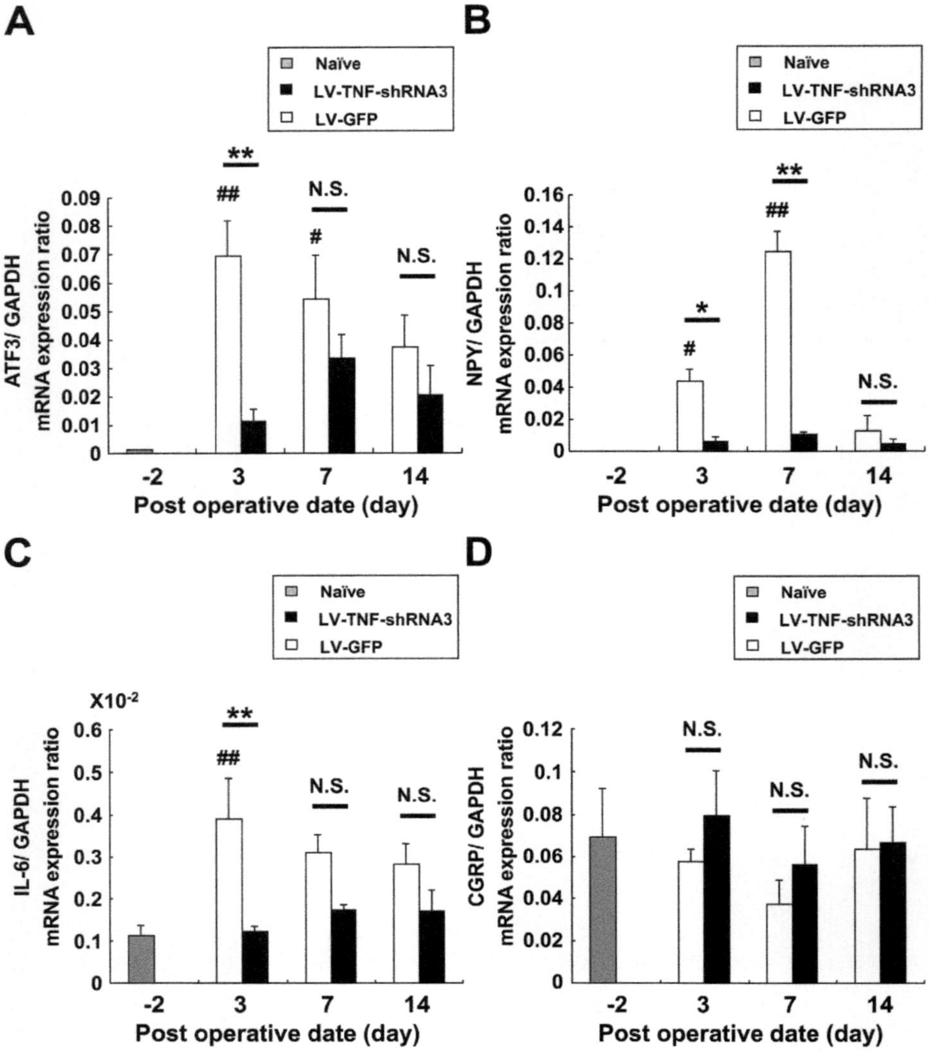

Figure 7. mRNA expression of neuropeptides, inflammatory and injury markers in SNT mice L5 DRG with treatment. ATF3 (**A**), NPY (**B**), IL-6 (**C**) and CGRP (**D**) mRNA expression were measured on day 3, 7 and 14 after SNT. The data are normalized to GAPDH. Gray bars - naïve DRG (on day −2); white bars - LV-GFP group; black bars - LV-TNF-shRNA3 group (n = 6–8 per group). Bars show means ± S.E. **p*<0.05, ***p*<0.01, #*p*<0.05 compared with naïve, ##*p*<0.01 compared with naïve. N.S. means "not significant".

DRG was also reported to be vastly superior to intraneural injection into sciatic nerve [66]. Lentiviral vectors have been delivered to either directly into DRG or indirectly via the sciatic nerve, which also ended up in the DRG [61,62]. In general, direct DRG injection appears to be the most effective and widely used approach. We note, however, that direct injection to DRG may induce additional tissue damage. Especially for the treatment of neuropathic pain, it is important to avoid further damage of the sensory nerve system, which by itself may induce neuropathic pain [67]. Here, we selected injection onto injury site of spinal nerve as a promising approach.

Unexpectedly, we found that spinal nerve injection led to high level transduction of the DRG. It was much higher than that reported in a previous study that utilized direct injection of lentiviral vectors into DRG in rats [62]. The administration method of injection onto injury site of spinal nerve seems to produce results from three different delivery methods, combining the effects of intrathecal injection, direct sciatic nerve or DRG injection. In fact, we demonstrated that GFP expression and silencing of TNF-α occurred in the ipsilateral as well as contralateral DRGs. The lentiviral vector might have spread through the cerebrospinal fluid to the contralateral DRG. This phenomenon is consistent with the expression pattern as transgene was found to be diffusely expressed at many spinal levels of DRG after intrathecal injection. At the same time, lentiviral vectors may be delivered to the DRG neurons by axonal transport because lentiviral vectors were injected onto spinal nerve in a manner similar to that following sciatic nerve injection as previously reports [56]. In our results, transgene was expressed diffusely in DRG neurons, which was different from the expression pattern immediately adjacent to the injection site following direct injection into DRG. Finally, it is possible that lentiviral vectors may access the ipsilateral DRG by direct infiltration. Here, we showed that lentiviral vectors injected onto the injury site of the spinal nerves led to high efficiency transduction of DRGs, constituting a promising approach for delivering transgenes to the DRG,

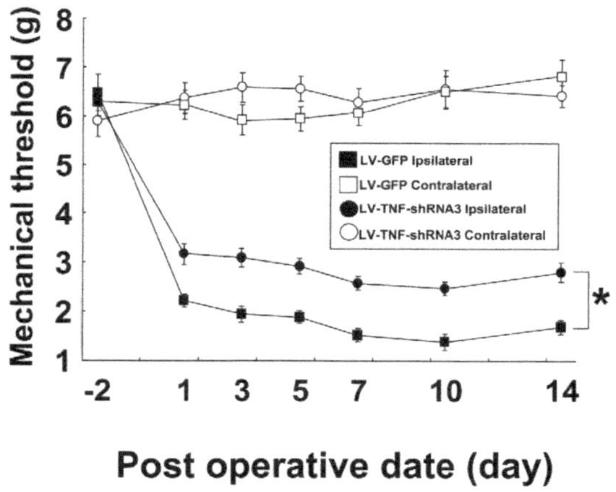

Figure 8. The effect of gene therapy with LV-TNF-shRNA3 for neuropathic pain in SNT mice. The threshold of mechanical allodynia was measured on the ipsilateral and contralateral sides in a neuropathic pain model for 14 days after SNT, in mice administered LV-TNF-shRNA3 or LV-GFP (as a control) (n = 6-7 per group). White circles - contralateral side of LV-TNF shRNA3 group; black circles - ipsilateral side of LV-TNF shRNA3 group; white squares - contralateral side of LV-GFP group; black squares - ipsilateral side of LV-GFP group. Data indicate means ± S.E. *$p<0.01$ between LV-TNF-shRNA3 ipsilateral and LV-GFP ipsilateral group.

although further studies should be needed to clarify the details of mechanism of their high efficiency.

Clinical relevance of lentiviral vector-mediated silencing of TNF-α

Clinical reports suggest that anti-TNF-α drugs, such as etanercept [7,28,29] and infliximab [25,30], have the potential to relieve neuropathic pain caused by sciatica or disc herniation. In addition, HIV chemotherapy may lead to peripheral neuropathy caused by the massive release of TNF-α in serum and TNF-α therapy for cancer was shown to cause peripheral neuropathy [68,69]. Thus, silencing TNF-α, an initiator of the immune cascade, could be a therapeutic target for different types of neuropathic pain. However, anti-TNF-α drugs administered systemically is associated with many side effects, e.g., general immunosuppression in patients. The strategy used in this study addresses this problem because the gene was selectively delivered locally to the injury site. There are many potential clinical applications for the treatment method developed in this study. On the other hand, we must also contend with potential lentiviral toxicity. Our data showed the TNF-α mRNA expression ratio increased slightly in the LV-GFP group compared with SNT only (no infection), which might be have been induced by the gene delivery of lentiviral vectors, GFP, and/or undesired proteins remaining in the preparation of lentiviral vectors after the purification processes.

Considering the gene therapy of sensory neuronopathy, we previously reported the intrathecal administration of DRG-targeting fiber-modified helper-dependent adenovirus (HDAd) vectors [70]. The fiber-modified vectors display high affinities for neurons compared to the wild type Ad vectors. However, injection onto spinal nerve of lentiviral vectors showed quite high transduction efficiency to DRG neurons, which seems to be as good as, if not better than, the fiber-modified HDAd vectors. As some psuedtyped lentiviral vectors generally have high tropism to neurons compared with adenoviral vectors, local injection of lentiviral vectors showed high performance without recombination like as the modification of fiber protein. Moreover, the target gene delivered by lentiviral vectors can be integrated into the nuclei of neuronal cells leading to stable and long-term expression of therapeutic genes [71]. It obviates the necessity for repeated injections which might lead to an immune response. Therefore, we believe that lentiviral vectors may be the optimal vector for long-term therapy and may be ideal for the treatment of sensory neuronopathies or chronic neuropathic pain as this study.

In conclusion, we presented a strategy to relieve neuropathic pain using lentiviral shRNA vectors. Our results support previous evidence for TNF-α in the pathogenesis of neuropathic pain. In addition, we showed that TNF-α silencing by lentiviral shRNA vectors protects injured DRG neurons from apoptosis. Silencing TNF-α by lentiviral vector-mediated gene transfer targeted to DRGs with injection onto injury site of spinal nerve may provide a novel therapeutic alternative for the treatment of neuropathic pain.

Acknowledgments

We thank Fumiko Kimura, Mayuko Shohi, Emiko Ioka and Central Research Laboratory of Shiga University of Medical Science for excellent technical assistance.

Author Contributions

Conceived and designed the experiments: NO TT H. Kawai H. Kojima KO HM. Performed the experiments: NO TT KO. Analyzed the data: NO TT H. Kojima. Wrote the paper: NO H. Kawai TT H. Kojima KO LC HM.

References

1. Merskey H, Bogduk N (1994) Classification of chronic pain: descriptions of chronic pain syndromes and definitions of pain terms. In IASP Task Force on Taxonomy. Seattle: IASP Press. pp.209–214.
2. Silas Weir Mitchell (1872) Injuries of nerves and their consequences. Philadelphia: JB Lippincott. 377p.
3. Woolf CJ, Mannion RJ (1999) Neuropathic pain: aetiology, symptoms, mechanisms, and management. Lancet 353: 1959–1964.
4. Kuntzer T, Antoine JC, Steck AJ (2004) Clinical features and pathophysiological basis of sensory neuronopathies (ganglionopathies). Muscle Nerve 30: 255–268.
5. André N, Carré M, Brasseur G, Pourroy B, Kovacic H, et al. (2002) Paclitaxel targets mitochondria upstream of caspase activation in intact human neuroblastoma cells. FEBS letters 532: 256–260.
6. Ghosh AK, Jana S, Das T, Sa G, Mandal N, et al. (1999) Protection by protein A of apoptotic cell death caused by anti-AIDS drug zidovudine. Biochem Biophys Res Commun 264: 601–604.
7. Leung L, Cahill CM (2010) TNF-alpha and neuropatihic pain - a review. J Neuroinflamation 7:27. doi: 10.1186/1742-2094-7-27.
8. Jaggi AS, Jain V, Singh N (2011) Animal models of neuropathic pain. Fundam Clin Pharmacol 25: 1–28.
9. Kim SH, Chung JM (1992) An experimental model for peripheral neuropathy produced by segmental spinal nerve ligation in the rat. Pain 50: 355–363.
10. Li Y, Dorsi MJ, Meyer RA, Belzberg AJ (2000) Mechanical hyperalgesia after an L5 spinal nerve lesion in the rat is not dependent on input from injured nerve fibers. Pain 85: 493–502.
11. Vallejo R, Tilley D, Vogel L, Benyamin R (2010) The role of glia and the immune system in the development and maintenance of neuropathic pain. Pain Pract: 167–184.
12. Miao P, Madec K, Gong Y, Shen H, Eisenstat D, et al. (2008) Axotomy-induced up-regulation of tumor necrosis factor-alpha in the dorsal root ganglia. Neurol Res 30: 623–631.
13. Schäfers M, Svensson CI, Sommer C, Sorkin LS (2003) Tumor necrosis factor-alpha induces mechanical allodynia after spinal nerve ligation by activation of p38 MAPK in primary sensory neurons. J Neuro Sci 23: 2517–2521.
14. Xu JT, Xin WJ, Zang Y, Wu CY, Liu XG (2006) The role of tumor necrosis factor-alpha in the neuropathic pain induced by Lumbar 5 ventral root transection in rat. Pain 123: 306–321.
15. Wells MR, Racis SP Jr, Vaidya U (1992) Changes in plasma cytokines associated with peripheral nerve injury. J Neuroimmunol 39: 261–268.

16. Zhang YH, Vasko MR, Nicol GD (2002) Ceramide, a putative second messenger for nerve growth factor, modulates the TTX-resistant Na+ current and delayed rectifier K+ current in rat sensory neurons. J Physiol 544: 385–402.
17. Sorkin LS, Doom CM (2000) Epineurial application of TNF elicits an acute mechanical hyperalgesia in the awake rat. J Peripher Nerv Syst 5: 96–100.
18. Wagner R, Myers RR (1996) Endoneurial injection of TNF alpha produces neuropathic pain behaviors. Neuroreport 7: 2897–2901
19. Joseph EK, Levine JD (2004) Caspase signalling in neuropathic and inflammatory pain in the rat. Eur J Neurosci 20: 2896–2902.
20. Terashima T, Kojima H, Chan L (2012) Bone marrow expression of poly(ADP-ribose) polymerase underlies diabetic neuropathy via hematopoietic-neuronal cell fusion. FASEB J 26: 295–308.
21. Yamakawa I, Kojima H, Terashima T, Katagi M, Oi J, et al. (2011) Inactivation of TNF-α ameliorates diabetic neuropathy in mice. Am J Physiol Endocrinol Metab 301: E844–852.
22. Sommer C, Lindenlaub T, Teuteberg P, Schäfers M, Hartung T, et al. (2001) Anti-TNF-neutralizing antibodies reduce pain-related behavior in two different mouse models of painful mononeuropathy. Brain Res 913: 86–89.
23. Lindenlaub T, Teuteberg P, Hartung T, Sommer C (2000) Effects of neutralizing antibodies to TNFalpha on pain-related behavior and nerve regeneration in mice with chronic constriction injury. Brain Res 866: 15–22.
24. Sommer C, Schäfers M, Marziniak M, Toyka KV (2001) Etanercept reduces hyperalgesia in experimental painful neuropathy. J Peripher Nerv Syst 6: 67–72.
25. Caroyer J, Manto M, Steinfeld S (2002) Severe sensory neuronopathy responsive to infliximab in primary Sjögren's syndrome. Neurology 59: 113–114.
26. Camussi G, Lupia E (1998) The future role of anti-tumour necrosis factor (TNF) products in the treatment of rheumatoid arthritis. Drugs. 55: 613–620.
27. Empl M, Renaud S, Erne B, Fuhr P, Straube A, et al. (2001) TNF-alpha expression in painful and nonpainful neuropathies. Neurology 56: 1371–1377.
28. Cohen SP, Bogduk N, Dragovich A, Buckenmaier CC 3rd, Griffith S, et al. (2009) Randomised, double-blind, placebo-controlled, dose-response, and preclinical safety study of transforaminal epidural etanercept for the treatment of Sciatica. Anesthesiology 110: 1116–1126.
29. Ohtori S, Miyagi M, Eguchi Y, Inoue G, Orita S, et al. (2012) Epidural administration of spinal nerves with the tumor necrosis factor-alpha inhibitor, etanercept, compared with dexamethasone for treatment of sciatica in patients with lumbar spinal stenosis: a prospective randomized study. Spine 37: 439–444.
30. Karppinen J, Korhonen T, Malmivaara A, Paimela L, Kyllönen E, et al. (2003) Tumor necrosis factor-alpha monoclonal antibody, infliximab, used to manage severe sciatica. Spine 28: 750–753; discussion 753–754.
31. Lai Y, Li D, Li C, Muehleisen B, Radek KA, et al. (2012) The antimicrobial protein REG3A regulates keratinocyte proliferation and differentiation after skin injury. Immunity 37: 74–84.
32. El Maarouf A, Kolesnikov Y, Pasternak G, Rutishauser U (2005) Polysialic acid-induced plasticity reduces neuropathic insult to the central nervous system. Proc Natl Acad Sci U S A 102: 11516–11520.
33. Latha M, Bangaru Y, Park F, Hudmon A, Mccallum JB, et al. (2013) Validation of Optimal Reference Genes. J Mol Neurosci 46: 497–504.
34. Campana WM, Myers RR (2003) Exogenous erythropoietin protects against dorsal root ganglion apoptosis and pain following peripheral nerve injury. Eur J Neurosci 18: 1497–1506.
35. Hansson PT, Fields HL, Hill RG, Marrchettini P (2001) Neuropathic Pain: Pathophysiology and Treatment. Seattle: IASP press 288p.
36. Hao S, Mata M, Glorioso JC, Fink DJ (2007) Gene transfer to interfere with TNFalpha signaling in neuropathic pain. Gene Ther 14: 1010–1016.
37. Sorkin LS, Xiao WH, Wagner R, Myers RR (1997) Tumour necrosis factor-alpha induces ectopic activity in nociceptive primary afferent fibres. Neuro Sci 81: 255–262.
38. Zhang JM, Li H, Liu B, Brull SJ (2002) Acute Topical Application of Tumor Necrosis Factor α Evokes Protein Kinase A-Dependent Responses in Rat Sensory Neurons. J Neurophysiol 88: 1387–1392.
39. Homma Y, Brull SJ, Zhang JM (2002) A comparison of chronic pain behavior following local application of tumor necrosis factor alpha to the normal and mechanically compressed lumbar ganglia in the rat. Pain 95: 239–246.
40. Murata Y, Onda A, Rydevik B, Takahashi I, Takahashi K, et al. (2006) Changes in pain behavior and histologic changes caused by application of tumor necrosis factor-alpha to the dorsal root ganglion in rats. Spine 31: 530–535.
41. Jin X, Gereau RW (2006) Acute p38-mediated modulation of tetrodotoxin-resistant sodium channels in mouse sensory neurons by tumor necrosis factor-alpha. J Neurosci 26: 246–255.
42. Czeschik JC, Hagenacker T, Schäfers M, Büsselberg D (2008) TNF-alpha differentially modulates ion channels of nociceptive neurons. Neurosci Lett 434: 293–298.
43. Marchand F, Perretti M McMahon SB (2005) Role in immune system in chronic pain. Nat Rev Neurosci 6: 521–532.
44. Janicke RU (1998) Caspase-3 is required for DNA fragmentation and morphological changes associated with apoptosis. J Biol Chem 273: 9357–9360.
45. Saito H, Kanje M, Dahlin LB (2009) Delayed nerve repair increases number of caspase 3 stained Schwann cells. Neurosci Lett 456: 30–33.
46. Andrade P, Visser-Vandewalle V, Hoffmann C, Steinbusch HW, Daemen MA, et al. (2011) Role of TNF-alpha during central sensitization in preclinical studies. Neurol Sci 32: 757–771.
47. Wei XH, Na XD, Liao GJ, Chen QY, Cui Y, et al. (2013) The up-regulation of IL-6 in DRG and spinal dorsal horn contributes to neuropathic pain following L5 ventral root transection. Exp Neurol 241: 159–168.
48. Arruda JL, Colburn RW, Rickman AJ, Rutkowski MD, DeLeo JA (1998) Increase of interleukin-6 mRNA in the spinal cord following peripheral nerve injury in the rat: potential role of IL-6 in neuropathic pain. Brain Res Mol Brain Res 62: 228–235.
49. Lee KM, Jeon SM, Cho HJ (2009) Tumor necrosis factor receptor 1 induces interleukin-6 upregulation through NF-kappaB in a rat neuropathic pain model. Eur J Pain 13: 794–806.
50. Tsujino H, Kondo E, Fukuoka T, Dai Y, Tokunaga A, et al. (2000) Activating transcription factor 3 (ATF3) induction by axotomy in sensory and motoneurons: A novel neuronal marker of nerve injury. Mol Cell Neurosci 15: 170–182.
51. Ossipov MH, Zhang ET, Carvajal C, Gardell L, Quirion R, et al. (2002) Selective mediation of nerve injury-induced tactile hypersensitivity by neuropeptide Y. J Neurosci 22: 9858–9867.
52. Fukuoka T, Yamanaka H, Kobayashi K, Okubo M, Miyoshi K, et al. (2012) Re-evaluation of the phenotypic changes in L4 dorsal root ganglion after L5 spinal nerve ligation. Pain 153: 68–79.
53. Decosterd I, Ji RR, Abdi S, Tate S, Woolf CJ (2002) The pattern of expression of the voltage-gated sodium channels Na(v)1.8 and Na(v)1.9 does not change in uninjured primary sensory neurons in experimental neuropathic pain models. Pain 96: 269–277.
54. Fukuoka T, Tokunaga A, Kondo E, Miki K, Tachibana T, et al. (1998) Change in mRNAs for neuropeptides and the GABA(A) receptor in dorsal root ganglion neurons in a rat experimental neuropathic pain model. Pain 78: 13–26.
55. Huang Y, Liu X, Dong L, Liu Z, He X, et al. (2011) Development of viral vectors for gene therapy for chronic pain. Pain Res Treat 2011: 968218.
56. Verma IM, Somia N (1997) Gene therapy-promises, problems and prospects. Nature 389: 239–42.
57. Bergelson JM, Cunningham JA, Droguett G, Kurt-Jones EA, Krithivas A, et al. (1997) Isolation of a Common Receptor for Coxsackie B Viruses and Adenoviruses 2 and 5. Science, 275: 1320–1323.
58. Greber U, Willetts M, Webster P, Helenius A (1993) Stepwise Dismantling of Adenovirus 2 durig Entry into Cells. Cell 75: 477–486.
59. Hotta Y, Honda T, Naito M, Kuwano R (2003) Developmental distribution of coxsackie virus and adenovirus receptor localized in the nervous system. Brain Res Dev Brain Res, 143: 1–13.
60. Mason MRJ, Ehlert EME, Eggers R, Pool CW, Hermening S, et al. (2010) Comparison of AAV serotypes for gene delivery to dorsal root ganglion neurons. Mol Ther 18: 715–724.
61. Yang P (2012) Lentiviral vector mediates exogenous gene expression in adult rat DRG following peripheral nerve remote delivery. J Mol Neurosci 47: 173–179.
62. Yu H, Fischer G, Jia G, Reiser J, Park F, et al. (2011) Lentiviral gene transfer into dorsal root ganglion of adult rats. Mol Pain 7:63. Available: http://www.molecularpain.com/content/7/1/63. Accessed on 2014 Feb 20.
63. Desmaris N, Bosch A, Salaün C, Petit C, Prévost M, et al. (2001) Production and Neurotropism of Lentivirus Vectors Pseudotyped with Lyssavirus Envelope Glycoproteins. 4: 149–156.
64. Nayak S, Herzog R (2009) Progress and prospects: immune responses to viral vectors. Gene Ther 17: 295–304.
65. Xu Y, Gu Y, Wu P, Li G-W, Huang L-YM (2003) Efficiencies of transgene expression in nociceptive neurons through different routes of delivery of adeno-associated viral vectors. Hum Gene Ther 14: 897–906. doi:10.1089/104303403765701187.
66. Glatzel M, Flechsig E, Navarro B, Klein MA, Paterna JC, et al. (2000) Adenoviral and adeno-associated viral transfer of genes to the peripheral nervous system. Proc Natl Acad Sci U S A 97: 442–447
67. Puljak L, Kojundzic S, Hogan Q, Sapunar D (2009) Lidocaine injection into the rat dorsal root ganglion causes neuroinflammation. Anesth Analg 108: 1021–1026.
68. Tonini G, Santini D, Vincenzi B, Borzomati D, Dicuonzo G, et al. (2002) Oxaliplatin may induce cytokine-release syndrome in colorectal cancer patients. J Biol Regul Homeost Agents 16: 105–109.
69. Drory VE, Lev D, Groozman GB, Gutmann M, Klausner JM (1998) Neurotoxicity of isolated limb perfusion with tumor necrosis factor. J Neurol Sci 158: 1–4.
70. Terashima T, Oka K, Kritz AB, Kojima H, Baker AH, et al. (2009) Adenoviruses mediate selective gene delivery for therapeutic rescue of sensory neuronopathies in mice. J Clin Invest 119: 2100–2112.
71. Blömer U, Naldini L, Kafri T, Trono D, Verma IM, et al. (1997) Highly efficient and sustained gene transfer in adult neurons with a lentivirus vector. J Virol 71: 6641–6649.

6

Involvement of EphB1 Receptors Signalling in Models of Inflammatory and Neuropathic Pain

Vincent Cibert-Goton[1]✉, Guanglu Yuan[1]✉, Anna Battaglia[1], Sarah Fredriksson[1], Mark Henkemeyer[2], Thomas Sears[1], Isabella Gavazzi[1]*

1 Wolfson Centre for Age-Related Diseases, The Wolfson Wing, King's College London, Guy's Campus, London, United Kingdom, **2** Department of Developmental Biology, Kent Waldrep Center for Basic Research on Nerve Growth and Regeneration, University of Texas Southwestern Medical Center, Dallas, Texas, United States of America

Abstract

EphB receptors tyrosine kinases and ephrinB ligands were first identified as guidance molecules involved in the establishment of topographical mapping and connectivity in the nervous system during development. Later in development and into adulthood their primary role would switch from guidance to activity-dependent modulation of synaptic efficacy. In sensory systems, they play a role in both the onset of inflammatory and neuropathic pain, and in the establishment of central sensitisation, an NMDA-mediated form of synaptic plasticity thought to underlie most forms of chronic pain. We studied wild type and EphB1 knockout mice in a range of inflammatory and neuropathic pain models to determine 1), whether EphB1 expression is necessary for the onset and/or maintenance of persistent pain, regardless of origin; 2), whether in these models cellular and molecular changes, e.g. phosphorylation of the NR2B subunit of the NMDA receptor, increased c-fos expression or microglial activation, associated with the onset of pain, are affected by the lack of functional EphB1 receptors. Differences in phenotype were examined behaviourally, anatomically, biochemically and electrophysiologically. Our results establish firstly, that functional EphB1 receptors are not essential for the development of normal nociception, thermal or mechanical sensitivity. Secondly, they demonstrate a widespread involvement of EphB1 receptors in chronic pain. NR2B phosphorylation, c-fos expression and microglial activation are all reduced in EphB1 knockout mice. This last finding is intriguing, since microglial activation is supposedly triggered directly by primary afferents, therefore it was not expected to be affected. Interestingly, in some models of long-term pain (days), mechanical and thermal hyperalgesia develop both in wild type and EphB1 knockout mice, but recovery is faster in the latter, indicating that in particular models these receptors are required for the maintenance, rather than the onset of, thermal and mechanical hypersensitivity. This potentially makes them an attractive target for analgesic strategies.

Editor: Claudia Sommer, University of Würzburg, Germany

Funding: This work was supported by Wellcome Trust Project Grant GR071663MA and Biotechnology and Biological Sciences Research Council Project Grant C505816 to IG and by National Institutes of Health grant 2R01 MH66332 to MH. The funders had no role in study design, data collection and analysis, decision to publish, or preparation of the manuscript.

Competing Interests: The authors have declared that no competing interests exist.

* E-mail: isabella.gavazzi@kcl.ac.uk

✉ These authors contributed equally to this work.

Introduction

The discovery that members of the EphB subfamily of receptor tyrosine kinases are involved in the formation of glutamatergic synapses [1] led rapidly to the finding that these molecules are not only required for axonal guidance and neuronal circuit assembly during development, but are also involved in synaptic plasticity during development and into adulthood. The majority of studies on adult plasticity have focused on EphB-ephrinB interactions in the onset and/or maintenance of long-term potentiation (LTP) in different areas of the hippocampus, and in the striatum [2,3], where significant advances in establishing mechanisms and functional significance of Eph and ephrin involvement in synaptic plasticity have been made using genetically modified mice [3]. The use of transgenic mice proved necessary to study these molecules for a variety of reasons, primarily linked to the binding promiscuity of the different EphB receptors, and the bidirectional signalling activated by EphB-ephrinB. There are 5 EphB receptors in mammals (EphB1-4 and EphB6), which bind promiscuously with 3 transmembrane ligands (ephrinB1-B3)(see e.g. [4–6]). Despite being conventionally called receptor and ligand, both EphBs and ephrinBs activate intracellular signalling cascades (forward and reverse signalling). The only tools currently available to interfere with EphB-ephrinB interaction, EphB-Fc or ephrinB-Fc chimeras, are not specific for a given receptor or ligand, and, whilst blocking the activation of EphB receptors or ephrinB respectively, can also bind to and activate ephrinBs or EphB receptors. The results obtained in rats and wild type mice are therefore unavoidably ambiguous, and studies in genetically modified animals are currently essential to clarify mechanisms.

Synaptic plasticity in which EphB-ephrinB interactions are involved has also been revealed at spinal cord level using models of chronic pain, thus providing an alternative model for the study of the link between molecular mechanisms and behavioural outcomes (see e.g. [7–10]).

In many models of chronic pain, a fundamental mechanism underlying enhanced responsiveness or spontaneous pain is central sensitisation, a mechanism which shares some features with hippocampal LTP, implying enhanced transmission at synapses formed by peripheral sensory afferents onto dorsal horn neurons; to what extent LTP itself contributes to central sensitisation and chronic pain is still debated (see e.g.[11,12,12–15]). Most, if not all, forms of central sensitisation are thought to be NMDA – mediated, but, despite three decades of research, controversy remains as to the specific molecular mechanisms and the role of NMDA receptor subunits, and even on the extent of NMDA receptor involvement (see e.g. [16–19]). Furthermore, there is a substantial body of evidence supporting the hypothesis that the mechanisms underlying the onset of different forms of chronic pain (e.g. inflammatory and neuropathic) as well as thermal and mechanical hyperalgesia, differ, even if there are contradictory findings also in relation to this issue (see e.g. [20–23]. It is clearly of importance therefore a), to establish in full the molecular mechanisms involved in the process of central sensitisation; b) to determine to what extent the same mechanisms are common to different types of chronic pain. This is essential to identify therapeutic targets for the development of effective mechanism-based analgesics hopefully with greater efficacy and fewer side effects than those currently available. Clarifying the contribution of EphB receptors to the spinal mechanisms of chronic pain would help achieving these goals.

Previous work carried out *in vivo* on adult rats in our laboratory demonstrated a requirement for spinal EphB receptor activation in NMDA-dependent increases in synaptic efficacy, using two models of chronic pain (formalin and carrageenan tests, [7]), and later EphB receptors were shown to be involved in neuropathic pain and the physical dependence on morphine [9,10,24]. Whereas in the hippocampus LTP is mainly dependent on EphB2, we suggested that in the spinal cord the primary receptor involved in chronic pain would be EphB1 [7], an hypothesis strongly supported by subsequent studies on EphB1 knockout (EphB1 KO) mice, which reported a lack of thermal hyperalgesia in KO mice in a model of neuropathic pain [25] and showed that EphB1 is essential for the generation of LTP between C-fibres afferents and dorsal horn neurons [26]. These findings suggest that a better understanding of the role of EphB1 receptor in chronic pain could, potentially, not only contribute to clarify the mechanisms underlying central sensitisation in different pain models, but provide an alternative therapeutic target for the treatment of chronic pain of different aetiology.

The aim of the present work was to advance understanding of the role played by EphB1 receptors in the onset of persistent pain, using EphB1 KO mice. We hypothesised that, if NMDA-mediated central sensitisation is indeed responsible for the onset of thermal and mechanical hyperalgesia, as well as spontaneous pain, in models of tissue injury, inflammatory and neuropathic pain, then EphB1 KO mice should display blunted pain responses in all these models. Furthermore, since NR2B phosphorylation and c-fos upregulation are thought to be downstream of EphB receptors activation ([27]; see also [7,8]), we hypothesised that we would observe a reduction in NR2B phosphorylation and c-fos expression in KO mice in models of inflammatory pain, as we had previously shown to occur in rats, if we blocked the interaction between EphB receptors and ephrinBs ligands in vivo. We also examined microglial activation in neuropathic pain. The mechanisms leading to microglial activation in neuropathic pain models are still incompletely understood, but they appear to involve direct activation by primary afferents, possibly via the release of ATP, followed by activation depending on release of fractalkine from neurons, cleaved by Cathepsin S of microglial origin [28]. None of these mechanisms should be affected by the absence of EphB1. Previous studies had not analysed normal sensory function in EphB1 KO mice; there are no findings available from studies on embryos suggesting a role for EphB1 in the development of primary sensory afferents, but we deemed nonetheless essential to ascertain anatomically, behaviourally, immunohistochemically and electrophysiologically whether EphB1 deficiency caused any major developmental alterations in the functional connectivity of the sensory system. We were able to demonstrate that functional EphB1 receptors are not essential for the development of normal nociception, thermal or mechanical sensitivity, whereas, in agreement with our hypothesis, they are required for the onset and/or maintenance of thermal and mechanical hyperalgesia and spontaneous pain behaviour in a variety of persistent pain models. Surprisingly, microglial activation following nerve injury was reduced in EphB1 KO mice. Of particular interest is the finding that in some models of long-term pain mechanical and thermal hyperalgesia develop both in wild type and EphB1 knockout mice, but recovery is faster in the latter. This implies that in these models EphB1 receptors are required for the maintenance, rather than the onset, of hyperalgesia, and may therefore be useful therapeutic targets for the development of new analgesics.

Materials and Methods

Ethical Approval

All experiments were undertaken in accordance with the United Kingdom Animals (scientific procedures) Act 1986 (Project Licence PPL 70/4774), and all efforts were made to minimize animal suffering, and to reduce the number of animals used, in accordance with the concept of "The Three Rs" (*replacement, reduction, refinement*).

Animals

This study has been conducted on EphB1 null mutant mice. Generation of the mutation has already been described [29]. We used EphB1−/− mutants backcrossed for several generation in the CD1 background to avoid possible confounding effects of background genetic differences, and EphB1 lacz/lacz mutants (expressing beta-galactosidase as a marker for EphB1 expression), backcrossed for several generations in a CD1/129 background. Aged-matched wild type (WT) littermates were used for comparison. Male and females mice were housed up to five per cage on a standard 12 hours light/dark cycle, with water and food pellets available ad lib except during the testing period. Animals were aged 12 to 15 weeks at the time of testing.

Animal Models

A number of models of acute and persistent pain were used, i.e. the formalin test (a model of tissue injury [30], the Carrageenan and Complete Freund's Adjuvant (CFA) models of inflammation and two models of neuropathic pain, chronic constriction injury (CCI) and partial nerve ligation (PNL).

For the formalin test, 20 μl of formalin at a 5% concentration (40% stock solution considered as 100%) were injected subcutaneously into the plantar surface of the right hind paw, using insulin syringes with 0.33 mm needles.

For the Carrageenan model of inflammation, each animal received a 20 μl injection of carrageenan (2% or 20 mg/ml Carrageenan Lambda, Type IV, Sigma-Aldrich, Gillingham, Dorset, UK) into the right hind paw.

For the CFA model of inflammation, 20 μl of CFA (Sigma F-5881, Sigma-Aldrich) were injected into the plantar surface of the right hind paw of the mouse.

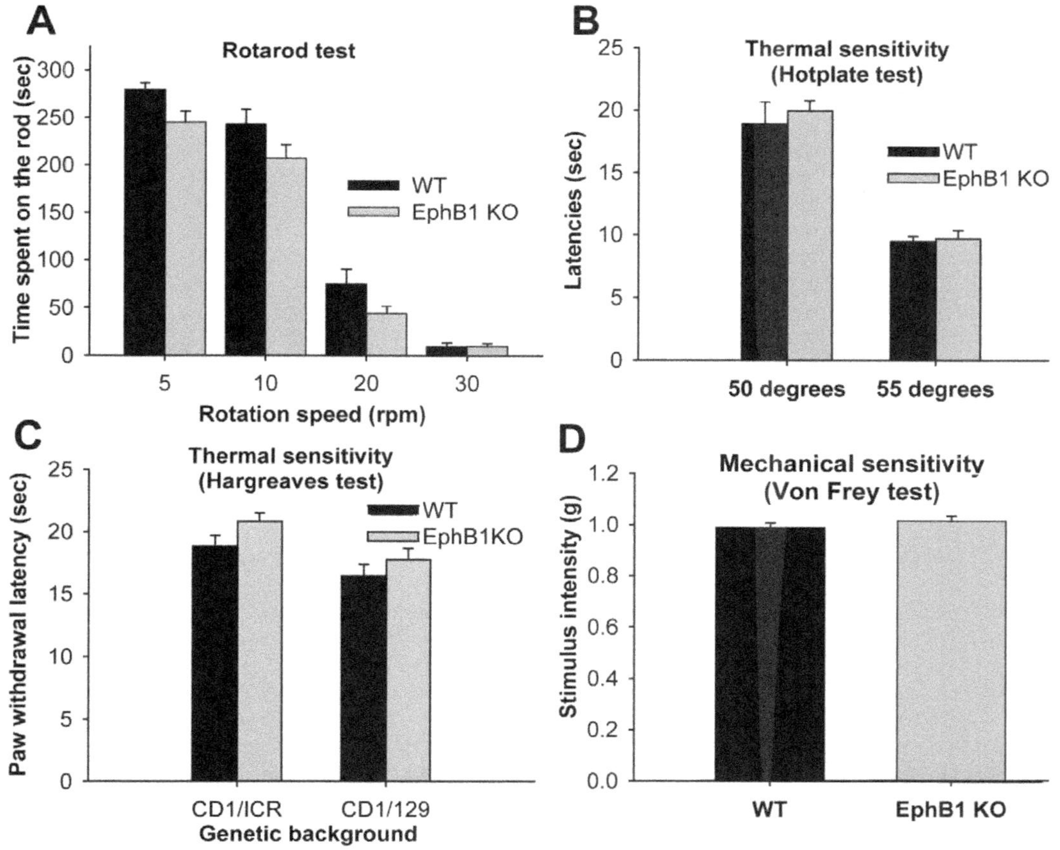

Figure 1. EphB1 KO mice have normal thermal and mechanical sensitivity. Bar charts illustrating the performance of EphB1 KO and WT mice in a range of behavioural tests designed to measure motor performance (rotarod, A) or acute thermal (hot plate and Hargreaves, B and C) or mechanical (von Frey, D) nociception. Behavioural analysis did not identify a significant difference between EphB1 KO and WT mice in any test. (t-test in A for 10 and 30 rpm, C and D; Mann-Whitney U-test in A for 5 and 20 rpm and in B) A) 5, 10, 20 rpm WT n = 19, EphB1 KO n = 29; 30 rpm WT n = 8, EphB1 KO n = 16; B) WT n = 16, EphB1 KO n = 25; C) CD1/ICR WT n = 24, EphB1 KO n = 17, CD1/129 WT n = 13, EphB1 KO n = 12. Bars represent mean +/ − SEM.

Chronic constriction injury (CCI or Bennett model) [31]: for all animals, anesthesia was induced and maintained with 3% isofluorane in 95% oxygen, 5% CO2 via a face-mask. The left common sciatic nerve was exposed at the mid-thigh level and proximal to the sciatic nerve's trifurcation, and four ligatures with chromic catgut were tied around it with about 1 mm spacing between ligatures. Each ligature was tightened in order to reduce the diameter of the nerve and retard, but not interrupt the epineural circulation.

Partial sciatic nerve ligation (PNL or Seltzer model) [32]: animals were anaesthetised as above. An incision was made in the skin of the upper left leg and blunt scissors were used to part the muscle layers to access the sciatic nerve. A tight ligation of between ½-⅓ of the nerve was made using 6-0 mersilk suture (Ethicon, Gargrave, North Yorkshire, UK). The skin was closed using 4-0 mersilk sutures (Ethicon). In sham animals, the surgery was performed as described above, but the nerve was not ligated.

Behavioural Testing

All experiments were done during the day portion of the circadian cycle only (06:00–18:00 h) and were performed blinded to all test paradigms.

The Rotarod test was used to measure the balance and the forced motor-coordination activity. We used a combination of both accelerating and staggered Rotarod procedures on an accelerating Rotarod (IITC Inc. Life Science, Woodland Hills, CA) with a 32 mm diameter rod. On the first day the mice were given a limited habituation of 5 min on a non rotating rod. Forty eight h later they were tested 3 times at a rotating speed of 5 rpm and the latency to fall was measured for up to 2 min, with a 30 min inter-trial interval back in their home cages, to limit the effects of physical exhaustion. Every time a mouse was tested it was placed on a non rotating rod, which was accelerated to a defined rotating speed (5, 10, 20 and 30 rpm) with a constant incremental slope. Any mice falling before the rod reached its full speed was given 2 more chances. In case of 3 consecutive failures the given score was 0. The test was performed on 4 different days, every 48 h.

The Hargreaves' Plantar test (IITC Inc. Life Science) was used to examine thermal sensitivity. Each mouse was housed separately, in a randomly chosen compartment. A glass heating system assured a standardized temperature of 22°C at the contact zone between the plantar surface of the paw and the glass (baseline temperature of the skin). Before the test, mice were habituated to the experimental set-up for 2 h minimum on 2 consecutive days prior and on the day of experiment. During the test, a heat source was applied to the plantar surface of the hind paw, from underneath and through the glass floor. The area tested was the mid-plantar hind paw, in the area supplied by the tibial nerve, avoiding the footpads, and was located by positioning a light spot on the plantar surface of the paw. The stimulus and a timer to record the reaction time were activated simultaneously. As soon as the mouse removed its paw, the stimulus and timer were stopped.

After preliminary testing on control mice (WT CD1-ICR and CD1/129), the light intensity was set at 18% of maximum, in order to achieve a baseline of 10 to 20 seconds. The minimum resting period between each successive exposure was 5 min for alternate paws or 10 min for the same paw, to minimize the effects of repeated exposures. Two to 4 measurements were collected for each paw, depending on their reproducibility. For the data presented in figure 1, control WT and EphB1 mice were tested 3 times on 3 different days, with at least 2 days rest between test days. To examine the development of thermal hyperalgesia in inflammatory and neuropathic pain, animals were tested before treatment, and 90 and 150 min after carrageenan or saline injection [33], on day 1, 2, 5, 7, 9 and 14 after CFA or saline injection and at 3, 5, 7, 10, 14, and 21 days after PNL.

For the Hotplate test for thermal sensitivity, on the previous day and just before testing, mice were habituated for 10 minutes in the Hot Plate Plexiglas box (IITC Inc. Life Science). Mice from the same rearing box were habituated together, to minimize stress. After habituation, mice were placed individually on the hot plate, heated at either 50 or 55°C, and the latency to first sign of paw licking or escape jumping was recorded as an index of the pain threshold. The experiment was performed 3 times with 48 h between two measurements. A stimulus cut-off of 45 s and 1 min were used respectively when testing at 55 and 50°C to avoid any paw damage.

Mechanical sensitivity was tested using von Frey Hairs. To determine the baseline threshold for mechanical sensitivity for the mice used in our experiments (baseline mechanical sensitivity varies considerably in mice depending on genetic background), we used a series of 6 calibrated nylon monofilaments (Touch-Test Sensory Evaluator, Semmes-Weinstein Monofilaments) chosen with equal spacing ($\sigma = 0.34$ on average) on the log-dose scale, ranging from 0.04 g to 4.56 g. The mice were placed in individual plastic compartments on a stand with a metal mesh floor, and the von Frey hair applied perpendicularly to the plantar surface of the paw until it buckled slightly (minimum 20%), and maintained for 6 seconds. The next stimulus was presented as soon as any behavioural response due to the previous one was resolved. A positive response was recorded when the mouse sharply removed its paw, often followed by shaking and even licking [34]. Flinching immediately upon application or removal of the hair was considered a positive response. When assessing the baseline paw withdrawal threshold, each monofilament was applied five times on each paw at 5 min interval. The withdrawal threshold corresponded to the force in g at which the mouse withdrew the paw in minimum 5 out of 10 trials (combining the results of contra- and ipsi- lateral paws). Data for figure 1 were collected using this method. For all subsequent experiments (carrageenan and CFA i.pl. injection, neuropathic pain models) we adopted instead the up-and down method described by Chaplan et al. [34], which allows interpolation of the mechanical threshold (stimulus intensity at which the mouse would respond 50% of the times) with fewer applications of the von Frey filaments, and was therefore more suitable for these tests, inducing less stress in the animals. The up-and-down method requires prior knowledge of baseline mechanical threshold, so it could not have been applied in our initial experiments. Animals were tested before treatment, and 90 and 150 min after carrageenan or saline injection [33], on day 1, 2, 5, 7, 9 and 14 after CFA or saline injection, at 3, 5, 7, 10, 14, and 21 days after PNL Mechanical and at 7, 14 and 21 days after CCI.

For the Formalin test mice were housed in a square test box, maintaining a constant temperature of 22°C at the plantar surface of the paw [35]. Three out of the four sides of the box were mirrors, to simplify the observation and characterisation of the different behaviours recorded. Mice were habituated to the experimental environment for 30 min on two different days, and 15 min on the day of experiment. After formalin injection, mice were immediately transferred into the box and nocifensive responses (Lifting/Favouring; Licking/Biting) related to the injected hind paw, recorded in 5 min blocks for 1 h. A 'painscore' was then calculated according to the formula PS = (Time spent in full weight bearing position * 0)+(time spent lifting or favouring * 1)+(time spent licking or Biting * 2)).

Immunohistochemistry

Mice were deeply anesthetized with pentobarbital (140 mg/kg, i.p.) and perfused transcardially with heparinised saline (0.9% NaCl) followed by 0.1M pH 7.4 phosphate buffer (PB) containing 4% paraformaldehyde (PFA). The left and right L4 and L5 lumbar dorsal root ganglia (DRGs) and/or lumbar spinal cords were then dissected and stored in 4% PFA overnight. The following day tissues were transferred in 20% sucrose in 0.1M PB, pH 7.4 for 24 h at at 4°C and then blocked in O.C.T. (Optimum Cutting Temperature) embedding matrix (BDH, Essex, UK) in liquid nitrogen and stored at −80°C. In all studies, 2–5 slides from each animal were used for the staining. 2 slides were randomly chosen as negative control for the staining process, 1 slide was coated only with primary antibody and the other with secondary antibody only. 15 μm thick transverse sections of L4 and L5 DRGs (perpendicular to the neuronal axis of the DRG) or 30 μm thick lumbar spinal cord section (L3-4, where afferents from the mouse hind limb preferentially terminate, see [36]) were cut on a Bright microtome 5040, mounted on slides (Superfrost Plus, BDH) sequentially, allowed to dry at room temperature for 30 min and then preserved in cryoprotectant (30% sucrose w/v, 30% ethylene glycol w/v in 0.01M phosphate buffer saline (PBS) at –20°C.

Lumbar DRG staining: three randomly chosen left or right DRGs from intact EphB1 KO mice and three randomly chosen left or right DRGs from intact WT mice were used, and slides were chosen from each animal so that 5 roughly equidistant sections taken from the entire length of the ganglion would be examined for each staining. The slides were then processed with conventional immunofluoscence techniques. To identify the proportion of peptidergic nociceptive neurons in the DRGs, the sections were stained for CGRP using primary antibodies rabbit anti-CGRP (Sigma c8198) at 1:1300 and, to stain all neurons, with the general neuronal marker mouse anti-βIII-tubulin (Promega, Southampton, UK, 1 mg/ml) at 1:1200 with secondary antibodies donkey anti-mouse CyIII (Jackson Immunochemicals, West Grove, PA, 1.3 mg/ml) and donkey anti-rabbit FITC (Jackson, 1.4 mg/ml). Non peptidergic nociceptive neurons were identified on the basis of their binding to isolectin B_4 (IB_4). IB_4-biotin (Sigma, 0.5 mg/ml) was used in the concentration 1:500 together with mouse βIII-tubulin (Promega, 1 mg/ml) at 1:1200. As secondary antibodies, donkey anti-mouse FITC (Jackson, 1.4 mg/ml) at 1:200 and anti-IB_4 TRITC (Sigma, 2 mg/ml) at 1:200 were used. Large, mainly proprio- or mechanoceptive, neurons were stained using mouse N52 antibody (Sigma) at 1:400 and the general neuronal marker rabbit protein gene product (PGP) 9.5 (Abcam, Cambridge, UK) at 1:400. The secondary antibodies used were donkey anti-rabbit FITC (Jackson, 1.5 mg/ml) at 1:200 and donkey anti-mouse CyIII (Jackson, 1.3 mg/ml) at 1:1000. The slides were then washed with 0.01M PBS (3×5 min) and covered with 22×50 mm Borosillicate glass cover slips (Calbiochem, San Diego, USA) using Flurosave^{TM} Reagent (Sigma, St. Louis, MO, USA). All antibodies were diluted using 0.01M PBS with 0.2% Triton X (w/v) and 0.1% (w/v) of sodium azide.

Spinal cord sections: to examine the anatomical integrity of nociceptive afferent terminals in the dorsal horn of the spinal cord, the spinal cords from 3 WT and 3 EphB1 KO mice were dissected. 3 slides were then randomly chosen from each animal and double-stained for CGRP and IB4. Sections were stained for CGRP using as primary antibody a rabbit anti-CGRP (Sigma c8198) at 1:1400 with secondary antibody Goat anti-rabbit Alexafluor 546 (Molecular Probes, Eugene, OR, USA). IB_4-biotin (Sigma, 0.5 mg/ml) was used in the concentration 1:500 and as secondary Extravidine FITC at 1:500. To examine the effect of inflammation or tissue injury on the expression of c-fos, the spinal cords of 12 WT and 12 EphB1 KO mice were dissected out. Both WT and KO mice had been assigned randomly to one of 4 treatment groups: 1) saline i.pl injection 1 h prior to culling; 2) formalin i.pl. injection 1 h prior to culling; 3) saline i.pl. injection 3 h prior to culling; 4) carrageenan i.pl injection 3 h prior to culling; all injections were performed as described previously. Two slides were randomly chosen from each animal, then coated with a primary antibody rabbit anti-c-fos (1:2500) (Invitrogen, Paisley, UK) and a secondary antibody Alexafluor 488 goat anti-rabbit IgG (1:1000) (Molecular Probes). For assessment of microglial activation following PNL, 4–5 sections of spinal cords from WT and KO mice were randomly collected 3,7,14 and 21 days after lesion. Sham operated animals acted as controls. Slides were coated with Rabbit anti Iba1 (Wako, Japan) 1:1000, followed by Goat anti rabbit IgG Alexa fluor 546 (Molecular Probes A11035) 1:1000. All antibodies were diluted to working concentrations with 0.01M PBS with 1% (w/v) TritonX and 0.01% (w/v) sodium azide.

Image Acquisition and Analysis

All images were acquired using a Zeiss fluorescence microscope (Axioplan 2 or Imager Z1) with a 20× objective with a Zeiss Axiocam HRm (Carl Zeiss, Goettingen, Germany), using Axiovision 40LE version 4.2 software (Carl Zeiss). All analysis was performed with the investigator blinded to genotype and treatment.

Lumbar DRGs: Two randomly chosen pictures were taken using a Zeiss Axioplan 2 microscope. All stained cells with visible nuclei were counted, first in sections stained with the general neuronal marker, then in sections stained with the subpopulation-specific marker. For each animal, 5 sections were counted for each staining, for a total of 15 sections per animal. A total of 43660 cells were counted for WT, and 47827 cells for EphB1 KO mice.

Spinal cords: to quantify nociceptive afferents in the dorsal horn, photomicrographs of sections stained for CGRP immunorectivity or IB4 binding were taken using a Zeiss Imager.Z1 microscope. The surface of the stained area was measured using the outlining application in Axiovision 40LE version 4.2 software (Carl Zeiss). Immunoreactive c-fos expressing cells were counted in Laminae I and II of the ipsilateral (injected) side of the lumbar spinal cord grey matter.

To study microglial activation, usually 5 (or a minimum of 4) sections from each animal were chosen at random. Four boxes measuring 10^4 μm^2 were placed onto areas of the lateral, central and medial dorsal horn. The mean number of Iba1 positive cells, morphologically identified as activated microglia, was determined within this area [37]. All spinal cord sections were examined using a Zeiss Axioplan 2 microscope.

Western Blot and Immunoprecipitation

Animals were divided into saline, CFA, carrageenan and formalin treated groups for both genotypes. The mice were culled and hemisected lumbar spinal cord tissues were rapidly removed at 60 minutes after formalin injection, 3 hours after carrageenan and 14 days after CFA. Saline controls were taken at the same time as their treated counterpart. Tissues were frozen in liquid nitrogen and stored at −80°C until use.

Each sample, obtained pooling the tissues from two mice, was homogenized on ice using an Ultraturax (IKA) homogeniser in 300 µl of NP-40 lysis buffer (1% Nonidet P-40, 150 mM NaCl, 500 mM Tris-HCl pH8, 1 mM EDTA, 0.5% SDS, adding 25× Protease inhibitor cocktail (Complete Roche), 100 µl leupetin (10 µg/ml), 100 µl phosphatase inhibitor cocktail 2 (Sigma), 200 µl NaF (250 mM stock) mix and 100 µl (1 mM final) PMSF to each 10 ml of buffer). 2×300 µl of lysis buffer was added to wash the Ultraturax to collect all the homogenate. The Ultraturax was also cleaned with ethanol and ddH_2O between each sample homogenization. The homogenates were placed in a carousel for 2 hours at 4°C before being centrifuged at 12000 rpm for 20 minutes at 4°C. The supernatants were collected and the protein concentrations were determined using a detergent-compatible assay (BCA-Pierce kit) with a bovine serum albumin (BSA) standard in a Dynex reader (Dynex Technologies, Inc. Chantilly, VA).

For immunoprecipitation, total lysates (1 mg) were incubated with 5 µl of goat anti-NR2B IgG (Santa Cruz Biotechnology, Santa Cruz, CA, 0.2 µg/µl) on a carousel overnight at 4°C, followed by incubation with 50 µl of Protein G- Sepharose slurry (1:1, Santa Cruz Biotechnology) at 4°C for 2 hours in agitation and further centrifugation at 5000 rpm for 2 minutes. Supernatants were discarded and Sepharose beads were washed 3 times with 1 ml of lysis buffer; with vigorous vortex and brief spin at 5000 rpm after each wash. 40 µl of 2 times SDS sample buffer was added to each sample, then vortexed and heated at 95°C for 5 minutes, before 5 minutes centrifugation at 12000 rpm. The immunoprecipitation samples were then kept at −20°C until loaded.

For western blot analysis, proteins (1 mg) were resolved on 8% SDS-PAGE gels run in migration buffer (3 g Tris-base, 14.4 g glycine, 1 g 1% SDS for 1litre) for 90 minutes at 90V and loaded along with controls (using normal goat serum) and full range rainbow recombinant marker (Amersham Biosciences, Arlington Heights, IL). Transfer was run in buffer (100 ml migration buffer (without SDS), 200 ml methanol, 700 ml H_2O for 1 litre) for an hour at 100V using nitrocellulose membranes (Amersham) and a Trans-Blot Transfer Cell system (Bio-Rad, Hercules, CA) to which an icebox was added to avoid overheating and damage to the membrane. The blots were blocked at room temperature for 1 hour on agitation with 4% BSA in TBS-T (2.42 g Tris base, 8 g NaCl, adjust PH = 7.6 with HCl, 0.5 ml Tween 20, adding H_2O for 1 litre) and the membrane incubated with two primary antibodies: mouse a-p-Tyr (1:2000 TBS-T; Santa Cruz Biotechnology) and rabbit anti-NR2B IgG (1:1000 TBS-T; Upstate 1 µg/µl) in a polythene container overnight at 4°C. The membrane was then washed 3 times for 10mins in TBS-T before being incubated with the secondary antibodies, goat anti-mouse IR680 and donkey anti-rabbit IR800 (both 1:15,000–20,000 in TBS-T) for 1 hour on agitation. Revelation was carried out using the Odyssey Lyca Scan.

Electrophysiology

Mice were given an initial dose of 1.8 g/kg urethane i.p. and 15 min later, 0.4 g/kg for sustained anaesthesia. Rectal temperature was maintained at a mean of 36–38°C. After tracheotomy, mice were supported prone by clamps at T13 and L3/4. L1-2 laminae were removed, the dura opened, and the tissues covered by 4% saline-agar which was subsequently removed over the SC and the pool filled with paraffin oil. The sciatic nerve was exposed for stimulation in-continuity in the popliteal fossa, and the sural nerve freed and sectioned distally for stimulation. Sciatic nerve stimulation involved low and medium threshold fibres from muscle and skin, whereas stimulation of the sural nerve provided solely a cutaneous input. We did not stimulate at C-fibre strengths for the comparison of WT and KO mice because preliminary experiments failed to reveal consistent reliable field potentials in recordings from the cord dorsum. In the rat, the antecedent volleys in the lower threshold A-fibres can inhibit C-fibre evoked field potentials which can be revealed better using TTX to block A-fibres leaving conduction intact for a group of TTX-resistant unmyelinated fibres [38]. However, the procedures were considered impractical to allow a valid comparison of WT and KO mice with the limited numbers of mice available for this part of the study.

Stimulation was via bipolar Platinum hook electrodes with 0.05 or 0.1 ms square wave voltage pulses (Digitimer DS2) at 2 Hz and the intensity set at 5 ×threshold (5T) for the systematic comparison of WT and KO mice. A plastic ensheathed 100 μm diameter Pt. wire was used for focal recording at the cord dorsum surface with the reference electrode on nearby muscle. The spatial distribution of the evoked potentials was then determined at the root entry zone (REZ) in 200 μm steps from the rostral end of T13 to the caudal end of L2 vertebral levels (the location of the epicentre of the hind limb representation; cf. [39]). At each site, 20 evoked responses were recorded through a FET-follower head stage and fed to a high-gain AC-couple differential amplifier (Digitimer DL150) with HF bandwith at 10 or 3 kHz and TC 30 ms. Signals were fed to a CED interface, sampled at 20 kHz and the average of 20 responses derived for each site using Spike2 software.

Statistical Analysis

Data are expressed as mean ± S.E.M. Behavioural, biochemical and immunohistochemical studies were statistically analyzed with one-way or two-way analysis of variance (ANOVA; for repeated measures for behavioural tests) followed by post-hoc multiple comparisons testing with the Holm-Sidack method. ANOVA on ranks was used when the data failed the normality or equal variance tests. t-test or Mann-Whitney U-test as appropriate were employed to compare two groups. A p value <0.05 was considered to be statistically significant. All statistical analyses were performed using "SigmaStat for Windows" (version 2.0; Jandel Corporation, San Rafael, CA, USA). For the electrophysiological data, a mixed design two-way ANOVA (SPSS statistical software) was used with the between factor set as WT or EphB1KO and the within factor as level of the spinal cord. Additional post-hoc analysis (independent t test or Mann-Whitney Rank Sum test) was done at each position along the rostro caudal axis.

Results

EphB1 KO Mice Respond Normally to Acute Pain Stimuli and their Small Diameter Primary Sensory Afferents are Anatomically Intact, Although Changes in Connectivity of Larger Diameter Cutaneous Fibres were Observed

Locomotor coordination. A prerequisite for any behavioural study of an animal's susceptibility to noxious and non-noxious stimulation in models of chronic pain is an intact functioning motor system. Therefore, prior to the systematic use of a number of established tests of acute nociception to assess the functional integrity of primary nociceptive afferents, we examined proprioception, coordination and tactile sensibility in WT and KO mice as an aspect of locomotion using the Rotarod test. (figure 1A). The scores revealed no clear differences between the two groups save perhaps for a slight trend towards a reduced performance in the KO mice at lower rotation speeds, but this did not reach significance.

Acute thermal nociception was assessed using a radiant heat source applied to the plantar surface of the hind paw (Hargreaves test) or a hot plate (figure 1B–C). *Mechanical sensory thresholds* were assessed manually using von Frey hairs (figure 1D). Neither acute thermal nociception or the response to mechanical stimulation differed significantly in WT and KO mice. These behavioural results confirmed our previous finding of a lack of involvement of EphB1 receptors in acute nociception, and indicated the functional integrity of nociceptive pathways, despite the absence of functional EphB1.

Immunohistochemical analysis of primary sensory afferents. We further confirmed the anatomical integrity of primary sensory afferents by immunohistochemical analysis of lumbar DRGs and nociceptive terminals in the dorsal horn of the spinal cord. DRGs were double-stained with a general neuronal marker (PGP9.5 or beta-tubulin) and a marker for either peptidergic or non-peptidergic nociceptive neurons, respectively, using anti-CGRP antibodies or the isolectin IB4. The proportions of DRG neurons stained with the different markers were calculated by counting both the total number of nucleated neurons, and the number of CGRP or IB4- positive neurons, present in randomly chosen sections. There were no differences between wild type and EphB1 KO mice in the proportion of DRG neurons stained with the two different markers (table 1). Similarly, nociceptive afferent terminations were examined after staining lumbar spinal cord sections with anti-CGRP antibodies and the isolectin IB4. Again there was no significant difference in the area occupied by nociceptive afferents in the dorsal horn of the spinal cord in wild type and EphB1 KO mice (table 1), suggesting anatomical integrity of these primary afferents terminations in the mutant mice, in agreement with their normal acute nociception (figure 1B–C).

Large mechanoceptive and proprioceptive DRG neurons were stained with N52 antibodies, which recognise high molecular weight neurofilament and again there was no difference in the proportion of neurons in the DRGs between WT and EphB1 KO mice (table 1) in agreement with their normal mechanical sensitivity and normal motor behaviour, which requires intact vestibular, propriospinal and tactile sensation (Figure 1A and 1D).

Electrophysiological comparison of afferent transmission in WT and KO Eph.B1 mice. Further evidence concerning the functional status of primary afferent pathways in these KO mice relates to the somatotopic organisation and synaptic transmission to 2nd or higher order neurones. This was determined electrophysiologically by measuring the spatial distribution and amplitudes of the compound action potentials (CAPs) and field potentials (FPs) evoked at the cord dorsum by electrical stimulation of the sciatic and sural nerves (figure 2). For comparison of the WT and KO mice the stimulus intensities were set at 5× T where T is the threshold of the lowest threshold fibre in the stimulated nerve conducted to the root entry zone. For the sciatic nerve this threshold is that of the fast conducting primary afferent fibres (Group1A) from muscle spindles in the calf and foot, whereas for the sural nerve the threshold is that of Aβ fibres cutaneous fibres innervating the lateral plantar surface of the foot. The epicentre of

Table 1. Lack of alteration in DRG neurons and dorsal horn immunoreactivity in EphB1 KO mice.

Table 1		WT (n = 3)	EphB1 KO (n = 3)
DRGs	% of CGRP positive neurons	31.8+/−0.01	30.6+/−0.04
	% of IB4 binding neurons	34.5+/−0.021	34.9+/−0.03
	% of N52 stained neurons	35.8+/−0.027	36.7+/−0.038
Dorsal Horn	Area covered by CGRP-immunoreactive terminals (μ^2)	38899.8+/−1528.489	39645.3+/−884.572
	Area covered by IB4-binding terminals (μ^2)	24026.1+/−1472.583	24325.3+/−440.958

Sections of lumbar L4 and L5 DRGs were double-stained with markers for the different subpopulation of neurons in the DRG and a general neuronal marker (PGP9.5 or beta-tubulin). Anti-CGRP antibodies and the isolectin IB4 bind respectively to peptidergic and non-peptidergic small and medium sized nociceptive neurons, whereas N52 antibodies bind to high molecular weight neurofilament present in large mechanoceptive and proprioceptive neurons. Quantification of the proportion of the total number of neurons (identified by the general neuronal marker), which also stained for a specific subpopulation marker, was carr ed out. No difference was observed between WT and EphB1KO mice. Sections of lumbar spinal cords were stained with anti-CGRP antibodies of the isolectin IB4, which bind respectively to the terminals of peptidergic and non-peptidergic nociceptive afferents. No difference was observed between WT and EphB1KO mice in the area covered by CGRP-positive and IB4-positive terminals in the dorsal horn of the spinal cord.

the hindlimb representation lay under the L1 vertebra. No significant differences between WT and EphB1KO mice were observed either in the spatial profile or peak amplitudes of the evoked-CAPs and FPs with stimulation of the sciatic nerve ($p>0.05$; data not shown), nor in the evoked-CAPs with stimulation of the sural nerve (figure 2A). Interestingly, however, with stimulation of the sural nerve the peak amplitudes of the FPs were highly significantly increased by approximately threefold in the KO as compared to WT ($P<0.001$; figure 2B) and this was manifest over the entire spatial array of recordings. This suggests that the lack of EphB1R during development resulted in changes in spinal connectivity of the large and medium-sized cutaneous Aβ/δ fibres in the superficial dorsal horn.

Persistent Pain Behaviour Following Tissue Injury is Significantly Reduced in EphB1 KO Mice

We then tested WT and EphB1 KO mice in a model of persistent pain, the formalin test. Spontaneous pain behaviour elicited by the injection of a diluted solution of formalin in the plantar surface (i. pl.) of the hind paw was recorded for 60 min. We recorded both licking and lifting/favouring of the injected paw, which we then combined to obtain a pain score (figure 3). The response following formalin injection can be divided in two phases. Phase I, corresponding to acute nociception, lasts about 10 minutes, and during this phase no significant difference was observed between WT and EphB1 KO mice. A short interval then occurs, during which the animal displays no signs of spontaneous pain, followed by Phase II, the resumption of pain behaviour, lasting for 30 or more minutes, depending on mouse strain. In part, Phase II is attributed to central sensitisation. EphB1 KO mice displayed significantly less spontaneous pain behaviour in Phase II of the formalin test as compared to their WT counterparts ($p<0.05$).

EphB1 Receptor Expression is Required for the Onset of Short-term Inflammatory Pain and EphB1 Deficient Mice Recover Significantly Faster from Thermal Hyperalgesia and Mechanical Allodynia in a Long-term Model of Inflammation

Peripheral tissue inflammation can lead to the onset of persistent (chronic) pain, mediated by mechanisms including peripheral and central sensitisation.

We used two tests of inflammatory pain, of shorter and longer duration (carrageenan and CFA injection in the hind paw respectively), to assess the role played by EphB1 receptor in the onset of inflammatory pain. Thermal and mechanical responses were measured before and after i.pl. injection with carrageenan and CFA (figure 4). The onset of both thermal hyperalgesia and mechanical allodynia was delayed and depressed in EphB1 KO mice in the carrageenan test (figure 4A). Thermal hyperalgesia was assessed in two strains of mice (CD1 and CD1/129), since it is well established that thermal and mechanical sensitivities depend on genetic background in mice. The results were similar, even if prevention of thermal hyperalgesia was more complete in the strain which developed a less pronounced hyperalgesia in the WT mice (CD1/129, figure 4A). The latency to paw withdrawal to thermal stimuli was significantly decreased already at 90 min after carrageenan injection in WT animals for both strains ($p<0.05$), whereas there was no significant decrease in EphB1 KO, again regardless of strain. In the CD1 strain of mice tested only the WT mice developed allodynia ($p<0.05$), none being present in the EphB1 KO.

In the longer duration CFA injection model, responses to thermal and mechanical stimuli were recorded at 1, 2, 5, 7, 9 and 14 days after CFA injection (figure 4B). Both WT and EphB1 KO mice developed thermal hyperalgesia, but whilst the latency to paw withdrawal remained significantly lower than baseline values for the duration of the experiment in WT ($p<0.05$), by day 9 in EphB1 KO mice these latencies had returned to values not significantly different from baseline. Both WT and EphB1 KO developed significant ($p<0.05$) and persistent mechanical allodynia, but the thresholds remained significantly lower for WT animals at 9 and 14 days ($p<0.05$), again indicating a faster recovery for EphB1 KO from day 9.

The Increase in the Number of c-fos Expressing Cells in Laminae I and II of the Dorsal Horn, which Follows i.pl. Injection with Formalin or Carrageenan, is Significantly Smaller in EphB1 KO Mice

C-fos expression in dorsal horn neurons is considered as an indicator of activation of nociceptive pathways. We counted the number of c-fos expressing neurons in laminae I and II of the dorsal horn in immunostained sections of spinal cord of animals, which had received a unilateral i.pl. injection of saline, formalin or carrageenan (figure 5). A large and significant ($p<0.05$) increase in the number of c-fos expressing neurons was observed in WT mice

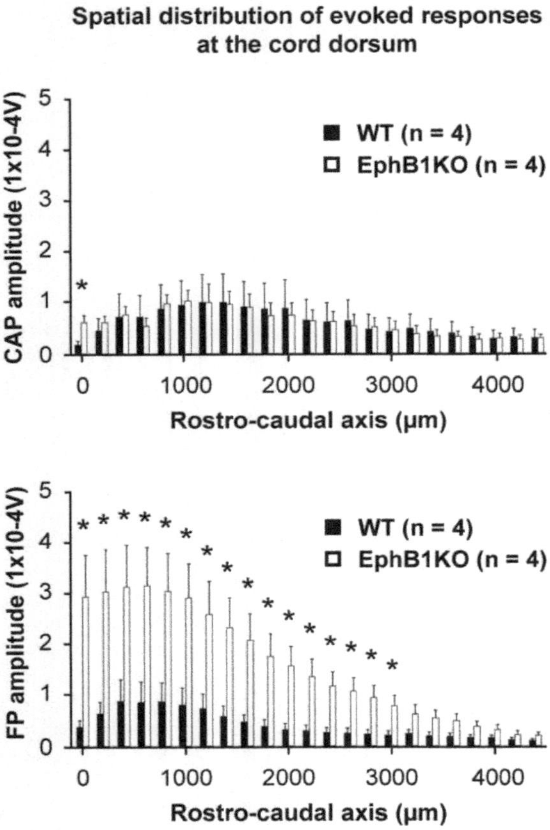

Figure 2. EphB1 KO mice display enhanced A-fibre evoked field potentials along the cord dorsum. Electrical stimulation of the central end of the cut sural nerve at 5T typically evoked a synchronous triphasic compound action potential (CAP), followed by a negative field potential (FP) at the root entry zone. Recordings were made systematically along the rostro-caudal axis 200 µm apart. At each site, 20 successive responses were averaged and the amplitudes (Voltsx10-4) plotted as a function of their rostro-caudal distribution. CAP values were normalised (amplitude and distribution) so allowing comparison of resulting FPs to inputs of similar strengths. Top and bottom panels respectively show the spatial distribution of the CAP and FP amplitudes, with the mean evoked-potentials at each successive position indicated by the paired histograms (WT: filled column; EphB1KO: empty column). While no statistical difference was found between genotypes in the amplitude of the evoked-CAPs (mixed design two-way ANOVA, between factors, $p>0.05$), the distribution of the evoked-FPs (bottom panel) along the rostro-caudal axis of the cord was significantly different between WT and EphB1KO mice (between factors, $p<0.001$), indicating that knocking out the EphB1 gene produced profound alterations in the amplitude of Aβ/Aδ fibre-mediated synaptic responses of the dorsal horn neurones in EphB1KO mice. For both types of evoked-potentials, a significant effect ($p<0.001$) was present for the within factor (level of the spinal cord) indicating that they differ along the rostro-caudal axis of the cord within each genotype. As indicated (stars), post-hoc analysis (independent t -test or non-parametric Mann-Whitney rank sum test) showed that, while it is only the case at the first rostral position for the CAPs, the majority of the FPs were significantly different between the two genotypes ($p<0.05$), except for the most caudal sites (3200 to 4000 µm) where the signals appeared greatly reduced both for WT and EphB1KO mice.

following formalin and carrageenan injection, as compared to saline treated WT mice. A significant increase in c-fos expression was also present in formalin or carrageenan treated EphB1 KO mice, but this was significantly smaller than in WT ($p<0.05$).

The NR2B Subunit of the NMDA Receptor is Phosphorylated in WT, but not EphB1 KO Mice following Formalin or Carrageenan Injection

To examine further the role of the NMDA receptor in EphB/ephrinB signalling, we measured the phosphorylation state of its NR2B subunit in spinal dorsal horn preparations of WT and EphB1 KO mice, after i.pl. injection with saline, formalin carrageenan (figure 6). NR2B was immunoprecipitated from the spinal cords, and western blotting was performed using anti-phosphotyrosine antibodies, followed by anti-NR2B antibodies to measure total NR2B. Levels of phosphorylation were calculated using densitometry. Both carrageenan and formalin injection caused a significant increase in tyrosine phosphorylation of the NR2B subunit in WT ($p<0.05$), but not in EphB1 KO mice.

Deletion of the EphB1 Receptor Gene Reduces, but does not Abolish, Mechanical Allodynia in Two Models of Neuropathic Pain and Thermal Hyperalgesia in the Seltzer Model

We examined the development of mechanical allodynia in two models of neuropathic pain, the PNL and CCI models (figure 7). The CCI model has a more marked inflammatory component.

Animals with PNL were tested 3, 5, 7, 10 14 and 21 days after injury. Both genotypes developed thermal hyperalgesia following injury, but its development was significantly less marked in EphB1 KO mice. In WT mice, thermal hyperalgesia developed from the first day of testing (3 days after injury) and persisted throughout the duration of the experiment. In EphB1 KO mice, the reduction in paw withdrawal latency was significantly smaller than in WT mice at all time points, except 5 days after injury. The mice also developed signs of mechanical allodynia with a marked decrease in the threshold of the response (lifting response to tactile stimulation) of the injured paw as compared to baseline (see figure 7). This increased mechanical sensitivity was markedly reduced in EphB1 KO mice when compared to WT at all time points ($p<0.05$).

A more complete prevention of development of mechanical allodynia was observed in the CCI model. Animals were tested at 7, 14 and 21 days after injury. WT mice developed a significant mechanical allodynia by 7 days ($p<0.05$), and this persisted throughout the experiment, whilst EphB1 KO mice failed to develop a significant mechanical allodynia. Note that autotomy was not observed in any of the animals. Sham operated animals did not develop significant hyperalgesia or allodynia in either genotype (results not shown).

For CCI injured mice, we verified that the behavioural difference between WT and KO mice was not due to differences in the extent to which the animals were affected by the injury: we stained DRG neurons with ATF3 (a marker of axonal injury), and IB4 (a marker for small, non peptidergic, nociceptors), and sections of dorsal horn were stained with IB4. In both genotypes, CCI caused a similar and significant ($p<0.05$) increase in the number of DRG neurons with ATF3+ nuclei in the injured compared to the uninjured side (uninjured, 0.09+/−.057 for WT and 0.109+/−.0711 for EphB1 KO; injured, 15.5+/−1.231 for WT and 12.1+/−4.113 for EphB1 KO). There was no change in the proportion of IB4+ neurons in the injured DRG, but a loss of IB4+ terminals in lamina II of the dorsal horn was observed, in a lateral position (data not shown). C-fos activation in the dorsal horn was absent at 28 days after injury in both genotypes (data not shown).

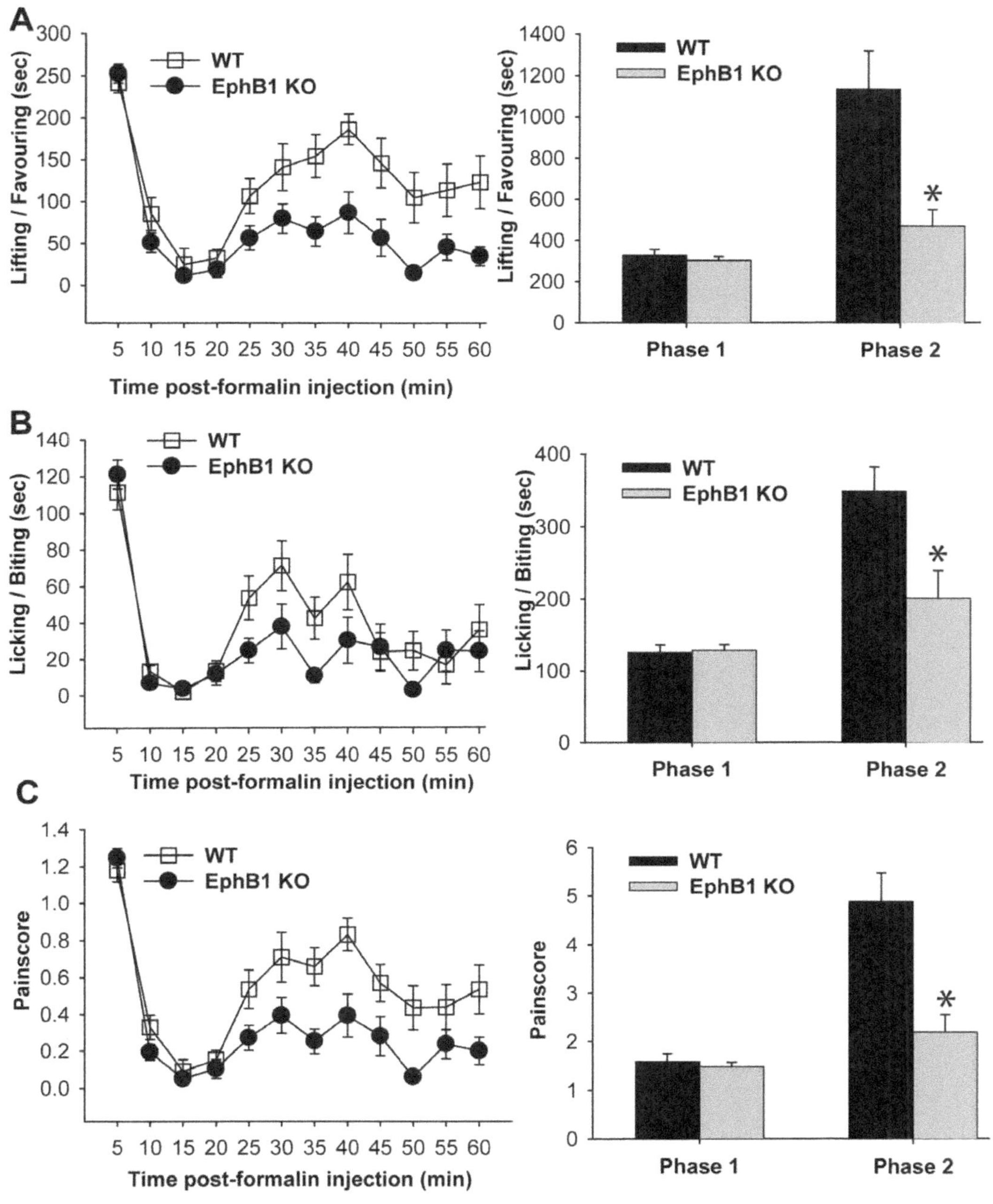

Figure 3. EphB1 KO mice display less spontaneous pain behaviour than WT mice in the formalin test. The behavioural responses of EphB1 KO and WT mice were examined in the formalin test. A formalin solution was injected in one of the hind paws, and the mice were observed for 60 minutes. Pain-related behaviours (lifting-favouring and licking of the injected paw) were recorded in 5 minutes intervals, and the results are graphically represented in panels A and B. A 'pain score' was calculated based on these data, and is represented in panel C. The animals displayed initially an acute response to the injection (Phase I), which is akin to acute nociception and depends upon activation of peripheral terminals of nociceptors. This phase lasted approximately 10 minutes. After a pause of a few minutes, during which little pain related behaviour was observed, the mice began again to lift or lick the affected paw (Phase II). When the cumulative results of EphB1 KO and WT mice for Phase I and Phase II were compared, there was no difference between WT and KO during Phase I. However, EphB1 KO mice displayed significantly less pain related behaviours (Lifting/favouring, licking and pain score) as compared to WT mice during Phase II. Bar charts represent mean +/− SEM Asterisks indicate a significant difference WT vs EphB1 KO with $p<0.05$ (t-test). WT n = 13, EphB1 KO n = 15.

Microglial Activation in the Spinal Cord following PNL is Attenuated in EphB1 KO Mice

Microglial cell activation has been shown to be associated with the onset of neuropathic pain. We identified microglial cells with Iba1 antibodies and manually counted the number of morphologically identified activated microglial cells in the dorsal horn of the spinal cord in control, sham animals, and in animals which had undergone PNL, both ipsilaterally and contralaterally to the lesion. In sham animals there was no difference in the number of activated microglial cells in WT or EphB1 KO mice (figure 8 A,

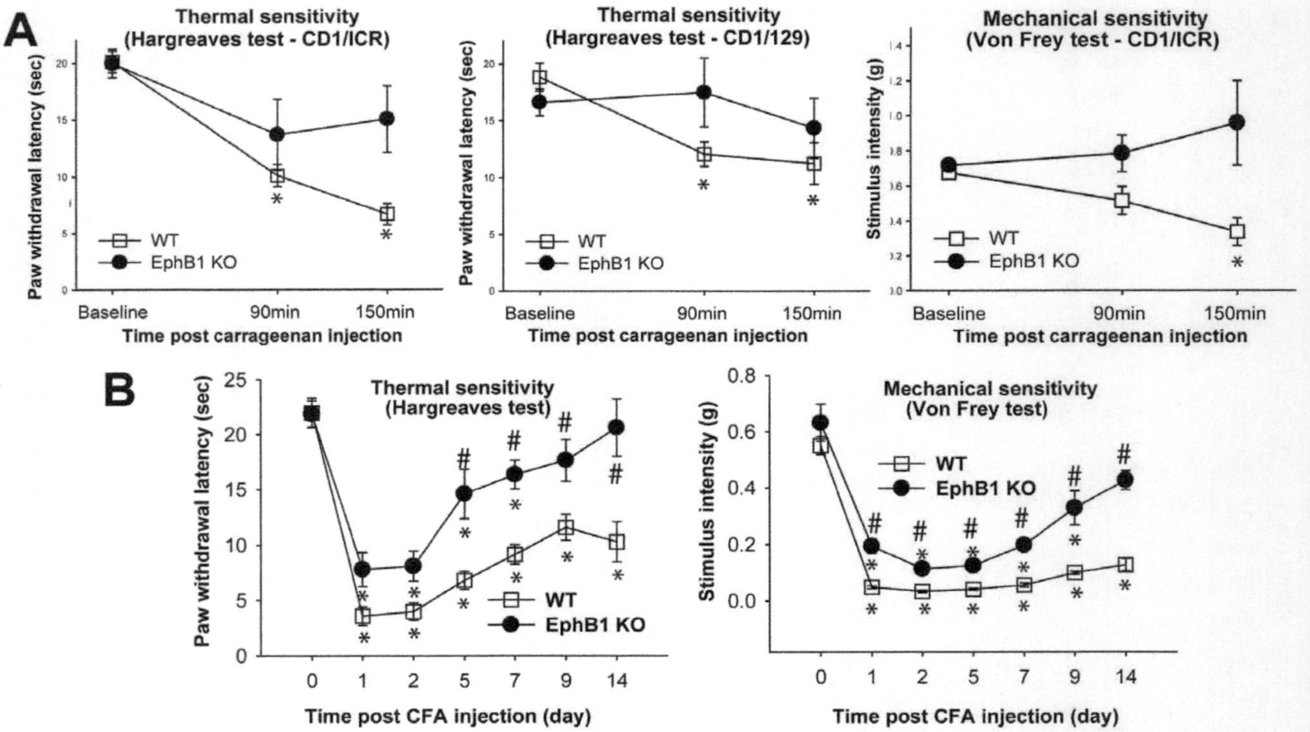

Figure 4. EphB1 KO mice display reduced thermal and mechanical hyperalgesia in inflammatory pain models. The behavioural responses of EphB1 KO and WT mice were examined in two test of inflammatory pain. Either carrageenan (A) or CFA (B) were injected in a hind paw, and responses to thermal (Hargreaves) and mechanical (von Frey) stimuli were recorded up to a maximum of 150 minutes (A) or 14 days (B). Thermal sensitivity following carrageenan injection was tested in mice of two genetic backgrounds, CD1/ICR and CD1/129, and mechanical allodynia was tested in CD1/ICR mice only. All WT mice developed thermal and mechanical hyperalgesia ($p<0.05$). EphB1 KO mice did not develop thermal or mechanical hyperalgesia. Following CFA injection, which elicits a greater and more prolonged inflammatory response as compared to carrageenan, both WT and EphB1 KO mice developed thermal and mechanical hyperalgesia (B). However, EphB1 KO mice displayed a faster recovery in terms of thermal hyperalgesia and a significantly smaller development of mechanical allodynia. * $p<0.05$ vs respective baseline, # $p<0.05$ comparing WT and EphB1 KO mice at equivalent time points (Repeated Measures ANOVA followed by Multiple Comparisons versus Control Group, Holm-Sidak method). A) CD1/ICR Hargreaves WT n = 9, EphB1 KO n = 9, von Frey WT n = 10, EphB1 KO n = 10; CD1/129 WT n = 8, EphB1 KO n = 6; B) n = 8 for all groups except EphB1 KO in the von Frey test, where n = 9.

B). Following nerve injury, increased microglia activation was observed in the ipsilateral dorsal horn of the spinal cord from day 3 onwards. This activation was present also in EphB1 KO mice, but to a significantly lesser extent, as compared to WT ($p<0.05$). By day 22, though, there was no significant microglial activation, as compared to sham animals, in either WT or KO mice. We did not observe a significant microglial activation on the contralateral side (average number of activated microglial cells/100 μm^2: day 3 WT 1.133+/−0.0726, EphB1 KO 1.117+/−0.0167; day 7 WT 1.083+/−0.209, EphB1 KO 1.400+/−0.277; day 14 WT 1.258+/−0.0902, EphB1 KO 1.175+/−0.142; day 22 WT 1.046+/−0.123, EphB1 KO 0.917+/−0.0928).

Discussion

In this study we characterised extensively EphB1 receptor KO mice in terms of their responses to acute noxious stimuli and susceptibility to persistent (chronic) pain, in a number of models in which spontaneous pain behaviour and/or thermal and mechanical hyperalgesia have been attributed at least in part to the development of central sensitisation, an activity-dependent alteration of synaptic connectivity within the spinal cord,. Our main findings are 1) the EphB1 receptor is not essential for the development of peripheral nociception, nor for thermal or mechanical sensitivity; 2) functional EphB1 receptors are required for the development and/or maintenance of thermal and mechanical hyperalgesia and spontaneous pain in a variety of pain models; 3) EphB1 receptors are necessary for the induction of phosphorylation of the NR2B subunit of the NMDA receptor and are involved in the increase of c-fos expression in models of inflammatory pain and tissue injury and in microglial activation following PNL.

EphB1 receptors, together with other Eph receptors, play an important role in neuronal development (see e.g. [40]), therefore it was important to establish that EphB1 KO mice were normal in terms of development of nociceptive pathways and nociception, in order to be suitable in models for the study of the modulation of pain processing. This had not been examined in previous studies using these mice. Since pain sensitivity in animal models is measured through behavioural tests dependent on a motor response, it was also important to test naïve KO mice in comparison to WT littermate in a motor test, particular in light of findings indicating that EphB1 KO exhibit neuronal loss in the substantia nigra [41]. We found no indication that this loss affected the response to acute noxious stimuli using a variety of tests, including thermal and mechanical stimuli, or to the first phase of the formalin test, reflecting acute tissue damage. Gross anatomical abnormalities were also absent from both the DRG and the dorsal

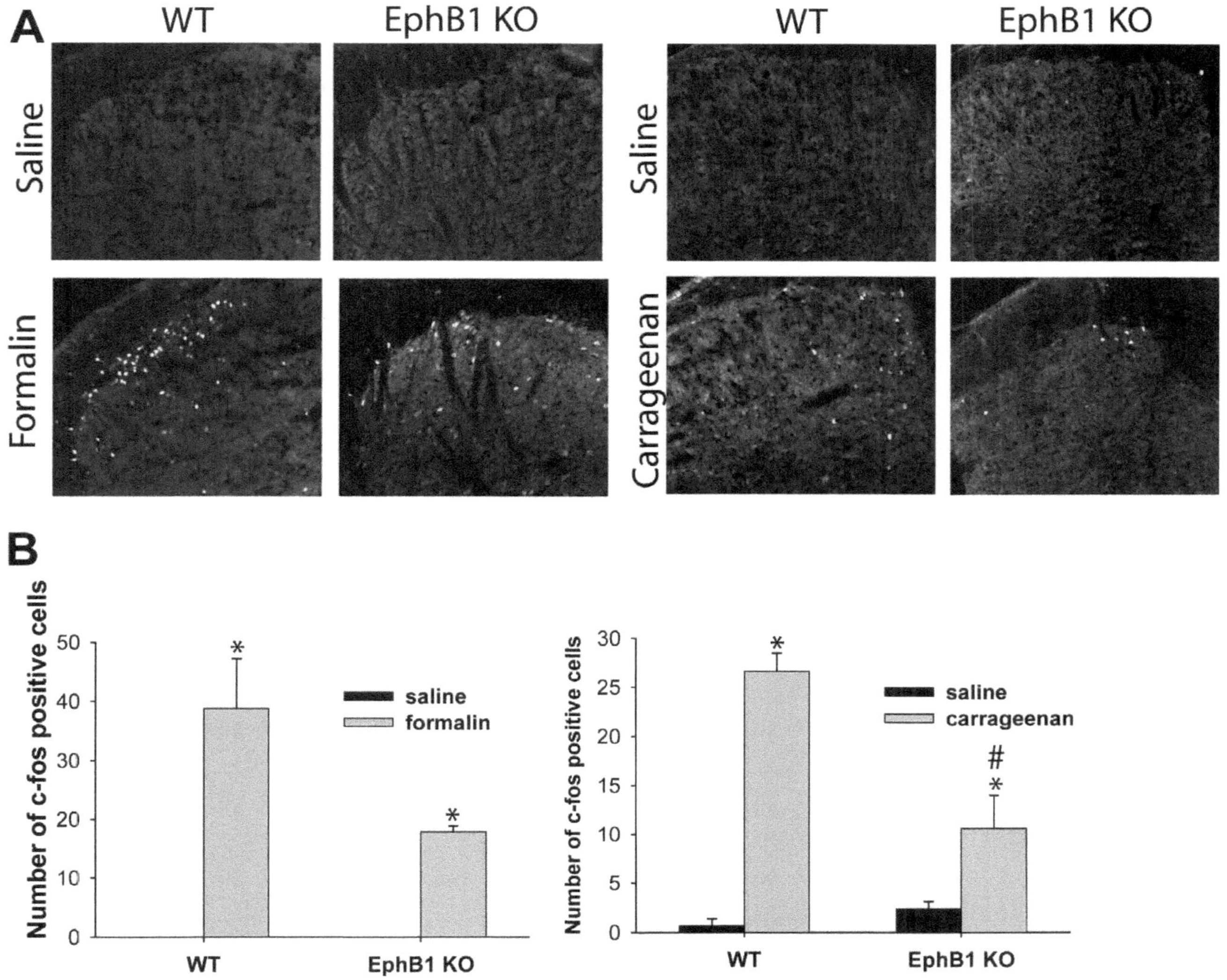

Figure 5. Upregulation of c-fos expression following formalin or carrageenan injection is reduced in EphB1 KO mice. C-fos immunoreactivity was examined in EphB1 KO and WT mice following formalin and carrageenan injection. Saline injected animals were used as controls. (A) photomicrographs of section of lumbar spinal cord of EphB1 KO and WT mice injected with formalin, carrageenan or saline as indicated, immunostained with anti c-fos antibodies. B) c-fos positive cells were counted in lumbar cord section of mice treated as in (A). Saline treated animals had none or few c-fos positive cells. Both formalin and carrageenan injection induced a significant increase in the number of c-fos positive cells in WT mice (two-way ANOVA followed by multiple comparisons, Holm-Sidak method, for carrageenan, t-test for formalin experiments), but carrageenan or formalin injection caused a significantly lower increase in EphB1 KO mice. * $p<0.05$ vs respective saline, # $p<0.05$ vs WT. For all experimental groups $n=3$.

horn of the spinal cord. Similarly electrophysiological recording at the cord dorsum, measuring the spatial distribution and amplitudes of the CAPs and FPs following sciatic nerve stimulation, did not reveal any difference between WT and EphB1 KO mice in terms of somatotopic organisation of sensory projections in the spinal cord. Although the presence of developmental defects in glutamatergic synapses in the hippocampus of transgenic EphB2 KO mice remains unclear [42,43], it is possible that in single mutants (EphB1 or EphB2 receptors KO) compensatory mechanisms, due to the presence of other EphB receptors, which bind promiscuously to the same ephrinB ligands, may allow a comparatively normal development. We cannot however exclude the presence of subtle changes, for example at the level of the glutamatergic synapses of sensory afferents onto dorsal horn neurons, below the level of detection behaviourally. In this respect our finding of enhanced sural nerve evoked superficial dorsal horn FPs is of relevance in that it indicates such a change in the connectivity of Aβ-fibres. Our simplest explanation for this finding draws on the changes observed early postnatally in the rat where the predominant A-fibre innervation of the superficial dorsal horn at birth undergoes a dramatic, activity-dependent withdrawal of the nerve terminals to deeper layers over the first postnatal weeks [44,45]. It is proposed here that such functional and structural reorganisation did not occur in EphB1KO mice. Further studies are needed to determine whether inhibitory or excitatory interneurons, projection neurons or both, are involved in this refinement process. Although this change in the connectivity of A fibres in the sural nerve is of considerable interest in view of the guidance role of Eph receptors during development, it had no demonstrable impact on the behavioural tests we employed, or on

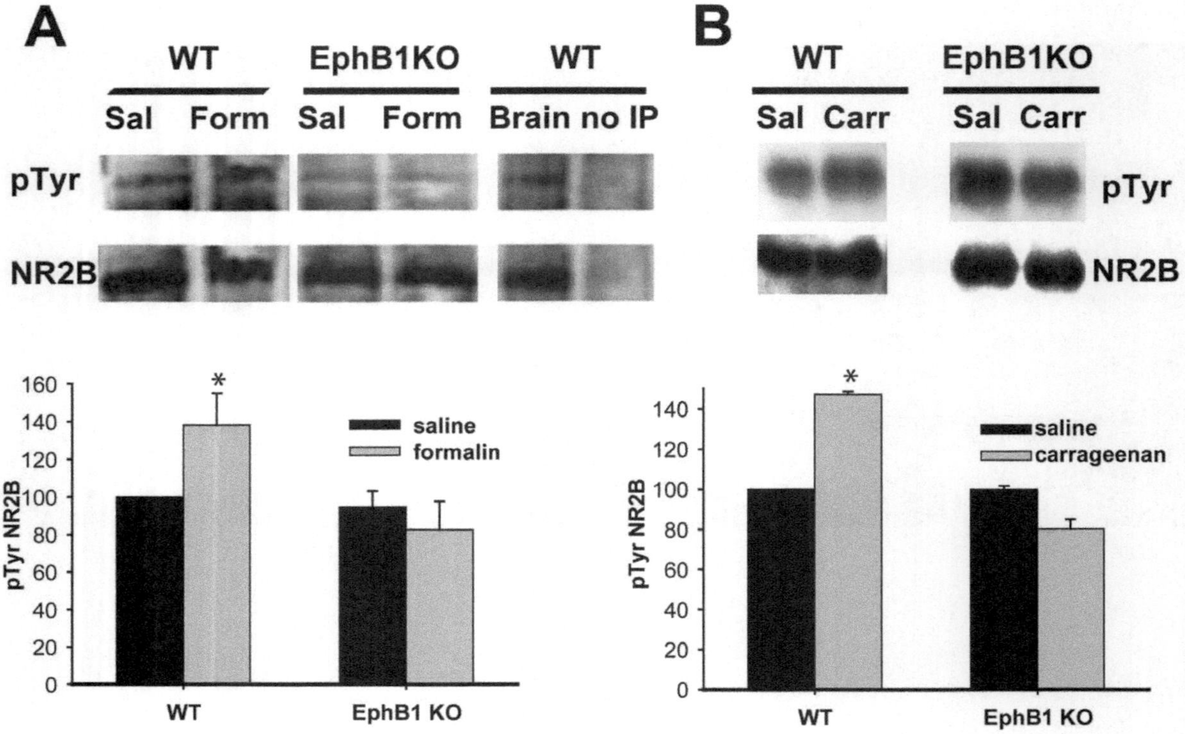

Figure 6. Lack of increase in NR2B phosphorylation in EphB1 KO mice following formalin or carrageenan injection. Tyrosine phosphorylation of the NR2B subunit of the NMDA receptor was analysed by immunoprecipitation followed by Western Blotting in WT and EphB1 KO mice after injection with formalin or carrageenan. Saline injected animals were used as controls. Spinal cords were dissected from injected animals 1 h (A) or 3 hours (B) after injection. Representative immunoblots are shown in the top part of panels A and B. In panel A, the last two columns represent positive (mouse brain tissue) and negative (immunoprecipitation of mouse brain tissue conducted in the absence of anti-NR2B antibodies) controls of the immunoprecipitation and Western blotting protocol. The blots were quantified, and the ratio of phosphoTyr to the total NR2B present was calculated. The bar charts in the bottom half of panels A and B show the mean and SEM of the levels of phosphoNR2B present in EphB1 KO and WT mice following injection with Formalin, Carrageenan or saline, as indicated. There was a significant increase in Tyrosine phosphorylation of NR2B in WT mice following formalin (A) and carrageenan injection (B), $p<0.05$. There was no change in the level of NR2B phosphorylation in EphB1 KO mice following either injection. Comparisons performed with t-test for WT in the formalin experiment and EphB1 KO in the carrageenan experiments, with Mann-Whitney U-test in the remaining experiments. * $p<0.05$ vs respective saline. For all experimental groups $n=3$, except in A) EphB1 KO saline $n=4$.

the gross anatomical connectivity of C and Aδ fibres. Another possible explanation for the enhanced synaptic transmission we observed could be a change in the electrophysiological properties of the large diameter Aβ-fibre, as described in DRG neurons for a rat model of osteoarthritic pain [46] and more recently in a neuropathic pain model [47].

Clearly indicated for future work would be a comparison of a), the cord dorsum CAP and field potentials evoked by fibres in the sural and saphenous nerves; b), their depth profiles in the dorsal horn as this would provide direct evidence of a developmentally – based shift in their sites of termination and/or or their synaptic strength.

Following our initial work demonstrating an involvement of EphB receptors-ephrins interaction in modulation of pain processing in the spinal cord [7], a growing number of other studies has provided evidence supporting a role of EphB receptors in a variety of short-term inflammatory and longer-term, chronic pain models (carrageenan and formalin injection in the hind paw, chronic constriction injury, pain induced by morphine withdrawal in dependent animals, cancer pain, see e.g. [9,24,48–52]). Initially, the unequivocal identification of the specific EphB receptor involved had been impossible, due to the lack of suitable reagents and in particular specific agonists and antagonists. A study by Han et al. [25], performed on one of the strains of EphB1 KO mice used here, confirmed the hypothesis of an involvement of EphB1 receptors in neuropathic pain (thermal hyperalgesia in the CCI model) and in physical dependence to morphine, comparing the behavioural responses of EphB1 KO, heterozygous and WT mice. In their study, a complete lack of development of thermal hyperalgesia was observed in EphB1 KO mice in the CCI model. Here, we examine the EphB1 KO mice studied by Han et al. in a number of other models, including short-term (carrageenan injection) and long-term (CFA injection) inflammation, tissue damage and PNL. Even if the molecular and cellular mechanisms underlying hypersensitivity in experimental models of pain have not been completely clarified, it is clear that different molecular and cellular mechanisms underlie hypersensitivity in different pain models (see e.g. [23]), and also mechanical and thermal hyperalgesia in the same model; for example, with regard to neuropathic pain, it has been shown that there are significant differences in the mechanisms leading to chronic pain in different models [53,54], and in the mechanisms leading to the induction of thermal and mechanical hyperalgesia. It is therefore important to establish if and to what extent EphB1 receptors contribute to thermal and mechanical hyperalgesia, as well as spontaneous pain behaviour, in pain states of different aetiology.

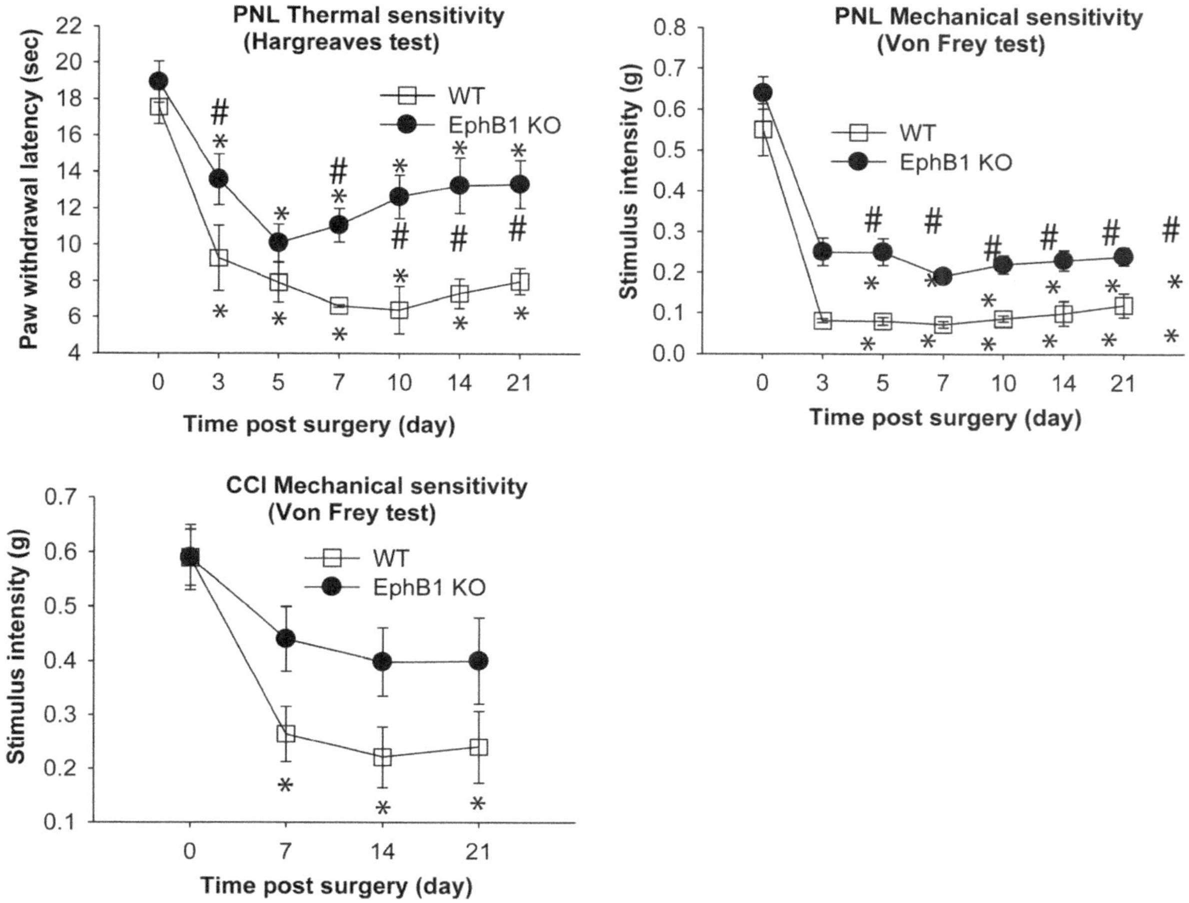

Figure 7. Accelerated recovery from mechanical and thermal hyperalgesia following nerve injury in EphB1 KO mice. Behavioural responses following peripheral nerve lesion were examined in EphB1 KO mice and WT mice. Two models of nerve injury were used, partial nerve lesion (PNL) and chronic constriction injury (CCI). Development of both thermal and mechanical hyperalgesia were studied after PNL, mechanical hyperalgesia only was examined after CCI. WT mice developed significant thermal hyperalgesia in both models. In WT mice with PNL, hyperalgesia developed by 3 days after injury and persisted throughout the duration of the experiment. This reduction in paw withdrawal latency was significantly smaller in EphB1 KO mice at all time points, except 5 days after injury. WT mice also developed mechanical allodynia with a marked decrease in stimulus intensity required to trigger a lifting response of the injured paw as compared to baseline. EphB1 KO mice displayed a less pronounced mechanical allodynia when compared to WT at all time points ($p<0.05$). In the CCI model mice responses to mechanical stimuli were tested at 7, 14 and 21 days after injury. WT mice developed a significant mechanical allodynia by 7 days ($p<0.05$), and this persisted throughout the experiment, whilst EphB1 KO mice failed to develop a significant mechanical allodynia.* $p<0.05$ vs respective baseline, # $p<0.05$ vs WT. Test: repeated measures ANOVA followed by multiple comparisons, Holm-Sidak method. PNL WT n = 6, EphB1 KO n = 9; CCI WT n = 7, EphB1 KO n = 5.

In a number of models (CCI and carrageenan injection) we observed a complete lack of development of mechanical and thermal hyperalgesia, as we expected on the basis of previous findings obtained in rats treated with the EphB receptor blocker EphB1-Fc (for carrageenan injection and thermal hyperalgesia in CCI; [7,9]) or in EphB1 KO mice (for thermal hyperalgesia in CCI; [25]).

However, in the CFA-induced inflammatory pain model hyperalgesia and allodynia developed almost normally in KO mice, but recovery was accelerated. This is particularly interesting because due to its duration the CFA model would arguably be one of the most clinically relevant. Furthermore, this finding was partially replicated in the PLN model of neuropathic pain where thermal hyperalgesia developed almost normally in KO mice, but recovery was accelerated. The results obtained in the CFA and PNL models indicate that EphB1 receptors play a significant role in maintaining sensitisation hence emphasising their importance as a potential therapeutic target.

The behavioural findings reported here are evidence of a crucial role of EphB1 receptors in the onset and/or maintenance of thermal and mechanical hypersensitivity in a variety of models of pain, but what are the specific cellular and molecular mechanisms involved? Notwithstanding the number of differences in the molecular and cellular changes they induce, in all of the models we have used, a supposed common mechanism is represented by classical central sensitisation, an activity-dependent increase in the strength of synaptic transmission between primary sensory afferents and dorsal horn neurons [12]. Although such sensitisation is thought to be an NMDA receptor-mediated process, its mode of modulation is not yet fully understood. LTP at C-fibre synapses on a subpopulation of nociceptive neurons in lamina I of the dorsal horn could also contribute to pain amplification [14,15]. Phosphorylation of NMDA receptor subunits has been proposed to lead to increased Ca^{++} entry through the receptor, both in central sensitisation and in NMDA dependent LTP [19,55]. Liu et al. [56] showed that uncoupling Src from the NMDA receptor

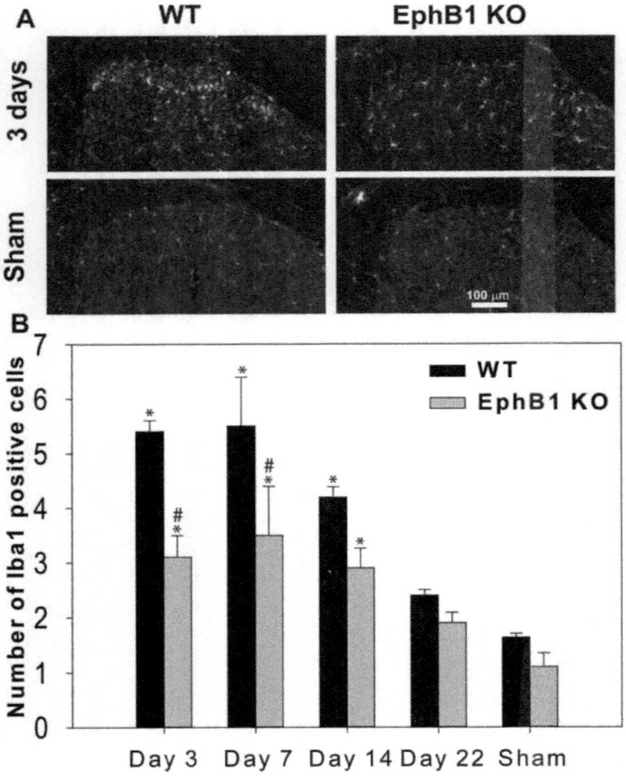

Figure 8. Microglial activation following PNL is attenuated in the spinal cord of EphB1 KO mice. In (A) representative immunostaining for Iba1 in the superficial laminae of the dorsal horn of the spinal cord 3 days after PNL, or in sham operated animals. The hemicord ipsilateral to the sciatic nerve partial ligation is shown. In (B) bar chart illustrating cell counting for Iba1 positive cells in the dorsal horn. An increase in microglia cell activation was shown after PNL in both WT and EphB1 KO mice at 3, 7 and 14 days after lesion ($p<0.05$). However, the increase of immunoreactivity for Iba1 was attenuated in EphB1 KO mice ($p<0.05$ overall, and at 3 and 7 days after lesion). Data shown as mean ± SEM. * $p<0.05$ vs respective sham, # $p<0.05$ vs WT. Test: two-way ANOVA followed by multiple comparisons, Holm-Sidak method. WT and EphB1 KO n = 3 for each timepoint.

complex, thus preventing NMDA tyrosine phosphorylation, suppresses inflammatory and neuropathic pain. Phosphorylation of the NR2B subunit has been claimed to be important for the onset of persistent pain, however there is evidence both in favour and against NR2B involvement, particularly in inflammatory pain (in favour [8,19,20,57,57,58] [59]; against [18,20,60]).

Guo et al. [19] were the first to propose that NMDA receptor phosphorylation in central sensitisation could be modulated by other receptors, rather than simply by activation of the NMDA receptor itself (with consequent activation of Src tyrosine kinases); and they were also the first to show NR2B tyrosine phosphorylation in CFA induced inflammatory pain. Work from our laboratory had suggested a role for EphB receptors in central sensitisation, showing that, in analogy with what had previously been demonstrated in cultures of embryonic cortical and hippocampal neurons [27], EphB receptor activation could lead to NR2B subunit phosphorylation in the spinal cord, a process mediated by the activation of the non-receptor tyrosine kinase Src [8]. Furthermore, in a model of acute inflammatory pain (carrageenan injection) in adult rats [8] and also in the formalin model in adult mice [49], we showed NR2B tyrosine phosphorylation in the spinal cord following injection, in contrast to the findings of Caudle et al. [18], who found that the NR2B receptor is not involved in inflammatory pain. Liu et al. [52] replicated our finding showing that EphB receptor activation in rats induces NR2B phosphorylation, but also showed that blocking receptor activation with EphB2-Fc chimera (which blocks the activation of all EphB receptors) prevented the increased phosphorylation of NR2B in a model of cancer pain. On the basis of the findings reported in the literature, and discussed above, and in particular [7,8,27,52], we hypothesised that in WT type mice inflammation or tissue injury may lead to activation of EphB1 in dorsal horn neurons, with consequent phosphorylation of NR2B; lack of functional EphB1 receptor would therefore abolish such increased phosphorylation. The findings reported here are consistent with the hypothesis that NR2B subunit phosphorylation is indeed downstream of EphB1 receptor activation in both the carrageenan model and in the formalin model, in which NR2B is tyrosine phosphorylated in WT but not in KO mice. However, our findings also provide support for the conflicting hypothesis [18],that NR2B phosphorylation is not required for the onset of chronic pain, since in some long-term models we observed the onset of hyperalgesia and allodynia also in EphB1 KO mice. We attempted to analyse NR2B phosphorylation in a longer duration model (CFA), using naive mice, and mice at 1, 7 and 14 days after injection of CFA or saline. Despite using 8 mice/genotype/timepoint (2 mice/sample), our results were inconclusive, with no obvious increase in NR2B phosphorylation in EphB1 KO mice, and a non-significant, 20% increase in phosphorylation in WT mice at 1 day only (data not shown). This would be consistent with the time course of NR2B phosphorylation in the spinal cord of rats, following CFA injection, reported by Guo et al. [19] but needs to be confirmed. The biochemical analysis of NR2B receptor phosphorylation in the mouse spinal cord is challenging, possibly due to low levels of the receptor as a proportion of total protein level; further investigations on the link between EphB1 receptors, NR2B phosphorylation and chronic inflammatory and neuropathic pain could probably more profitably investigated with genetic manipulation, for example by crossing EphB1 mutants with mice in which NR2B cannot be phosphorylated on tyr1472, which have been shown to develop attenuated neuropathic pain [20], or by developing a spatially and time restricted NR2B knockout, similar to the one generated for NR1 [17,61]. This second alternative may give different results from those obtained in mutants in which tyr 1472 cannot be phosphorylated, since there are two other tyrosine phosphorylation sites on NR2B (tyr1252 and tyr 1336), which may play a role. It is however worth noting that NMDA-dependent synaptic plasticity in the hippocampus was shown to be independent of EphB2 receptor kinase activity, despite requiring the extracellular portion of the receptor [42,43], in contrast to the requirement for kinase activity shown by Takasu et al. [27] in embryonic neurons in culture. It is therefore possible that EphB1 receptors may mediate alterations in spinal cord processing of pain independent of their kinase activity.

The immediate early gene c-fos has been shown to be expressed in neurons of the dorsal horn following activation of nociceptive pathways [62,63], and Takasu et al. [27] showed increased c-fos expression following EphB receptor activation in cultured embryonic cortical and hippocampal neurons. We previously showed increase in c-fos-positive cells in the superficial laminae of the dorsal horn in carrageenan treated rats, an increase which was not present when EphB1-Fc was injected intrathecally prior to carrageenan injection, thus linking EphB1 receptor activation to c-fos expression also in vivo. Liu et al. [26] demonstrated increased c-fos expression in the dorsal horn of mice following high frequency stimulation of C fibres in vivo. This was prevented by EphB2-Fc pre-treatment and in EphB1 KO mice. Furthermore, Liu et al. [10] showed NR2B phosphorylation and increased c-fos expression in the dorsal horn in a morphine withdrawal model. Both increases were prevented by blocking EphB receptor activation with EphB2-Fc. Here, we show that both formalin and carrageenan injection induce an increase in c-fos expression in WT but a significantly smaller increase in EphB1 KO mice. This suggests that c-fos upregulation may mediate some of the effect of EphB1 activation on pain sensitivity. We cannot directly link the increase in c-fos expressing neurons to NR2B phosphorylation, since we cannot demonstrate that the neurons expressing c-fos are the same in which NR2B is phosphorylated. Hopefully technical improvement in immunohistochemical approaches will allow doing so in the future. However the findings by Takasu et al [27] in culture, together with the indirect evidence from the in vivo studies cited above, would suggest that c-fos upregulation is likely to be linked, at least in part, to increased NMDA receptor activity.

We did not comprehensively investigate c-fos expression in neuropathic pain models, since published results on c-fos expression in neuropathic pain models, particularly in the chronic phase, have been extremely inconsistent, even in the rat, which has been studied fairly extensively [64]. However, instead, we did examine one of the potential cellular mechanism, through which EphB1 deficiency may modulate neuropathic pain, based on a growing body of evidence implicating microglial activation in neuropathic pain, which would lead to pro-inflammatory responses with pathological effects [28,65]. We therefore counted activated microglia in the dorsal horn of the spinal cord of WT and EphB1 KO mice following PNL. Possibly due to the fact that many of the studies on the molecular mechanism regulating microglial activation have been conducted in vitro, the precise nature of the cellular and molecular mechanisms regulating this activation in vivo is still poorly understood, but the current consensus is that activation is triggered by signals coming from primary afferents, with prominent candidates being ATP and monocyte chemoattractant protein-1 (MCP-1), followed by neuronal factalkine, cleaved by Cathepsin S of microglial origin [28,66], Furthermore, input from A fibres has been shown to be important for microglial activation in the spared nerve model [67]. None of these mechanisms should be affected by lack of EphB1 receptors. However, microglial activation was attenuated in EphB1 KO mice from day 3, in parallel with the observed attenuation of thermal and mechanical hyperalgesia. This would suggest that the EphB1 receptor is implicated in the mechanisms leading to microglia activation in neuropathic pain, even though other mechanisms, independent of EphB1 receptor expression, must be involved, since some level of microglial activation was present also in KO mice. We had observed an analogous reduction in microglial activation in a conditional knockout (generated in a different mouse strain), lacking ephrinB2 specifically in a subpopulation (largely nociceptive) of DRG neurons [49], confirming that the observations made here in EphB1 KO mice cannot be due to the lack of presumptive pre-synaptic EphB1 receptors. This would indicate that microglial activation must be at least in part mediated by post-synaptic mechanisms. Daulhac et al. [68] observed, in a model of diabetic neuropathy, that microglia activation was dependent on NMDA receptor activity. The findings presented here would suggest that a similar mechanism may also be at work in our injury model of neuropathic pain, since lack of EphB1 receptors can affect NMDA receptor function. Further studies should be carried out on these potential post-synaptic mechanisms, also to determine if they contribute to microglial activation in all types of pain. In contrast to Dauhlac et al. findings in diabetic neuropathy, Cheng et al, [69] observed NMDA-independent microglia activation in CFA-induced inflammatory pain.

Interestingly, both thermal and mechanical hyperalgesia are still present at day 21 in WT, and to a lesser extent in EphB1 KO mice, when microglial activation is no longer detectable, supporting the hypothesis that microglial activation is important for the early phases of neuropathic pain, rather than long-term maintenance.

Our findings can be explained in their entirety by postulating an exclusively post-synaptic site of action for EphB1 receptors. Nevertheless two of the studies by Song's group [9,25] would suggest that, at least in the CCI model, there may be an involvement of pre-synaptic EphB1 receptors in the behavioural responses observed. They demonstrated hyperexcitability of DRG neurons following CCI, which was not present in EphB1 KO mice and which could be blocked by EphB1-Fc. Also in rats CCI led to increased expression of EphB1 in DRG neurons. Kobayashi et al. [24] suggested the presence of ephrin B2 in spinal cord neurons, and this could potentially activate EphB1 receptors on DRG neurons. Any pre-synaptic role of EphB1 receptors is however likely to be in addition to, rather than in alternative, to a post-synaptic role, since both EphB1 and NMDA receptors have been shown to be present in dorsal horn neurons, and can be immunoprecipitated together from the spinal cord. Crucially, in a nociceptor-specific ephrinB2 deficient mouse we showed a reduced phosphorylation of NR2B in the formalin and PNL models [49]. This reduction could not be mediated by pre-synaptic EphB1 receptors, since their potential ephrinB2 ligands in the spinal cord are still present in the ephrin B2 nociceptive specific KO. Also, the findings we reported with ephrin B2 nociceptive specific KO mice allow us to exclude that the results we report here may be due to EphB1 receptors in the dorsal horn acting by activating reverse signalling via pre-synaptic ephrinB2; as mentioned in the introduction, EphB receptor-ephrinB interactions may activate both forward signalling via the receptor, and reverse signalling via the transmembrane ligand, and there is evidence, mainly in the hippocampus, that ephrin signalling may modulate synaptic function [6].

Moreover, it is not clear whether any possible role played by EphB1 receptors in DRG neurons would be at the level of central synapses, or rather in the periphery, where at least in the case of tissue damage models (formalin), peripheral EphB receptors appear to be important [70]. It is however worth noticing that the role identified by Cao et al. [70] for EphB receptors in the periphery may not be mediated entirely (or at all) by EphB1 receptors, but by another EphB receptor. Intraplantar injection of EphB1-Fc (which would block any EphB receptor) reduced pain-related behaviour in both phase I and phase II in Cao et al.'s experiments, whereas in EphB1 KO mice the response in Phase I is not affected. A peripheral site of action for EphB1 receptors on DRG neurons could still explain the differences in excitability observed by Han et al. [25] in injured EphB1 KO mice.

Conclusions

Independently of the differences we observed in the extent of the effect of the lack of functional EphB1 receptors in a variety of inflammatory, tissue and nerve injury models, in all cases we found that the lack of EphB1 protein led to a blunted or absent thermal and mechanical hyperalgesia, or spontaneous pain behaviour. It would therefore appear likely that the induction and/or maintenance of central sensitisation require the presence of EphB1 receptors, regardless of cause and sensory modality examined. Cellular and molecular mechanisms that mediate the role of EphB1 in leading to increased sensitivity/spontaneous pain are likely to include NR2B phosphorylation,increased c-fos expression and microglial activation. Our present findings confirm the identity of the EphB receptors involved in the onset of various types of persistent, chronic pain as the EphB1 receptors, extend the involvement of EphB receptors to models of long term inflammation and the Seltzer neuropathic pain model, suggesting that this receptor is probably involved in all forms of allegedly NMDA-dependent persistent pain. Intriguingly, in models of persistent pain we observed that EphB1 KO mice developed hyperalgesia/allodynia, but recovered faster as compared to WT mice, suggesting that the EphB1 receptor may be an attractive target for the development of analgesic strategies.

Author Contributions

Critically revised the manuscript: VC-G GY AB SF MH. Conceived and designed the experiments: IG TS AB VC-G. Performed the experiments: VC-G GY SF AB TS. Analyzed the data: VC-G GY SF TS IG. Contributed reagents/materials/analysis tools: MH TS. Wrote the paper: IG TS.

References

1. Dalva MB, Takasu MA, Lin MZ, Shamah SM, Hu L, et al. (2000) EphB receptors interact with NMDA receptors and regulate excitatory synapse formation. Cell 103: 945–956.
2. Calo L, Cinque C, Patane M, Schillaci D, Battaglia G, et al. (2006) Interaction between ephrins/Eph receptors and excitatory amino acid receptors: possible relevance in the regulation of synaptic plasticity and in the pathophysiology of neuronal degeneration. J Neurochem 98: 1–10.
3. Klein R (2009) Bidirectional modulation of synaptic functions by Eph/ephrin signaling. Nat Neurosci 12: 15–20.
4. Drescher U (1997) The Eph family in the patterning of neural development. Curr Biol 7: R799–R807.
5. Pasquale EB (2008) Eph-ephrin bidirectional signaling in physiology and disease. Cell 133: 38–52.
6. Hruska M, Dalva MB (2012) Ephrin regulation of synapse formation, function and plasticity. Mol Cell Neurosci 50: 35–44.
7. Battaglia AA, Sehayek K, Grist J, McMahon SB, Gavazzi I (2003) EphB receptors and ephrin-B ligands regulate spinal sensory connectivity and modulate pain processing. Nat Neurosci 6: 339–340.
8. Slack S, Battaglia A, Cibert-Goton V, Gavazzi I (2008) EphrinB2 induces tyrosine phosphorylation of NR2B via Src-family kinases during inflammatory hyperalgesia. Neuroscience 156: 175–183.
9. Song XJ, Zheng JH, Cao JL, Liu WT, Song XS, et al. (2008) EphrinB-EphB receptor signaling contributes to neuropathic pain by regulating neural excitability and spinal synaptic plasticity in rats. Pain 139: 168–180.
10. Liu WT, Li HC, Song XS, Huang ZJ, Song XJ (2009) EphB receptor signaling in mouse spinal cord contributes to physical dependence on morphine. FASEB J 23: 90–98.
11. Costigan M, Scholz J, Woolf CJ (2009) Neuropathic pain: a maladaptive response of the nervous system to damage. Annu Rev Neurosci 32: 1–32.
12. Latremoliere A, Woolf CJ (2009) Central sensitization: a generator of pain hypersensitivity by central neural plasticity. J Pain 10: 895–926.
13. Ji RR, Kohno T, Moore KA, Woolf CJ (2003) Central sensitization and LTP: do pain and memory share similar mechanisms? Trends Neurosci 26: 696–705.
14. Sandkuhler J (2007) Understanding LTP in pain pathways. Mol Pain 3: 9.
15. Sandkuhler J (2010) Central sensitization versus synaptic long-term potentiation (LTP): a critical comment. J Pain 11: 798–800.
16. Inturrisi CE (2005) The role of N-methyl-D-aspartate (NMDA) receptors in pain and morphine tolerance. Minerva Anestesiol 71: 401–403.
17. Weyerbacher AR, Xu Q, Tamasdan C, Shin SJ, Inturrisi CE (2010) N-Methyl-D-aspartate receptor (NMDAR) independent maintenance of inflammatory pain. Pain 148: 237–246.
18. Caudle RM, Perez FM, Del Valle-Pinero AY, Iadarola MJ (2005) Spinal cord NR1 serine phosphorylation and NR2B subunit suppression following peripheral inflammation. Mol Pain 1: 25.
19. Guo W, Zou S, Guan Y, Ikeda T, Tal M, et al. (2002) Tyrosine phosphorylation of the NR2B subunit of the NMDA receptor in the spinal cord during the development and maintenance of inflammatory hyperalgesia. J Neurosci 22: 6208–6217.
20. Matsumura S, Kunori S, Mabuchi T, Katano T, Nakazawa T, et al. (2010) Impairment of CaMKII activation and attenuation of neuropathic pain in mice lacking NR2B phosphorylated at Tyr1472. Eur J Neurosci 32: 798–810.
21. Otsubo Y, Satoh Y, Kodama M, Araki Y, Satomoto M, et al. (2012) Mechanical allodynia but not thermal hyperalgesia is impaired in mice deficient for ERK2 in the central nervous system. Pain. S0304–3959(12)00431–9 [pii];10.1016/j.pain.2012.07.020 [doi].
22. Seal RP, Wang X, Guan Y, Raja SN, Woodbury CJ, et al. (2009) Injury-induced mechanical hypersensitivity requires C-low threshold mechanoreceptors. Nature 462: 651–655.
23. Xu Q, Yaksh TL (2011) A brief comparison of the pathophysiology of inflammatory versus neuropathic pain. Curr Opin Anaesthesiol 24: 400–407. 10.1097/ACO.0b013e32834871df [doi].
24. Kobayashi H, Kitamura T, Sekiguchi M, Homma MK, Kabuyama Y, et al. (2007) Involvement of EphB1 receptor/EphrinB2 ligand in neuropathic pain. Spine 32: 1592–1598.
25. Han Y, Song XS, Liu WT, Henkemeyer M, Song XJ (2008) Targeted mutation of EphB1 receptor prevents development of neuropathic hyperalgesia and physical dependence on morphine in mice. Mol Pain 4: 60.
26. Liu WT, Han Y, Li HC, Adams B, Zheng JH, et al. (2009) An in vivo mouse model of long-term potentiation at synapses between primary afferent C-fibers and spinal dorsal horn neurons: essential role of EphB1 receptor. Mol Pain 5: 29.
27. Takasu MA, Dalva MB, Zigmond RE, Greenberg ME (2002) Modulation of NMDA receptor-dependent calcium influx and gene expression through EphB receptors. Science 295: 491–495.
28. Zhuo M, Wu G, Wu LJ (2011) Neuronal and microglial mechanisms of neuropathic pain. Mol Brain 4: 31. 1.
29. Williams SE, Mann F, Erskine L, Sakurai T, Wei S, et al. (2003) Ephrin-B2 and EphB1 mediate retinal axon divergence at the optic chiasm. Neuron 39: 919–935.
30. Saddi G, Abbott FV (2000) The formalin test in the mouse: a parametric analysis of scoring properties. Pain 89: 53–63.
31. Bennett GJ, Xie YK (1988) A peripheral mononeuropathy in rat that produces disorders of pain sensation like those seen in man. Pain 33: 87–107.
32. Seltzer Z, Dubner R, Shir Y (1990) A novel behavioral model of neuropathic pain disorders produced in rats by partial sciatic nerve injury. Pain 43: 205–218.
33. Sammons MJ, Raval P, Davey PT, Rogers D, Parsons AA, et al. (2000) Carrageenan-induced thermal hyperalgesia in the mouse: role of nerve growth factor and the mitogen-activated protein kinase pathway. Brain Res 876: 48–54.
34. Chaplan SR, Bach FW, Pogrel JW, Chung JM, Yaksh TL (1994) Quantitative assessment of tactile allodynia in the rat paw. J Neurosci Methods 53: 55–63.
35. Tjolsen A, Berge OG, Hunskaar S, Rosland JH, Hole K (1992) The formalin test: an evaluation of the method. Pain 51: 5–17.
36. Rigaud M, Gemes G, Barabas ME, Chernoff DI, Abram SE, et al. (2008) Species and strain differences in rodent sciatic nerve anatomy: implications for studies of neuropathic pain. Pain 136: 188–201.
37. Clark AK, Yip PK, Grist J, Gentry C, Staniland AA, et al. (2007) Inhibition of spinal microglial cathepsin S for the reversal of neuropathic pain. Proc Natl Acad Sci U S A 104: 10655–10660.
38. Steffens H, Hoheisel U, Eek B, Mense S (2001) Tetrodotoxin-resistant conductivity and spinal effects of cutaneous C-fibre afferents in the rat. Neurosci Res 39: 413–419.
39. Graham BA, Brichta AM, Callister RJ (2007) Pinch-current injection defines two discharge profiles in mouse superficial dorsal horn neurones, in vitro. J Physiol 578: 787–798.
40. Wilkinson DG (2001) Multiple roles of EPH receptors and ephrins in neural development. Nat Rev Neurosci 2: 155–164.
41. Richards AB, Scheel TA, Wang K, Henkemeyer M, Kromer LF (2007) EphB1 null mice exhibit neuronal loss in substantia nigra pars reticulata and spontaneous locomotor hyperactivity. Eur J Neurosci 25: 2619–2628.
42. Henderson JT, Georgiou J, Jia Z, Robertson J, Elowe S, et al. (2001) The receptor tyrosine kinase EphB2 regulates NMDA-dependent synaptic function. Neuron 32: 1041–1056.
43. Grunwald IC, Korte M, Wolfer D, Wilkinson GA, Unsicker K, et al. (2001) Kinase-independent requirement of EphB2 receptors in hippocampal synaptic plasticity. Neuron 32: 1027–1040.
44. Fitzgerald M, Butcher T, Shortland P (1994) Developmental changes in the laminar termination of A fibre cutaneous sensory afferents in the rat spinal cord dorsal horn. J Comp Neurol 348: 225–233.
45. Beggs S, Torsney C, Drew LJ, Fitzgerald M (2002) The postnatal reorganization of primary afferent input and dorsal horn cell receptive fields in the rat spinal cord is an activity-dependent process. Eur J Neurosci 16: 1249–1258.
46. Wu Q, Henry JL (2010) Changes in Abeta non-nociceptive primary sensory neurons in a rat model of osteoarthritis pain. Mol Pain 6: 37.
47. Zhu YF, Henry JL (2012) Excitability of Abeta sensory neurons is altered in an animal model of peripheral neuropathy. BMC Neurosci 13: 15.
48. Song XJ, Cao JL, Li HC, Zheng JH, Song XS, et al. (2008) Upregulation and redistribution of ephrinB and EphB receptor in dorsal root ganglion and spinal dorsal horn neurons after peripheral nerve injury and dorsal rhizotomy. Eur J Pain 12: 1031–1039.

49. Zhao J, Yuan G, Cendan CM, Nassar MA, Lagerstrom MC, et al. (2010) Nociceptor-expressed ephrin-B2 regulates inflammatory and neuropathic pain. Mol Pain 6: 77.
50. Orikawa Y, Kato H, Seto K, Kobayashi N, Yoshinaga K, et al. (2010) Z-360, a novel therapeutic agent for pancreatic cancer, prevents up-regulation of ephrin B1 gene expression and phosphorylation of NR2B via suppression of interleukin-1 beta production in a cancer-induced pain model in mice. Mol Pain 6: 72.
51. Dong Y, Mao-Ying QL, Chen JW, Yang CJ, Wang YQ, et al. (2011) Involvement of EphB1 receptor/ephrinB1 ligand in bone cancer pain. Neurosci Lett 496: 163–167.
52. Liu S, Liu WT, Liu YP, Dong HL, Henkemeyer M, et al. (2011) Blocking EphB1 receptor forward signaling in spinal cord relieves bone cancer pain and rescues analgesic effect of morphine treatment in rodents. Cancer Res 71: 4392–4402.
53. Lee BH, Yoon YW, Chung K, Chung JM (1998) Comparison of sympathetic sprouting in sensory ganglia in three animal models of neuropathic pain. Exp Brain Res 120: 432–438.
54. Dowdall T, Robinson I, Meert TF (2005) Comparison of five different rat models of peripheral nerve injury. Pharmacol Biochem Behav 80: 93–108.
55. Macdonald JF, Jackson MF, Beazely MA (2006) Hippocampal long-term synaptic plasticity and signal amplification of NMDA receptors. Crit Rev Neurobiol 18: 71–84.
56. Liu XJ, Gingrich JR, Vargas-Caballero M, Dong YN, Sengar A, et al. (2008) Treatment of inflammatory and neuropathic pain by uncoupling Src from the NMDA receptor complex. Nat Med 14: 1325–1332.
57. Abe T, Matsumura S, Katano T, Mabuchi T, Takagi K, et al. (2005) Fyn kinase-mediated phosphorylation of NMDA receptor NR2B subunit at Tyr1472 is essential for maintenance of neuropathic pain. Eur J Neurosci 22: 1445–1454.
58. Qu XX, Cai J, Li MJ, Chi YN, Liao FF, et al. (2009) Role of the spinal cord NR2B-containing NMDA receptors in the development of neuropathic pain. Exp Neurol 215: 298–307.
59. Tan PH, Yang LC, Shih HC, Lan KC, Cheng JT (2005) Gene knockdown with intrathecal siRNA of NMDA receptor NR2B subunit reduces formalin-induced nociception in the rat. Gene Ther 12: 59–66.
60. Vikman KS, Rycroft BK, Christie MJ (2008) Switch to Ca2+-permeable AMPA and reduced NR2B NMDA receptor-mediated neurotransmission at dorsal horn nociceptive synapses during inflammatory pain in the rat. J Physiol 586: 515–527.
61. South SM, Kohno T, Kaspar BK, Hegarty D, Vissel B, et al. (2003) A conditional deletion of the NR1 subunit of the NMDA receptor in adult spinal cord dorsal horn reduces NMDA currents and injury-induced pain. J Neurosci 23: 5031–5040.
62. Hunt SP, Pini A, Evan G (1987) Induction of c-fos-like protein in spinal cord neurons following sensory stimulation. Nature 328: 632–634.
63. Harris JA (1998) Using c-fos as a neural marker of pain. Brain Res Bull 45: 1–8.
64. Coggeshall RE (2005) Fos, nociception and the dorsal horn. Prog Neurobiol 77: 299–352.
65. Graeber MB, Christie MJ (2012) Multiple mechanisms of microglia: a gatekeeper's contribution to pain states. Exp Neurol 234: 255–261.
66. Gao YJ, Ji RR (2010) Chemokines, neuronal-glial interactions, and central processing of neuropathic pain. Pharmacol Ther 126: 56–68.
67. Suter MR, Berta T, Gao YJ, Decosterd I, Ji RR (2009) Large A-fiber activity is required for microglial proliferation and p38 MAPK activation in the spinal cord: different effects of resiniferatoxin and bupivacaine on spinal microglial changes after spared nerve injury. Mol Pain 5: 53.
68. Daulhac L, Mallet C, Courteix C, Etienne M, Duroux E, et al. (2006) Diabetes-induced mechanical hyperalgesia involves spinal mitogen-activated protein kinase activation in neurons and microglia via N-methyl-D-aspartate-dependent mechanisms. Mol Pharmacol 70: 1246–1254.
69. Cheng HT, Suzuki M, Hegarty DM, Xu Q, Weyerbacher AR, et al. (2008) Inflammatory pain-induced signaling events following a conditional deletion of the N-methyl-D-aspartate receptor in spinal cord dorsal horn. Neuroscience 155: 948–958.
70. Cao JL, Ruan JP, Ling DY, Guan XH, Bao Q, et al. (2008) Activation of peripheral ephrinBs/EphBs signaling induces hyperalgesia through a MAPKs-mediated mechanism in mice. Pain 139: 617–631.

7

Brain Signature of Chronic Orofacial Pain: A Systematic Review and Meta-Analysis on Neuroimaging Research of Trigeminal Neuropathic Pain and Temporomandibular Joint Disorders

Chia-shu Lin*

Department of Dentistry, School of Dentistry, National Yang-Ming University, Taipei, Taiwan (ROC)

Abstract

Brain neuroimaging has been widely used to investigate the bran signature of chronic orofacial pain, including trigeminal neuropathic pain (TNP) and pain related to temporomandibular joint disorders (TMD). We here systematically reviewed the neuroimaging literature regarding the functional and structural changes in the brain of TNP and TMD pain patients, using a computerized search of journal articles via PubMed. Ten TNP studies and 14 TMD studies were reviewed. Study quality and risk of bias were assessed based on the criteria of patient selection, the history of medication, the use of standardized pain/psychological assessments, and the model and statistics of imaging analyses. Qualitative meta-analysis was performed by examining the brain regions which showed significant changes in either brain functions (including the blood-oxygen-level dependent signal, cerebral blood flow and the magnetic resonance spectroscopy signal) or brain structure (including gray matter and white matter anatomy). We hypothesized that the neuroimaging findings would display a common pattern as well as distinct patterns of brain signature in the disorders. This major hypothesis was supported by the following findings: (1) TNP and TMD patients showed consistent functional/structural changes in the thalamus and the primary somatosensory cortex, indicating the thalamocortical pathway as the major site of plasticity. (2) The TNP patients showed more alterations at the thalamocortical pathway, and the two disorders showed distinct patterns of thalamic and insular connectivity. Additionally, functional and structural changes were frequently reported in the prefrontal cortex and the basal ganglia, suggesting the role of cognitive modulation and reward processing in chronic orofacial pain. The findings highlight the potential for brain neuroimaging as an investigating tool for understanding chronic orofacial pain.

Editor: Michael Costigan, Boston Children's Hospital and Harvard Medical School, United States of America

Funding: This study was funded by National Science Council of Taiwan (NSC 102-2314-B-010-049). The funders had no role in study design, data collection and analysis, decision to publish, or preparation of the manuscript.

Competing Interests: The author has declared that no competing interests exist.

* E-mail: winzlin@ym.edu.tw

Introduction

Trigeminal neuropathic pain (TNP) and pain related to temporomandibular disorders (TMD) have been the challenging issues in chronic orofacial pain [1,2]. Effective management of the pain has not been established. Unlike acute orofacial pain (e.g., toothache), TNP and TMD pain may persist when the peripheral lesions have been treated, or even without peripheral abnormalities being found [3,4]. In addition, the degree of TNP and TMD pain is associated with the cognitive and emotional factors, such as anxiety and depression [5]. Since pain is a multidimensional experience, consisting of sensory-discriminative and cognitive-affective experiences [6], TNP and TMD pain may be closely associated with the abnormality in the central pathophysiological process [7]. Therefore, the understanding of how the brain shapes pain experience would be critical to manage the pain of TNP and TMD patients.

Brain neuroimaging has been widely used to investigate the changes in brain function and structure associated with chronic orofacial pain (TNP: [8–17]; TMD: [10,11,18–29]). However, the conclusions drawn from a single study could be limited by its specific research conditions, including the criteria of patient selection, the experimental design and the approach of neuroimaging data analysis. And statistically, the imaging results from a single study can also be compromised by the small number of participants. The small sample size may lead to a lower statistical power, thus influencing the reproducibility of the results [30]. Therefore, in the current study we systematically reviewed the literature regarding TNP/TMD pain-related changes in brain structure (including gray matter and white matter anatomy [31]) and brain function (including the blood-oxygen-level-dependent [BOLD] signal, the cerebral blood flow and the magnetic resonance spectroscopy signal [32]). Previous investigation on the other types of chronic pain has revealed that changes in the pain-related network (including the thalamus, the primary and secondary somatosensory cortices, the mid/anterior cingulate cortex, and the insula) were associated with chronic pain [33,34]. In the pain-related network, the alterations in the thalamocortical pathway of somatosensation are associated with pain with a central nature [35–37]. In addition, cognitive-affective factors, such as cognitive reappraisal, anxiety and depression, are critical to shape the experience of chronic pain [6,38]. Based on the previous evidence, we here hypothesized that (1) both TNP and TMD would show a common pattern of functional and structural changes within the pain-related network. (2) As a central pain, TNP would show more changes in the thalamocortical pathway, compared to TMD pain, which is predominantly associated with the abnormality within the peripheral musculoskeletal system (e.g., the masticatory muscle and the joint). (3) The prefrontal cortex, the limbic system and the circuitry of reward processing (including the basal ganglia) would show functional or structural changes related to chronic orofacial pain [33,34].

Methods

Procedures of Literature Search

The current review was performed according to the guide of Preferred Reporting Items for Systematic Reviews and Meta-Analyses (PRISMA) for reporting in systematic reviews and meta-analyses [39]. To identify relevant neuroimaging studies on pain related to TNP and TMD, a computerized search of journal articles via PubMed (http://www.ncbi.nlm.nih.gov/pubmed) was conducted with several sets of keyword combinations, including "trigeminal", "temporomandibular disorder", "pain", "brain" and "MRI" as the keywords (see Table 1 for the complete search strategy). We deliberately used a broad range of keyword combinations to avoid missing studies. The search was restricted to the journal articles published during the period from 1994 Jan. 1 to 2013 Aug. 31. Review articles and case reports were excluded (Figure 1).

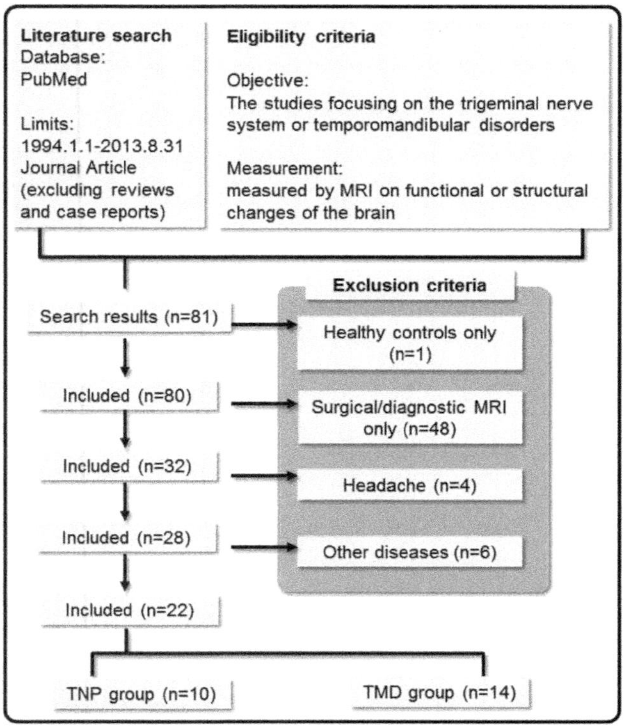

Figure 1. Flow diagram describing the process of review and study selection.

Eligibility Criteria and Study Selection

The studies retrieved according to the above-stated search strategy (Figure 1) were further screened according to the inclusion and exclusion criteria listed in Table 1B. In this review, we only focused on the findings associated with the following five major neuroimaging approaches: (1) BOLD signal-based functional MRI (fMRI), (2) arterial spin labelling (ASL), (3) magnetic resonance spectroscopy (MRS), (4) T1-weighted structural MRI (sMRI), and (5) diffusion-weighted imaging (DWI). Note that we considered MRS signal changes here as a signature of brain function, because it reflects the metabolic changes of biochemical molecules, which underlie the transduction of neural signals. All the five imaging modalities have been widely used in investigating the brain signature of chronic diseases. For detailed introduction of the methodology about each approach, see [34,40–42]. The studies that potentially used the same patient cohort with different imaging analyses were included. The eligibility assessment was performed by the first author (C-S.L.), primarily according to the title and the abstract of the selected articles.

Data Collection and Extraction of Data Items

The full text of all the selected studies, together with the online supporting materials, was retrieved from the Internet. The following data items were manually extracted from the full text version of the original articles and classified into two categories:

(1) Demographic and clinical characteristics (6 items), including the diagnosis of orofacial disorders (including subtypes), the number of participants of each sex and mean age (for both the patient and the control groups), pain severity (including the ratings of intensity and/or unpleasantness), and the duration of pain (Table 2)

(2) Experimental design and neuroimaging findings (6 items), including the type of imaging modality, the type of stimuli and the site of stimulation, the covariate (e.g., pain severity) considered in imaging analysis, the signals measured by neuroimaging, and the major imaging findings (Table 3 and Table 4).

In addition, five data items related to study quality and risk of bias were extracted (see Table 5 and Table 6). In total 17 data items were extracted.

Assessment of Study Quality and Risk of Bias

In the current PRISMA guideline, the assessment of risk of bias and study quality has been clearly distinguished [39]. For the assessment of risk of bias, we considered the heterogeneity of diagnosis and symptomatology as the major factor that would introduce bias in research outcomes. Therefore we focused on the inclusion/exclusion criteria for patient selection, the patients' history of medication and the use of standardized clinical assessments (i.e., the items 1–3). For the assessment of study quality, we applied the recently proposed guideline on reporting functional MRI studies [43], focusing on the statistical model for comparison and imaging statistics (i.e., the items 4–5):

(1) Criteria of patient selection: whether established criteria (e.g., the Research Diagnostic Criteria [RDC], [44]) or detailed inclusion/exclusion criteria were applied for patient selection.

(2) Statuts of medication: whether the history of prescription has been recorded and the medication was temporally discontinued before the MRI scan.

(3) Standardized assessment: whether standardized pain/psychological assessments were applied to assess the patients.

Table 1. Search strategy and study selection.

Search strategy:			
Search	**Query**	**Filters**	**Items found**
#1	trigeminal (neuralgia OR neuropathy OR neuropathic) NOT (Case Reports[ptyp] OR Review[ptyp])	Journal Article; Publication date from 1994/01/01 to 2013/08/31	1949
#2	temporomandibular disorder NOT (Case Reports[ptyp] OR Review[ptyp])		5176
#3	pain (central nervous system OR brain) MRI		5042
#4	(#1 OR #2) AND #3		81
Inclusion and exclusion criteria of study selection:			
Inclusion criteria			
1. The studies which performed on either TNP or TMD patients.			
2. The MRI-related studies, including structural MRI (sMRI), functional (BOLD-based) MRI (fMRI), MRS, and diffusion-weighted MRI (DWI).			
Exclusion criteria			
1. The studies which investigated only healthy controls.			
2. The studies which applied MRI as a diagnostic tool for surgery or clinical assessment, i.e., not focusing on the long-term changes in brain signatures.			
3. The studies which focused on the trigeminal system-related disorders other than TNP and TMD, such as dental pain or headache.			

(4) Statistical model: whether the type of group-wise statistical inference (e.g., random or fixed effect) was reported.

(5) Imaging statistics: whether correction of multiple comparison was applied to the resulted images.

Each item was scored as 1 if the related details were reported in the study, otherwise as 0. The total score of a study ranged from 0 to 5.

Qualitative Meta-Analysis

In the current review, we did not perform a quantitative imaging meta-analysis because of the heterogeneity of imaging modalities and analysis approaches, and the small number of participants in some studies. Instead, we performed a qualitative meta-analysis by identifying the brain regions that showed significant functional or structural changes in patients, compared to the healthy control participants, or within the patients between the affected and the unaffected sites. The reported brain regions were categorized into 14 regions of interest (ROIs) that are associated with pain processing [33]: the thalamus, the primary and secondary somatosensory cortices (S1/S2), the anterior and mid-cingulate cortices (ACC/MCC), the anterior and posterior insular cortices (aINS/pINS), the superior, middle, inferior and orbitofrontal part of the prefrontal cortex (PFC), the basal ganglia (BG), the medial temporal lobe (including the hippocampus and the amygdala, MT), and the periaqueductal gray (PAG). Categorization was performed separately for the positive changes (e.g., increased BOLD activity or increased GMV in patients vs. healthy control participants) and the negative changes (e.g., decreased BOLD activity or decreased GMV in patients vs. healthy control participants).

The anatomical labels of the ROIs were surveyed using FSLView (http://fsl.fmrib.ox.ac.uk/fsl/fslview/). The Oxford thalamic connectivity atlas [45] was consulted for specifying the functional role of the thalamic sub-regions, according to their patterns of cortical connections. The Jülich histological atlas (http://www.fz-juelich.de/inb/inb-3/Home) was consulted for specifying the Brodmann area of the S1.

Statistical Analysis

Quantifying the similarity and distinctiveness of brain signature pattern. Our main hypothesis focused on the similarity and distinctiveness of the pattern of brain signature related to TNP and TMD pain. We quantified the *brain signature pattern* based on the changes in the pain-related ROIs, according to the following definitions:

(A) For each ROI, we defined the number of the studies that reported significant changes, as shown in the qualitative meta-analysis, as the index *regional change* of that ROI. This index was calculated respectively for positive and negative changes and for different imaging modalities. For example, in the functional studies about TNP and TMD, the positive regional change for S1 was '3' and '4', respectively (Table 7).

(B) For the positive and negative changes of different imaging modalities, the brain signature pattern of the TNP or the TMD group was represented as a set of regional changes from the nine ROIs: THA, S1, S2, PFC, BG, MT, PAG, the cingulate cortex (CC, including ACC and MCC), and the insula (INS, including aINS and pINS).

Notably, we here focused on the studies that applied whole-brain analysis. The findings derived from ROI-specific analyses were excluded (e.g., [9]). It should be clarified that an analysis was here considered as 'whole-brain', if a greater mask was applied to restrict the search in the cortical area (e.g., [17]). The findings from the MRS studies ([10–12]) were also excluded, because all the studies applied ROI-specific analyses. The analyses were performed separately for functional and structural studies and for the reports of positive and negative changes. Because there were very few findings from the functional studies with negative changes and the structural studies with positive changes (for descriptive data see Figure S1), we focused only on (1) the functional studies with positive changes and (2) the structural studies with negative changes. Similarity or distinctiveness of the brain signature patterns related to TNP and TMD was judged by the following two conditions: (1) there is a significant association in the regional changes between the two groups, and (2) there is no significant difference in the regional changes between the two groups.

Table 2. Demographic and clinical profiles of the included studies.

Source	Diagnosis	Patient					Control		
		F	M	Age	Severity (0–10)	Duration (Year)	F	M	Age
Trigeminal neuropathic pain									
Becerra 2006	TNP	5	1	48.8[1]	>4[3]	N/A	-		
Blatow 2009	TN	14	4	48–73	N/A	N/A	8	5	25–70
		6	4	44–76	N/A	N/A			
Scrivani 2010	TNP	4	2	48.3	>3–4[3]	N/A	-		
Gustin 2011	TNP[6]	17	4	54.7	3.5/3.4[4]	8.5	24	6	53.6
Moisset 2011	TNP-i	6	9	67.2	4–6	8.3			
Gustin 2012	TNP	12	3	50	3.8/3.6[4]	4.7	27	26	41
Henderson 2013	TNP	19	4	49.8	3.9	5.8	31	12	49.8
Obermann 2013	TN[7]	36	24	62	7.7	8.3	28	21	61.8
DeSouza 2013	TN-i	15	9	48.5	N/A	6.3	15	9	47.6
DeSouza 2014	TN	11	7	54.1	N/A	N/A	11	7	49.6
Temporomandibular joint disorder pain									
Jiang 2006	TMD-s	6	1	26.9	N/A	1–6(mo)	5	5	31
Younger 2010	TMD-m	15	0	38	4.3[1]	4.4	15	0	N/A[5]
Abrahamsen 2010	TMD-m	18	1	40.7	4.8	12.4	-		
Nebel 2010	TMD	13	0	28.7	2.4	N/A	12	0	28.8
Zhao 2011	TMD-s	12	4	33.7	≥5	N/A	7	7	23.7
Gerstner 2011	TMD-m	9	0	25.4[1]	2.2	2.5	9	0	24.8[2]
Gustin 2011	TMD	16	4	45.7	4.7/3.2[4]	11.5	25	6	46.8
Moayedi 2011	TMD-i	17	0	33.1	4.3/5.4[2]	9.8	17	0	32.2
Weissman-Fogel 2011	TMD	17	0	35.2[1]	4.2	9.3	17	0	N/A[5]
Gerstner 2012	TMD	10	1	25.8	3.8	0.5–7	10	1	24.8
Ichesco 2012	TMD	8	0	25.4	2.2	2.5	8	0	24.9
Moayedi 2012	TMD-i	17	0	33.1	4.3/5.4[2]	9.8	17	0	32.8
Salomons 2012	TMD	17	0	33.1	4.3/5.4[2]	9.8	17	0	32.2
Gustin 2012	TMD	13	4	44	4.2/4.5[4]	10.7	27	26	41

i, idiopathic; m, myofascial; s, synovitis; F, number of female participants; M, number of male participants; N/A, not available from the full text; TNP, trigeminal neuropathic pain; TMD, temporomandibular joint disorder.

[1]Mean age is calculated based on the data revealed in the original table; [2]average pain intensity/unpleasantness over the last month; [3]brushing-evoked/spontaneous pain; [4]pain a week before/pain before scanning; [5]age matched with the patient group; [6]including TN patients; [7]including TN patients with concomitant chronic facial pain.

Analysis on the association of regional changes. We considered the brain signature patterns related to TNP and TMD as similar, if the brain signature changes of one group were associated with those in another group. We performed the non-parametric Spearman rank correlation analysis on the regional changes, between TNP and TMD. A significantly positive correlation indicated that the brain signature pattern between the two groups was associated. The correlation coefficient with a p value <0.05 was considered statistically significant.

Analysis on the overall difference of regional changes. To claim that the patterns are similar between the two groups, we considered that the overall degree of regional changes (e.g., the mean regional changes over the nine ROIs) not to be significantly different. It should be noted that a direct comparison in regional change could be biased by the total number of articles related to TNP and TMD. Therefore, we compared the *normalized regional change*, i.e., the original index (i.e., regional change) divided by the total number of articles. We performed the two-tailed paired Wilcoxon test on the normalized regional changes between TNP and TMD. The resulting W statistics quantifies the difference in the overall brain signatures pattern between the two groups. Note that the null hypothesis referred to 'no difference between the two groups'. The W statistics with a p value <0.05 was considered statistically significant.

Decision-making on the similarity and distinctiveness of brain signature. The pattern of brain signature between TNP and TMD was categorized as 'common' if the Spearman rank correlation coefficient was significant AND the paired Wilcoxon test failed to reject the null hypothesis. In contrast, it was categorized as 'different' if the Spearman rank correlation coefficient was not significant AND the paired Wilcoxon test rejected the null hypothesis.

Table 3. Experimental design and neuroimaging findings of the included studies: Trigeminal neuropathic pain.

Source	Experimental design					Major neuroimaging findings on the pain-related brain regions
	Modality	Stimuli	Site	Covariate	Signal	
Becerra 2006	fMRI	Mechanical	R V2 area	-	BOLD	AF>UF: THA/SI/R aINS/R ACC
		Thermal	(with allodynia)			
Blatow 2009	fMRI	Mechanical	R/L fingers and lips	-	BOLD	Pre-OP<HC (finger and lip): [B S1/B S2]
Scrivani 2010	fMRI	Mechanical Thermal	R/L V2 or V3 area	-	BOLD	Medication<Placebo (Thermal): R THA/R MCC/R S1
						Medication>Placebo (Mechanical): R INS/R S1
Gustin 2011	sMRI	-	-	age/sex/TBV	GMV	TNP>HC: CL pINS
						TNP<HC: B THA/IL S1/IL aINS
	fMRI	Mechanical	R bottom lips	-	BOLD	(for localizing ventroposterior THA)
	MRS	-	-	-	NAA/Cr	TNP<HC: [THA]
Moisset 2011	fMRI	Mechanical	AF/UF V2/V3 area, R hand	-	BOLD	AF>UF (evoked pain): L S1/R THA/L aINS/R ACC/L MCC
Gustin 2012	fMRI	Mechanical	IL lower lip/fingers	-	BOLD	Functional reorganization: [CL S1]
	DWI	-	-	age/sex	FA	TNP<HC: [CL S1]
	ASL	-	-	age/sex	CBF	TNP<HC: [CL S1]
Henderson 2013	sMRI	-	-	age/sex/TBV	GMV	TNP<HC: IL aINS/IL S1/B THA
	fMRI	Mechanical	lower lip	-	BOLD	(for localizing ventroposterior THA)
		Resting-state		-	FC	Negative correlation with thalamic GABA level
	ASL	-	-	age/sex	CBF	TNP<HC: [CL THA/CL S1]
	MRS	-	-		GABA	TNP<HC: [THA]
Obermann 2013	sMRI	-	-	age	GMV	TN<HC: L S1/B INS/B ACC/L THA/L S2
DeSouza 2013	sMRI	-	-	age	GMV	TN>HC: [IL THA]
				age	CT	TN>HC: [CL S1]
						TN<HC: [B ACC/IL pINS/IL aINS]
DeSouza 2014	DWI	-	-	-	FA	TN<HC: CC/cingulum/CL SLF/B pCOR

ACC, anterior cingulate cortex; AF, affected side; aINS, anterior insula; ASL, arterial spin labeling; B, bilateral; BOLD, blood-oxygen-level-dependent; CBF, cerebral blood flow; CC, corpus callosum; CL, contralateral; COR, corona radiate; CT, cortical thickness; DWI, diffusion-weighted imaging; FA, fractional anisotropy; FC, functional connectivity; fMRI, functional magnetic resonance imaging; GMV, gray matter volume; IL, ipsilateral; L, left side; MCC, mid-cingulate cortex; MRS, magnetic resonance spectrum; pINS, posterior insula; R, right side; S1, primary somatosensory cortex; S2, secondary somatosensory cortex; SC, structural connectivity (probabilistic tractography); SLF, superior longitudinal fasciculus; sMRI, structural magnetic resonance imaging; TBV, total brain volume; THA, thalamus; TNP, trigeminal neuropathic pain; UF, unaffected side; V2, the maxillary nerve; V3, the mandibular nerve; WMV, white matter volume.

Results

Included Studies

According to the strategy of literature search (Table 1), in total 81 studies were included as the original set of studies (Figure 1). Among this set, 59 studies were excluded according to the pre-defined exclusion criteria (Table 1B): (1) one study investigating only the healthy control participants; (2) 48 studies applying MRI as a diagnostic tool (e.g., for surgical assessment [46] or examination of vascular pathology [47]); (3) 10 studies focusing on the disorders other than TNP and TMD, including 4 studies of headache (mostly about migraine) and 6 studies of other disorders (Table 1B). In total, 22 studies were included as the final set for qualitative meta-analysis (Figure 1). Full text was retrieved from all the studies. Twenty studies were originally published in English and two in Chinese ([20,27]). Within the final set (n = 22), 8 studies exclusively recruited TNP patients; 12 studies exclusively recruited TMD pain patients, and two studies recruited both TNP and TMD pain patients ([10,11]). In total 10 TNP-related and 14 TMD pain-related studies were included.

Demographic and Clinical Profiles

Diagnosis. The studies under review diverted in the diagnostic categories (Table 2). In the TNP studies, 4 out of 10 studies focused exclusively on trigeminal neuralgia (TN), an episodic form of neuropathic pain [48]. The other 6 studies included TNP with a variety of etiologies (e.g., trauma or post-herpetic infection, [8]). The heterogeneity of diagnosis was also found in the TMD studies. Three out of 14 TMD studies focused exclusively on the myofascial-type TMD ([18,26,28]), two on idiopathic (non-traumatic) TMD ([21,22]), and 2 on inflammatory-type TMD (synovitis, [20,27]).

The demographic profiles of the patients. The sample size of the patient group was relatively small (n<12) in two TNP studies [8,14] and in 4 TMD studies [19,20,28,29] (Table 2). There were more females patients recruited than male patients (Table 2). In the TNP studies, the ratio of female to male patients was approximately 2:1. In the TMD studies, the number of female patients was even overwhelmingly higher than the number of the male patients, with eight studies exclusively recruiting only female patients ([13,19,22–26,28]). The age range of the patients in the TNP and the TMD studies was approximately 45–55 y/o and 25–45 y/o, respectively (Table 2). The patients in the TNP studies

Table 4. Experimental design and neuroimaging findings of the included studies: Temporomandibular joint disorder pain.

Source	Experimental design					Major neuroimaging findings on the pain-related brain regions
	Modality	Stimuli	Site	Covariate	Signal	
Jiang 2006	fMRI	Clenching	N/A	-	BOLD	TMD (clenching > resting): R S1/L ACC
Younger 2010	sMRI	-	-	-	GMV	TMD>HC: R aINS/B THA
						TMD<HC: R S1
Abrahamsen	fMRI	Mechanical	L V3 area	-	BOLD	Stim > No stim: R pINS/R S1
2010		Hypnosis				Hyperalgesia>Hypoalgesia: L IPL
Nebel 2010	fMRI	Mechanical	R index finger	-	BOLD	TMD>HC: B THA/CL S1/B S2/CL INS/B ACC
						TMD<HC: CL INS/CL S1/CL S2
Zhao 2011	fMRI	Clenching	R molars	-	BOLD	TMD (CL clenching>resting): B ACC
Gerstner 2011	sMRI	-	-	age	GMV	TMD<HC: L ACC/R aINS
					WMV	TMD>HC: B STG
						TMD<HC: B ACC
Gustin 2011	sMRI	-	-	age/sex/TBV	GMV	TMD v. HC: n.s.
	fMRI	Mechanical	R bottom lips	-	BOLD	(for localizing ventroposterior THA)
	MRS	-	-	-	NAA/Cr	[THA]: TMD v. HC n.s.
Moayedi 2011	sMRI	-	-	age/TIV	GMV	[THA]: TMD v. HC n.s.
				age	CT	TMD>HC: [R S1]
Weissman- Fogel 2011	fMRI	Stroop task		-	BOLD	TMD>HC (cognitive interference): ACC/L S1
						TMD>HC (emotional interference): L ACC
Gerstner 2012	MRS	Pressure	R anterior temporalis	-	Glu/Gln/	TMD>HC (NAA/Cho): [L pINS]
			R thumb		NAA/Cho level	
Ichesco 2012	fMRI	Pressure	L anterior temporalis	age	FC	TMD>HC: L aINS-R ACC/R aINS-R ACC
		Resting-state				TMD>HC: L aINS-R ACC/L pINS-L PHG/R aINS-R THA
Moayedi 2012	DWI	-	-	age	FA	TMD<HC: [R THA/R S1](nearby)
					SC	TMD>HC: CC-L FP
Salomons 2012	sMRI	-	-	-	CT	Correlated with helplessness- positive: [L SMA], negative: [L MCC/ L PCC]
	DWI				FA	Correlated with helplessness-positive: [cingulum], negative: [CC/ CST]
Gustin 2012	fMRI	Mechanical	IL lower lip/fingers	age/sex	BOLD	No functional reorganization at CL S1
	DWI	-	-	-	FA	[CL SI]: TMD v. HC n.s.
	ASL	-	-	age/sex	CBF	[CL SI]: TMD v. HC n.s.

ACC, anterior cingulate cortex; aINS, anterior insula; ASL, arterial spin labeling; B, bilateral; BOLD, blood-oxygen-level-dependent; CBF, cerebral blood flow; CC, corpus callosum; CL, contralateral; CST, cortical spinal tract; CT, cortical thickness; DWI, diffusion-weighted imaging; FA, fractional anisotropy; FC, functional connectivity; fMRI, functional magnetic resonance imaging; GMV, gray matter volume; IL, ipsilateral; L, left side; MCC, mid-cingulate cortex; MRS, magnetic resonance spectrum; pINS, posterior insula; R, right side; S1, primary somatosensory cortex; S2, secondary somatosensory cortex; SC, structural connectivity (probabilistic tractography); SLF, superior longitudinal fasciculus; sMRI, structural magnetic resonance imaging; STPI, State Trait Personality Inventory; TBV, total brain volume; THA, thalamus; TIV, total intracranial volume; TMD, temporomandibular disorder; V3, the mandibular nerve; WMV, white matter volume.

were, in general, older than the patients in the TMD studies. One study has patients with a mean age >65 y/o ([13]), which were considered the older population. The sex and age profiles of the patients, in general, were consistent with the previous epidemiological findings of the disorders [48].

The clinical profiles of the patients. Most studies set minimal severity of pain as the inclusion criteria, such as a score greater than 4 on a 0–10 visual analogue scale (VAS). The definition of pain severity, however, varied across studies. While some studies defined it as the current pain intensity (e.g., [18,28]), other studies defined it as the average pain over a month (e.g., [21,22,24]) or the pain a week before scanning (e.g., [10,11]). In general, both the TNP and TMD studies showed pain severity at the moderate level (mean pain intensity <5 on a 0–10 VAS, Table 2). In the TMD studies, the patients with mild pain were included in two studies ([19,23]). The duration of pain, on contrary, varied significantly between studies and between patients (Table 2). In the TNP studies, the mean duration of pain ranged from 4.7 to 8.5 years, across 6 studies. In the TMD studies, the mean duration of pain ranged from 2.5 to 12.4 years, across 11 studies.

Table 5. Results of assessments of risk of bias and study quality: Trigeminal neuropathic pain.

Source	Criteria of patient selection		Status of medication		Standardized assessment		Statistical model		Imaging statistics		Total score
Becerra 2006	Inclusion/Exclusion[1]	1	[Y], 1-dose interval	1	QST, BDI[2]	1	FE	1	Generalized mixture model	1	5
Blatow 2009	-	0	[Y]	1	-	0	-	0	Bonferroni correction	1	2
Scrivani 2010	Inclusion/Exclusion	1	[Y], drug screening	1	QST, MADRS	1	RE[3]	1	Gaussian mixture model	1	5
Gustin 2011	Liverpool Criteria	1	[Y]	1	BDI, STAI, MPQ	1	RE	1	FDR	1	5
Moisset 2011	Inclusion/Exclusion	1	[Y], 12 hrs	1	QST, NPSI	1	RE	1	uncorrected	0	4
Gustin 2012	Liverpool Criteria	1	[Y]	1	MPQ	1	RE	1	FWE	1	5
Henderson 2013	Liverpool Criteria	1	[Y]	1	MPQ	1	RE	1	FDR	1	5
Obermann 2013	Inclusion/Exclusion	1	[Y]	1	-	0	-	0	FWE	1	3
DeSouza 2013	Inclusion/Exclusion	1	[Y]	1	-	0	Permutation testing	1	corrected based on permutation testing	1	4
DeSouza 2014	Inclusion/Exclusion	1	[Y]	1	-	0	Permutation testing	1	TFCE	1	4

BDI, Beck Depression Inventory; BPI, Brief Pain Inventory; FDR: control for false discovery rate; FWE: control for family-wise error; MADRS, Montgomery-Asberg Depression Rating Scale; (s)MPQ, (short-form) McGill Pain Questionnaire; NPSI, neuropathic pain symptom inventory; STAI: State-Trait Anxiety Inventory; TFCE; Threshold-Free Cluster Enhancement [85].

[1]Details about the criteria were not found; [2]The use of BDI was only noted in Figure S1; [3]using FMRIB's local analysis of mixed effects; [Y] denotes that the status of medication was reported.

Experimental Design

Imaging modalities. The TNP studies included 6 investigations on the structural changes (sMRI/DWI = 4/2) and 9 investigations on the functional changes (fMRI/ASL/MRS = 5/2/2). The TMD studies included 8 investigations on the structural changes (sMRI/DWI = 5/3) and 10 investigations on the functional changes (fMRI/ASL/MRS = 7/1/2) (Table 4). In two studies, the fMRI investigations were performed mainly for functionally localizing a specific ROI ([11,12]). These investigations were not included in the subsequent meta-analysis.

Stimulation models and tasks. In the TNP studies, 7 studies have applied mechanical stimuli (brushing) to the subjects ([8–14]) (Table 3). Two studies additionally applied thermal (cold and heat) stimuli ([8,14]) to evoke pain or allodynia. In the TMD studies, 4 studies applied mechanical stimuli to the subjects ([10,11,18,23]) and one study applied pressure stimuli ([19]) to evoke pain. Two studies used a clenching task to evoke pain [20,27]. Behavioral tasks were applied in two studies: one study applied hypnotic modulation to modulate pain experience ([18]) and another study applied the Stroop task to assess the attentional interference related to pain ([25]).

Assessment of Study Quality and Risk of Bias

In general, the included 22 studies showed a moderate to high score of study quality and risk of bias assessment. The score (mean±standard deviation) of the TNP studies is 4.2±1.0 and that of the TMD studies is 3.7±1.2. There was no significant difference in the assessment score between the two groups (two-tailed independent t-test $p = 0.3$).

Criteria of patient selection. Twenty-two studies have reported the detailed criteria about patient selection (TNP: 9/10; TMD: 13/14). In the TMD studies, the Research Diagnostic Criteria (RDC) [44] was the most frequently adopted diagnostic criteria [11,18,19,21,23,25,28,29].

Status of medication. Nineteen studies have reported the status of medication of the patients (TNP: 10/10; TMD: 9/14). However, only 9 studies have reported that the medications were temporally discontinued before MRI scanning. Among these studies, the duration of medications discontinuation varied from 2 weeks to only one drug interval.

Standardized assessment. Standardized assessments of pain, such as the McGill Pain Questionnaire [49,50] or Quantitative Sensory Testing (QST) [51], were performed in some of the studies (TNP: 6/10; TMD: 6/14). The psychological assessments regarding the chronic pain-related moods, such as the Beck Depression Inventory (BDI, [52]) for depression and the State-Trait Anxiety Inventory (STAI) for anxiety, were not widely used.

Statistical model. Twelve studies applied the random-effect (RE) model for the group-wise comparison. With this model, a conclusion drawn from the imaging results can be inferred to the population [53]. The fixed-effect (FE) model was suggested for a study with a small sample size [54]; however, it was only applied in one of the small-sample-size studies [8]. The permutation testing [55], a non-parametric approach for imaging analysis, was applied in four studies [16,17,22,28].

Imaging statistics. Twenty studies have applied some form of correction of multiple comparison in the imaging results (TNP: 9/10; TMD: 11/14). This item of assessment was not applied to one study [29], which only reported findings from an ROI-based but not a whole-brain analysis.

Findings from the Qualitative Meta-analysis

Changes in brain function. The results on brain function included the investigations on BOLD/CBF and MRS studies (Table 7 and Table 8). For both TNP and TMD patients, the S1, the ACC/MCC and the PFC are the most consistently reported regions (S1: 7 studies; ACC/MCC: 8 studies; PFC: 8 studies) (Table 7, Table 8 and Figure S1), while the S2 activation was only reported in 2 studies (Table 7). These findings from BOLD/CBF/MRS changes have revealed predominantly positive changes. The pattern of changes is more consistent in the TNP studies, where three studies have consistently reported an increased BOLD activation at the thalamus, S1, ACC/MCC and PFC [8,13,14]. In contrast, the pattern in the TMD group was less consistent across studies. Notably, concurrent increased/decreased activation was found between the thalamus and the S1 [8,12–14,23], and

Table 6. Results of assessments of risk of bias and study quality: Temporomandibular joint disorder pain.

Source	Criteria of patient selection		Status of medication		Standardized assessment		Statistical model		Imaging statistics		Total score
Jiang 2006	-	0	-	0	-	0	RE	1	uncorrected	0	1
Younger 2010	Inclusion/Exclusion criteria	1	[Y]	1	-	0	-	0	FDR	1	3
Abrahamsen 2010	RDC	1	-	0	SCL, HGSH:A	1	RE	1	FWE	1	4
Nebel 2010	RDC	1	-	0	sMPQ	1	RE[2]	1	Cluster-corrected	1	4
Zhao 2011	CDC	1	-	0	SCL-90	1	-	0	-	0	2
Gerstner 2011	RDC	1	3 days[3]	1	sMPQ, BPI, STPI	1	Permutation testing	1	corrected based on permutation testing	1	5
Gustin 2011	RDC	1	[Y]	1	BDI, STAI, MPQ	1	RE	1	FDR	1	5
Moayedi 2011	RDC	1	[Y], 24 hrs	1	NEO-FFI	1	-	0	FDR, Bonferroni correction	1	4
Weissman- Fogel 2011	RDC	1	[Y], 24 hrs	1	-	0	-	0	FDR	1	3
Gerstner 2012	RDC	1	2 wks	1	sMPQ, STPI	1	RE	1	-[3]	0	4
Ichesco 2012	RDC	1	3 days[1]	1	sMPQ, BPI, STPI	1	RE	1	Cluster-corrected	1	5
Moayedi 2012	Inclusion/Exclusion criteria	1	-	0	-	0	Permutation testing	1	TFCE or cluster-mass corrected	1	3
Salomons 2012	Inclusion/Exclusion criteria	1	[Y], 24 hrs	1	PCS	1	-	0	FWE	1	4
Gustin 2012	RDC	1	[Y]	1	MPQ	1	RE	1	FWE	1	5

BDI, Beck Depression Inventory; BPI, Brief Pain Inventory; CDC, Clinical Diagnostic Criteria [84]; FDR: control for false discovery rate; FWE: control for family-wise error; HGSHS:A, Harvard Group Scale of Hypnotic Susceptibility Form A; (s)MPQ, (short-form) McGill Pain Questionnaire; PCS: Pain Catastrophizing scale; RDC: Research Diagnostic Criteria [44]; SCL, Symptom Check List; STAI: State-Trait Anxiety Inventory; STPI, State-Trait Personality Inventory; TFCE; Threshold-Free Cluster Enhancement [85].

[1]Nonsteroidal anti-inflammatory drugs; [2]using FMRIB's local analysis of mixed effects; [3]the study directly compared the metabolite level resulted from the selected ROIs. [Y] denotes that the status of medication was reported.

Table 7. The findings of meta-analysis on functional changes by pain-related regions: BOLD/CBF.

Source	Positive changes									Negative changes								
	THA	S1	S2	CC	INS	PFC	BG	MT	PAG	THA	S1	S2	CC	INS	PFC	BG	MT	PAG
Trigeminal neuropathic pain																		
Becerra 2006[1]	PM	2		a	a	mi	↑			↓					↓	↓	↓	
Blatow 2009											*	*						
Scrivani 2010[2]	PF	1		m		smio	↑				↓			a	i			
Moisset 2011[1]	PM	3b		am	a	i	↑	↑		N/A	N/A	N/A	N/A	N/A	N/A	N/A	N/A	N/A
Gustin 2012[3]											*							
Henderson 2013[3]										*	*							
Temporomandibular joint disorder pain																		
Jiang 2006		2		a		o	↑			N/A	N/A	N/A	N/A	N/A	N/A	N/A	N/A	N/A
Abrahamsen 2010		2			p	m				N/A	N/A	N/A	N/A	N/A	N/A	N/A	N/A	N/A
Nebel 2010	PF	1/3b		m	p			↑			2/1	↓		p				
Zhao 2011				a		mi				N/A	N/A	N/A	N/A	N/A	N/A	N/A	N/A	N/A
Weissman-Fogel 2011[4]		1		a		sm	↑	↑		N/A	N/A	N/A	N/A	N/A	N/A	N/A	N/A	N/A
Ichesco 2012[5]	PF			a		s		↑		N/A	N/A	N/A	N/A	N/A	N/A	N/A	N/A	N/A

See Table 3 for the abbreviations of the brain regions. N/A: The study did not report the findings of negative changes. The asterisk denotes that the finding was derived from a ROI-specific analysis. Upward and downward arrows denote positive and negative changes, respectively (without showing the sub-region of the change). a, anterior; m, mid; p, posterior; i, inferior; s, superior; o, oribitofrontal; PM, connection with the premotor cortex; PF, connection with the prefrontal cortex.
[1]Affected side > Unaffected side; [2]the findings shown in 'Decreased activation' represents 'placebo>drug'; [3]baseline cerebral blood flow; [4]effect of cognitive and emotional interference; [5]increased resting-stated/pain-evoking functional connectivity between the insula and these regions.

between the PFC and the basal ganglia [8,13,14,20,25]. Within the PFC, the superior or middle frontal gyrus (i.e., the dorsolateral PFC) was more frequently reported than the medial or orbital part of the PFC.

For the negative changes, a decreased NAA/Cr/GABA level was found in the thalamus only in the TNP but not the TMD patients [11,12]. In contrast, a decreased NAA/Cho level was found in the TMD patients [29] (Table 8). The TNP patients also showed decreased baseline CBF in the thalamus and the S1, which were not reported in the TMD patients [10,12].

Changes in brain structure. The results on brain structure included the investigations on gray matter and white matter (Table 9 and Table 10). For both TNP and TMD studies, there were more findings on negative changes than positive changes (Figure S1I). Again, the brain regions with significant changes were predominantly the pain-related regions, including the thalamus, S1, ACC/MCC, and the insula. Concurrent changes were found between the thalamus and the S1 [11,15,17,22], and additionally between the ACC/MCC and the insula [15,17,28]. Changes on white matter were exclusively negative changes. Three studies have consistently reported decreased FA nearby the S1 [10,16,22] (Table 10).

Statistical Analysis

The correlation analysis and the paired Wilcoxon test were performed on the regional changes of the pain-related ROIs between the TNP and the TMD groups, separately for the functional studies with positive changes and the structural studies with negative changes. In the functional studies with positive changes, the paired Wilcoxon test failed to reject the null hypothesis ($W = 1.56$, $p = 0.12$), and the correlation analysis showed a significant correlation (Spearman's $rho = 0.70$, $p = 0.035$) (Figure 2A–B). In contrast, in the structural studies with negative changes, the paired Wilcoxon test rejected the null hypothesis ($W = 2.28$, $p = 0.023$), and the correlation analysis did not show a significant correlation (Spearman's $rho = 0.61$,

Table 8. The findings of meta-analysis on functional changes by pain-related regions: MRS.

Source	Positive changes									Negative changes								
	THA	S1	S2	CC	INS	PFC	BG	MT	PAG	THA	S1	S2	CC	INS	PFC	BG	MT	PAG
Trigeminal neuropathic pain																		
Gustin 2011[1]										*								
Henderson 2013[2]										*								
Temporomandibular joint disorder pain																		
Gerstner 2012[3]					p*													

See Table 3 for the abbreviations of the brain regions. The asterisk denotes that the finding was derived from a ROI-specific analysis. p, posterior.
[1]NAA/Cr level; [2]GABA level; [3]NAA/Cho level.

Table 9. The findings of meta-analysis on structural changes by pain-related regions: Gray matter.

Source	Positive changes									Negative changes								
	THA	S1	S2	CC	INS	PFC	BG	MT	PAG	THA	S1	S2	CC	INS	PFC	BG	MT	PAG
Trigeminal neuropathic pain																		
Gustin 2011					p					PF	3b			a		↓		
Obermann 2013										TP	1	↓	a	a	dlo	↓		
DeSouza 2013[1]	PF[2]	2/1				pl	↑	↑	↑				a	p	o			
Temporomandibular joint disorder pain																		
Younger 2010	PF				a	i	↑				3b							
Gerstner 2011													m	a	i		↓	
Moayedi 2011[1]		3b*				vl*												

See Table 3 for the abbreviations of the brain regions. The asterisk denotes that the finding was derived from a ROI-specific analysis. Upward and downward arrows denote positive and negative changes, respectively (without showing the sub-region of the change). a, anterior; m, mid; p, posterior; i, inferior; oribitofrontal; vl, ventrolateral; dl, dorsolateral; PF, connection with the prefrontal cortex; TP, connection with the temporal cortex.
[1]cortical thickness; [2]gray matter volume.

p = 0.083) (Figure 2C–D). Therefore, according to our criteria, the regional changes from the functional studies with positive changes showed similar brain signature pattern between TND and TMD, and the regional changes from the structural studies with negative changes showed distinct brain signature pattern between TND and TMD.

Discussion

Common Brain Signature related to TNP and TMD pain

We hypothesized that the two chronic orofacial pain disorders are associated with a common pattern of brain signature. This hypothesis was partially supported. The statistical analysis revealed similar pattern of brain signature only in the functional studies with positive changes (Table 7–10 and Figure 2A–B). In contrast, the structural studies with negative changes showed distinct pattern (Table 7–10 and Figure 2C–D). Among the major pain-related ROIs, changes at the thalamus, the S1, the ACC/MCC, and the insula were frequently reported. In contrast, changes at the S2 were relatively fewer. The significance of each of the regions was discussed as follows.

The thalamus and the S1. Both the thalamus and the S1 are critical regions of the trigeminal nerve system [56] and play a major role in the thalamocortical pathway [12]. In line with these findings, we found that the thalamus and S1 were the most frequently reported brain regions in functional and structural investigations. Notably, the thalamus and the S1 showed a higher frequency of concurrent changes. In the 11 studies that showed functional or structural changes in the thalamus, 8 studies showed concurrent changes in the S1 (positive changes: [8,13,14,17,23]; negative changes: [11,12,15]). The findings highlight the role of the thalamocortical pathway in chronic pain [12,34].

The S2. Compared to the other pain-related brain regions, the S2 showed a lesser degree of changes in both brain function and structure. The S2, together with the insula and the mid-cingulate cortex, is considered as the key brain region evoked by noxious stimuli [57]. Its activation reliably predicted the experience of acute pain [58,59]; however, its role in chronic pain is more elusive[33]. Animal studies have shown that both the S1 and S2 show reorganization after peripheral lesioning [60]. Human fMRI findings revealed that changes in individual perceptual threshold is linearly correlated with the degree of re-organization of the S1, but not the S2 [61]. Therefore, the S2 changes may predominantly reflect a transient change of pain experience (e.g., acute evoked pain), rather than a long-term alteration in pain processing.

The ACC/MCC and the insula. Both the ACC/MCC and the insular activation is frequently associated with noxious stimuli

Table 10. The findings of meta-analysis on structural changes by pain-related regions: White matter.

Source	Positive changes									Negative changes								
	THA	S1	S2	CC	INS	PFC	BG	MT	PAG	THA	S1	S2	CC	INS	PFC	BG	MT	PAG
Trigeminal neuropathic pain																		
Gustin 2012											↓							
DeSouza 2014[1]											↓	↓	m		↓			
Temporomandibular joint disorder pain																		
Gerstner 2011[2]													a		smi			
Moayedi 2012										*	*							

See Table 3 for the abbreviations of the brain regions. The asterisk denotes that the finding was derived from a ROI-specific analysis. Downward arrows denote negative changes (without showing the sub-region of the change). a, anterior; m, mid; i, inferior; s, superior.
[1]The brain regions affected by the white matter tracts, inferred from the Discussion; [2]white matter volume.

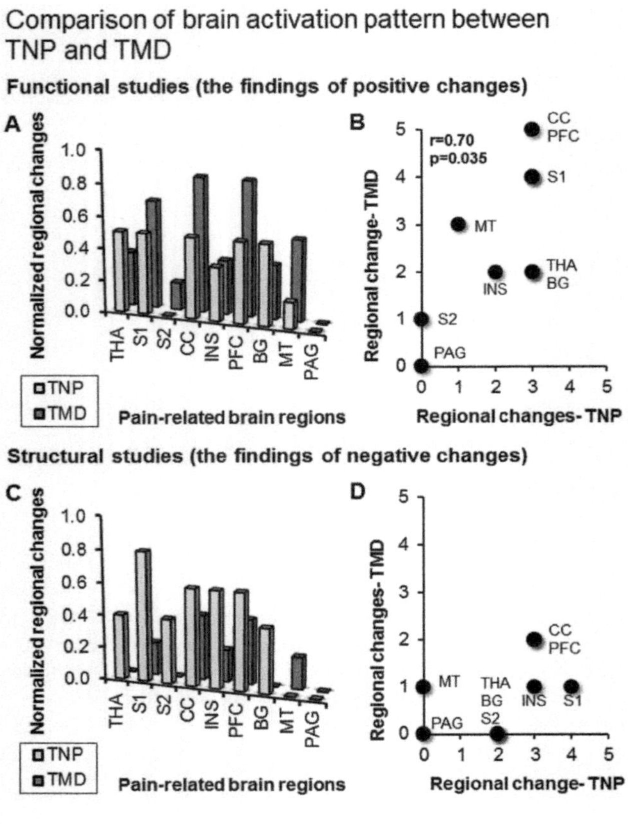

Figure 2. Results of the statistical analysis. Panel (A) and (B) show the pattern of brain signature from the functional studies with positive changes. Between TNP and TMD, the overall pattern did not significantly differ (A), and the pattern across each ROI was significantly correlated (B). Panel (C) and (D) show the pattern of brain signature from the structural studies with negative changes. Between TNP and TMD, the overall pattern significantly differed (C), and the pattern across each ROI was not significantly correlated (D). See Table 3 for the abbreviations.

and encodes pain experience [57,59]. The ACC activation was associated with the magnitude of subjective pain, while the MCC activation was associated with the magnitude of stimuli intensity [34,62]. In terms of brain connectivity, the ACC and the insula are the major regions of the salience network [63]. Recent evidence has revealed that altered activity of the salience network is associated with the endogenous and self-sustaining nature of chronic pain [64]. In migraine patients, the salience network showed aberrant intrinsic connectivity [65]. In terms of brain structure, the pain sensitizers showed significant reduction in gray matter density in the ACC and the insula [66]. In line with the findings, in the patients with chronic orofacial pain, we found predominantly positive changes in brain function and negative changes in brain structure in the regions. The finding may suggest an altered subjective experience of pain in the chronic orofacial pain patients.

Distinct Brain Signature related to TNP and TMD pain

In contrast to the similarity of activation pattern from the functional studies with positive changes, in the structural studies with negative changes, we found distinct brain signature, which may be specific to the TNP and TMD patients. Firstly, the TMD patients showed overall fewer negative changes in brain structure than the TNP patients (Figure 2C). In the TNP patients, the negative changes may indicate a loss-of-inhibition mechanism in modulating the thalamocortical pathway [12]. In addition, there were more concurrent changes in brain function between the thalamus and the S1 in the TNP studies (Table 7–10), suggesting that in the TNP patients, pain are more associated with the thalamocortical pathway, compared to the TMD patients. A recent meta-analysis has shown that, in the patients with neuropathic pain, the thalamus showed hypoactivity during resting but hyperactivity during allodynia [67]. The resting hypoactivity may be associated with sensory deafferentation related to neuropathy [67]. Our findings supported the proposal by showing decreased baseline activity (including CBF and MRS signals) and increased stimuli-evoked activity at the thalamus and the S1 ([10–12], see Table 7 and Table 8).

The functional studies showed that activation at the aINS was seen mainly in the TNP group, while activation at the pINS was seen in the TMD group (Table 7). It has been widely established that the anterior and the posterior sub-division of the insula play a different role in pain processing. The aINS and the pINS, respectively, showed a greater degree of functional and structural connection with the cognitive-affective network (e.g., the PFC) and the sensory discriminative network related to pain (e.g., the S1 and S2) [68,69]. The segregation could be explained based on each etiology and symptomatology. In TNP patients, pain would like to emerge spontaneous and continuously, and therefore the aINS would play a major role in shaping such a salient experience. By contrast, in TMD patients, pain is more likely to be triggered from the peripheral tissue, and therefore a sensory-discriminative network, including the pINS, would be involved.

It should be noted that both the patterns of insula and thalamus connectivity were indirectly concluded by relatively small samples. Still, the findings strengthen the general hypothesis that plasticity in connectional pattern, rather than regional activity, would account for the difference in pain experience [70,71]. The findings therefore highlight the importance for investigation the chronic orofacial pain at the level of brain connectome.

The Role of Cognitive-Affective Network

Supporting our third hypothesis, we found profound functional and structural changes in the PFC, including the dorsolateral PFC (the superior or middle frontal gyrus), the ventrolateral PFC (the inferior frontal gyrus) and the orbitofrontal cortex (Table 7 and Figure 2). The orbitofrontal cortex plays a critical role in coping with pain and shows deficit activation in the neuropathic pain patients [67]. The dorsolateral and ventrolateral PFC play a key role in modulating pain, particularly via cognitive re-appraisal [6]. The consistent engagement of the PFC in both TNP and TMD pain highlights the role of psychological factors in chronic orofacial pain [38].

Notably, we found concurrent functional and structural changes between the PFC and the basal ganglia, and partly with the limbic system. The basal ganglia are the neural substrates critical for motivation and reward learning [72], and the basal ganglia-cortical loop is associated with the prediction of future reward [73]. The experience of pain relief, as a reward, is particularly important to chronic pain patients. The changes of the basal ganglia-PFC pathways may be associated with the transition from acute to chronic pain [34].

Further Considerations and Clinical Implications

The current review showed a great variation in the criteria of patient selection and the study designs across the studies (Table 5 and Table 6). Either TNP or TMD can be categorized into different sub-types, which differ in etiology and symptomatology. For example, trigeminal neuralgia is associated with an episodic shooting and sharp pain, while the painful trigeminal neuropathy is associated with a continuous dull or sharp pain [48]. Therefore, it is crucial to systematically investigate the signs and symptoms presented by the patient group. For example, the thalamic hypoactivity may be associated with sensory deafferentation [67], and QST would be a critical tool for investigating the thalamic changes associated with the neuropathic pain. In addition, the changes in brain function and structure can be influenced by a variety of factors, such as age [74–76] and chronic distress [77]. Therefore, to sharpen the association between symptoms and brain changes, it would be important to clarify the effect from these confounding factors.

A general theme underlying the disease-related alterations in brain signature is neuroplasticity, which refers to the changes in brain organization that account for various forms of behavioral modifiability [78]. Brain neuroplasticity related to pain may represent the somatic memories of pain, that are sculpted by injury (e.g., peripheral noxious stimuli) or experience (e.g., pain-related distress) [79]. Therefore, investigations on neuroplasticity of brain function and structure may help explain how the experience of chronic orofacial pain is shaped. Plasticity referred to 'an intrinsic property of the nervous system retained throughout a lifespan', which can be molded by environmental changes and experiences [80]. In contrast, the term *neuroelasticity* referred to an adaptive process of plastic effect, in which functional or structural plasticity of the brain occurs dynamically in accordance with the addition or removal of stimuli [81]. From the clinical perspective, the concept of adaptive neuroelasticity could be useful, because it regards the brain reorganization as a dynamic course, which corresponds to the exacerbation or relief of the illness status. For example, in patients with chronic low back pain, the pain-related decrease in cortical thickness was reversed after surgical treatment [82]. In the patients with painful osteoarthritis, the pain-related decrease in GMV was reversed to the level observed in healthy controls, after successful surgery [81,83]. The neural mechanisms of such elastic and adaptive changes in brain organization are still unclear. However, these recent findings suggest that the plastic changes in brain functions and structure, as a brain marker, would help the clinicians not only in prognosis but also in assessing the effect of the treatment of chronic orofacial pain.

Conclusions

The current review has revealed that TNP and TMD patients showed a common pattern of brain signature regarding changes in brain function. In contrast, the pattern of structural changes differed from each other. The alterations in the thalamocortical pathway differed between the TNP and the TMD pain patients. In addition, changes in the PFC and the basal ganglia suggested the role of cognitive modulation and reward processing in chronic orofacial pain. The findings highlight the potential for brain neuroimaging as an investigating tool for understanding chronic orofacial pain.

Supporting Information

Figure S1 Results of qualitative meta-analysis. The charts revealed the number of studies that showed significant changes in each of the pain-related regions. Figure S1A–C showed both functional and structural changes; Figure S1D–F showed functional changes, and Figure S1G–I showed structural changes, in trigeminal neuropathic pain (TNP), temporomandibular joint disorder (TMD) pain, and both disorders (TNP+TMD).

Checklist S1 PRISMA checklist.

Author Contributions

Conceived and designed the experiments: CSL. Analyzed the data: CSL. Contributed reagents/materials/analysis tools: CSL. Wrote the paper: CSL.

References

1. Pan HC, Sheehan J, Huang CF, Sheu ML, Yang DY, et al. (2010) Quality-of-life outcomes after Gamma Knife surgery for trigeminal neuralgia. J Neurosurg 113 Suppl: 191–198.
2. Rener-Sitar K, Celebic A, Mehulic K, Petricevic N (2013) Factors related to oral health related quality of life in TMD patients. Coll Antropol 37: 407–413.
3. Auvenshine RC (2007) Temporomandibular disorders: associated features. Dent Clin North Am 51: 105–127, vi.
4. DaSilva AF, DosSantos MF (2012) The role of sensory fiber demography in trigeminal and postherpetic neuralgias. J Dent Res 91: 17–24.
5. Murray GM, Peck CC (2007) Orofacial pain and jaw muscle activity: a new model. J Orofac Pain 21: 263–278; discussion 279–288.
6. Wiech K, Ploner M, Tracey I (2008) Neurocognitive aspects of pain perception. Trends Cogn Sci 12: 306–313.
7. Sarlani E, Greenspan JD (2005) Why look in the brain for answers to temporomandibular disorder pain? Cells Tissues Organs 180: 69–75.
8. Becerra L, Morris S, Bazes S, Gostic R, Sherman S, et al. (2006) Trigeminal neuropathic pain alters responses in CNS circuits to mechanical (brush) and thermal (cold and heat) stimuli. J Neurosci 26: 10646–10657.
9. Blatow M, Nennig E, Sarpaczki E, Reinhardt J, Schlieter M, et al. (2009) Altered somatosensory processing in trigeminal neuralgia. Hum Brain Mapp 30: 3495–3508.
10. Gustin SM, Peck CC, Cheney LB, Macey PM, Murray GM, et al. (2012) Pain and plasticity: is chronic pain always associated with somatosensory cortex activity and reorganization? J Neurosci 32: 14874–14884.
11. Gustin SM, Peck CC, Wilcox SL, Nash PG, Murray GM, et al. (2011) Different pain, different brain: thalamic anatomy in neuropathic and non-neuropathic chronic pain syndromes. J Neurosci 31: 5956–5964.
12. Henderson LA, Peck CC, Petersen ET, Rae CD, Youssef AM, et al. (2013) Chronic pain: lost inhibition? J Neurosci 33: 7574–7582.
13. Moisset X, Villain N, Ducreux D, Serrie A, Cunin G, et al. (2011) Functional brain imaging of trigeminal neuralgia. Eur J Pain 15: 124–131.
14. Scrivani S, Wallin D, Moulton EA, Cole S, Wasan AD, et al. (2010) A fMRI evaluation of lamotrigine for the treatment of trigeminal neuropathic pain: pilot study. Pain Med 11: 920–941.
15. Obermann M, Rodriguez-Raecke R, Naegel S, Holle D, Mueller D, et al. (2013) Gray matter volume reduction reflects chronic pain in trigeminal neuralgia. Neuroimage 74: 352–358.
16. Desouza DD, Hodaie M, Davis KD (2014) Abnormal Trigeminal Nerve Microstructure and Brain White Matter in Idiopathic Trigeminal Neuralgia. Pain.
17. Desouza DD, Moayedi M, Chen DQ, Davis KD, Hodaie M (2013) Sensorimotor and Pain Modulation Brain Abnormalities in Trigeminal Neuralgia: A Paroxysmal, Sensory-Triggered Neuropathic Pain. PLoS One 8: e66340.
18. Abrahamsen R, Dietz M, Lodahl S, Roepstorff A, Zachariae R, et al. (2010) Effect of hypnotic pain modulation on brain activity in patients with temporomandibular disorder pain. Pain 151: 825–833.
19. Ichesco E, Quintero A, Clauw DJ, Peltier S, Sundgren PM, et al. (2012) Altered functional connectivity between the insula and the cingulate cortex in patients with temporomandibular disorder: a pilot study. Headache 52: 441–454.
20. Jiang T, Li J, Jin Z, Wang YW, Feng HL, et al. (2006) [Comparison of atypical orofacial pain and temporomandibular disorders synovitis pain processing in the human brain using functional magnetic resonance imaging]. Zhonghua Kou Qiang Yi Xue Za Zhi 41: 670–673.
21. Moayedi M, Weissman-Fogel I, Crawley AP, Goldberg MB, Freeman BV, et al. (2011) Contribution of chronic pain and neuroticism to abnormal forebrain gray matter in patients with temporomandibular disorder. Neuroimage 55: 277–286.
22. Moayedi M, Weissman-Fogel I, Salomons TV, Crawley AP, Goldberg MB, et al. (2012) White matter brain and trigeminal nerve abnormalities in temporomandibular disorder. Pain 153: 1467–1477.
23. Nebel MB, Folger S, Tommerdahl M, Hollins M, McGlone F, et al. (2010) Temporomandibular disorder modifies cortical response to tactile stimulation. J Pain 11: 1083–1094.

24. Salomons TV, Moayedi M, Weissman-Fogel I, Goldberg MB, Freeman BV, et al. (2012) Perceived helplessness is associated with individual differences in the central motor output system. Eur J Neurosci 35: 1481–1487.
25. Weissman-Fogel I, Moayedi M, Tenenbaum HC, Goldberg MB, Freeman BV, et al. (2011) Abnormal cortical activity in patients with temporomandibular disorder evoked by cognitive and emotional tasks. Pain 152: 384–396.
26. Younger JW, Shen YF, Goddard G, Mackey SC (2010) Chronic myofascial temporomandibular pain is associated with neural abnormalities in the trigeminal and limbic systems. Pain 149: 222–228.
27. Zhao YP, Ma XC, Jin Z, Li K, Liu G, et al. (2011) Cerebral activation during unilateral clenching in patients with temporomandibular joint synovitis and biting pain: an functional magnetic resonance imaging study. Chin Med J (Engl) 124: 2136–2143.
28. Gerstner G, Ichesco E, Quintero A, Schmidt-Wilcke T (2011) Changes in regional gray and white matter volume in patients with myofascial-type temporomandibular disorders: a voxel-based morphometry study. J Orofac Pain 25: 99–106.
29. Gerstner GE, Gracely RH, Deebajah A, Ichesco E, Quintero A, et al. (2012) Posterior insular molecular changes in myofascial pain. J Dent Res 91: 485–490.
30. Button KS, Ioannidis JP, Mokrysz C, Nosek BA, Flint J, et al. (2013) Power failure: why small sample size undermines the reliability of neuroscience. Nat Rev Neurosci 14: 365–376.
31. Zatorre RJ, Fields RD, Johansen-Berg H (2012) Plasticity in gray and white: neuroimaging changes in brain structure during learning. Nat Neurosci 15: 528–536.
32. Poldrack RA (2000) Imaging brain plasticity: conceptual and methodological issues—a theoretical review. Neuroimage 12: 1–13.
33. Apkarian AV, Bushnell MC, Treede RD, Zubieta JK (2005) Human brain mechanisms of pain perception and regulation in health and disease. Eur J Pain 9: 463–484.
34. Apkarian AV, Hashmi JA, Baliki MN (2011) Pain and the brain: specificity and plasticity of the brain in clinical chronic pain. Pain 152: S49–64.
35. Cauda F, Sacco K, Duca S, Cocito D, D'Agata F, et al. (2009) Altered resting state in diabetic neuropathic pain. PLoS One 4: e4542.
36. Schaible HG (2012) Mechanisms of chronic pain in osteoarthritis. Curr Rheumatol Rep 14: 549–556.
37. Walton KD, Dubois M, Llinas RR (2010) Abnormal thalamocortical activity in patients with Complex Regional Pain Syndrome (CRPS) type I. Pain 150: 41–51.
38. Gustin SM, Wilcox SL, Peck CC, Murray GM, Henderson LA (2011) Similarity of suffering: equivalence of psychological and psychosocial factors in neuropathic and non-neuropathic orofacial pain patients. Pain 152: 825–832.
39. Liberati A, Altman DG, Tetzlaff J, Mulrow C, Gotzsche PC, et al. (2009) The PRISMA statement for reporting systematic reviews and meta-analyses of studies that evaluate health care interventions: explanation and elaboration. PLoS Med 6: e1000100.
40. Ellingson BM, Mayer E, Harris RJ, Ashe-McNally C, Naliboff BD, et al. (2013) Diffusion tensor imaging detects microstructural reorganization in the brain associated with chronic irritable bowel syndrome. Pain 154: 1528–1541.
41. Feraco P, Bacci A, Pedrabissi F, Passamonti L, Zampogna G, et al. (2011) Metabolic abnormalities in pain-processing regions of patients with fibromyalgia: a 3T MR spectroscopy study. AJNR Am J Neuroradiol 32: 1585–1590.
42. Wasan AD, Loggia ML, Chen LQ, Napadow V, Kong J, et al. (2011) Neural correlates of chronic low back pain measured by arterial spin labeling. Anesthesiology 115: 364–374.
43. Poldrack RA, Fletcher PC, Henson RN, Worsley KJ, Brett M, et al. (2008) Guidelines for reporting an fMRI study. Neuroimage 40: 409–414.
44. Dworkin SF, LeResche L (1992) Research diagnostic criteria for temporomandibular disorders: review, criteria, examinations and specifications, critique. J Craniomandib Disord 6: 301–355.
45. Behrens TE, Johansen-Berg H, Woolrich MW, Smith SM, Wheeler-Kingshott CA, et al. (2003) Non-invasive mapping of connections between human thalamus and cortex using diffusion imaging. Nat Neurosci 6: 750–757.
46. Zahra H, Teh BS, Paulino AC, Yoshor D, Trask T, et al. (2009) Stereotactic radiosurgery for trigeminal neuralgia utilizing the BrainLAB Novalis system. Technol Cancer Res Treat 8: 407–412.
47. Yang J, Simonson TM, Ruprecht A, Meng D, Vincent SD, et al. (1996) Magnetic resonance imaging used to assess patients with trigeminal neuralgia. Oral Surg Oral Med Oral Pathol Oral Radiol Endod 81: 343–350.
48. Leeuw d (2008) Orofacial Pain: Guidelines for Assessment, Diagnosis, and Management: Quintessence Pub Co.
49. Melzack R (1987) The short-form McGill Pain Questionnaire. Pain 30: 191–197.
50. Melzack R (1975) The McGill Pain Questionnaire: major properties and scoring methods. Pain 1: 277–299.
51. Rolke R, Baron R, Maier C, Tolle TR, Treede RD, et al. (2006) Quantitative sensory testing in the German Research Network on Neuropathic Pain (DFNS): standardized protocol and reference values. Pain 123: 231–243.
52. Beck AT, Ward CH, Mendelson M, Mock J, Erbaugh J (1961) An inventory for measuring depression. Arch Gen Psychiatry 4: 561–571.
53. Mumford JA, Poldrack RA (2007) Modeling group fMRI data. Soc Cogn Affect Neurosci 2: 251–257.
54. Friston KJ, Holmes AP, Worsley KJ (1999) How many subjects constitute a study? Neuroimage 10: 1–5.
55. Nichols TE, Holmes AP (2002) Nonparametric permutation tests for functional neuroimaging: a primer with examples. Hum Brain Mapp 15: 1–25.
56. DaSilva AF, Becerra L, Makris N, Strassman AM, Gonzalez RG, et al. (2002) Somatotopic activation in the human trigeminal pain pathway. J Neurosci 22: 8183–8192.
57. Duerden EG, Albanese MC (2013) Localization of pain-related brain activation: a meta-analysis of neuroimaging data. Hum Brain Mapp 34: 109–149.
58. Brodersen KH, Wiech K, Lomakina EI, Lin CS, Buhmann JM, et al. (2012) Decoding the perception of pain from fMRI using multivariate pattern analysis. Neuroimage 63: 1162–1170.
59. Wager TD, Atlas LY, Lindquist MA, Roy M, Woo CW, et al. (2013) An fMRI-based neurologic signature of physical pain. N Engl J Med 368: 1388–1397.
60. Tandon S, Kambi N, Lazar L, Mohammed H, Jain N (2009) Large-scale expansion of the face representation in somatosensory areas of the lateral sulcus after spinal cord injuries in monkeys. J Neurosci 29: 12009–12019.
61. Pleger B, Villringer A (2013) The human somatosensory system: from perception to decision making. Prog Neurobiol 103: 76–97.
62. Baliki MN, Geha PY, Apkarian AV (2009) Parsing pain perception between nociceptive representation and magnitude estimation. J Neurophysiol 101: 875–887.
63. Taylor KS, Seminowicz DA, Davis KD (2009) Two systems of resting state connectivity between the insula and cingulate cortex. Hum Brain Mapp 30: 2731–2745.
64. Otti A, Guendel H, Wohlschlager A, Zimmer C, Noll-Hussong M (2013) Frequency shifts in the anterior default mode network and the salience network in chronic pain disorder. BMC Psychiatry 13: 84.
65. Xue T, Yuan K, Zhao L, Yu D, Dong T, et al. (2012) Intrinsic brain network abnormalities in migraines without aura revealed in resting-state fMRI. PLoS One 7: e52927.
66. Stankewitz A, Valet M, Schulz E, Woller A, Sprenger T, et al. (2013) Pain sensitisers exhibit grey matter changes after repetitive pain exposure: A longitudinal voxel-based morphometry study. Pain 154: 1732–1737.
67. Garcia-Larrea L, Peyron R (2013) Pain matrices and neuropathic pain matrices: a review. Pain.
68. Augustine JR (1996) Circuitry and functional aspects of the insular lobe in primates including humans. Brain Res Brain Res Rev 22: 229–244.
69. Deen B, Pitskel NB, Pelphrey KA (2011) Three systems of insular functional connectivity identified with cluster analysis. Cereb Cortex 21: 1498–1506.
70. Bolwerk A, Seifert F, Maihofner C (2013) Altered Resting-State Functional Connectivity in Complex Regional Pain Syndrome. J Pain.
71. Mansour AR, Baliki MN, Huang L, Torbey S, Herrmann KM, et al. (2013) Brain white matter structural properties predict transition to chronic pain. Pain 154: 2160–2168.
72. Yin HH, Ostlund SB, Balleine BW (2008) Reward-guided learning beyond dopamine in the nucleus accumbens: the integrative functions of cortico-basal ganglia networks. Eur J Neurosci 28: 1437–1448.
73. Tanaka SC, Doya K, Okada G, Ueda K, Okamoto Y, et al. (2004) Prediction of immediate and future rewards differentially recruits cortico-basal ganglia loops. Nat Neurosci 7: 887–893.
74. Mahncke HW, Bronstone A, Merzenich MM (2006) Brain plasticity and functional losses in the aged: scientific bases for a novel intervention. Prog Brain Res 157: 81–109.
75. Moayedi M, Weissman-Fogel I, Salomons TV, Crawley AP, Goldberg MB, et al. (2012) Abnormal gray matter aging in chronic pain patients. Brain Res 1456: 82–93.
76. Ceko M, Bushnell MC, Fitzcharles MA, Schweinhardt P (2013) Fibromyalgia interacts with age to change the brain. Neuroimage Clin 3: 249–260.
77. McEwen BS, Morrison JH (2013) The brain on stress: vulnerability and plasticity of the prefrontal cortex over the life course. Neuron 79: 16–29.
78. Berlucchi G, Buchtel HA (2009) Neuronal plasticity: historical roots and evolution of meaning. Exp Brain Res 192: 307–319.
79. Melzack R, Coderre TJ, Katz J, Vaccarino AL (2001) Central neuroplasticity and pathological pain. Ann N Y Acad Sci 933: 157–174.
80. Pascual-Leone A, Amedi A, Fregni F, Merabet LB (2005) The plastic human brain cortex. Annu Rev Neurosci 28: 377–401.
81. Gwilym SE, Filippini N, Douaud G, Carr AJ, Tracey I (2010) Thalamic atrophy associated with painful osteoarthritis of the hip is reversible after arthroplasty: a longitudinal voxel-based morphometric study. Arthritis Rheum 62: 2930–2940.
82. Seminowicz DA, Wideman TH, Naso L, Hatami-Khoroushahi Z, Fallatah S, et al. (2011) Effective treatment of chronic low back pain in humans reverses abnormal brain anatomy and function. J Neurosci 31: 7540–7550.
83. Rodriguez-Raecke R, Niemeier A, Ihle K, Ruether W, May A (2009) Brain gray matter decrease in chronic pain is the consequence and not the cause of pain. J Neurosci 29: 13746–13750.
84. Truelove EL, Sommers EE, LeResche L, Dworkin SF, Von Korff M (1992) Clinical diagnostic criteria for TMD. New classification permits multiple diagnoses. J Am Dent Assoc 123: 47–54.
85. Smith SM, Nichols TE (2009) Threshold-free cluster enhancement: addressing problems of smoothing, threshold dependence and localisation in cluster inference. Neuroimage 44: 83–98.

8

$Ca_V3.2$ T-Type Calcium Channels in Peripheral Sensory Neurons Are Important for Mibefradil-Induced Reversal of Hyperalgesia and Allodynia in Rats with Painful Diabetic Neuropathy

Aleksandar Lj. Obradovic[1,2], Sung Mi Hwang[1,3], Joseph Scarpa[1], Sung Jun Hong[1,4], Slobodan M. Todorovic[1,5,6], Vesna Jevtovic-Todorovic[1,5,6]*

1 Department of Anesthesiology, University of Virginia Health System, Charlottesville, Virginia, United States of America, **2** Department of Physiology, Faculty of Pharmacy University of Belgrade, Belgrade, Serbia, **3** Department of Anesthesiology and Pain Medicine, Chuncheon Sacred Heart Hospital, College of Medicine, Hallym University, Chuncheon, South Korea, **4** Department of Anesthesiology and Pain Medicine, Kangdong Sacred Heart Hospital, College of Medicine, Hallym University, Seoul, South Korea, **5** Department of Neuroscience, University of Virginia Health System, Charlottesville, Virginia, United States of America, **6** Neuroscience Graduate Program, University of Virginia Health System, Charlottesville, Virginia, United States of America

Abstract

We recently showed that streptozotocin (STZ) injections in rats lead to the development of painful peripheral diabetic neuropathy (PDN) accompanied by enhancement of $Ca_V3.2$ T-type calcium currents (T-currents) and hyperexcitability in dorsal root ganglion (DRG) neurons. Here we used the classical peripherally acting T-channel blocker mibefradil to examine the role of $Ca_V3.2$ T-channels as pharmacological targets for treatment of painful PDN. When administered intraperitoneally (i.p.), at clinically relevant doses, mibefradil effectively alleviated heat, cold and mechanical hypersensitivities in STZ-treated diabetic rats in a dose-dependent manner. We also found that $Ca_V3.2$ antisense (AS)-treated diabetic rats exhibit a significant decrease in painful PDN compared with mismatch antisense (MIS)-treated diabetic rats. Co-treatment with mibefradil (9 mg/kg i.p.) resulted in reversal of heat, cold and mechanical hypersensitivity in MIS-treated but not in AS-treated diabetic rats, suggesting that mibefradil and $Ca_V3.2$ AS share the same cellular target. Using patch-clamp recordings from acutely dissociated DRG neurons, we demonstrated that mibefradil similarly blocked T-currents in diabetic and healthy rats in a voltage-dependent manner by stabilizing inactive states of T-channels. We conclude that antihyperalgesic and antiallodynic effects of mibefradil in PDN are at least partly mediated by inhibition of $Ca_V3.2$ channels in peripheral nociceptors. Hence, peripherally acting voltage-dependent T-channel blockers could be very useful in the treatment of painful symptoms of PDN.

Editor: J. David Spafford, University of Waterloo, Canada

Funding: This work was supported in part by grants from National Institutes of Health DA 029342 to SMT and VJT, American Diabetes Association Basic Research Grant 7-09-BS-190 to SMT, UVA Diabetes Launch Pad Grant to VJT, funds from Hallym University to SJH and SMH, and the Harold Carron Endowment to VJT. The funders had no role in study design, data collection and analysis, decision to publish, or preparation of the manuscript.

Competing Interests: The authors have declared that no competing interests exist.

* E-mail: vj3w@virginia.edu

Introduction

Systemic administration of streptozotocin (STZ) has been shown to induce type 1 diabetes in rodents, resulting in peripheral diabetic neuropathy (PDN) often manifested as heat and mechanical hyperalgesia [1]. It is well known that $Ca_V3.2$ T-type calcium channels (T-channels) contribute to the hyper-excitability of sensory neurons manifested as hyperalgesia and allodynia in rats with PDN [2,3]. Blockade of $Ca_v3.2$ T-type channels in STZ models of neuropathy, either by pharmacological means or by gene silencing using antisense technology, significantly reduces nociception in diabetic rats and mice *in vivo* [1–4]. Although several T-channel blockers exhibit effective antinociceptive activity in different animal models of neuropathic pain, due to the questionable selectivity of these agents, it remains unclear whether the observed effects are specific to T-channels or could be caused by the modulation of some off-targets. It is noteworthy that some new pharmacological agents, like 3, 5-dichloro-N-[1-(2, 2-dimethyl-tetrahydro-pyran-4-ylmethyl)-4-fluoro-piperidin-4-ylmethyl]-benzamide (TTA-P2) that are very selective T-channel blockers are effective analgesics in diabetic rats [5]. The studies with selective agents like TTA-P2 and related compounds are important to establish proof of concept for the use of T-channel blockers in the treatment of PDN. However, TTA-related drugs clearly exhibit sedation in animal models, likely due to the effects on T-channels in the central nervous system (CNS) [6]. This effect makes them unsuitable for long-term use in patients with chronic pain disorders [7]; thus there is need to examine the role of peripherally acting T-channel blockers in order to avoid side effects resulting from blockade of T-channels in the CNS. Hence, in our focus on T-channels in peripheral nociceptors as potential targets for PDN, we examined the role of the classical peripherally acting T-channel blocker mibefradil in combination with $Ca_V3.2$-specific antisense oligonucleotides.

Materials and Methods

Chemicals and animals

All experimental protocols were approved by the University of Virginia Animal Care and Use Committee. All experiments were conducted in accordance with the *Guide for the Care and Use of Laboratory Animals* adopted by the U.S. National Institute of Health. Every effort was made to minimize animal suffering and the number of animals used. Using standard batteries of behavioral tests for mechanical and thermal hyperalgesia and allodynia, we established that retired breeder female and male rats exhibit similar pain sensitivity [8]. Thus, we used adult female Sprague–Dawley rats (retired breeders, 10–12 months old, weight 259±8 g) for the present study. Streptozotocin (STZ) was purchased from Sigma, St. Louis, MO. Previously published sequences [1,9] of antisense Cav3.2 oligonucleotides (AS) and mismatched Cav3.2 oligonucleotides (MIS) were purchased from Eurofins MWG Operon. Morphine sulphate (administered i.p. at a dose of 10 mg/kg in sterile solution) was obtained from the University of Virginia pharmacy. Mibefradil (Sigma-Aldrich, St. Louis, MO), AS-$Ca_V3.2$ and MIS-$Ca_V3.2$ oligonucleotides where dissolved in appropriate sterile pH 7.4 buffer solution.

Peripheral diabetic neuropathy model

To induce PDN, we intraperitoneally (i.p.) injected freshly dissolved STZ solution at pH 4.5 at a dose of 50 mg/kg, which causes severe hyperglycemia and pain-like behavior by the 4th week after injection [1]. Control rats received the same volume/kg i.p. of sterile saline (SAL). Heat and mechanical hypersensitivities and cold allodynia pharmacological and oligonucleotide testing were performed during the 4th week following STZ injections. All drug injections were performed in a blinded manner.

Intrathecal Injections

We initiated intrathecal injections of either AS or MIS after we established stable heat and mechanical hyperalgesia concomitantly with elevated glucose blood levels (>600 mg/dl), at which point STZ-injected rats had developed PDN (day 21 post-STZ injection). Rats were maintained under isoflurane anesthesia (2% in oxygen delivered via nose cone) during the injection procedure. We injected into the L5–6 region of the spinal cord 12.5 μg/25 μl of either AS or MIS every 12 h for 4 consecutive days (total of 8 injections). All solutions were adjusted to pH 7.4 to avoid spinal cord irritation.

Behavioral Assessment of Heat Nociception

The nociceptive response to heat stimulation was measured using a paw thermal stimulation system. Briefly, the system consists of a clear plastic chamber (10×20×24 cm) that sits on a clear elevated glass floor and is temperature regulated at 30°C using a paw thermal stimulation system [10]. Each animal is placed in the plastic chamber for 15 min to acclimate. A radiant heat source mounted on a movable holder beneath the glass floor is positioned to deliver a thermal stimulus to the plantar side of the hind paw. When the animal withdraws the paw, a photocell detects interruption of a light beam reflection and the automatic timer shuts off. This method has a precision of ±0.05 s for measurement of paw withdrawal latency in seconds (PWL). To prevent thermal injury, the light beam is automatically discontinued at 20 s if the rat fails to withdraw its paw. Pain testing was done before STZ or vehicle injection (normal baseline) and at the end of the third week after injection (peripheral neuropathy baseline) to establish development of PDN. The PWLs were noted after AS or MIS injections (marked as AS/MIS) to confirm the effect of knock-down treatment and just before the pharmacological studies with mibefradil or morphine (marked as 0 hr).

Behavioral Assessment of mechanical sensitivity

To measure mechanical sensitivity, rats were placed in a clear plastic cage with a wire-mesh-bottom. The cage permits rats freedom of movement while allowing investigators access to their paws [11]. Von Frey filaments (Stoelting, Wood Dale, IL) were used to assess the mechanical threshold for paw withdrawal. These filaments are designated as the log10 (milligram weight required to cause bending ×10). We have found that applying the 5.18 filaments to the plantar surface of the foot causes a noxious response in female rats that results in an average of 4–5 paw withdrawal responses (PWRs) in 10 trials. Baseline withdrawal scores were determined in both paws to establish development of neuropathic pain prior to injections of AS, MIS, mibefradil or morphine using the same paradigm as for heat testing.

Behavioral Assessment of cold allodynia

The procedure was described in detail in [12,13]. Briefly, after a drop (50 μl) of acetone was sprayed onto the ventral side of the hind paw, we started to time the rats' reaction over the ensuing 20 s. No response (score = 0) was recorded if the rat did not withdraw, flick or stamp its paw. However, our observation period was increased to 40 s if the animal responded so that pain-related responses *per se* could be recorded. The scoring system was instituted following the criteria published by Flatters and Bennett [13]: 0, no response; 1, quick withdrawal, flick or stamp of the paw; 2, prolonged withdrawal or repeated flicking (at least two) of the paw; 3: repeated flicking of the paw with licking directed at the ventral side of the paw. The responses were obtained after acetone was applied alternately three times to each paw. Cumulative scores were generated with the minimum score being 0 (no response to any of the six trials) and the maximum possible score being 18 (repeated flicking and licking of paws on each of the six trials). Baseline cold scores were determined prior to and 3 weeks after injections of STZ. To assess the cooling effect of acetone we measured skin temperature post-acetone application and determined that there is about 3°C drop (from approximately 29.5°C to 26.5°C in SAL rats and from 28.0°C to 25.0°C in STZ rats over the course of 20 seconds; data not shown, n = 4 animals in each group). This is in accordance with previously published findings suggesting about a 4°C drop in skin temperature post-acetone application [14].

Computerized analyses of the areas under the curve

To analyze the areas under the curves, we first plotted the combined mean values from right and left paws. Once the computerized graphs were created, we calculated the mean areas under the curve so that we could perform *vis-à-vis* comparisons of either heat or mechanical responses in SAL- and STZ- rats. The superimposed areas under the curve were calculated using ImageJ (NIH) software.

Statistical analysis

Statistical analyses where performed using GraphPad Prism® software. We used two-way analysis of variance (ANOVA) to analyze within-subject variables, test session (before the administration of STZ or vehicle versus each post-treatment day) and between-subject variables (AS- or MIS-treated groups before and

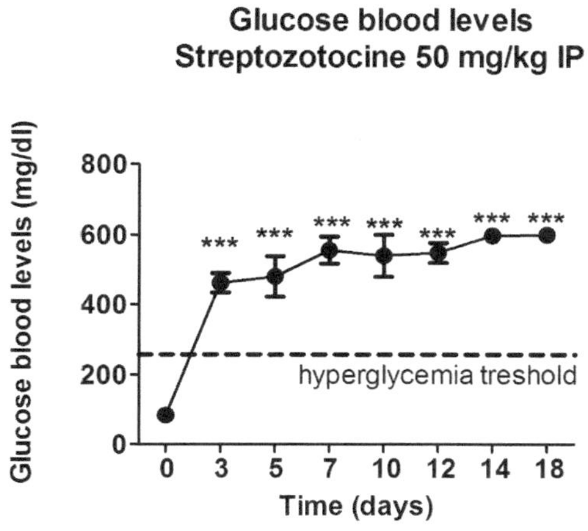

Figure 1. Systemically administered streptozotocine (STZ) induces severe hyperglycemia in adult female rats. Intraperitoneally (IP) injected STZ, at 50 mg/kg, resulted in high blood glucose levels within the first three days. The blood glucose levels reached 600 mg/dl (the limits of the glucometer) within two weeks post-treatment and remained elevated thereafter (***, $p<0.001$ compared to the baseline glucose level; dashed line marks the hyperglycemia threshold in rats; n = 5 rats per data point).

after administration of mibefradil or morphine). On the raw data, we used one-way ANOVA to confirm the efficacy of AS vs. MIS treatment. Relevant pair-wise comparisons were made and alpha levels were adjusted using the Bonferroni procedure when appropriate. We considered $p<0.05$ as being statistically significant. All data are presented as means ± SEM.

Western Blot Analysis of $Ca_V3.2$ channel protein expression

For the collection of lumbar DRGs, STZ-rats were deeply anesthetized with isoflurane and decapitated. Both right and left lumbar DRGs were rapidly extracted and dissected in phosphate buffer with a protease inhibitor cocktail (Roche, Germany), at which point they were rapidly frozen in liquid nitrogen. Tissue samples were homogenized in a phosphate buffer with protease inhibitor cocktail, sonicated and centrifuged at 12000 rpm for 10 min at 4°C to remove cell debris. Supernatants were collected and protein concentrations were determined using the Lowry method. Samples were combined with 2× Laemmli buffer (Sigma-Aldrich, St. Louis, MO, USA), boiled for 5 minutes, loaded into a 7.5% polyacrylamide gel and electrophoresed. Separated proteins were transferred to nitrocellulose membranes and blocked with 5% non-fat milk at room temperature for 1 hour. The membranes were incubated overnight in primary goat polyclonal antibodies directed at the C-terminus of the $Ca_V3.2$ channel (sc-16263, Santa Cruz Biothechology Inc, CA) or at the house-keeping protein actin (Sigma-Aldrich) at respective dilutions of 1:100 and 1:11,000, respectively. Appropriate horseradish peroxidase–conjugated secondary antibodies (anti-rabbit IgG, 1:10,000 for actin and 1:5000 for the $Ca_V3.2$ channel; Santa Cruz Biotechnology Inc, CA) were applied for 1 hour. The membranes were developed using enhanced chemiluminescence (ECL) detection reagents (GE Healthcare Life Sciences, Piscataway, NJ) and band density was quantified using Syngene Gel documentation, G-box analysis software (Syngene, USA). Densities for $Ca_V3.2$ channel bands were normalized to bands for actin, which was used as a housekeeping protein. Since saline and MIS treatments caused no changes in the expression of $Ca_V3.2$ channel protein expression, the data were combined and are presented as the MIS-control group. To determine the specificity of anti-$Ca_V3.2$ antibody, we performed Western Blot experiments under identical conditions with human embryonic kidney (HEK-293) cells stably transfected with either human $Ca_V3.1$ or $Ca_V3.2$ isoforms of T-channels. A main band of strong immunoreactivity at approximately 250 KD in the membrane fraction was present only in $Ca_V3.2$-transfected HEK-293 cells, not $Ca_V3.1$-transfected HEK-293 cells (n = 4 experiments in each group, data not shown).

Electrophysiological recordings

DRG cells from adolescent rats were prepared as previously described [15]. For recording, cells were plated onto uncoated glass coverslips, placed in a culture dish, and perfused with external solution. All *in vitro* experiments were done at room temperature.

Recording electrodes were pulled from borosilicate glass microcapillary tubes (Drummond Scientific, Broomall, PA); when filled with solution, they had resistances between 1 and 4 MΩ. We made recordings using an Axopatch 200B patch-clamp amplifier (Molecular Devices, Foster City, CA). Digitization of membrane voltages and currents was controlled using a Digidata 1322A interfaced with Clampex 8.2 or 9.0 (Molecular Devices). We analyzed data using Clampfit 8.2 or 9.0 (Molecular Devices) and Origin 7.0 (Microcal Software, Northampton, MA). Currents were low pass-filtered at 2–5 kHz. We took series resistance and capacitance values directly from readings of the amplifier after electronic subtraction of the capacitive transients. Series resistance was compensated to the maximum extent possible (usually 50%–80%). Multiple independently controlled glass syringes served as reservoirs for a gravity-driven perfusion system.

The external solution contained (in mM) 152 TEA-Cl, 2 $CaCl_2$, and 10 HEPES, adjusted to pH 7.4 with TEA-OH. For studies of well-isolated and well-clamped T-currents in acutely isolated DRG cells, we used only fluoride (F^-)-based internal solution to facilitate high voltage-activated (HVA) Ca^{2+} current rundown; this internal solution contained (in mM) 135 TMA-OH, 40 HEPES, 10 EGTA, and 2 $MgCl_2$, adjusted to pH 7.2 with hydrogen fluoride (HF). The amplitude of the T-current at any given potential was measured from the end of the pulse to its peak. Mibefradil was prepared as a 100 mM stock solution and freshly diluted to the final concentrations in the external solution at the time of experiments.

The percent reductions in peak T-current at various concentrations of mibefradil were used to generate concentration-response curves. Mean values were fit to the following Hill-Langmuir function:

$$PI([\text{Mibefradil}]) = PI_{max}/(1 + (IC_{50}/[\text{Mibefradil}])^h) \quad (1)$$

where PI_{max} is the maximal percent inhibition of peak current by mibefradil, IC_{50} is the concentration that produces 50% inhibition, and *h* is the apparent Hill-Langmuir coefficient for inhibition. The fitted values are reported with >95% linear confidence limits.

To study the effects of mibefradil on steady-state inactivation of T-channels, currents are evoked every 7 seconds by test steps to −40 mV after 3.5-sec pre-pulses to potentials ranging from −110 mV to −45 mV in 5 mV increments.

The voltage dependence of steady-state inactivation was described with a single Boltzmann distribution of the following form:

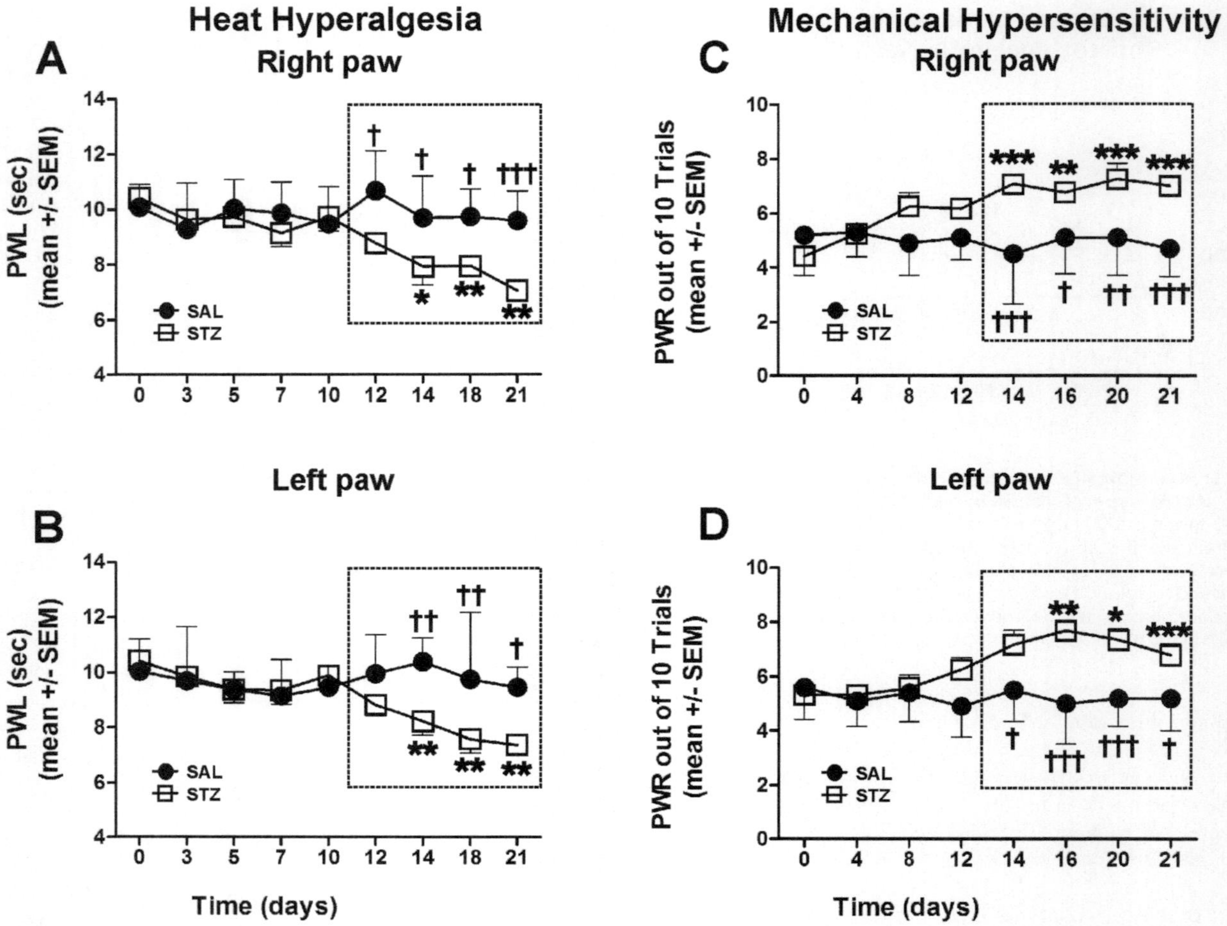

Figure 2. Diabetic rats develop significant heat hyperalgesia (A, C) and mechanical hypersensitivity (B, D). PWLs and PWRs were recorded starting with assessment of the baseline before STZ administration (0 day) followed by periodical assessment for the next 21 days (A, Right paw, B, Left paw). Although a decline in PWL was noted first on day 12, it did not reach significance until day 14 when it approached a steady state (marked with dashed rectangle) of heat hyperalgesia as compared with the baseline recordings (*, $p<0.05$; **, $p<0.01$). The PWLs recorded in SAL animals revealed no change compared with the baseline but a significant change compared with those of STZ animals from day 12 (A) and day 14 (B) (†, $p<0.05$; ††, $p<0.01$; †††, $p<0.001$). Note similar latencies recorded in left and right paws indicating the systemic nature of the disease (A and B). The steady rise in PWRs indicative of mechanical hypersensitivity started on day 12; PWRs became significant from 14 days post-STZ treatment as compared with the baseline PWR recordings (*, $p<0.05$; **, $p<0.01$; ***, $p<0.001$). The PWRs recorded in SAL animals revealed no changes compared with the baseline but a significant change compared with STZ animals from day 14 (†, $p<0.05$; ††, $p<0.01$; †††, $p<0.001$; n = 5 STZ rats and n = 5 SAL rats per data point in A and B; n = 6 STZ rats and n = 5 SAL rats per data point in C and D).

$$I(V) = I_{max}/(1 + \exp[(V - V_{50})/k]) \quad (2)$$

where I_{max} is the maximal activatable current, V_{50} is the voltage at which half the current is inactivated, and k is the voltage dependence (slope) of the distribution.

Results

Metabolic parameters

Body weights were assessed daily after SZT- or saline (SAL) injection. While body weights of control animals injected i.p. with saline (pH = 7.4) did not fluctuate much, there was about 10–18% weight loss in STZ-injected animals (data not shown).

Before assigning rats to either STZ (experimental) or SAL (control) groups, we determined their baseline blood glucose to be about 80 mg/dl. While blood glucose levels in the SAL group remained around that level throughout the experimental period (data not shown), STZ-animals developed severe hyperglycemia (over 400 mg/dl) within the first three days and it continued to worsen, exceeding 600 mg/dl (the limitation of the glucometer) in about two weeks (Figure 1). In addition, STZ-animals had increased water and food consumption during the first three weeks as well as an increase in urine output (thus mimicking clinical signs of diabetes, e.g. polydipsia, polyphagia and polyuria), but without any signs of general sickness due to ketoacidosis. Hence, we chose to conduct our behavioral tests during the 4th week (21 days post-STZ injection) when the clinical picture of poorly controlled diabetes was confirmed and yet general well-being of the animals was acceptable so as not to confound the studies of neuropathic pain behavior.

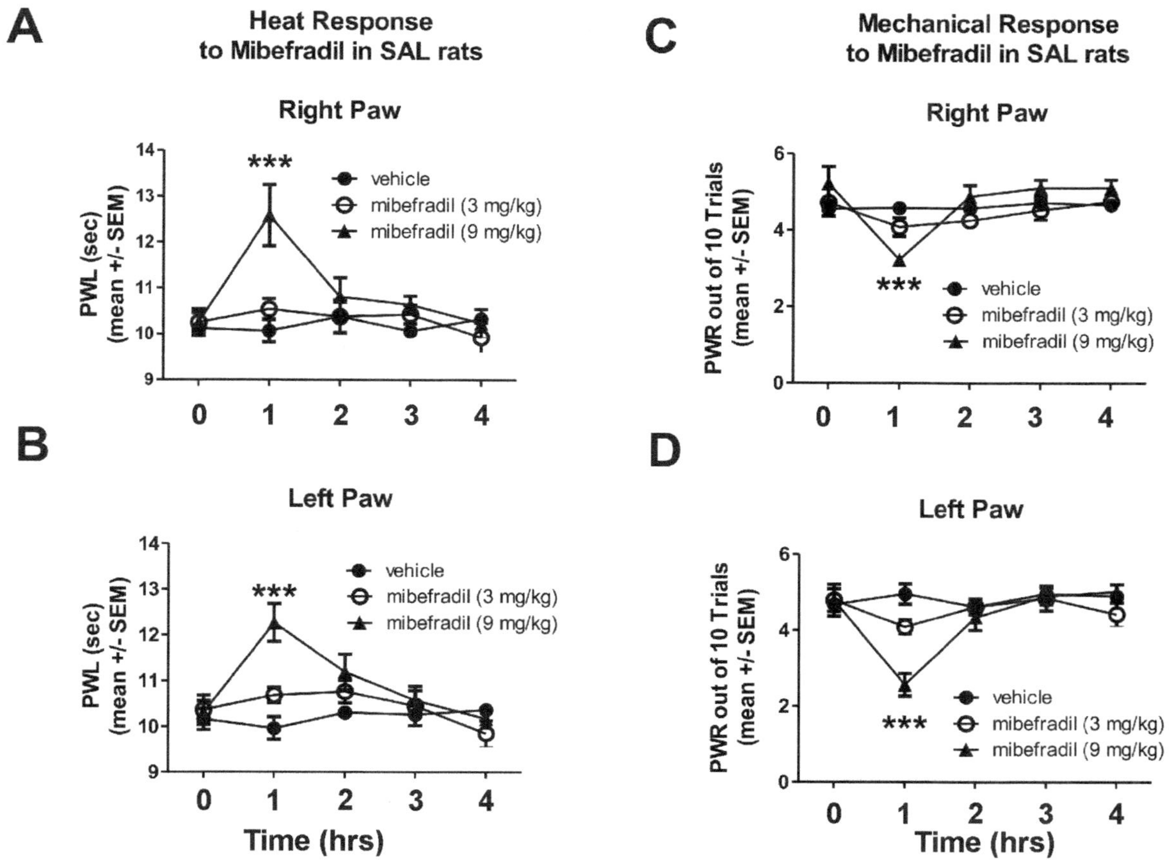

Figure 3. Mibefradil induces transient alleviation of heat and mechanical sensitivity in non-diabetic rats. Mibefradil at 9 mg/kg but not at 3 mg/kg causes significant, although transient, decrease in heat (***, $p<0.001$ at 1 hr compared to vehicle in both left and right paws; Panel A, right paw; B, left paw) and mechanical sensitivity (***, $p<0.001$ at 1 hr compared to vehicle in both paws; Panel C, right paw; D, left paw) in control (SAL)-rats (n = 3–9 rats per data point).

STZ-induced painful diabetic neuropathy is manifested by heat and mechanical hyperalgesia that is alleviated with mibefradil and $Ca_V3.2$ antisense

To study the development of PDN *in vivo*, we examined heat (PWLs; Figure 2A and B) and mechanical (PWRs; Figure 2C and D) sensitivities in STZ- and SAL-rats. Baseline heat and mechanical sensitivities were assessed before the assigned treatment (marked as day 0). Note similar responses recorded in the right (A and C) and left paws (B and D). As shown in Fig. 2A and B, PWLs started to decline approximately two weeks post STZ-injection (by about 20–25% compared with the baseline, *, $p<0.05$; **, $p<0.01$) and remained significantly decreased throughout the testing period, suggesting the development of heat hyperalgesia. Note that significant heat hyperalgesia (outlined with dashed rectangle) occurs about a week after the development of severe hyperglycemia (as shown in Fig. 1). The PWLs recorded from the SAL-rats during the same time period reveled minimal changes compared with the baseline and consequently, significant changes compared with PWLs in STZ-rats (†, $p<0.05$; ††, $p<0.01$; †††, $p<0.001$ starting from day 12- right paw and day 14- left paw).

Likewise, PWRs started to increase soon after STZ treatment and became significantly elevated in about 2 weeks (around 40–60% increase compared with the baseline PWRs; *, $p<0.05$; **, $p<0.01$; ***, $p<0.001$), suggesting the development of significant mechanical hypersensitivity (dashed rectangle; Fig. 2C and D). The PWRs recorded from the SAL-rats during the same time period reveled minimal changes compared with the baseline and consequently, significant changes compared with PWRs in STZ-rats (†, $p<0.05$; ††, $p<0.01$; †††, $p<0.001$ starting from day 14).

We conclude that the onsets of heat hyperalgesia and mechanical hypersensitivity, the hallmarks of PDN, coincide with the development of severe hyperglycemia (Fig. 1) although (as expected) the development of the behavioral indices of PDN lagged behind the development of metabolic indices of diabetes.

To investigate the role of peripheral T-channels in the development of painful PDN, we used two clinically relevant doses, 3 and 9 mg/kg, of mibefradil injected intraperitoneally (i.p.). At these two doses, mibefradil was shown previously to have transient analgesic effects in healthy rats without affecting their sensorimotor ability [16]. Furthermore, it has been shown that at these doses, mibefradil exhibits beneficial cardiovascular protective effects in rats [17–19]. Here we show that mibefradil at 9 mg/kg but not 3 mg/kg causes a significant, although transient, decrease in heat (***, $p<0.001$ at 1 hr compared with vehicle in both left and right paws; Fig. 3A, right paw; 3B-left paw) and mechanical (***, $p<0.001$ at 1 hr compared with vehicle in both paws; Fig. 3C, right paw; 3D, left paw) sensitivity in control (SAL)-rats.

However, in diabetic STZ-treated rats (Figure 4) with confirmed PDN (note the 0 h time point PWLs and PWRs compared to 0 h time point in Figure 3), mibefradil had a dose-dependent and more

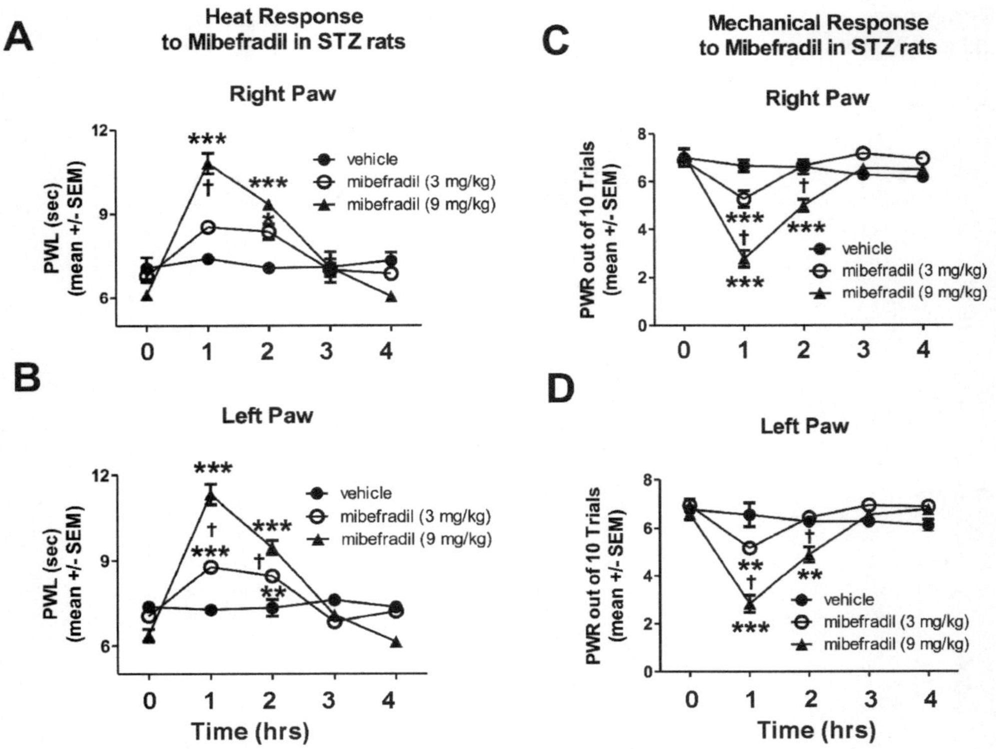

Figure 4. Mibefradil induces longer-lasting alleviation of heat hyperalgesia and mechanical hypersensitivity in diabetic rats. Mibefradil treatment was performed on day 21 when PDN was confirmed (see Figure 2). Mibefradil causes a dose-dependent profound effect on heat (**A**, right paw; **B**, left paw) and mechanical (**C**, right paw; **D**, left paw) hypersensitivity. The lower dose of mibefradil (3 mg/kg) caused a significant alleviation of heat hyperalgesia for the first couple of hours compared with a vehicle treatment (*, $p<0.05$; **, $p<0.01$; *** $p<0.001$). A higher dose (9 mg/kg) of mibefradil induced an even more profound effect (***, $p<0.001$ compared with vehicle); (†, $p<0.05$, ††† $p<0.001$, in mibefradil at 3 mg/kg compared to mibefradil at 9 mg/kg). Similarly, mibefradil induced dose-dependent, significant (both at lower and higher doses) alleviation of mechanical hypersensitivity in diabetic rats that lasted a couple of hours (**, $p<0.01$ and ***, $p<0.001$ compared with vehicle; †††, $p<0.001$ mibefradil at 3 mg/kg compared with mibefradil at 9 mg/kg) (n = 3–6 rats per data point).

profound effect on heat and mechanical hypersensitivity. For example, the lower dose of mibefradil (3 mg/kg) that was ineffective in SAL-rats caused significant alleviation of heat hyperalgesia in STZ-rats for the first couple of hours compared with a vehicle treatment (*, $p<0.05$, **, $p<0.01$ and ***, $p<0.001$; Fig. 4-A, right paw; 4-B, left paw) whereas at a higher dose (9 mg/kg), mibefradil induced even more profound and longer lasting effect (***, $p<0.001$ compared with vehicle in both paws; †, $p<0.05$ and †††, $p<0.001$, mibefradil at 3 mg/kg compared with mibefradil at 9 mg/kg). Note that PWLs and PWRs recordings at 0 h time point are as shown in Fig. 2 on day 21 post-STZ injection.

Similarly, mibefradil induced significant and dose-dependent alleviation of mechanical hypersensitivity in diabetic rats that was more pronounced and longer lasting than that observed in SAL-rats (Fig. 4- C, right paw; 4-D, left paw; **, $p<0.01$ and ***, $p<0.001$ compared with vehicle; †††, $p<0.001$ mibefradil at 3 mg/kg compared with mibefradil at 9 mg/kg).

These findings suggest that mibefradil is more effective in alleviating thermal and mechanical sensitivity in STZ- compared with SAL-rats in terms of duration and dose required to achieve the desired effect. To confirm this notion we conducted computerized analyses of the average areas under the curve for both paws and compared the thermal and mechanical response in SAL- and STZ-rats to either 3 or 9 mg/kg of mibefradil. As shown in schematic representation (Fig. 5), we found that a lower dose of mibefradil was about 3- to 4-fold more effective in STZ- compared with SAL-rats, both in terms of alleviating heat (A) and mechanical hyperalgesia (C). Interestingly, at a higher dose, the effectiveness of mibefradil (B and D) was somewhat less impressive (slightly less than 3-fold difference between SAL- and STZ-rats), presumably due to a ceiling effect.

To further validate the $Ca_V3.2$ T-channel as an important cellular target for pain-alleviating effects of mibefradil in PDN, we administered intrathecally every 12 hrs for a total of 4 doses an antisense oligodeoxynucleotide (AS) specific for the $Ca_v3.2$ T-channel or a mismatch oligodeoxynucleotide (MIS) as a control. At the end of the antisense/mismatch treatment we established two important elements: first, that the AS application resulted in a significant down-regulation of $Ca_V3.2$ T-channel protein expression in lumbar DRGs compared with MIS-Control (Fig. 6, *, $p<0.05$, n = 5 rats in MIS-control group and 4 rats in AS group), and second, that the AS-treated diabetic rats exhibited a significant decrease in heat and mechanical hypersensitivity as compared with MIS-treated diabetic rats (Fig. 7; 0 h time point marked as AS/MIS). Once the hypersensitivity was confirmed (**, $p<0.01$; ***, $p<0.001$ AS vs. MIS in both paws), mibefradil was administered (indicated with an arrow) and pain phenotype was assessed on an hourly basis. As illustrated in Fig. 7 (A, right paw; B, left paw) co-treatment with mibefradil (9 mg/kg i.p.) in AS-treated STZ-rats had no further effect on heat sensitivity, i.e., PWLs' recordings remained stable throughout the four-hour period post-

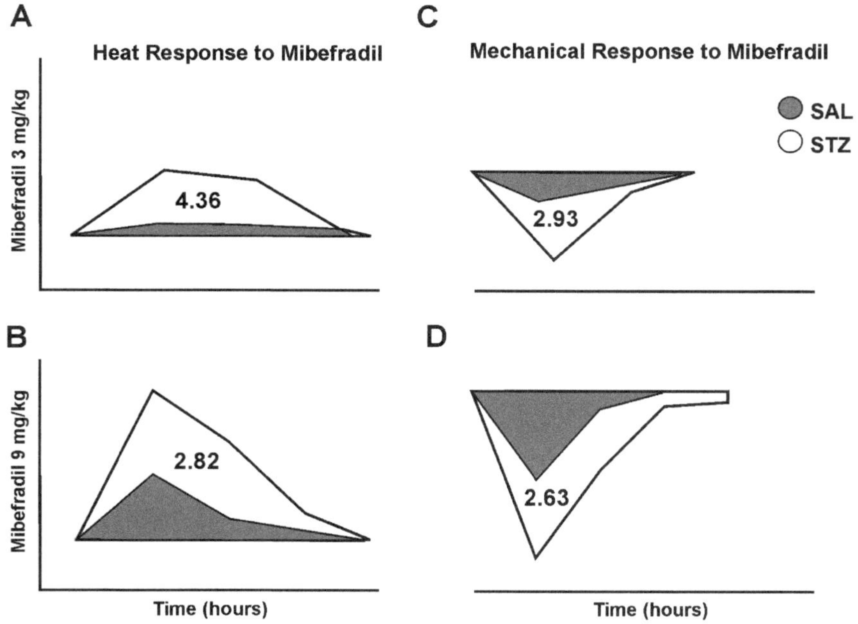

Figure 5. Schematic representation of the areas under the curves calculated from the thermal and mechanical responses to mibefradil recorded from SAL- and STZ-rats. Using computerized analyses of the actual data presented in Figs. 3 and 4, we calculated the average area under the curve for right and left paws in SAL- (shaded area) and STZ-rats (open area) in order to quantify and compare the antinociceptive effectiveness of mibefradil in SAL- and STZ-rats. At lower dose (3 mg/kg) we report higher effectiveness of mibefradil in alleviating heat (4.36-fold) (A) and mechanical sensitivity (2.93-fold) (C) in STZ-rats compared with SAL-rats. At a higher dose (9 mg/kg), we also report higher effectiveness of mibefradil [2.82-fold for heat sensitivity (B) and 2.63-fold for mechanical sensitivity (D)], although the effect is somewhat less impressive than that with the lower dose, most likely due to a ceiling effect.

mibefradil administration, suggesting that mibefradil and AS likely share the same cellular target. On the other hand, MIS-treated STZ-rats responded to mibefradil similarly to what we observed in

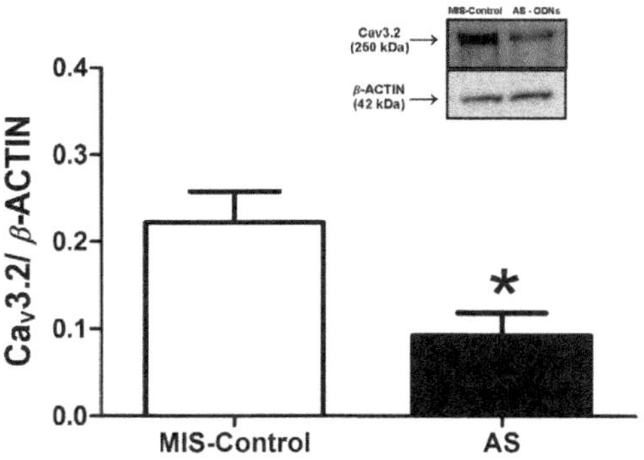

Figure 6. Intrathecal lumbar administration of AS induces significant down-regulation of the $Ca_V3.2$ channel protein expression in lumbar DRGs of STZ rats. Protein expression of $Ca_V3.2$ channel was analyzed and expressed as a ratio to that of the housekeeping protein β-actin. The bar graph shows that in AS-$Ca_V3.2$-treated rats (closed bar) we detected, on average, about a 60% decrease in $Ca_V3.2$ channel expression as compared with that of the MIS-control group (open bar; *, $p<0.05$). The protein measurement was performed 10 hours after the last AS-$Ca_V3.2$ injection. (n = 5 rats in MIS-control group; n = 4 rats in AS group). The insert illustrates original immunoblots from the representative experiments. (Since there was no difference in protein expression of $Ca_V3.2$ channel in STZ rats treated with either MIS or saline, the findings are compiled and presented as MIS-Control).

STZ-rats that did not receive either AS or MIS treatment (as shown in Fig. 4 A-right paw; B-left paw), i.e., mibefradil induced a significant increase in PWLs (†††, $p<0.001$ at 1 hr post-mibefradil injection in MIS STZ-rats compared to 0 h), further suggesting that the $Ca_V3.2$ T-channel is mibefradil's cellular target for alleviating thermal hypersensitivity in PDN (*, $p<0.05$ and ***, $p<0.001$ in AS vs. MIS rats post-mibefradil injection). Similarly, when mechanical sensitivity was assessed (Fig. 7; C, right paw; D, left paw), we observed significant alleviation of mechanical hypersensitivity in AS-treated diabetic rats (**, $p<0.01$; ***, $p<0.001$ in AS vs. MIS rats) and the effect was unchanged with mibefradil treatment. However, in MIS-treated diabetic rats in which mechanical hypersensitivity was unchanged compared with the baseline, mibefradil caused a significant decrease in PWRs (***, $p<0.001$, right paw; **, $p<0.01$, left paw), suggesting that $Ca_V3.2$ T-channels play an important role in mechanical hypersensitivity and are a likely cellular target of mibefradil's anti-PDN effects. Note that the assessment of mechanical sensitivity was initiated 1 h post mibefradil treatment when the effect was shown to be most significant (Fig. 3C and D).

Although not included in Fig. 7, our previously published work with SAL-AS-rats confirmed the importance of $Ca_V3.2$ T-channels in the development of thermal and mechanical hyperalgesia while showing a complete lack of pain phenotype in SAL-MIS-rats [1].

To probe further the mechanism of PDN in AS- or MIS-treated diabetic animals, we examined the antinociceptive response to a prototype opioid agent, morphine (10 mg/kg, i.p.). We found that morphine provided a similar decrease in heat nociceptive responses (Fig. 8A, right paw; 8B, left paw; †††, $p<0.001$ at 1–2 h after morphine injection) and mechanical nociceptive

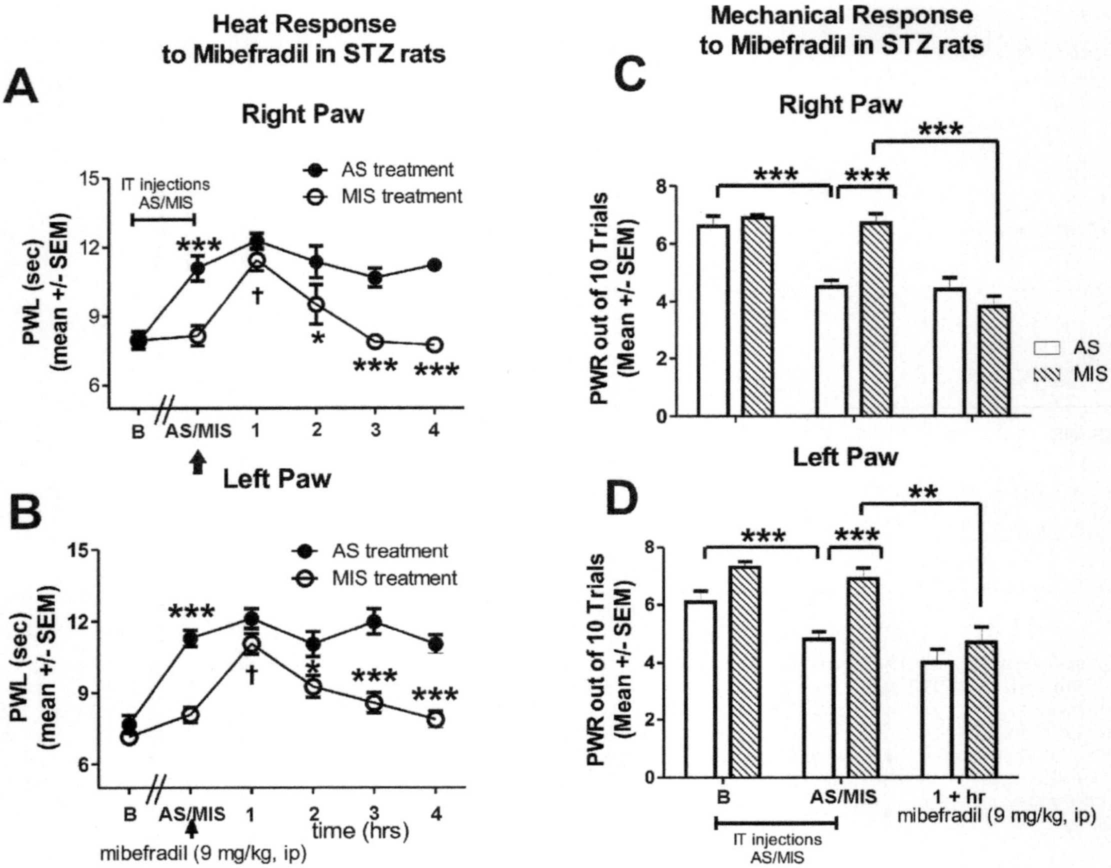

Figure 7. Knock-down of Ca$_V$3.2 abolishes mibefradil-induced alleviation of heat hyperalgesia and mechanical hypersensitivity in diabetic rats. Ca$_V$3.2 T-channels in sensory neurons were knocked-down with intrathecal administration (every 12 hrs for a total of 4 doses) of oligodeoxynucleotide (AS) specific for the Ca$_V$3.2 T-channels. Controls were given mismatch oligodeoxynucleotide (MIS). Heat hyperalgesia was quantified with PWLs (A, right paw; B, left paw) and mechanical hypersensitivity was measured using PWRs (C, right paw; D, left paw). Compared with baseline recordings (marked as B), AS-treated diabetic rats exhibited a significant increase in PWLs (***, $p<0.001$) and a significant decrease in PWRs (***, $p<0.001$; marked as AS/MIS). At that point, mibefradil was administered (indicated with an arrow) and heat hyperalgesia was assessed hourly. Mibefradil (at 9 mg/kg i.p.) had no further effect to alleviate heat hyperalgesia; i.e., PWLs recordings remained stable (and significantly elevated compared with the MIS-treated STZ rats; *, $p<0.05$; ***, $p<0.001$) throughout the four-hour period post-mibefradil administration (closed circles). In MIS-treated diabetic rats, mibefradil induced a transient increase in PWLs (†, $p<0.05$ at 1 hr post-injection). Mechanical sensitivity assessment was initiated 1 h post mibefradil treatment when the effect was shown to be most significant (as indicated in Fig. 3C and D). PWRs in AS-treated diabetic rats post-mibefradil injection remain unchanged whereas in MIS-treated diabetic rats there was a significant effect of mibefradil marked by a decrease in PWRs (***, $p<0.001$, right paw; **, $p<0.01$, left paw; n = 5 rats per data point).

responses (Fig. 8C, right paw, †, $p<0.05$; and 8D, left paw, †, $p<0.05$; ††, $p<0.01$) in both AS- and MIS-treated diabetic groups, indicating that morphine's anti-nociceptive effects most likely are not mediated through Ca$_v$3.2 T-channels. Note the significant upward shift in PWLs (A and B) and a significant downward shift in PWRs (C and D) in AS- compared with MIS-treated diabetic rats, indicating the shift in pain baseline due to Ca$_V$3.2 T-channel knock-down (*, $p<0.05$; **, $p<0.01$; ***, $p<0.001$).

STZ-induced painful diabetic neuropathy is manifested by cold allodynia that is alleviated by mibefradil and Ca$_V$3.2 antisense but not by morphine

Since cold allodynia is another important symptom of PDN [20,21] and the importance of T-channels in its development remains unknown, we explored the putative roles of T-channels in cold allodynia in STZ-treated rats. Unlike SAL-treated rats that do not have any response to cold stimulus, STZ-rats when tested on the 21st post-STZ treatment day, show obvious signs of cold allodynia [baseline (B) cold scores around 10 noted at 0 hrs; Fig. 9]. Once cold allodynia was confirmed, we performed AS/MIS and pharmacological experiments with mibefradil or morphine during the 4th week (starting from the 21st day post-STZ injection) as described for heat and mechanical testing. We found that mibefradil induced dose-dependent alleviation of cold allodynia in diabetic rats as compared with vehicle treatment. For instance, mibefradil, at 9 mg/kg i.p., caused an approximate 45% decrease in pain scores (**, $p<0.01$) compared with vehicle treatment, an effect that lasted a couple of hours (Fig. 9A). Similar to the effects of mibefradil on heat and mechanical hypersensitivity, the antiallodynic effect of mibefradil was not detected in AS-treated STZ-rats, but was significant in MIS-treated STZ rats (†, $p<0.05$ before mibefradil vs. 1+ post-treatment; Fig. 9B), again suggesting that AS and mibefradil share the same cellular target for alleviation of cold allodynia. Note a significant decrease in cold allodynia in AS-treated STZ rats when compared to baseline recordings (†††, $p<0.001$) and compared with MIS-treated STZ-

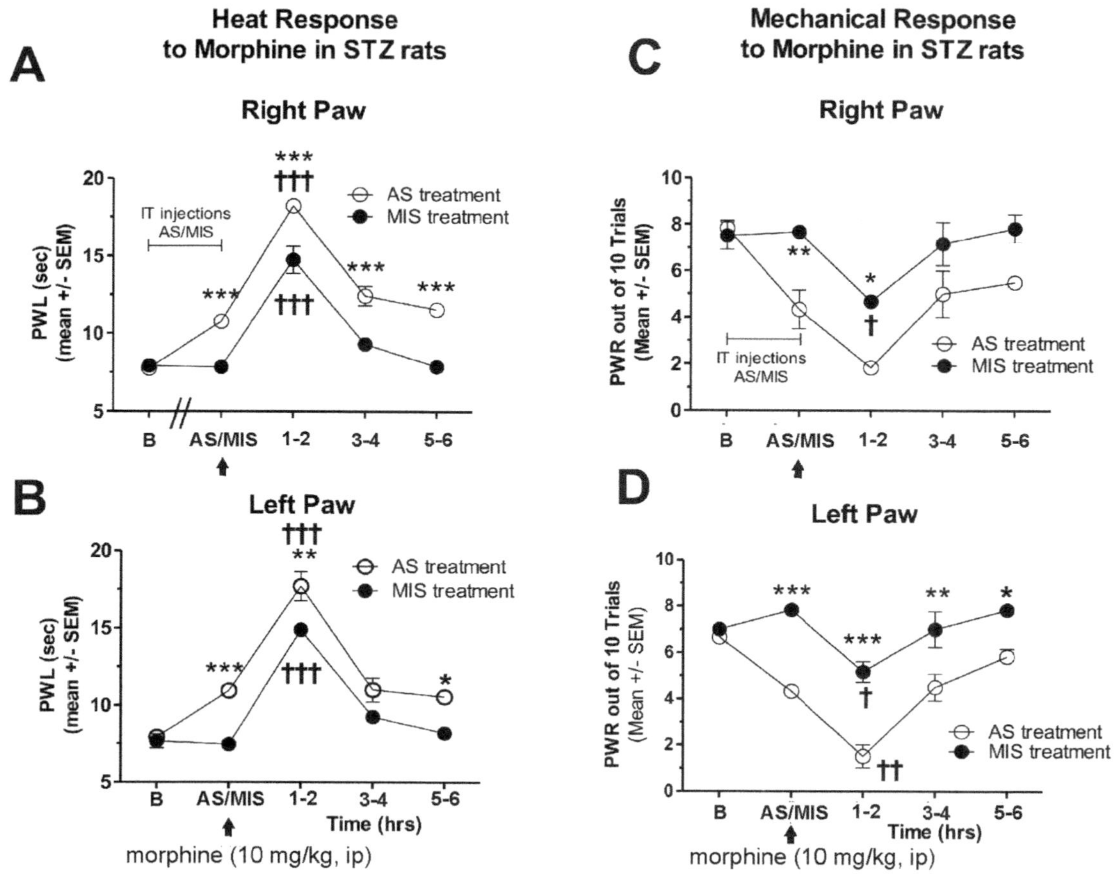

Figure 8. Knock-down of Cav3.2 has no effect on morphine-induced alleviation of heat and mechanical hypersensitivity. $Ca_V3.2$ T-channels in sensory neurons were knocked down with intrathecal administration (every 12 hrs for a total of 4 doses) of oligodeoxynucleotide (AS) specific for the $Ca_V3.2$ T-channels. Controls were given mismatch oligodeoxynucleotide (MIS). Heat hyperalgesia was quantified with PWLs (A, right paw; B, left paw) and mechanical hypersensitivity was measured using PWRs (C, right paw; D, left paw). The response to morphine (10 mg/kg, i.p.) in AS-treated diabetic rats mimicked the response in MIS-treated diabetic rats in that both groups exhibited change of PWLs and PWRs at around 1–2 hrs post morphine injection (†, $p<0.001$ compared with before injection in A and B; †, $p<0.05$ compared to before injection in C and D) except that there was a notable upward shift in the PWLs and a downward shift in the PWRs in AS-treated diabetic rats due to $Ca_V3.2$ T-channel knock down (*, $p<0.05$; **, $p<0.01$; ***, $p<0.001$ in AS vs. MIS treatment; n = 3 rats per data point).

rats (***, $p<0.001$). Finally, we show that unlike mibefradil, morphine was completely ineffective in alleviating cold allodynia in both AS- and MIS-diabetic rats (Fig. 9C). Note that there was a similar decrease in cold allodynia in AS-treated STZ rats compared to baseline recordings (††, $p<0.01$) and compared to MIS-treated STZ-rats (***, $p<0.001$).

Mibefradil inhibits isolated DRG T-currents in diabetic rats in a voltage-dependent manner

We have demonstrated previously that mibefradil blocks isolated DRG T-currents in healthy rats in a voltage-dependent manner [15]. To examine whether mibefradil also inhibits T-currents in a voltage-dependent manner in diabetic rats, we performed voltage-clamp experiments using acutely dissociated DRG neurons (<35 μm) (Figure 10). Representative T-current traces before and after application of 1 μM mibefradil are shown in Fig. 10A and average currents are shown in Fig. 10B. For these studies we used our standard double pulse protocols wherein pre-pulses at different voltages serve to remove inactivation of T-channels (see Materials and Methods). A fit of the average data points with a Boltzmann function (solid lines in Fig. 10B) revealed that mibefradil shifted the steady-state inactivation from a pre-drug value of −71 mV (black solid line) to −87 mV (gray solid line). We next used escalating concentrations (0.1–3 μM) of mibefradil under identical recording conditions to determine its potency in blocking DRG T-currents in healthy and diabetic rats. Fig. 10C summarizes these experiments. The solid lines are best fits of a Hill function to average data points and yield an IC_{50} for T-current inhibition in healthy rats of 0.6 μM and in diabetic rats of 0.3 μM. Even though mibefradil was somewhat more potent in blocking T-currents from diabetic than from healthy rats, there was no statistically significant difference in the amplitudes of blocked currents with 1 μM and 0.3 μM mibefradil between the two groups (Fig. 10C). Thus, we conclude that mibefradil is a more effective blocker of T-channels at depolarized membrane potential and that it inhibits with similar potency DRG T-currents in healthy and diabetic rats.

Discussion

In this study we confirm that peripheral $Ca_V3.2$ T-channels are important cellular targets for the development of drugs effective in PDN. Using *in vivo* antisense technology and pharmacological

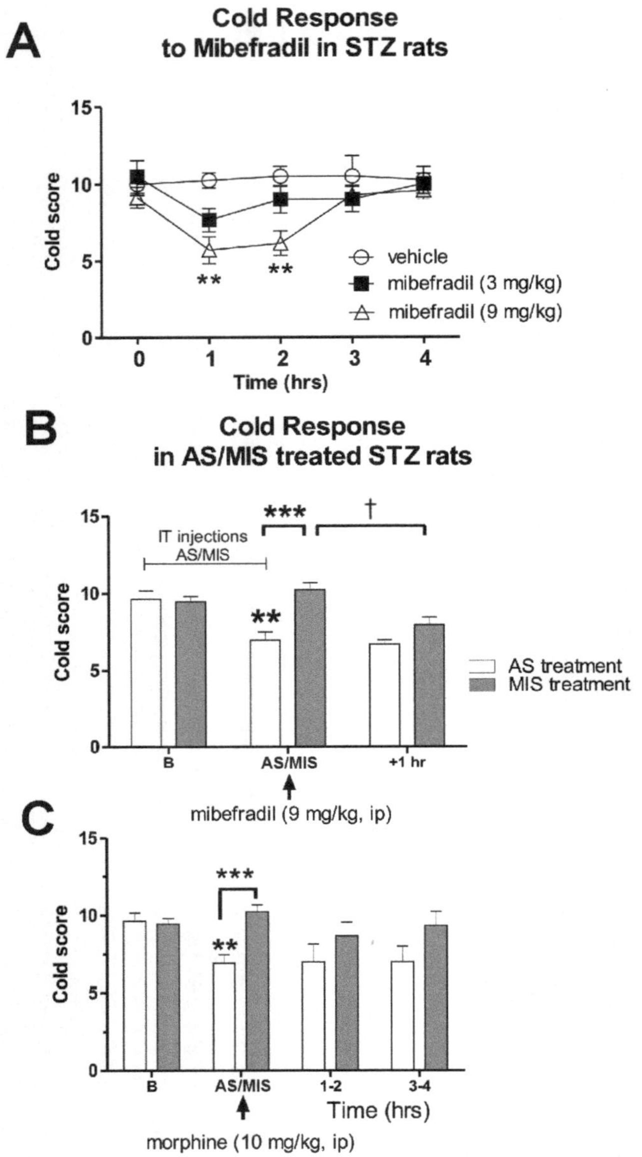

Figure 9. Mibefradil and Cav3.2 antisense are effective in alleviating diabetic cold allodynia. $Ca_v3.2$ T-channels in sensory neurons were knocked down with intrathecal administration (every 12 hrs for a total of 4 doses) of oligodeoxynucleotide (AS) specific for the $Ca_v3.2$ T-channels. Controls were given mismatch oligodeoxynucleotide (MIS). Cold allodynia was quantified using cold score (see Methods). **A**) Mibefradil induced dose-dependent alleviation of cold allodynia in diabetic rats compared with vehicle treatment. At 9 mg/kg, i.p., it caused approximately a 45% decrease in pain scores (**, $p<0.01$) compared with vehicle treatment, an effect that lasted a couple of hours. Although mibefradil, at 3 mg/kg, i.p., induced a slight decrease in cold scores, the effect was very transient and non-significant. **B**) AS-$Ca_V3.2$ treatment had significant antiallodynic effect compared with the baseline (†††, $p<0.001$) and MIS-treatment (***, $p<0.001$). The antiallodynic effect of mibefradil was blocked with AS-$Ca_V3.2$ (i.e., cold scores in AS-treated animals before and after mibefradil injection were not different), but not with MIS-$Ca_V3.2$ (i.e. there was a significant decrease in cold scores in MIS-treated animals after mibefradil treatment compared with cold scores before the treatment; †, $p<0.01$). **C**) Unlike mibefradil, morphine was completely ineffective in alleviating cold allodynia in both AS- and MIS-diabetic rats at any of the time points. (††, $p<0.01$ in AS-treated diabetic animals compared with the baseline; ***, $p<0.001$ compared with MIS-treated diabetic animals) (n = 3–11 rats per data point).

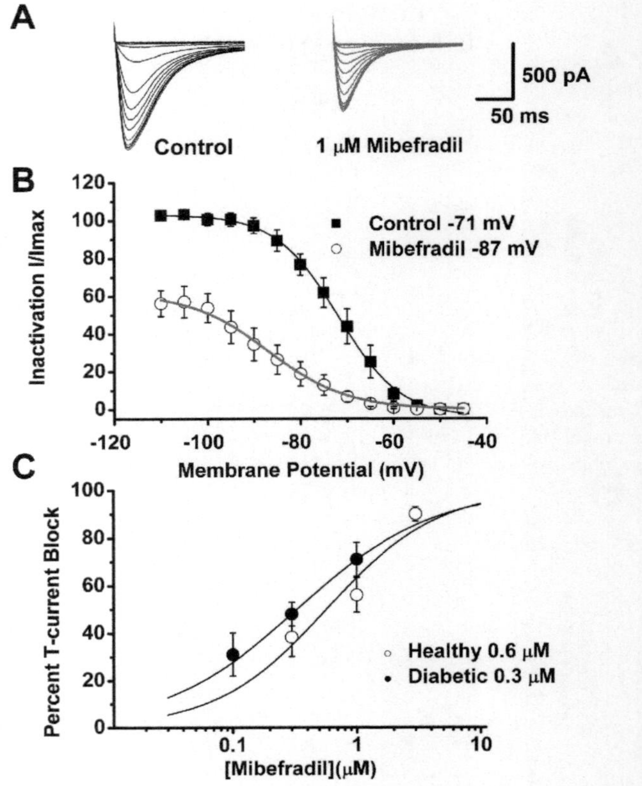

Figure 10. Voltage-dependent blockade of DRG T-currents in diabetic rats by mibefradil. A: Original traces from the same representative DRG cell from a diabetic rat. We used our standard double-pulse protocol (currents are evoked every 7 seconds by test steps to −40 mV after 3.5-sec pre-pulses to potentials ranging from −110 mV to −45 mV in 5 mV increments) to generate steady-state inactivation curves under control conditions (black traces) and after 5 minutes of application of 1 μM mibefradil (gray traces). Calibration bars pertain to both panels. **B**: Averaged data from 6 cells obtained before (■) and after applications of 1 μM mibefradil (○) in the same cells. Data points are averages of multiple determinations with vertical bars representing ± SEM. Solid lines are best fits using the Boltzmann equation (2) for control (solid black line) and mibefradil (solid gray line). Peak currents are normalized to the values of T-currents at pre-pulses of −110 mV in control (predrug) conditions. Mibefradil induced a hyperpolarizing shift in steady-state inactivation curves of about 16 mV (control V_{50} −87±1 mV versus mibefradil V_{50} −71±1 mV). There was a smaller change in the slope of the curve from 6.6±0.3 mV to 8.5±0.8 mV in the presence of mibefradil. **C**: This panel summarizes the average percent inhibition of T-currents in DRG cells by escalating concentrations of mibefradil (holding potential of −90 mV and test potential of −40 mV every 7 seconds) in healthy (○) and diabetic (●) rats. Solid lines are best fits of data points using the Hill equation (1) yielding IC_{50} and slope (n) values as follows for control rats (IC_{50} = 0.6±0.2 μM, n = 1.0±0.4) and for diabetic rats (IC_{50} = 0.3±0.1 μM, n = 0.8±0.1). All fits are constrained to 100% maximal inhibition. Each data point is averaged from at least 5 different cells (control rats total of 24 cells; diabetic rats total of 20 cells). Short vertical black bars indicate ± SEM.

inhibition with mibefradil, we have shown that down-regulation of $Ca_V3.2$ T-channels has significant therapeutic effects on the most important and the most difficult-to-treat signs of PDN – heat and mechanical hypersensitivity and cold allodynia. In addition, using *in vitro* patch-clamp recordings, we show that mibefradil inhibits T-currents in a voltage-dependent manner and with similar potency in control DRG neurons from control SAL-treated rats and DRG neurons from diabetic STZ-treated rats.

Recent studies have implicated pharmacological agents that target $Ca_V3.2$ T-channels as important regulators of the cellular excitability of nociceptors and have suggested their usefulness in treating neuropathic pain in different animal models (reviewed in [22]). One such drug, mibefradil, has been used extensively for functional studies of T-channels including studies of their role in nociceptive transmission. Mibefradil was marketed by Hoffmann-LaRoche primarily as a peripherally acting antihypertensive drug. We studied mibefradil since, to our knowledge, it is the only peripherally-acting T-channel blocker that is widely available. Mibefradil has been shown to block preferentially T-currents at low micro- and nanomolar concentrations in vascular smooth muscle [23,24] and cerebellar Purkinje cells [25]. Hence, it was considered, for a while, to be a promising selective and potent T-channel blocker. Further studies have shown that mibefradil exhibits voltage- and use-dependent inhibition of T-currents in acutely dissociated small DRG neurons *in vitro*. These properties could be beneficial for its use in pain disorders, given that the drug is more active in affecting channels in depolarized and actively firing neurons [15]. Indeed, ensuing *in vivo* studies have shown that mibefradil has mild analgesic properties in healthy rats [16] and prominent antihyperalgesic properties in rats with neuropathic pain from chronic constrictive injury (CCI) of the sciatic nerve [26]. Particularly exciting was the fact that when marketed in Europe as an antihypertensive agent, mibefradil was well tolerated, presumably due to its poor penetration into the CNS – although it consequently was withdrawn from the market due to unwanted drug-drug interactions. Studies have since indicated that mibefradil blocks not only low-voltage activated-type calcium T-currents, but also high-voltage-activated (HVA)-type calcium and other voltage-gated currents (e.g., I_{Na+} and I_{K+}) at low μM concentrations, thus casting doubt on its usefulness as a selective T-channel blocker [27–29].

The intriguing possibility that the analgesic properties of mibefradil that we and others have reported may not be related to its blockade of T-channels in peripheral nociceptors must be raised, since its selectivity in blocking T-channels in DRG neurons is questionable. However, several lines of evidence in our present study strongly suggest that the analgesic actions of mibefradil are, indeed, mediated by peripheral T-channel blockade. First, we show that the antihyperalgesic effect of mibefradil in PDN was fully mimicked by knock-down of $Ca_V3.2$ channels in DRG cells using specific AS; second, we show that in animals pretreated with $Ca_V3.2$ AS, mibefradil was completely ineffective in further affecting thermal and mechanical sensitivities, while its antihyperalgesic properties in $Ca_V3.2$ MIS animals was maintained, thus suggesting that mibefradil shares the same cellular target as $Ca_V3.2$ AS. In contrast, we show that the anti-hyperalgesic effect of morphine, a prototype opioid analgesic, was not affected by $Ca_V3.2$ AS or MIS pretreatment. Consistent with these results, it has been shown that T-currents in small DRG cells are insensitive to opiod agonists [30] and that the response of Cav3.2 knock-out mice to morphine was essentially identical to that of wild type mice [31]. Since mibefradil poorly penetrates the CNS and its effects are mostly confined to peripheral targets [23,24], its use is not known to cause the sedation that is often encountered with pain killers commonly used in PDN (such as gabapentin and related drugs) [32,33]. Indeed, we have demonstrated previously that systemic administration of mibefradil at 9 mg/kg i.p. did not affect sensorimotor performance of rats [16]. Hence, we suggest that peripheral analogs of mibefradil that are more selective and perhaps more potent should be developed since they may prove useful not only in the functional studies of T-channels, but in the development of clinical analgesics for patients with painful PDN and other chronic pain disorders. Collectively, our data strongly suggest that $Ca_V3.2$ channels in sensory neurons are important target for the prominent analgesic effects of mibefradil. However, the possible contribution of other ion channels to its analgesic effects cannot be excluded. Future biophysical and molecular studies employing knock-down of other nociceptive ion channels in DRG cells from diabetic rats will be needed to address this issue.

Another important novel finding of this study is that both mibefradil treatment and $Ca_V3.2$ AS, but not morphine, greatly attenuated cold allodynia scores in diabetic rats. Similar to our observations with heat hyperalgesia and mechanical hypersensitivity, mibefradil failed to modulate cold allodynia scores in diabetic animals pretreated with $Ca_V3.2$ AS but it was still effective in animals pretreated with $Ca_V3.2$ MIS, further suggesting that mibefradil and $Ca_V3.2$ AS share the same cellular target. This finding also points at T-channels as a promising cellular target for treating hypersensitivity to cold stimuli in patients with PDN. Cold allodynia is a common sign of neuropathic pain in patients and in animal models of PDN [20,21] but its underlying mechanisms remain poorly understood. This poor understanding is, at least in part, due to the fact that ion channels involved in cold transduction are not fully characterized. Recent data with agents targeting transient receptor potential (TRP) channels (especially TRPA1 and TRPM8) suggest that these channels are promising targets in developing treatments for cold allodynia [21]. However, very little is known about the role of T-channels in cold transduction pathways in the context of PDN. *In vitro* studies with small DRG neurons have shown that cold, similarly to heat, evokes inward currents in sensory neurons such that the somas fire multiple action potentials, which resemble burst firing [33]. This multiple firing is relevant to our study since T-channels are key regulators of cellular excitability and burst firing in small DRG neurons [34,35]. Although T-currents have been recorded in cold-sensitive sensory neurons [36], their role in excitability of cold-sensitive neurons has not been studied. Our *in vivo* data strongly suggest a supportive role of T-channels in cold-induced neuronal transduction. Further cellular and molecular studies are needed to investigate this notion, especially since T-channel blockers may be very effective in treating cold allodynia in diabetic patients, a debilitating condition very refractive to conventional treatment.

In conclusion, our data indicate that blocking T-channels with the peripherally-acting, voltage-dependent agent mibefradil strongly attenuates diabetes-induced heat, cold and mechanical hypersensitivity in STZ-treated rats. These results suggest that further experimental and clinical studies can open avenues for the pharmacological development of novel and more specific therapies targeting ion channels in peripheral nociceptors. This approach could be useful for pain control in patients with diabetic neuropathy while minimizing side effects.

Acknowledgments

Parts of this study were presented at the 41th Annual Society for Neuroscience Meeting, Washington DC, November 2011. We thank Dr. Nathan Poiro and Dr. Benjamin Messenger for technical assistance.

Author Contributions

Conceived and designed the experiments: ALJO SMT VJT. Performed the experiments: ALJO SMH JS SJH. Analyzed the data: ALJO VJT SMT. Wrote the paper: ALJO SMT VJT.

References

1. Messinger RB, Naik AK, Jagodic MM, Nelson MT, Lee WY, et al. (2009) In-vivo silencing of the Cav3.2 T-type calcium channels in sensory neurons alleviates hyperalgesia in rats with streptozocin-induced diabetic neuropathy. Pain 145: 184–195.
2. Jagodic MM, Pathirathna S, Nelson MT, Mancuso S, Joksovic PM, et al. (2007) Cell-specific alterations of T-type calcium current in painful diabetic neuropathy enhance excitability of sensory neurons. J Neurosci 27: 3305–3316.
3. Khomula EV, Viatchenko-Karpinski VY, Borisyuk AL, Duzhyy DE, Belan PV, et al. (2013) Specific functioning of Cav3.2 T-type calcium and TRPV1 channels under different types of STZ-diabetic neuropathy. Biochim Biophys Acta 1832: 636–649.
4. Latham JR, Pathirathna S, Jagodic MM, Choe WJ, Levin ME, et al. (2009) Selective T-type calcium channel blockade alleviates hyperalgesia in ob/ob mice. Diabetes 58: 2656–2665.
5. Choe WJ, Messinger RB, Leach E, Eckle V-S, Obradovic A, et al. (2011) TTA-P2 is a potent and selective blocker of T-type calcium channels in rat sensory neurons and a novel antinociceptive agent. Mol Pharm 80: 900–910.
6. Kraus RL, Li Y, Gregan Y, Gotter AL, Uebele VN, et al. (2010) In vitro characterization of T-type calcium channel antagonist TTA-A2 and in vivo effects on arousal in mice. J Pharmacol Exp Ther 335: 409–17.
7. Uebele VN, Gotter AL, Nuss CE, Kraus RL, Doran SM, et al. (2009) Antagonism of T-type calcium channels inhibits high-fat diet-induced weight gain in mice. J Clin Invest 119: 1659–67.
8. Naik AK, Pathirathna S, Jevtovic-Todorovic V (2008) $GABA_A$ receptor modulation in dorsal root ganglia in vivo affects chronic pain after nerve injury. Neuroscience 154: 1539–1553.
9. Bourinet E, Alloui A, Monteil A, Barrere C, Couette B, et al. (2005) Silencing of the Cav3.2 T-type calcium channel gene in sensory neurons demonstrates its major role in nociception. EMBO J 24: 315–324.
10. Hargreaves K, Dubner R, Brown F, Flores C, Joris J (1988) A new and sensitive method for measuring thermal nociception in cutaneous hyperalgesia. Pain 32: 77–88.
11. Chaplan SR, Bach FW, Pogrel JW, Chung JM, Yaksh TL (1994) Quantitative assessment of tactile allodynia in the rat paw. J Neurosci Methods 53: 55–63.
12. Choi Y, Yoon YW, Na HS, Kim SH, Chung JM (1994) Behavioral signs of ongoing pain and cold allodynia in a rat model of neuropathic pain. Pain 59: 369–76.
13. Flatters SJ, Bennett GJ (2004) Ethosuximide reverses paclitaxel- and vincristine-induced painful peripheral neuropathy. Pain 109: 150–61.
14. Hulse RP, Donaldson LF, Wynick D (2012) Differential roles of galanin on mechanical and cooling responses at the primary afferent nociceptor. Mol Pain 6: 8–41
15. Todorovic SM, Lingle CJ (1998) Pharmacological properties of T-type Ca^{2+} current in adult rat sensory neurons: Effects of anticonvulsant and anesthetic agents. J Neurophysiol 79: 240–252.
16. Todorovic SM, Meyenburg A, Jevtovic-Todorovic V (2002) Mechanical and thermal antinociception in rats following systemic administration of mibefradil, a T-type calcium channel blocker. Brain Research 951: 336–340.
17. Karam H, Clozel JP, Bruneval P, Gonzalez MF, Ménard J (1999) Contrasting effects of selective T- and L-type calcium channel blockade on glomerular damage in DOCA hypertensive rats. Hypertension 34: 673–8.
18. Paquette F, Jasmin G, Dumont L (1999) Cardioprotective efficacy of verapamil and mibefradil in young UM-X7.1 cardiomyopathic hamsters. Cardiovasc Drugs Ther 13: 525–30.
19. Sandmann S, Claas R, Cleutjens JP, Daemen MJ, Unger T (2001) Calcium channel blockade limits cardiac remodeling and improves cardiac function in myocardial infarction-induced heart failure in rats. J Cardiovasc Pharmacol 37: 64–77.
20. Barrière DA, Rieusset J, Chanteranne D, Busserolles J, Chauvin MA, et al. (2012) Paclitaxel therapy potentiates cold hyperalgesia in streptozotocin-induced diabetic rats through enhanced mitochondrial reactive oxygen species production and TRPA1 sensitization. Pain 153: 553–61.
21. Szallasi A (2013) Targeting TRP channels for pain relief. Eur J Pharmacol Epub 716: 61–76.
22. Todorovic SM, Jevtovic-Todorovic V (2011) T-type voltage-gated calcium channel as targets for the developments of novel pain therapies. Brit J Pharmacol 163: 484–495.
23. Clozel J-P, Ertel EA, Ertel I (1997) Discovery and main pharmacological properties of mibefradil (R0 40-5967), the first selective T-type calcium channel blocker. J Hypertension Suppl 15: S17–S25.
24. Ertel SI, Ertel EA, Clozel J (1997) T-type Ca^{2+} channels and pharmacological blockade: potential pathophysiological relevance. Cardiovascular Drugs and Therapy 11:723–739.
25. McDonough SI, Bean BP (1998) Mibefradil inhibition of T-type calcium channels in cerebellar purkinje neurons. Mol Pharm 54:1080–1087.
26. Dogrul A, Gardell LR, Ossipov MH, Tulunay FC, Lai J, et al. (2003) Reversal of experimental neuropathic pain by T-type calcium channel blockers. Pain 105:159–168.
27. Jimenez C, Bourinet E, Leuranguer V, Richard S, Snutch TP, et al. (2000) Determinants of voltage-dependent inactivation affect Mibefradil block of calcium channels. Neuropharmacology 39: 1–10.
28. McNulty MM, Hanck DA (2004) State-dependent mibefradil block of Na+ channels. Mol Pharmacol 66:1652–1661.
29. Viana F, Van den Bosch L, Missiaen L, Vandenberghe W, Droogmans G, et al. (1997) Mibefradil (Ro 40-5967) blocks multiple types of voltage-gated calcium channels in cultured rat spinal motoneurones. Cell Calcium 22: 299–311.
30. Wu ZZ, Chen SR, Pan HL (2004) Differential sensitivity of N- and P/Q-type Ca2+ channel currents to a mu opioid in isolectin B4-positive and -negative dorsal root ganglion neurons. J Pharmacol Exp Ther 311: 939–47.
31. Barbara G, Alloui A, Nargeot J, Lory P, Eschalier A, et al. (2009) T-type calcium channel inhibition underlies the analgesic effects of the endogenous lipoamino acids. J Neurosci 29: 13106–14.
32. Edwards JL, Vincent AM, Cheng HT, Feldman EL (2008) Diabetic neuropathy: Mechanisms to management. Pharmacology & Therapeutics 120: 1–34.
33. Reid G, Flonta ML (2001) Physiology. Cold current in thermoreceptive neurons. Nature 413: 480.
34. Nelson MT, Joksovic PM, Perez-Reyes E, Todorovic SM (2005) The endogenous redox agent L-cysteine induces T-type Ca2+ channel-dependent sensitization of a novel subpopulation of rat peripheral nociceptors. J Neurosci 25: 8766–8775.
35. Nelson MT, Woo J, Kang H-W, Barrett PQ, Vitko J, et al. (2007) Reducing agents sensitize C-type nociceptors by relieving high-affinity zinc inhibition of T-type calcium channels. J Neurosci 27: 8250–8260.
36. Viana F, de la Pena E, Belmonte C (2002) Specificity of cold thermotransduction is determined by differential ionic channel expression. Nat Neurosci 5: 254–260.

9

Central Pain Processing in Chronic Chemotherapy-Induced Peripheral Neuropathy: A Functional Magnetic Resonance Imaging Study

Elaine G. Boland[1,2]*, Dinesh Selvarajah[3], Mike Hunter[4], Yousef Ezaydi[5], Solomon Tesfaye[3], Sam H. Ahmedzai[2], John A. Snowden[5], Iain D. Wilkinson[1]

1 Academic Unit of Radiology, Faculty of Medicine, Dentistry & Health, University of Sheffield, Sheffield, United Kingdom, **2** Academic Unit of Supportive Care, Department of Oncology, University of Sheffield, Sheffield, United Kingdom, **3** Department of Diabetes, Sheffield Teaching Hospitals NHS Foundation Trust, Sheffield, United Kingdom, **4** Academic Clinical Psychiatry, Department of Neuroscience, University of Sheffield, Sheffield, United Kingdom, **5** Department of Haematology, Sheffield Teaching Hospitals NHS Foundation Trust, Sheffield, United Kingdom

Abstract

Life expectancy in multiple myeloma has significantly increased. However, a high incidence of chemotherapy induced peripheral neuropathy (CIPN) can negatively influence quality of life during this period. This study applied functional magnetic resonance imaging (fMRI) to compare areas associated with central pain processing in patients with multiple myeloma who had chemotherapy induced peripheral neuropathy (MM-CIPN) with those from healthy volunteers (HV). Twenty-four participants (n = 12 MM-CIPN, n = 12 HV) underwent Blood Oxygen Level-Dependent (BOLD) fMRI at 3T whilst noxious heat-pain stimuli were applied to the foot and then thigh. Patients with MM-CIPN demonstrated greater activation during painful stimulation in the precuneus compared to HV (p = 0.014, FWE-corrected). Patients with MM-CIPN exhibited hypo-activation of the right superior frontal gyrus compared to HV (p = 0.031, FWE-corrected). Significant positive correlation existed between the total neuropathy score (reduced version) and activation in the frontal operculum (close to insular cortex) during foot stimulation in patients with MM-CIPN (p = 0.03, FWE-corrected; adjusted $R^2 = 0.87$). Painful stimuli delivered to MM-CIPN patients evoke differential activation of distinct cortical regions, reflecting a unique pattern of central pain processing compared with healthy volunteers. This characteristic activation pattern associated with pain furthers the understanding of the pathophysiology of painful chemotherapy induced peripheral neuropathy. Functional MRI provides a tool for monitoring cerebral changes during anti-cancer and analgesic treatment.

Editor: Andrea Antal, University Medical Center Goettingen, Germany

Funding: The University of Sheffield, The Royal Hallamshire Hospital Leukaemia and Myeloma Research Fund and the NAPP Research Bursaries 2009 from the Association of Palliative Medicine funded this study. The funders had no role in study design, data collection and analysis, decision to publish, or preparation of the manuscript.

Competing Interests: The authors have declared that no competing interests exist.

* E-mail: elaine.boland@nhs.net

Introduction

Modern cancer treatments may be associated with chemotherapy-induced peripheral neuropathy (CIPN), a potentially devastating side effect. Multiple myeloma (MM) is a haematological malignancy that has a particularly high incidence of CIPN following the administration of thalidomide, bortezomib or vincristine [1,2]. Neuropathy due to chemotherapy in myeloma may be painful and disabling. Moreover CIPN development may necessitate chemotherapy dose reduction or cessation [3,4]. Although some resolution of CIPN is possible, there is increasing recognition of the progressive chronicity of painful neuropathy in many patients. In addition, this frequently leads to the need for long-term administration of analgesic drugs with their attendant side effect profiles. Even with current analgesics, therapeutic response is often very poor [5]. Moreover, early diagnosis and objective assessment of CIPN and its symptomatic treatments are unsatisfactory. Overall, CIPN can result in reduced quality of life and impact on survival. This runs counter to the recent achievements linked to improved life expectancy from modern anti-cancer drugs [6].

Chemotherapy-induced peripheral neuropathy is thought to be caused by drug-induced damage to components of the peripheral nervous system (PNS) [7]. Neuropathy associated with thalidomide is thought to arise from Wallerian degeneration of the peripheral nerve fibres contributing to the development of pain via production of cytokines such as tumour necrosis factor-α and nerve growth factors [8]. Bortezomib-induced neuropathy is associated with deficits in Aβ, Aδ and C primary afferent fibres. There could potentially be a dysregulation of the neurotrophic factors since bortezomib inhibits the activation of the transcription factor, nuclear factor-kappa B and blocks the transcription of the trophic nerve growth factor [2]. Vincristine acts by binding on intracellular tubulin, which interferes with axonal transport. It is thought that it induces alterations in the cellular microtubule structure in the PNS and this might be a mechanistic link to neuropathic development [9,10]. Neuropathic symptoms are usually more common and severe in the lower extremities than in the upper extremities as the longest nerves are thought to be the first affected. Sensory changes affecting the toes, finally progress proximally to the ankles in a glove and stocking distribution [11]. Structural damage to the PNS results in abnormal somatosensory processing in the central and peripheral nervous systems [12]. Most of the current ideas regarding the pathophysiology of neuropathic pain originated from experimental work in animal models indicating peripheral and spinal cord reorganization of nociceptive pathways [13]. Animal models of neuropathic injuries that result in persistent pain suggest that peripheral and spinal cord impulses transmitting nociceptive signals towards the cortex undergo remarkable reorganization [14,15]. Although peripheral abnormalities are prominent, the central nervous system (CNS) appears to show concomitant involvement. Abnormalities in pain processing as shown on neuroimaging rather than just damage or inflammation to the peripheral nerves, seem to play an important part in chronic painful conditions such as trigeminal neuralgia, post-herpetic neuralgia, chronic low back pain and diabetic neuropathy [16–20]. Areas of brain activation that have been reported in chronic pain include the frontal lobe, insular cortex, somatosensory cortex, thalamus, periaquedactal grey and precuneus [21–23].

Our understanding of the pathological mechanisms underlying CIPN and identification of possible future treatment target areas for this debilitating complication may be significantly enhanced by the application of functional magnetic resonance imaging (fMRI). To our knowledge, to date there have been no reported fMRI studies in patients with multiple myeloma who have developed treatment emergent CIPN, that have attempted to document pain processing within the brain.

The aim of this work was to assess any alterations to the brain's cortical and sub-cortical pain matrix in MM-CIPN due to factors including: chemotherapy, chronicity of painful neuropathy and psychological adaptation. In light of previous pain-related functional studies, we hypothesised that regions such as the frontal cortex, insula, and postcentral gyrus, known to be involved in cognition and emotion processing and sensory perception, would be modulated by the presence of post-chemotherapeutic chronic neuropathy. To test this hypothesis, we used Blood Oxygenation Level Dependent (BOLD) fMRI to study central pain processing during noxious thermal stimulation in patients with MM who had already developed CIPN and to compare these findings to those from healthy volunteers (HV).

Material and Methods

Ethics statement

The study was granted ethical approval by the Sheffield Research Ethics Committee (REC no: 08/H1308/276) and the participants' written informed consent was obtained in accordance with the Declaration of Helsinki.

Subjects

The study sample comprised MM-CIPN patients and healthy volunteers. Myeloma patients had been treated with at least one of the anti-myeloma therapies commonly associated with CIPN (i.e; thalidomide, bortezomib or vincristine) and had experienced neuropathic pain of at least six months duration. Exclusion criteria included history of any major neurological or psychiatric disorder, contraindications to MRI, claustrophobia, left hand dominance, and neuropathy caused by other medical conditions. In addition, MM-CIPN patients who could not discontinue their tricyclics, noradrenaline reuptake inhibitors and/or calcium channel blocker analgesic medication for at least 48 hours prior to scanning were excluded. Patients who were on a long term, stable dose of opioids were included. Subjects did not receive any financial incentive for their participation. For each subject, demographic data collection, neuropathy assessment, chronic pain assessment and MR imaging were all undertaken on the same day.

Neuropathy assessment

All subjects underwent detailed clinical and neurophysiological assessments to diagnose and quantify the presence of neuropathy. This included a detailed clinical history and examination, quantitative sensory testing and peripheral nerve conduction assessment. Sensory testing using Computer Assisted Sensory Evaluation IV equipment comprised vibration perception, cooling and heating detection threshold of the right foot (CASE IV) (W.R. Electronics, Stillwater, MN, USA). Peripheral nerve conduction studies were performed at a stable skin temperature of 31°C (Medelec electrophysiological system, Synergy Oxford Instruments, Oxford, U.K.). A total neuropathy score reduced version (TNS-reduced version) was used, as has previously been used to stage neuropathy in MM patients [24]. This score evaluates motor and sensory symptoms and signs, quantitates pinprick and vibration perception threshold, and includes neurophysiological examination of one motor and one sensory nerve in the leg. The TNS-reduced version composite score ranges from 0 to 32; and the presence of neuropathy was defined as having a TNS-reduced version score >2.

Chronic pain assessment

To cover the psychosocial consequences of the pain experienced by the MM-CIPN patients, additional assessment tools were used. The chronic pain acceptance questionnaire (CPAQ) provides information on how chronic pain affects patients and is rated on a 0 (never true) to 6 (always true) scale [25]. The CPAQ total score ranges from 0 to 120, with a higher score indicating higher acceptance of pain. It shows the level of acceptance of chronic pain and focuses on participation in activities, the pursuit of personally relevant goals and the relative absence of attempts to control or avoid pain.

The pain catastrophizing scale (PCS) is a 13-item self-report test whose items are rated on a 5-point Likert-type scale. Ratings range from 0 (not at all) to 4 (always) representing the degree to which the subject experienced each of 13 thoughts or feelings when in pain [26]. The PCS total scores range from 0–52. The items fall within three different categories to assess negative thinking styles related to pain: rumination, magnification, and helplessness.

Heat-pain stimulation protocol

All heat-pain stimulation was applied to the right hand side of the body for each participant. The experimental thermal stimulus was delivered using a computer-controlled, MR-compatible, contact heat evoked potential device (CHEPS), which rapidly delivers heat with controllable temperatures (Medoc Pathway System, Medoc Ltd, Ramat Yishai, Israel). The foot was chosen as the primary stimulation area as this is the anatomical location where patients with CIPN develop pain-related symptomatology. The thigh was the secondary stimulation site and it was chosen as a potential control site, not being associated with neuropathic pain.

Prior to each subject entering the MR scanner, a simple heat pain-rating test was performed to determine the temperature threshold necessary to elicit a score of at least 7 on an 11-point numeric rating scale (with reference to a 0–10 point numeric rating scale; where 0 represented no pain and 10 represented the most extreme pain). This was performed separately for stimulation

Table 1. Baseline characteristics (median [IQR]) of the subjects recruited.

	Multiple Myeloma patients	Healthy Volunteers	p-value
Group Size	12	12	0
Age (Years)	63 [56–67]	53 [35–58]	0.04
Sex	8 Males; 4 Females	6 Males; 6 Females	0.42
Duration of MM (Years)	4.1 [2.0–7.7]	Not applicable	0
Duration of neuropathic pain (Years)	2 [0.9–3.2]	Not applicable	0

at both foot and thigh. The pain rating protocol started with a temperature application of 44.9°C at the foot and 42.9°C at the thigh. At these and subsequent temperature iterations, each subject reported their subjective pain status. The temperature was increased or decreased by 0.5–2°C until a pain score of 7/10 was identified. The maximum temperature at either site was set at 47.9°C. Thermal stimulation has been consistently used in other fMRI studies and has been shown to be an effective way to describe brain activity maps in response to thermal pain [27].

Each fMRI run comprised the presentation of 7 blocks of heat-pain stimuli (duration 30 seconds), at the pre-determined 7/10 pain-inducing temperature, interspersed with 7 blocks at a baseline temperature of 32°C (each baseline block duration was pseudo-randomised to 55, 60 or 65 seconds). Timing of the applied temperature protocol was controlled by the pre-programmed thermode-device computer. At the end of the imaging session, all participants rated their overall pain when the heat-pain stimulus was delivered to the foot and to the thigh. This was done by asking subjects to verbally rate the intensity of the pain on a numerical scale from zero (no pain) to ten (maximum imaginable pain).

Scanning protocol and fMRI acquisition

A fixed scanning protocol was used for every subject. Magnetic Resonance data were acquired at 3 Tesla (Achieva 3.0T, Philips Healthcare, Best, Holland). The scanning protocol included acquisition of standard T1-weighted, 3-dimensional and T2-weighted, 2-dimensional anatomical images prior to two fMRI runs. The fMRI datasets were acquired using a single-shot, T2*-weighted, gradient-recalled, echo planar imaging (EPI) sequence (Time to echo (TE) = 35 ms; Time to repeat (TR) = 3000 ms; SENSE encoding factor = 1.5). For each dataset, 35 contiguous transaxial slices of 4 mm thickness, with an in-plane resolution of 1.8 mm×1.8 mm were acquired at each imaging time-point or temporal dynamic (phase encoding in the anterior-posterior direction). Synchronicity was maintained between the scanner fMRI acquisition and the thermode-device PC control.

fMRI analysis

Imaging data analysis was carried out using statistical parametric mapping software (SPM5: www.fil.ion.ucl.ac.uk/spm). Blood oxygen level dependent response was modelled using a box-car waveform convolved with a canonical haemodynamic response function. Following spatial pre-processing, which included re-alignment, spatial normalisation and spatial smoothing, images were analysed using the General Linear Model. First-level functional images were produced comparing the BOLD response under the heat pain condition with the BOLD signal obtained at the baseline temperature. These contrast estimate maps were produced for every functional run at each of the two anatomical stimulation sites (foot and thigh) for each subject. Therefore, the first-level analysis yielded 2 contrast images per subject, comparing BOLD response under the heat-pain condition with baseline at (i) foot and (ii) thigh stimulation sites.

The resultant first-level contrast images were combined at the group level in a flexible factorial model with factors of subject, group (MM-CIPN and healthy volunteers) and site (foot and thigh). This appropriately modelled the independence of observations between subjects and groups, and the inequality of variance across all factors.

Within-group images of all pain (foot and thigh) response versus baseline were produced for each of the MM-CIPN and healthy volunteer groups. The statistical threshold for reporting within-group pain contrast activation was $p<0.05$, family-wise error (FWE) corrected across the whole spatial brain volume.

A functional anatomical mask of voxels activated in response to all heat-pain stimuli (compared with baseline) in both groups of

Table 2. Group median [IQR] temperature for pain stimulation and pain rating.

	Healthy Volunteers	MM patients	p-value
Foot stimulation			
Temperature (°C)	46.7 [45.5–47.8]	47.2 [46.6–47.9]	0.23
Pre-scan pain rating (0–10)	7.5 [6.6–8.0]	7.0 [7.0–8.0]	0.74
Post-scan pain rating (0–10)	7.7 [6.6–8.7]	7.7 [7.0–8.0]	0.95
Thigh stimulation			
Temperature (°C)	45.9 [45.6–47.9]	46.7 [45.5–47.9]	0.88
Pre-scan pain rating (0–10)	7.7 [5.9–8.0]	8.0 [7.6–8.0]	0.28
Post-scan pain rating (0–10)	8.0 [6.2–8.9]	8.0 [8.0–9.0]	0.29

Table 3. Anatomical regions showing areas where statistical significant BOLD fMRI response to heat-pain stimuli were greater than baseline temperature for Healthy Volunteers and myeloma patients with CIPN.

Region	BA	Talairach co-ordinates	Peak t	p (FWE-corr)	Voxels*
Healthy volunteers: Pain>Baseline					
R anterior cingulate	32	4 24 23	7.47	<0.001	1643
L superior temporal gyrus	38	−50 13 −8	7.19	<0.001	1491
L posterior cerebellar lobe	-	−30 −67 −20	6.56	0.002	2917
R inferior frontal gyrus	47	44 20 −9	6.52	0.002	1151
R supramarginal gyrus	40	64 −41 34	6.36	0.004	687
L superior temporal gyrus	42	−60 −30 18	6.13	0.007	709
L superior frontal gyrus	10	−32 48 20	5.80	0.018	469
R middle frontal gyrus	46	42 44 24	5.73	0.02	390
R superior frontal gyrus	8	6 39 48	5.68	0.025	216
L postcentral gyrus	7	−20 −41 68	5.66	0.026	212
CIPN-myeloma patients: Pain>Baseline					
Region	**BA**	**Talairach co-ordinates**	**Peak t**	**p (FWE-corr)**	**Voxels***
R superior temporal gyrus	22	56 4 0	8.10	<0.001	1356
R supramarginal gyrus	40	62 −41 35	7.65	<0.001	735
L middle frontal gyrus	46	−34 40 22	6.25	0.005	544
L area opercularis	44	−54 2 12	6.07	0.008	2228
L posterior cerebellar lobe	-	−34 −58 −24	6.00	0.01	2535

*Voxels = number of voxels exceeding threshold p<0.001, uncorrected

subjects (MM-CIPN and healthy volunteers) was created at a voxel-level statistical threshold p<0.001, uncorrected. This masking approach was used in order to reflect any variance in functional-anatomical location resulting from disease-specific pathogenesis. The mask was used as a volume-of-interest for correction for multiple comparisons in subsequent between-group contrasts.

The statistical threshold for reporting between-group differences in pain-evoked activation was p<0.05 FWE corrected (voxel-level) or p<0.05 corrected for extent of activation (cluster level) in either the whole brain volume or functionally defined region-of-interest (above). All activation results were displayed in the anatomical space as defined by the Montreal Neurological Institute (MNI) with stereotactic co-ordinates converted to the standard space of Talairach and Tournoux for the purposes of neuroanatomical labelling [28,29].

Behavioural data statistical analysis

Quantitative data were analysed using PASW Statistics version 18 [30]. Because of the asymmetric distribution of the cohort, a non-parametric (Mann-Whitney U test) was used for group comparisons. A linear regression analysis of fMRI signal response to heat-pain stimulation at the foot (i.e., neuropathic site) within the MM-CIPN patient group with TNS-reduced version and with the CPAQ and the PCS questionnaire scores was performed.

Results

Baseline characteristics

Twenty-four subjects were recruited (table 1): twelve MM-CIPN patients (8 males) and 12 healthy volunteers (6 males). The median age of the myeloma group was 63 years whilst that of the healthy volunteers was 53 years. Myeloma patients had the disease for a median [inter-quartile range (IQR)] of 4 [2–7.7] years and had neuropathic pain for a median of 2 [0.9–3.2] years. The anti-myeloma therapy that these patients received, which are known to cause peripheral neuropathy, varied between patients: n = 5 (42%) vincristine, n = 9 (75%) thalidomide and n = 8 (67%) bortezomib. All participants completed the study and none were excluded.

Neurological assessment and pain stimulation

Neurophysiological tests showed abnormality in each MM-CIPN subject indicative of peripheral neuropathy in the feet. The median [IQR] of the TNS-reduced version for MM-CIPN patients was 14 [11–17]. A length-dependent sensory axonal, large fibre neuropathy was evident from the nerve conduction studies. This showed smaller amplitudes and longer latencies and also impaired vibration and cooling thresholds on quantitative sensory testing.

The subject-reported rating for pain intensity was recorded before and after MRI scanning as shown in table 2. There were no significant group differences (p>0.05) in median temperatures applied to either the foot or thigh. There were no significant differences (p>0.05) between pre-scanning and post-scanning pain intensity rating in either healthy volunteers or MM-CIPN groups.

Chronic pain assessment

The total median CPAQ score in the MM group was 75. The median sum score for activities engagement was 45 and that of pain willingness was 31.

The total median catastrophisation score on the PCS was 11 (range 0–52) with the median scores (ranges) for magnification, rumination and helplessness being 2.5 (0–12), 5 (0–16) and 4.5 (0–24) respectively.

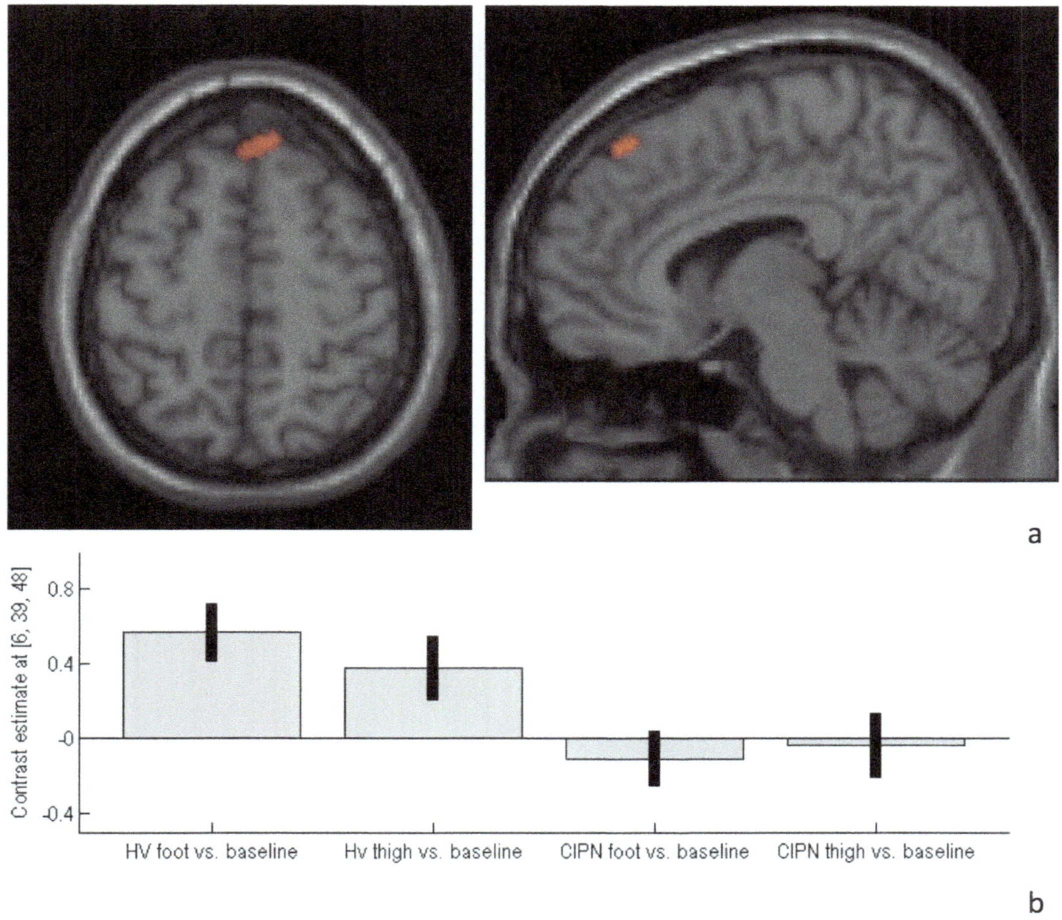

Figure 1. CIPN-myeloma patients demonstrated a) hypo-activation of superior frontal gyrus during heat-pain stimulation, compared with healthy volunteers. Functional imaging data are shown overlaid on both axial (z = 48 mm) and sagittal (x = 6 mm) slices through a canonical single-subject T1-weighted image. For display purposes, the statistical threshold is $p<0.001$, uncorrected, at the voxel-level. **b) Contrast estimates and 90% CI at co-ordinate 6, 39, 48 for both healthy volunteer and CIPN-myeloma patient groups.**

Brain activation in response to heat-pain stimulation in both healthy volunteers and MM-CIPN patients

Individual group analysis. Separate statistical parametric activation maps were constructed for the MM-CIPN group and the healthy volunteers group. Compared with baseline, heat-pain stimulation evoked a BOLD response or 'activation' in both healthy volunteers and patients with MM- CIPN (Table 3).

Comparison between groups. Patients with MM-CIPN demonstrated significantly less activation in the right superior frontal gyrus, close to the midline, than the healthy volunteer group (Figure 1a; Brodmann area 8; Talairach co-ordinates: 6, 39, 48; peak $t = 4.87$; $p = 0.03$, FWE-corrected within the volume-of-interest; 97 voxels exceeded height threshold $p<0.001$, uncorrected). Contrast estimates for pain stimulation at this focus, according to group and stimulation site, are presented (Figure 1b).

Compared with healthy volunteers, MM-CIPN patients demonstrated significantly greater activation in left precuneus (Figure 2a; Brodmann area 31; Talairach co-ordinates: −18, −61, 27; peak $t = 4.82$; 244 voxels exceeded height threshold $p< 0.001$, uncorrected; $p = 0.01$, corrected for extent of activation). This can be visualised in the plots for the contrast estimates for pain stimulation at this focus, according to group and stimulation site (Figure 2b).

Correlation of brain activation with the total neuropathy score, reduced version

A linear regression analysis of fMRI signal response to heat-pain stimulation at the foot (i.e., neuropathic site) within the MM-CIPN patient group indicated significant correlation of BOLD response with TNS-reduced version in the left operculo-insular cortex (Figure 3a, 3b, Talairach co-ordinates: −58, 2 4; peak $t = 8.02$; $p = 0.03$ FWE-corrected in the volume-of-interest for MM-CIPN foot activation).

No significant correlations were identified in the MM-CIPN patient group between BOLD response and CPAQ and/or the PCS questionnaire scores.

Discussion

This is the first report of a fMRI study exploring central pain processing in myeloma patients with chemotherapy-induced peripheral neuropathy. In this initial study, a thermal stimulus was applied to probe the subjects' BOLD-fMRI response to acute heat-pain. This type of stimulus was chosen since 'burning pain sensations' often feature strongly in CIPN clinical symptomatology. Our findings in patients who had this complex pathology mirror and underpin the central changes in other neuropathic

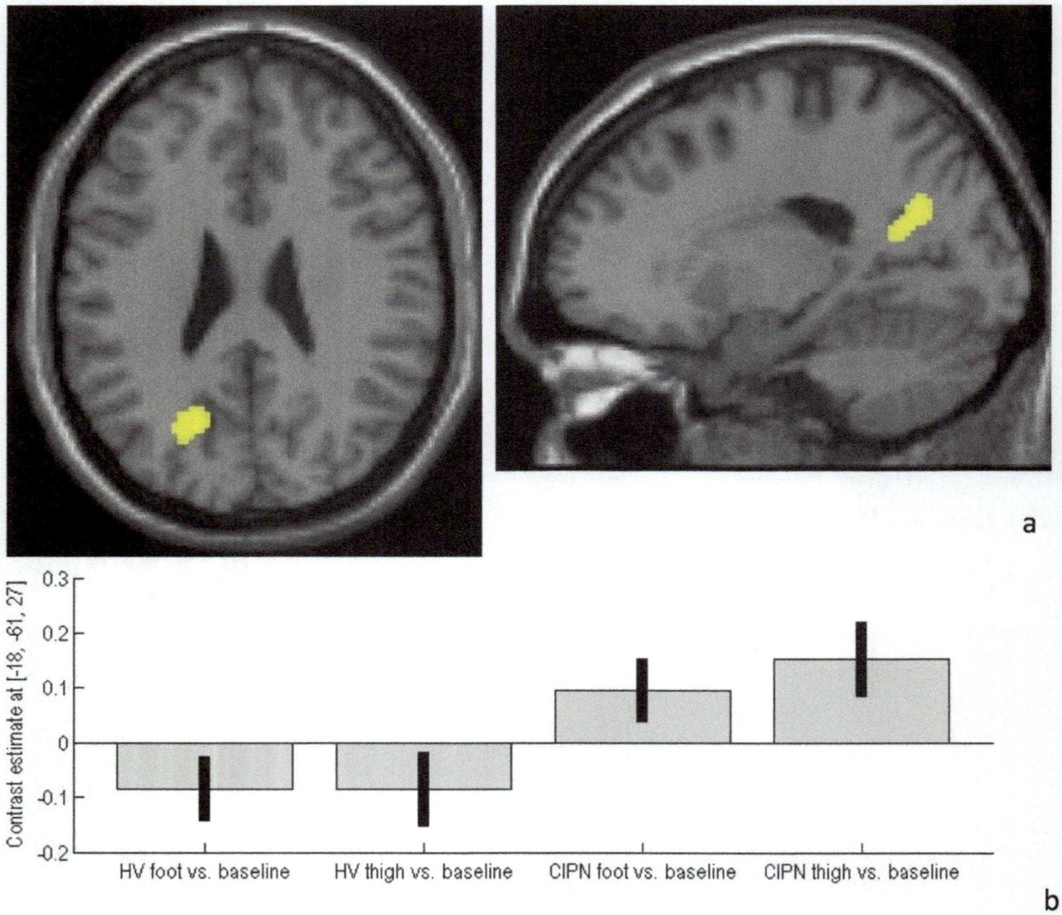

Figure 2. CIPN-myeloma patients demonstrated a0 hyper-activation of precuneus during heat-pain stimulation, compared with healthy volunteers. Functional imaging data are shown overlaid on both axial (z = 27 mm) and sagittal (x = −18 mm) slices through a canonical single-subject T1-weighted image. For display purposes, the statistical threshold is $p<0.001$, uncorrected, at the voxel-level. **b) Contrast estimates and 90% CI at co-ordinate −18, −61, 27 for both healthy volunteer and CIPN-myeloma patient groups.**

pain conditions reported in the literature. There was significant activation of the precuneus in the MM-CIPN group during heat-pain stimulation whilst there was significantly less response observed in this area in healthy volunteers. The precuneus, which lies on the posteromedial aspect of the parietal lobe, is thought to play a role in conscious pain perception and is involved in a broad range of higher order cognitive functions. Activation of the posterior precuneus exhibits the strongest correlation with successful retrieval of remembered episodes [31]. In MM-CIPN patients, the enhanced precuneus response to painful stimulation could imply that pain stimulates episodic pain memory retrieval. This is consistent with the literature in normal individuals [32,33]. It has also been shown in patients with other chronic neuropathic conditions [23,34–36].

In the MM-CIPN patients, there was a significant positive correlation between increasing neuropathy score (TNS-reduced version) and BOLD response in the operculo-insular cortex. This region includes parts of the insula deep inside the lateral sulcus. It also includes parts of the frontal and parietal lobes that cover the insula, called the opercula. The operculum is known to play a part in the cortical processing of painful stimuli [37]. There is evidence to show that the intensity of activation of the operculo-insular cortex correlates with perceived pain intensity in the human brain [38].

Interestingly, in our cohort of MM-CIPN patients, no functional anatomical response was identified in the superior frontal gyrus. This could result from adaptation due to the chronic presence of painful neuropathy of at least two years duration. Patients reported high scores in the chronic pain acceptance questionnaire and low scores in the pain catastrophizing questionnaire, which supports the hypothesis that reduction in BOLD fMRI response to acute heat-pain stimulation follows from long-term neuropathy-related pathophysiology. Previous studies have highlighted deactivation of the prefrontal cortex in response to pain in cluster headaches [39]. Repetitive transcranial magnetic stimulation has also been linked to deactivation in capsaicin-induced pain [40]. Activation in the right superior frontal gyrus has been previously reported in studies applying painful stimuli to healthy volunteers and activation in this area has been attributed to both the subjective experience of pain and other general unpleasant experiences [41].

We identified regions that are known components of the brain's pain matrix, during painful stimulation in both healthy volunteers and MM-CIPN patients. These functional areas are comparable to those found in other disease groups [23,42–44].

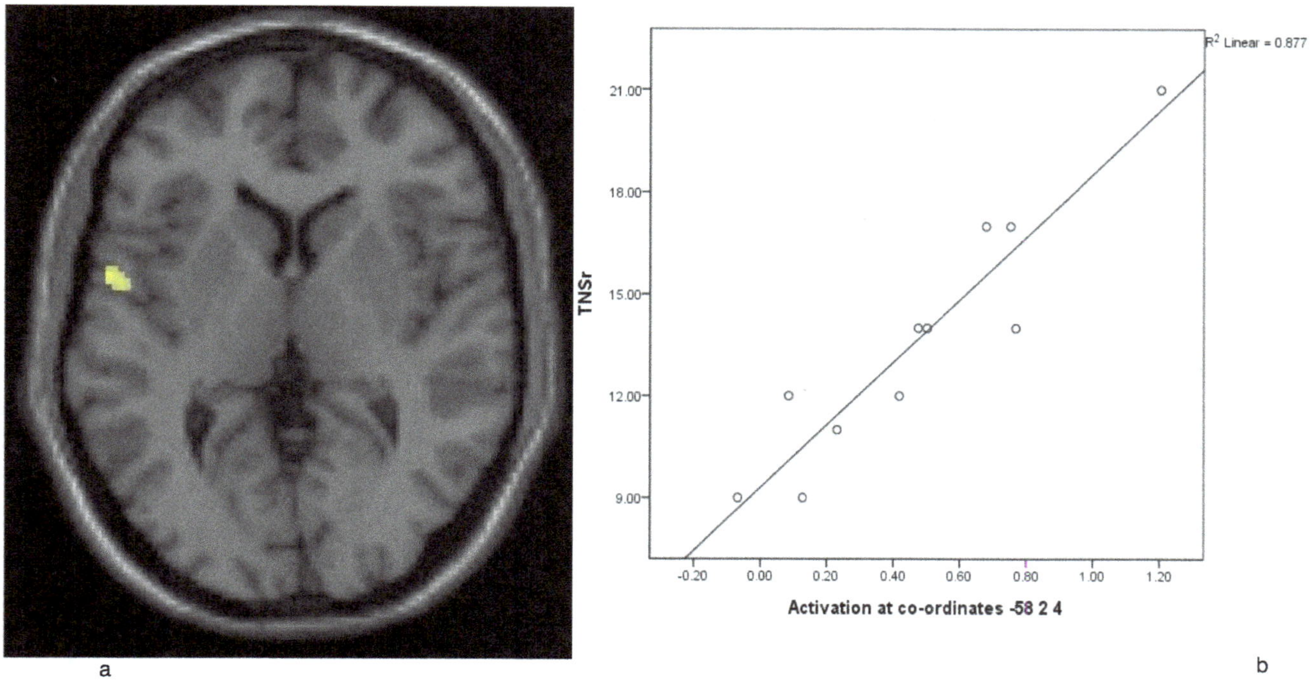

Figure 3. a: CIPN-myeloma patients demonstrated activation in the operculo-insular cortex. This activation was during painful heat stimulation, the degree of which correlated with TNS-reduced version. For display purposes, the statistical threshold is $p<0.001$, uncorrected, at the voxel-level. **b: Linear correlation between the TNS-reduced version and BOLD response within the operculo-insular cortex.**

There are numerous factors that may influence the overall *in-vivo* fMRI experiment [45]. In the current 'box-car' design, the BOLD effect is based on changes in MR signal between functional states, the source of which is assumed to be dominated by the net haemodynamic change linked to localised differences in synaptic and neuronal firing. It is not a direct measure of neuronal activity; rather it is an indirect physiological response. The vascular coupling is currently not fully understood, particularly in the context of pathophysiology. One potential limitation of this study was that the median age of the MM-CIPN group was greater than that of the healthy volunteers (albeit similar, approximately 10 years). The reported influences of age on BOLD fMRI response for non-pain-specific studies appear complex including overall intracranial increases, increases in frontal regions and decreases in the anterior regions, all with increasing age (a proposed posterior-anterior shift with age reported between 22- year and 69- year old normal volunteer groups) [46]. It must also be noted that chemotherapeutic agents themselves may alter vascular function and thus results should be interpreted in the light of these potential modulatory factors. However, as effects caused by alterations in cardiac output are likely to be systemic in nature and the group age difference in this study being comparatively small, it is assumed that potential effects between different intra-cranial functional areas are secondary to the proposed neuropathic effects. The significant correlation found with increasing neuropathic severity supports this hypothesis. Additionally, in terms of group response to pain-provoking stimulation, there were no significant differences between median temperatures that were delivered and their resultant pain ratings to either of the groups.

This was a cross-sectional screening study, with myeloma patients having already developed neuropathy in the context of receiving different anti-myeloma therapies. Some therapeutic regimens included more than one possible CIPN-inducing agent. Since no other known major risk factors for peripheral neuropathy were identified, such as diabetes, human immunodeficiency virus infection, chronic alcoholism, amyloidosis or renal failure, it would seem that a chemo-therapeutic response was the major overall causal factor linked to differences in both peripheral and central nervous systems. In addition, although peripheral neuropathy is seen at presentation in a small minority of patients with untreated MM, in our study, neuropathic pain started only after having received one of the anti-myeloma therapies described above. Most drugs used as an anti-myeloma treatment cannot permeate the blood–brain barrier [47]. The blood-nerve barrier protecting the peripheral system does however appear to be sensitive to the aforementioned agents. The PNS is thus more readily affected by circulating drug neurotoxicity than CNS structures [48]. In the light of this, the observed cerebral differences in BOLD response to heat stimulation may result from changes in sensory input to the brain or feedback circuitry via the spinal cord/brainstem. Longitudinal data from patients with myeloma embarking on chemotherapy would help to identify that CNS alterations do not occur prior to peripheral changes and thus the primary effect-site being the PNS. Such data would also help elucidate whether CNS and PNS changes occur concurrently or whether alterations in cerebral response follow a time lag suggestive of, for example, brain function accustomisation. This preliminary study compared a MM-CIPN cohort to findings in a healthy control group. Further data obtained from disease-control groups, consisting of patients with MM who have not developed symptoms or signs associated with peripheral neuropathy and those in the acute phase who have recently developed neuropathy, will add to our understanding of neuropathic pathogenesis. Patients receiving long-term opioid medication were not excluded and their medication was not withdrawn, to facilitate involvement and to sample the patients in their clinically relevant, chronic CIPN-state. It should be noted that future studies might reveal the potentially interesting modulatory effects of this psychoactive agent.

In conclusion, our results indicate that fMRI is capable of providing novel information with respect to the processing of pain within the CNS in CIPN. The results show that painful stimuli delivered to neuropathy-affected and symptom-free sites in our patients with CIPN evoked differential activation of distinct cortical regions. From this, we infer that the nociceptive system may undergo plastic changes, which appear to reflect abnormal central pain processing. Larger patient cohorts are needed to ensure that the current findings represent those of CIPN in general. Further identification and understanding of pathology-specific CNS involvement may provide an objective, in-vivo-based measure of pain experience and perception in patients with CIPN. This may aid in diagnosis and may also provide adjunctive information with which to steer targeting of novel pain-relieving therapies.

Acknowledgments

We would like to acknowledge Andrea Foster who helped in identifying the patients for this study and all the functional radiographers and radiologists of the University MRI Unit. Permission was granted from the Johns Hopkins University (copyright Cornblath and Chaudhry) for the use of the total neuropathy score, reduced version.

Author Contributions

Conceived and designed the experiments: EGB DS MH YE ST SHA JAS IDW. Performed the experiments: EGB DS YE JAS IDW. Analyzed the data: EGB DS MH IDW. Contributed reagents/materials/analysis tools: DS SHA JAS IDW MH ST. Wrote the paper: EGB JAS SHA IDW. Contributed to specific areas of expertise: IDW JAS ST SHA.

References

1. Verstappen CC, Koeppen S, Heimans JJ, Huijgens PC, Scheulen ME, et al. (2005) Dose-related vincristine-induced peripheral neuropathy with unexpected off-therapy worsening. Neurology 64: 1076–1077.
2. Mohty B, El-Cheikh J, Yakoub-Agha I, Moreau P, Harousseau JL, et al. (2010) Peripheral neuropathy and new treatments for multiple myeloma: background and practical recommendations. Haematologica 95: 311–319.
3. Richardson PG, Sonneveld P, Schuster MW, Stadtmauer EA, Facon T, et al. (2009) Reversibility of symptomatic peripheral neuropathy with bortezomib in the phase III APEX trial in relapsed multiple myeloma: impact of a dose-modification guideline. Br J Haematol 144: 895–903.
4. Bird JM, Owen RG, D'Sa S, Snowden JA, Pratt G, et al. (2011) Guidelines for the diagnosis and management of multiple myeloma 2011. Br J Haematol 154: 32–75.
5. Cata JP, Weng HR, Burton AW, Villareal H, Giralt S, et al. (2007) Quantitative sensory findings in patients with bortezomib-induced pain. J PAIN 8: 296–306.
6. Cavaletti G, Alberti P, Frigeni B, Piatti M, Susani E (2011) Chemotherapy-induced neuropathy. Curr Treat Options Neurol 13: 180–190.
7. Balayssac D, Ferrier J, Descoeur J, Ling B, Pezet D, et al. (2011) Chemotherapy-induced peripheral neuropathies: from clinical relevance to preclinical evidence. Expert Opin Drug Saf 10: 407–417.
8. Xu JT, Xin WJ, Zang Y, Wu CY, Liu XG (2006) The role of tumor necrosis factor-alpha in the neuropathic pain induced by Lumbar 5 ventral root transection in rat. Pain 123: 306–321.
9. Polomano RC, Bennett GJ (2001) Chemotherapy-evoked painful peripheral neuropathy. Pain Med 2: 8–14.
10. Quasthoff S, Hartung HP (2002) Chemotherapy-induced peripheral neuropathy. J Neurol 249: 9–17.
11. Wolf SL, Barton DL, Qin R, Wos EJ, Sloan JA, et al. (2011) The relationship between numbness, tingling, and shooting/burning pain in patients with chemotherapy-induced peripheral neuropathy (CIPN) as measured by the EORTC QLQ-CIPN20 instrument, N06CA. Support Care Cancer.
12. Bhagra A, Rao RD (2007) Chemotherapy-induced neuropathy. Curr Oncol Rep 9: 290–299.
13. Baliki MN, Geha PY, Apkarian AV (2007) Spontaneous pain and brain activity in neuropathic pain: functional MRI and pharmacologic functional MRI studies. Curr Pain Headache Rep 11: 171–177.
14. Apkarian AV, Baliki MN, Geha PY (2009) Towards a theory of chronic pain. Prog Neurobiol 87: 81–97.
15. Woolf CJ, Salter MW (2006) Plasticity and pain: role of the dorsal horn. In: K. M. McMahon SB, editors. Wall and Melzack's textbook of pain. London: Elsevier. pp. 91–105.
16. Selvarajah D, Wilkinson ID, Gandhi R, Griffiths PD, Tesfaye S (2011) Microvascular perfusion abnormalities of the Thalamus in painful but not painless diabetic polyneuropathy: a clue to the pathogenesis of pain in type 1 diabetes. Diabetes Care 34: 718–720.
17. Selvarajah D, Wilkinson ID, Emery CJ, Shaw PJ, Griffiths PD, et al. (2008) Thalamic neuronal dysfunction and chronic sensorimotor distal symmetrical polyneuropathy in patients with type 1 diabetes mellitus. Diabetologia 51: 2088–2092.
18. Giesecke T, Gracely RH, Grant MA, Nachemson A, Petzke F, et al. (2004) Evidence of augmented central pain processing in idiopathic chronic low back pain. Arthritis Rheum 50: 613–623.
19. Moisset X, Villain N, Ducreux D, Serrie A, Cunin G, et al. (2011) Functional brain imaging of trigeminal neuralgia. Eur J Pain 15: 124–131.
20. Geha PY, Baliki MN, Chialvo DR, Harden RN, Paice JA, et al. (2007) Brain activity for spontaneous pain of postherpetic neuralgia and its modulation by lidocaine patch therapy. Pain 128: 88–100.
21. Apkarian AV, Bushnell MC, Treede RD, Zubieta JK (2005) Human brain mechanisms of pain perception and regulation in health and disease. European Journal of Pain 9: 463–484.
22. Jaggi AS, Singh N (2011) Role of different brain areas in peripheral nerve injury-induced neuropathic pain. Brain Res 1381: 187–201.
23. Albuquerque RJ, de Leeuw R, Carlson CR, Okeson JP, Miller CS, et al. (2006) Cerebral activation during thermal stimulation of patients who have burning mouth disorder: an fMRI study. Pain 122: 223–234.
24. Cavaletti G, Frigeni B, Lanzani F, Piatti M, Rota S, et al. (2007) The Total Neuropathy Score as an assessment tool for grading the course of chemotherapy-induced peripheral neurotoxicity: comparison with the National Cancer Institute-Common Toxicity Scale. Journal of the Peripheral Nervous System 12: 210–215.
25. Vowles KE, McCracken LM, McLeod C, Eccleston C (2008) The Chronic Pain Acceptance Questionnaire: confirmatory factor analysis and identification of patient subgroups. Pain 140: 284–291.
26. Sullivan MJL, Bishop SR (1995) The Pain Catastrophizing Scale: Development and Validation. Psychological Assessment 7: 524–532.
27. Friebel U, Eickhoff SB, Lotze M (2011) Coordinate-based meta-analysis of experimentally induced and chronic persistent neuropathic pain. Neuroimage 58: 1070–1080.
28. Ashburner J, Friston KJ (2005) Unified segmentation. Neuroimage 26: 839–851.
29. Talairach J, Tournoux P (1988) Co-Planar Stereotaxic Atlas of the Human Brain. New York: Thieme Medical Publishers.
30. SPSS (2009) PASW STATISTICS 18.0 SPSS Inc, Chicago.
31. Cavanna AE, Trimble MR (2006) The precuneus: a review of its functional anatomy and behavioural correlates. Brain 129: 564–583.
32. Koyama T, McHaffie JG, Laurienti PJ, Coghill RC (2005) The subjective experience of pain: where expectations become reality. Proc Natl Acad Sci U S A 102: 12950–12955.
33. Kong J, Loggia ML, Zyloney C, Tu P, Laviolette P, et al. (2010) Exploring the brain in pain: activations, deactivations and their relation. Pain 148: 257–267.
34. Hsieh JC, Belfrage M, Stone-Elander S, Hansson P, Ingvar M (1995) Central representation of chronic ongoing neuropathic pain studied by positron emission tomography. Pain 63: 225–236.
35. Buvanendran A, Ali A, Stoub TR, Kroin JS, Tuman KJ (2010) Brain activity associated with chronic cancer pain. Pain Physician 13: E337–342.
36. Witting N, Kupers RC, Svensson P, Arendt-Nielsen L, Gjedde A, et al. (2001) Experimental brush-evoked allodynia activates posterior parietal cortex. Neurology 57: 1817–1824.
37. Baumgartner U, Iannetti GD, Zambreanu L, Stoeter P, Treede RD, et al. (2010) Multiple somatotopic representations of heat and mechanical pain in the operculo-insular cortex: a high-resolution fMRI study. J Neurophysiol 104: 2863–2872.
38. Iannetti GD, Zambreanu L, Cruccu G, Tracey I (2005) Operculoinsular cortex encodes pain intensity at the earliest stages of cortical processing as indicated by amplitude of laser-evoked potentials in humans. Neuroscience 131: 199–208.
39. Hsieh JC, Hannerz J, Ingvar M (1996) Right-lateralised central processing for pain of nitroglycerin-induced cluster headache. Pain 67: 59–68.
40. Tamura Y, Okabe S, Ohnishi T, N Saito D, Arai N, et al. (2004) Effects of 1-Hz repetitive transcranial magnetic stimulation on acute pain induced by capsaicin. Pain 107: 107–115.
41. Fulbright RK, Troche CJ, Skudlarski P, Gore JC, Wexler BE (2001) Functional MR imaging of regional brain activation associated with the affective experience of pain. AJR Am J Roentgenol 177: 1205–1210.
42. Becerra LR, Breiter HC, Stojanovic M, Fishman S, Edwards A, et al. (1999) Human brain activation under controlled thermal stimulation and habituation to noxious heat: an fMRI study. Magn Reson Med 41: 1044–1057.

43. Gelnar PA, Krauss BR, Sheehe PR, Szeverenyi NM, Apkarian AV (1999) A comparative fMRI study of cortical representations for thermal painful, vibrotactile, and motor performance tasks. Neuroimage 10: 460–482.
44. Coghill RC, McHaffie JG, Yen YF (2003) Neural correlates of interindividual differences in the subjective experience of pain. Proc Natl Acad Sci U S A 100: 8538–8542.
45. The Oxford Centre for Functional MRI of the Brain NDoCN, University of Oxford (2014) Introduction to fMRI.
46. Davis SW, Dennis NA, Daselaar SM, Fleck MS, Cabeza R (2008) Que PASA? The posterior-anterior shift in aging. Cerebral cortex 18: 1201–1209.
47. Nieuwenhuizen L, Biesma DH (2008) Central nervous system myelomatosis: review of the literature. Eur J Haematol 80: 1–9.
48. Balayssac D, Cayre A, Authier N, Bourdu S, Penault-Llorca F, et al. (2005) Patterns of P-glycoprotein activity in the nervous system during vincristine-induced neuropathy in rats. J Peripher Nerv Syst 10: 301–310.

10

A Retrospective Study of Chronic Post-Surgical Pain following Thoracic Surgery: Prevalence, Risk Factors, Incidence of Neuropathic Component, and Impact on Qualify of Life

Zhiyou Peng[1], Huiling Li[1], Chong Zhang[2], Xiang Qian[3], Zhiying Feng[1]*, Shengmei Zhu[1]

1 Department of Anesthesiology, First Affiliated Hospital, School of Medicine, Zhejiang University, Hangzhou, Zhejiang Province, China, **2** Department of Thoracic Surgery, First Affiliated Hospital, School of Medicine, Zhejiang University, Hangzhou, Zhejiang Province, China, **3** Department of Anesthesiology, Perioperative and Pain Medicine, Stanford University School of Medicine, Stanford, California, United States of America

Abstract

Background: Thoracic surgeries including thoracotomy and VATS are some of the highest risk procedures that often lead to CPSP, with or without a neuropathic component. This retrospective study aims to determine retrospectively the prevalence of CPSP following thoracic surgery, its predicting risk factors, the incidence of neuropathic component, and its impact on quality of life.

Methods: Patients who underwent thoracic surgeries including thoracotomy and VATS between 01/2010 and 12/2011 at the First Affiliated Hospital, School of Medicine, Zhejiang University were first contacted and screened for CPSP following thoracic surgery via phone interview. Patients who developed CPSP were then mailed with a battery of questionnaires, including a questionnaire referenced to Maguire's research, a validated Chinese version of the ID pain questionnaire, and a SF-36 Health Survey. Logistic regression analyses were subsequently performed to identify risk factors for CPSP following thoracic surgery and its neuropathic component.

Results: The point prevalence of CPSP following thoracic surgery was 24.9% (320/1284 patients), and the point prevalence of neuropathic component of CPSP was 32.5% (86/265 patients). CPSP following thoracic surgery did not improve significantly with time. Multiple predictive factors were identified for CPSP following thoracic surgery, including age<60 years old, female gender, prolonged duration of post-operative chest tube drainage (≥4 days), options of post-operative pain management, and pre-existing hypertension. Furthermore, patients who experienced CPSP following thoracic surgery were found to have significantly decreased physical function and worse quality of life, especially those with neuropathic component.

Conclusions: Our study demonstrated that nearly 1 out of 4 patients underwent thoracic surgery might develop CPSP, and one third of them accompanied with a neuropathic component. Early prevention as well as aggressive treatment is important for patients with CPSP following thoracic surgery to achieve a high quality of life.

Editor: Ruth Landau, University of Washington, United States of America

Funding: This study was supported by the grants from the Zhejiang Provincial Natural Science Foundation of China (Grant No. Y12H030053). The funders had no role in study design, data collection and analysis, decision to publish, or preparation of the manuscript.

Competing Interests: The authors have declared that no competing interests exist.

* E-mail: fzy1972@zju.edu.cn

Introduction

A surgical incision produces tissue injury, inflammation, and subsequent acute post-operative pain. Subsequent modulation of the peripheral and central nervous system can lead to chronic pain. Acute pain management including multimodal analgesia techniques aspires to stop the transition from acute pain to chronic pain, yet a significant reduction in the occurrence rate and severity of chronic pain has not occurred [1].

Thoracic surgeries including thoracotomy and video-assisted thoracoscopic surgery (VATS) are some of the highest risk procedures that often lead to chronic post-surgery pain (CPSP) [2–6]. Previous studies have shown that the prevalence of CPSP following thoracic surgery varies from 14% to 83% [2,4,6–11], while the prevalence of CPSP following thoracic surgery with neuropathic component varies from 22% to 66% [4,6,8,11,12]. Failure in proper management of CPSP following thoracic surgery is associated with higher morbidity and mortality, worse physical function and pain interference, and overall poor quality of life [13,14]. Consequently, an increasing emphasis and effort has been focused on the mechanisms underlying the transition from acute pain to chronic pain, as well as aggressive prevention and management of CPSP following thoracic surgery.

In spite of the devastating nature of CPSP, the current understanding of CPSP following thoracic surgery and its potential neuropathic component remains poor. Based on the diagnosis criteria from the International Association for the Study of Pain (IASP) [10] and recent studies [9], CPSP following thoracic surgery is defined as "pain persisting for at least 3 months after surgery, pain is different from pre-operative pain, and pain caused by other conditions such as continuing malignancy or chronic infection should be excluded". Some patients with CPSP following thoracic surgery also experience neuropathic component, which was recently redefined as "pain caused by a lesion or disease of the somatosensory system" [15]. According to the Assessment Committee of the Neuropathic Pain Special Interest Group (NeuPSIG) [16], diagnosis of neuropathic pain should be possible from history and clinical examination alone without the need for laboratory tests. Though a gold standard for neuropathic pain diagnosis is still lacking, some validated screening tools for neuropathic pain have become available, including a recently validated screening and diagnosis tool for neuropathic pain in Chinese patients [18]. In addition, a Chinese version of the Medical Outcomes Study Short Form-36 (SF-36) has also been validated and widely used to evaluate health-related quality of life (HRQOL) for patients who suffer from chronic post-operative pain or neuropathic pain [1].

This study aims to investigate the prevalence of CPSP following thoracic surgery and its neuropathic component, to identify risk factors, and to determine the effect of chronic pain on HRQOL following thoracic surgery. This information may be used to reduce the incidence of CPSP following thoracic surgery, guide the optimal post-operative pain management, and ultimately improve patients' qualify of life.

Methods

Ethics Statement

The study was approved by the ethics committee of the First Affiliated Hospital, School of Medicine, Zhejiang University. All subjects in this study were given verbal informed consent for their participation and the oral informed consent process was approved by the research ethical committee of the Department of Anesthesiology at the First Affiliated Hospital, School of Medicine, Zhejiang University. All participants received written information about the survey prior to the obtained consent. Written consent was deemed impractical in this large low risk survey and verbal consent was obtained by the interviewers and audited by the Department of Anesthesiology at the First Affiliated Hospital, School of Medicine, Zhejiang University.

Subjects

A retrospective questionnaire survey was undertaken on patients who had undergone thoracotomy and VATS between 01/2010 and 12/2011 at the First Affiliated Hospital of School of Medicine, Zhejiang University, China. Criteria for exclusion include: age <18 years old, history of pre-operative chemotherapy, history of previous thoracic surgery, history of neurological disorders or thoracic trauma, emergent operation, and surgical site infection. The survey was conducted between 3/2012 and 6/2012, more than 3 months after the initial surgery. A total of 1624 patients were identified and contacted.

Definitions and Questionnaire Design

According to the IASP [10] and recent studies [9], CPSP following thoracic surgery is defined as "persistent pain for at least 3 months after thoracic surgery, the pain differs in character from the pre-operative pain, and other causes for chronic pain such as continuing malignancy or chronic infection have been excluded.".

The ID Pain questionnaire is a six-item, patient-completed screening tool designed to help differentiate nociceptive and neuropathic pain. Patients scoring greater than or equal to 2 on a Chinese version for ID pain questionnaire are considered to have neuropathic component [17].

The HRQOL was measured using a Chinese version of SF-36, which is a standardized and validated tool and has been widely used to evaluate patient's health. The SF-36 assesses eight scales: physical function (PF), role limitations due to physical problems (role physical, RP), body pain (BP), general health (GH), vitality (VT), social function (SF), role limitations due to emotional problems (role emotional, RE), and mental health (MH). The raw scores of each subscale were converted to a range from 0 to 100, with higher scores indicating better levels of functioning or well-being.

Telephone interview and flow diagram

A total of 1624 patients were contacted. Patients with CPSP following thoracic surgery were identified if they answered yes to both of the following questions: 1) "Have you experienced any pain along the scar after surgery, different from what you had before the surgery?" 2) "Has the pain persisted for at least 3 months?". Patients were then asked for permission to mail them a battery of questionnaires, including a questionnaire referenced to Maguire's research [1,12], a validated Chinese version of the ID pain questionnaire [17], and a SF-36 Health Survey (Chinese version). Those patients who failed to respond within 1 month were reminded by telephone, and if necessary, were mailed the questionnaire again. Two months after sending the first questionnaire, the investigation was closed.

To identify potential risk factors for CPSP following thoracic surgery, patient demographics, past medical history, and clinical characteristics including anesthesia, surgery, and peri-operative pain management were collected from the electronic medical records system. Similar to a previous investigation [18], the following data were recorded: age, gender, presence of diabetes mellitus or hypertension, history of smoking, diagnosis of underlying thoracic disease, date of surgery, duration of the operation, surgical approach (VATS versus thoracotomy), surgeon, post-operative pain management (PCA regimen versus non-PCA regimen), the number of draining chest tube, duration of chest tube placement, surgical complications, cancer recurrence, and post-operative radiation and chemotherapy. Time since surgery was defined as the period between operation date and the telephone interview date. The operation time was defined from the moment of the incision to suture completion.

Surgery, anesthesia, and post-operative analgesia

Four different surgical teams were involved in this study, with both thoracotomy and VATS. The thoracotomy approach used a conventional protocol without rib resection during the operation. Skin incision was parallel to the ribs at the lateral or posterior-lateral part of the intercostal space. After placement of an intercostal chest tube (JINGLE®, China, 30-Fr, straight thoracic catheter), the intercostal space was closed by pericostal sutures with extreme precautions applied to avoid the injury of intercostal nerves. The VATS approach used a uniform anterior three-port technique with standardized port placements regardless of the lobe to be resected or not. The camera port was made in the 7th intercostal space at the middle axillary line, while the main port was placed in the 4th inter-costal space at the anterior axillary line, and the third port was placed in the 9th inter-costal space at the posterior axillary line. At the end of surgery, a draining chest tube (JINGLE®, China, 30-Fr, straight thoracic catheter) was inserted in the Camera port. The draining chest tube was removed as soon as no air leakage was detected for more than 24 hours, total amount of pleural effusion was less than 200 ml per day, and no chylothorax was present.

A total intravenous anesthesia (TIVA) technique composed of propofol, fentanyl or remifentanil, and intermittent rocuronium was used to maintain adequate anesthesia after induction. No paravertebral or epidural block was administrated preoperatively.

Under the current State Health Insurance Policy in Mainland China, cost related to PCA pump is not reimbursable. Many patients opted to choose the non-PCA regimen due to their willingness and capability for self-pay. As a result, 833 patients in our study chose PCA regimen for post-operative pain management. The PCA regimen included a patient controlled infusion pump (the Hospira GemStar® Pump, Hospira Inc., USA) programmed to deliver sufentanil with a continuous dose of 1–2 micrograms per hour, along with patient controlled bolus of 2–3 micrograms at a lockout interval of 10 minutes. The bolus dosage was subsequently adjusted and titrated for optimal analgesia (visual analogue scale (VAS) score less than 3). In addition, patients received intravenous Flurbiprofen at 50 mg every 12 hours for total 3 days, unless contradicted due to bleeding concerns or renal insufficiency. The non-PCA regimen included intravenous Flurbiprofen at 50 mg every 12 hours and tramadol 100 mg intramuscularly every 6 hours as needed (when VAS score more than 7). Those non-PCA option patients were managed by surgical teams from the Department of Thoracic Surgery, in contrast to the patients with PCA option who were managed by a dedicated Acute Pain Service (APS) team from the Department of Anesthesiology.

Statistical analysis

Data was analyzed using SPSS 16.0 software (SPSS, Inc., Chicago, IL, USA). Continuous variables were presented as mean ± standard deviations and categorical data were shown as numbers and percentages. Comparison of continuous data was performed by Student's *t* test with normal distribution and by the Mann-Whitney U test for variables with non-normal distribution. The Chi-square test was used to compare groups with categorical variables. P value less than 0.05 was considered significant. Univariate analyses and multiple forward stepwise logistic regression analyses were performed to identify risk factors predicting CPSP following thoracic surgery and its neuropathic component. After univariate analyses, variables with *p* value less than 0.05 were included in a multivariate logistic regression analysis to identify the independent factors of CPSP following thoracic surgery and its neuropathic component.

Results

Characteristics of responders

As shown in the overall flow diagram of Fig. 1, 1624 total patients were contacted and evaluated for enrollment. After phone interviews, 340 patients were excluded because they were either deceased (n = 84), not answering phone calls (n = 186), refusing to participate (n = 19), or being diagnosed with a tumor recurrence at the time of interview (n = 51). We were able to collect and analyze the data from the rest 1284 patients, whose baseline characteristics were summarized in Table 1.

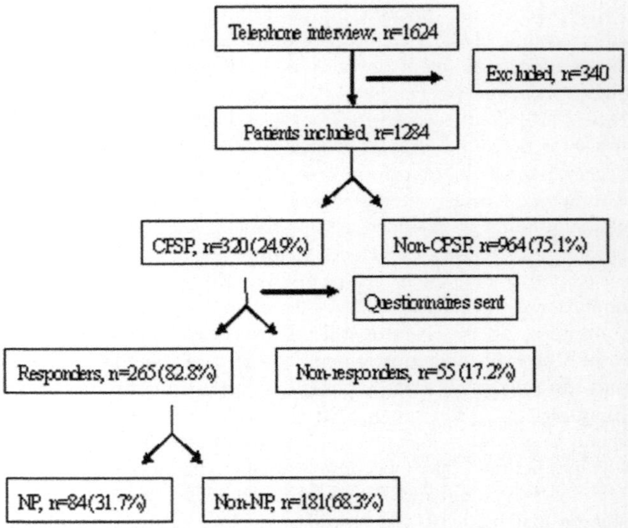

Figure 1. Flow diagram. CPSP, chronic post-surgical pain; NP, neuropathic pain.

Prevalence and properties of CPSP following thoracic surgery and its neuropathic component

At the time of phone interview, the point prevalence of CPSP following thoracic surgery was 24.9% (320/1284 patients). Those 320 patients were then mailed with the questionnaire referred to Maguire's research to further explore the nature of chronic pain. 265 patients subsequently sent back the form, of which the point prevalence of neuropathic component of CPSP following thoracic surgery was found to be at 32.5% (86/265 patients). Figure 2 displayed the trend for the prevalence of CPSP following thoracic surgery and its neuropathic component as a function of the 3-month length of time after operation. As time elapsed after operation, it has a trend to fall for the prevalence of CPSP following thoracic surgery and its neuropathic component.

To assess the properties of chronic pain, the questionnaires referred to Maguire's research were sent to 320 patients with CPSP following thoracic surgery, and 265 replies were sent back. Among them, 73.5% of patients reported their pain being mild, 22.3% moderate, and only 4.2% severe. The most frequent descriptions of the pain include dull, throbbing, pressure, rebound tenderness, and needle-like and electric shock-like sensations around the surgical site and the chest tube placement sites. In addition, 67.3% patients did not feel improvement in their pain over time, while 25.7% reported that the pain was worse, especially when there is a rapid weather change, including cloudy or rainy days.

Significant differences were noted in terms of pain characteristics between CPSP patients with and without neuropathic component (Table 2). CPSP following thoracic surgery with neuropathic component have higher prevalence of moderate and severe pain than those without neuropathic component ($p<0.05$), as well as statistically significant increases in the incidence of unpleasant skin sensation ($p<0.05$), hyperalgesia ($p = 0.013$), and skin temperature change ($p = 0.021$)

Risk factors for developing CPSP following thoracic surgery

Table 1 contains a list of the risk factors determined to be statistically significant for developing chronic post-thoracic pain,

Table 1. Principle Characteristics of Patients with or without CPSP following thoracic surgery.

Participants	CPSP($n=320$)	Non-CPSP ($n=964$)	p value
Age (<60 ys)	225 (70.3%)	619 (64.2%)	0.046
Female	147(45.9%)	305(31.6%)	<0.001
ASA physical status (I/II/III)	92/213/15 (29.0/66.6/4.7%)	277/630/54 (28.7/65.4/5.6%)	0.897
Smoking history	110(34.4%)	382(39.6%)	0.094
Hypertension	80(25%)	154(16.0%)	<0.001
Diabetes	14(4.4%)	26(27.0%)	0.134
Type of postoperative analgesia (PCIA/non-PCIA)	192/128 (60/40%)	641/323 (66.5/33.5%)	0.036
Type of pathology (cancer)	167(52.2%)	495(51.3%)	0.795
Type of procedure (Lung/Esophagus/Mediastinal)	256/28/36 (80/8.8/11.3%)	781/111/72 (81/11.5/7.5%)	0.055
Type of procedure (Thoracotomy/VATS)	239/81 (74.7/25.3%)	724/239 (75.1/24.8%)	0.859
Duration of operation (min)	143.02±70.76	141.11±75.26	0.690
Duration of chest tube drainage (≥4 days)	249(77.8%)	682(70.7%)	0.014
Number of pleural drains One	279(87.2%)	836(86.7%)	0.831
Two	41(12.8%)	128(13.3%)	
Follow-up (months)	11.75±5.373	11.57±5.834	0.627

Results are expressed as (n) or mean ± SD. CPSP, chronic post-surgical pain; NP, neuropathic pain, ASA indicates American Society of Anesthesiologists; PCIA, patient-controlled intravenous analgesia.

including age<60 years old, female gender, history of hypertension, lack of PCA regimen for post-operative analgesia, and prolonged duration of chest tube drainage (≥4 days). The prevalence of CPSP following thoracic surgery was significantly higher in patients below 60 years (225 patients, 70.3% versus 609 patients, 63.2%, $p<0.05$). In addition, women (147 patients, 32.5%) experienced more CPSP following thoracic surgery than men (173 patients 20.8%, $p<0.01$). CPSP prevalence in patients who had medical history of hypertension was also significantly higher than those without hypertension ($p<0.01$). The prevalence of CPSP in patients who were offered post-operative PCA based pain management was significantly less than those patients who did not receive PCA ($p=0.035$). Finally, duration of chest tube drainage (≥4 days) was found to be a significant risk factor for CPSP after thoracic surgery ($p<0.01$).

No statistically significant difference was found between the CPSP group and non-CPSP group including ASA physical status, history of smoking, past medical history of diabetes, diagnosis of cancer, type of procedure (thoracotomy versus VATS), and the duration of the procedure (Table 1). In addition, no significant difference of CPSP prevalence was found among the four surgical teams (data not shown).

Based on logistic regression analysis, risk factors for developing chronic pain after thoracic surgery include age below 60 years old (OR: 1.51, 95% CI: 1.13–2.02), female gender (OR: 1.77, 95% CI: 1.36–2.31), hypertension (OR: 1.86, 95% CI: 1.35–2.57), lack of PCA for post-operation analgesia (OR: 1.31, 95% CI: 1.00–1.71), and prolonged duration of chest tube drainage (≥4 days) (OR: 1.55, 95% CI: 1.14–2.10).

Predictive factors for the prevalence of neuropathic pain after thoracic surgery

Logistic regression was also used to determine the risk factor for neuropathic pain occurrence in patients who developed CPSP following thoracic surgery, including age, gender, ASA physical status, type of surgery, medical history of hypertension or diabetes, type of cancer, adjunct radiation and chemotherapy, number of chest tube drains, and duration of chest tube drainage. Interestingly, only the duration of chest tube drainage (≥4 days) was identified to correlate (positively) with neuropathic pain ($p<0.05$, OR: 0.421, 95% CI: 0.187–0.952).

The impact of CPSP following thoracic surgery and neuropathic pain on daily living and quality of life

As shown in Table 2, the presence of a neuropathic component in patients with CPSP following thoracic surgery was associated with more severe pain. This subset of patients rate pain as one of their worst medical problems, has greatly limited their quality of life and has led to various sleep disorders ($p<0.05$). Interestingly, there was no significant difference in the proportion of patients with or without neuropathic component, in terms of visit to pain clinic and seeking additional pain medications ($p>0.05$).

In order to confirm whether CPSP following thoracic surgery and its neuropathic component negatively impacts quality of life, SF-36 Health Survey (Chinese version) questionnaires were mailed to both CPSP patients and non-CPSP patients (n = 600). Total 467 replies were received, among which 202 were non-CPSP patients, 179 were CPSP patients without neuropathic component, and 86 patients were CPSP patients with neuropathic component, respectively (Figure 3). Compared to non-CPSP patients, there was a significant decrease in PF score and BP score for CPSP patients ($p<0.05$). In addition, compared to CPSP patients without neuropathic component, there was a significant decrease in PF for CPSP patients with neuropathic component ($p<0.05$).

Discussion

Our study found that one out of four patients undergoing thoracic surgery would develop characteristics consistent with persistent post-thoracic surgery chronic pain (CPSP), with one third of them reporting signs and symptoms consistent with neuropathic pain. Furthermore, our study has identified multiple risk factors for the development of CPSP following thoracic surgery, including age<60 years old, female gender, preoperative

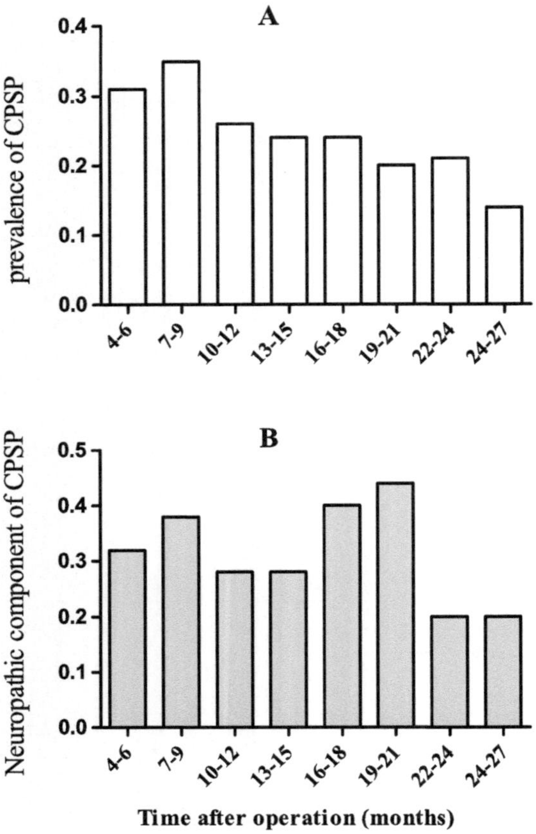

Figure 2. The trend for the prevalence of CPSP following thoracic surgery and neuropathic component of CPSP as a function of the length of time after operation. A: the trend for the prevalence of CPSP following thoracic surgery as a function of the length of time after operation, expressed in 3-month intervals. B: the trend for prevalence of neuropathic component of CPSP as a function of the length of time after operation, expressed in 3-month intervals. CPSP, chronic post-surgical pain; NP, neuropathic pain.

hypertension, post-operative non-PCA pain management regimen, and prolonged duration of post-operative chest tube drainage (≥4 days). In addition, the duration of post-operative chest tube drainage (≥4 days) was the only variable found to play a role for development of CPSP with neuropathic component. In our study, patients with CPSP have much worse quality of life, especially those with neuropathic component, suggesting the importance of preventing CPSP from development following thoracic surgery, as well as the need for aggressive treatment once it has developed. To our knowledge, this is the first study to investigate the prevalence of CPSP and its neuropathic component after thoracic surgery using a combined validated Chinese version of the ID pain questionnaire and a Short Form-36 (SF-36) Health Survey.

The reported prevalence of CPSP following thoracic surgery varies from 14% to 83% [2,4,6,7,10,19] and the prevalence of its neuropathic component varies from 22% to 66% [4,6,8,11,12]. This wide range may be explained by discrepancies among studies in methodology, timing of assessment, surgical procedure details, and varying definitions used to assess CPSP following thoracic surgery or neuropathic pain [3,4,9,20]. Unfortunately, it still lacks a standardized and universally accepted definition of CPSP following thoracic surgery [4,9,21]. The incidence of CPSP from our study appears lower in comparison with those reported in the literature [2,4,6–8,11,22,23]. Possible reasons include different sample size (1284 total patients in our study, largest among all studies in the literature), different definitions of CPSP following thoracic surgery (≥3 months duration in our study compared to 2 months duration in studies from Deumens and Macare et al [9,21]), different anesthesia techniques used for surgery [24] (TIVA in our study versus inhalational anesthesia in others) and different postoperative pain management [20,25] (PCA versus non-PCA regimen).

In contrast, the prevalence of CPSP following thoracic surgery with a neuropathic component identified from our study (32.5%) is similar to findings in literatures [4,8,11]. Neuropathic pain, defined as "pain arising as a direct consequence of a lesion or disease affecting the somatosensory system" [15] can be a debilitating symptom. Several patient-reported measures of neuropathic pain have been developed, including the ID Pain questionnaire, Neuropathic Pain Scale (NPS), the Neuropathic Pain Diagnostic Questionnaire (DN4), the Leeds Assessment of Neuropathic Symptoms and Signs (LANSS), the Neuropathic Pain Questionnaire (NPQ) and others. Among these questionnaires, the ID pain questionnaire appears to accurately detect the presence of a neuropathic pain [17,26,27]

Although most of the patients who undergo thoracic surgery will experience some tissue and nerve injuries, not all will develop CPSP following thoracic surgery. A number of studies have attempted to identify potential risk factors for the development of CPSP and its neuropathic component, but come to variable results [10,16,27]. The pathogenesis of CPSP following thoracic surgery remains poorly defined, partially due to its multifactorial etiology. Consistent with previous studies [2,3,6,8,22,23,28], some of the reported preoperative 'vulnerability factors' have been confirmed in our study, including young age and female gender, which could have contributed to CPSP following thoracic surgery due to an exaggerated stress, inflammatory, and immune system response [9]. Young age is considered to be related to higher requirements for post-operative analgesia, stronger inflammatory and immune reaction, and increased neuroplastic responses [9,23]. Gender related influences on pain and pain management have also been extensively studied in both basic and clinical researches [18,29–32]. Compared to men, women not only have greater pain sensitivity to most experimental pain modalities displaying a higher level of acute postoperative pain, but also seem to be associated with a higher prevalence of chronic postoperative pain [18,29–32]. In addition, no study has shown an increased risk of chronic postoperative pain in male patients [9]. Women are at particular risk for sensitization of their nervous system, as their neural circuitry tends to more readily detect pain and to attenuate it less than men [33].

Our study also for the first time demonstrated that pre-operative hypertension is a risk factor for CPSP following thoracic surgery. It is well known that there are adverse physiological effects of acute pain on cardiovascular systems by increasing sympathetic activity and stress response, which could be further exaggerated in hypertensive patients.

The trajectory for CPSP following thoracic surgery is not clear. Consistent to Steegers et al [8], we have found that the prevalence of CPSP following thoracic surgery did not decrease over time. The exact mechanism underlying the transition from acute to chronic pain is not clear, with possible mechanisms including central never system (CNS) reorganization and sensitization [9]. The etiology of CPSP following thoracic surgery is multifactorial with well-accepted predictors including intensity of acute post-operative pain [1,2,5,9,26,27] and concurrent perioperative nerve

Table 2. Responses to the questionnaire refer to the Maguire's research partially.

Question NO.	Question (in brief)	Answered 'yes' Total (n,%)	Answered 'yes' of Non-NP patients (n,%)	Answered 'yes' NP patients (n,%)	P value
2	Strange, unpleasant skin sensations	157(59.2%)	89 (49.7%)	68(79.1%)	0.000
3	Skin looks different	59 (22.3%)	42(23.5%)	17(19.8%)	0.498
4	Abnormally sensitive skin	137(51.7%)	83(46.4%)	54(62.8%)	0.012
5	Pain in sudden bursts	87(32.8%)	49(27.4%)	38(44.2%)	0.006
6	Skin temperature has changed	51(19.2%)	28(15.6%)	23(26.7%)	0.032
12	Improved with time	178(67.2%)	119(66.5%)	59(68.6%)	0.730
13	Pain severity mild	194(65.1%)	146(81.6%)	48(55.8%)	0.000
	moderate	59(29.1%)	28(15.6%)	31(36.0%)	
	severe	11(5.7%)	5(2.8%)	6(7.0%)	
14	Taking analgesia	56(17.7%)	43(24.0%)	13(15.1%)	0.096
15	Attended pain clinic	110(43.0%)	71(39.7%)	39(45.3%)	0.379
16	Pain the worst problem	104 (45.3%)	60(33.5%)	44(51.2%)	0.010
17	Pain limits daily activities	61(28.3%)	32(17.9%)	29(33.7%)	0.008
18	Pain limits sleep	72(32.5%)	39(21.8%)	33(38.4%)	0.008

NP, neuropathic pain.

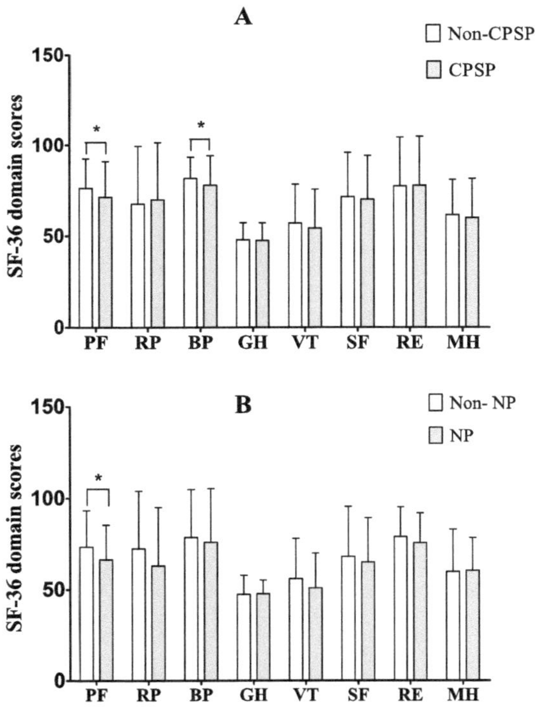

Figure 3. SF-36 domain scores of patients after thoracic surgery. Values of SF-36 domain scores represent mean ± SD in the respective group, whereas A show the result of SF-36 domain scores for the patients with CPSP or not, the B show the result of SF-36 domain scores for the patients with neuropathic pain or not. CPSP, chronic post-surgical pain; NP, neuropathic pain; PF, physical function; RP, role limitations due to physical problems; BP, body pain; GH, general health; VT, vitality; SF, social function; RE, role limitations due to emotional problems; MH, mental health.

injury [6,18,34]. A great deal of investigations found that the severity of acute postoperative pain was related to CPSP following thoracic surgery [1,2,5,7,9,35–37], while others found no association [19,23,38,39]. The underlying cause of this difference may lie in study design, using analgesic consumption instead of the acute pain scores [40], the different duration for acute pain evaluation [18], or a significant recall bias in retrospective investigations [18]. Our study found that post-operative non-PCA pain management regimen is a risk factor for CPSP. Possible reasons include improved post-operative pain relief when PCA regimen was used with systemic opioid [41]. The patients with the non-PCA regime usually were administered with tramadol intramuscularly at least every 6 hours as VAS score more than 7 except intravenous flurbiprofen 50 mg every 12 hours in our hospital. Multimodal pain management therapy with NSAIDs, COXIBs, or acetaminophen, regional blockade and/or opioid should be used and suggested strongly by the consultants and the American Society of Anesthesiologists because of its complicated mechanism and development of a chronic pain state after surgery [28,41]. In these survey, the patients was not used with regional blockade or ketamine or pregabalin for acute pain management, and it was not well demonstrated that they can reduce the intensity of acute pain or the incidence of CPSP consistently [18,23,42]. The further investigation of multimodal post-operative pain management combined with NSAIDs, regional blockade and opioids should be taken in the future.

Intercostal nerve damage is well known as a main cause of CPSP following thoracic surgery [18,43]. Both surgical incision and post-operation chest drain insertion are associated with nerve injury [44]. Consistent to previous studies [1,2,5,6,26], our investigation showed that the duration of chest tube drainage (≥4 days) (but not the different surgical procedures thoracotomy versus VATS, or different surgical site) was one of risk factors for CPSP following thoracic surgery. Chest drains are especially associated with movement-related pain which play a significant role in and lengthen the trajectory of acute post-operative pain until their removal [45]. Prolonged chest tube placement or inadequate post-operative pain management (the patient with non-PCA regimen) can be associated with more persistent pain, leading to continued stimulation to CNS and subsequent hypersensitivity and CNS reorganization. Moreover, Miyazaki demonstrated that chest tube insertion is also clearly harmful to both myelinated fibers (Aδ and Aβ fibers) and unmyelinated C fibers of the intercostal nerve and could result in post-thoracotomy pain by using current perception threshold testing recently [44]. This may explain why prolonged chest tube drains (≥4 days) were found to be not only a predictor for CPSP, but also the only predictor we identified for developing a neuropathic component of CPSP following thoracic surgery, which has not been reported before [4,8,11]. We should thus recognize that the draining chest tube would be removed as soon as possible, and more flexible drains should be applied and expected to eliminate or decrease the intercostal nerve injury and CPSP post-operatively [46].

Based on the SF-36 scores combined with scores from questionnaire referenced to Maguire's research, our study has found that CPSP patients in general have mild symptoms, with similar overall health vitality and mental health compared to patients who did not develop CPSP, though CPSP patients do have increased pain intensity and decreased physical functioning. Few CPSP patients needed to take pain medications. In contrast, the presence of neuropathic symptoms was associated with more severe pain, decreased daily activity, poorer sleep, and overall worse quality of life, which are consistent to findings from Steegers et al [8].

The retrospective study design is a limitation, and the shortcomings of self-reported pain on phone interview and in questionnaire surveys need to be kept in mind. We also could not rule out tumor recurrence and metastasis at the time point of phone interview and paper survey, which could complicate pain presentation. In addition, this is a single-center study; additional data from multi-center studies will be needed to verify our findings. Other potential risk factors including preoperative psychosocial comorbidity and genetic predisposition were omitted in this study as they could not be assessed or measured in retrospective study. Future studies are needed to address these limitations with well designed protocol [18,20].

Chronic pain is a common complication from thoracic surgery, which can significantly impact patient's daily life. Our study showed that about one out of four patients who received thoracic surgery will develop persistent post-thoracic surgery chronic pain, with about one third of them has neuropathic component. There are several predicting risk factors identified from our study, of which the duration of chest tube drainage (≥4 days) seems to be essential for both CPSP following thoracic surgery with and without neuropathic component. Patients with the neuropathic component have significantly worse quality of life, suggesting the importance of preventing CPSP following thoracic surgery from developing as well as aggressive treatment of CPSP once it has developed. Further studies are needed to investigate the impact of minimizing risk factors on the incidence of CPSP, especially a multifaceted approach to shorten the chest tube drainage.

Author Contributions

Conceived and designed the experiments: ZP HL CZ ZF SZ. Performed the experiments: ZP HL CZ ZF SZ. Analyzed the data: ZP HL CZ XQ ZF SZ. Contributed reagents/materials/analysis tools: ZP HL ZF SZ. Wrote the paper: ZP HL ZF SZ.

References

1. Kinney MA, Hooten WM, Cassivi SD, Allen MS, Passe MA, et al. (2012) Chronic postthoracotomy pain and health-related quality of life. Ann Thorac Surg 93: 1242–1247.
2. Buchheit T, Pyati S (2012) Prevention of chronic pain after surgical nerve injury: amputation and thoracotomy. Surg Clin North Am 92: 393–407, x.
3. Enck RE (2010) Postsurgical chronic pain. Am J Hosp Palliat Care 27: 301–302.
4. Haroutiunian S, Nikolajsen L, Finnerup NB, Jensen TS (2013) The neuropathic component in persistent postsurgical pain: a systematic literature review. Pain 154: 95–102.
5. Van de Ven TJ, John Hsia HL (2012) Causes and prevention of chronic postsurgical pain. Curr Opin Crit Care 18: 366–371.
6. Guastella V, Mick G, Soriano C, Vallet L, Escande G, et al. (2011) A prospective study of neuropathic pain induced by thoracotomy: incidence, clinical description, and diagnosis. Pain 152: 74–81.
7. Katz J, Jackson M, Kavanagh BP, Sandler AN (1996) Acute pain after thoracic surgery predicts long-term post-thoracotomy pain. Clin J Pain 12: 50–55.
8. Steegers MA, Snik DM, Verhagen AF, van der Drift MA, Wilder-Smith OH (2008) Only half of the chronic pain after thoracic surgery shows a neuropathic component. J Pain 9: 955–961.
9. Deumens R, Steyaert A, Forget P, Schubert M, Lavand'homme P, et al. (2013) Prevention of chronic postoperative pain: cellular, molecular, and clinical insights for mechanism-based treatment approaches. Prog Neurobiol 104: 1–37.
10. International Association for the Study of Pain Committee. ASP Taxonomy. Pain terms — Changes in the 2011 list. Available from www.iasp-pain.org/Content/NavigationMenu/GeneralResourceLinks/PainDefinitions/default.htm. Accessed 2012 Feb 18
11. Searle RD, Simpson MP, Simpson KH, Milton R, Bennett MI (2009) Can chronic neuropathic pain following thoracic surgery be predicted during the postoperative period? Interact Cardiovasc Thorac Surg 9: 999–1002.
12. Maguire MF, Ravenscroft A, Beggs D, Duffy JP (2006) A questionnaire study investigating the prevalence of the neuropathic component of chronic pain after thoracic surgery. Eur J Cardiothorac Surg 29: 800–805.
13. Salati M, Brunelli A, Xiume F, Refai M, Sabbatini A (2009) Quality of life in the elderly after major lung resection for lung cancer. Interact Cardiovasc Thorac Surg 8: 79–83.
14. Brunelli A, Socci L, Refai M, Salati M, Xiume F, et al. (2007) Quality of life before and after major lung resection for lung cancer: a prospective follow-up analysis. Ann Thorac Surg 84: 410–416.
15. Jensen TS, Baron R, Haanpaa M, Kalso E, Loeser JD, et al. (2011) A new definition of neuropathic pain. Pain 152: 2204–2205.
16. Haanpaa M, Attal N, Backonja M, Baron R, Bennett M, et al. (2011) NeuPSIG guidelines on neuropathic pain assessment. Pain 152: 14–27.
17. Li J, Feng Y, Han J, Fan B, Wu D, et al. (2012) Linguistic adaptation, validation and comparison of 3 routinely used neuropathic pain questionnaires. Pain Physician 15: 179–186.
18. Wildgaard K, Ravn J, Kehlet H (2009) Chronic post-thoracotomy pain: a critical review of pathogenic mechanisms and strategies for prevention. Eur J Cardiothorac Surg 36: 170–180.
19. Perttunen K, Tasmuth T, Kalso E (1999) Chronic pain after thoracic surgery: a follow-up study. Acta Anaesthesiol Scand 43: 563–567.
20. VanDenKerkhof EG, Peters ML, Bruce J (2013) Chronic pain after surgery: time for standardization? A framework to establish core risk factor and outcome domains for epidemiological studies. Clin J Pain 29: 2–8.
21. Macrae WA (2001) Chronic pain after surgery. Br J Anaesth 87: 88–98.
22. Wang HT, Liu W, Luo AL, Ma C, Huang YG (2012) Prevalence and risk factors of chronic post-thoracotomy pain in Chinese patients from Peking Union Medical College Hospital. Chin Med J (Engl) 125: 3033–3038.
23. Mongardon N, Pinton-Gonnet C, Szekely B, Michel-Cherqui M, Dreyfus JF, et al. (2011) Assessment of chronic pain after thoracotomy: a 1-year prevalence study. Clin J Pain 27: 677–681.
24. Song JG, Shin JW, Lee EH, Choi DK, Bang JY, et al. (2012) Incidence of post-thoracotomy pain: a comparison between total intravenous anaesthesia and inhalation anaesthesia. Eur J Cardiothorac Surg 41: 1078–1082.
25. Lavand'homme P (2011) The progression from acute to chronic pain. Curr Opin Anaesthesiol 24: 545–550.
26. Portenoy R (2006) Development and testing of a neuropathic pain screening questionnaire: ID Pain. Curr Med Res Opin 22: 1555–1565.
27. Reyes-Gibby C, Morrow PK, Bennett MI, Jensen MP, Shete S (2010) Neuropathic pain in breast cancer survivors: using the ID pain as a screening tool. J Pain Symptom Manage 39: 882–889.
28. Wu CL, Raja SN (2011) Treatment of acute postoperative pain. Lancet 377: 2215–2225.
29. Ochroch EA, Gottschalk A, Troxel AB, Farrar JT (2006) Women suffer more short and long-term pain than men after major thoracotomy. Clin J Pain 22: 491–498.
30. Puolakka PA, Rorarius MG, Roviola M, Puolakka TJ, Nordhausen K, et al. (2010) Persistent pain following knee arthroplasty. Eur J Anaesthesiol 27: 455–460.

31. Wildgaard K, Ravn J, Nikolajsen L, Jakobsen E, Jensen TS, et al. (2011) Consequences of persistent pain after lung cancer surgery: a nationwide questionnaire study. Acta Anaesthesiol Scand 55: 60–68.
32. Racine M, Tousignant-Laflamme Y, Kloda LA, Dion D, Dupuis G, et al. (2012) A systematic literature review of 10 years of research on sex/gender and pain perception - part 2: do biopsychosocial factors alter pain sensitivity differently in women and men? Pain 153: 619–635.
33. Mogil JS, Bailey AL (2010) Sex and gender differences in pain and analgesia. Prog Brain Res 186: 141–157.
34. Kehlet H, Jensen TS, Woolf CJ (2006) Persistent postsurgical pain: risk factors and prevention. Lancet 367: 1618–1625.
35. Pluijms WA, Steegers MA, Verhagen AF, Scheffer GJ, Wilder-Smith OH (2006) Chronic post-thoracotomy pain: a retrospective study. Acta Anaesthesiol Scand 50: 804–808.
36. Gotoda Y, Kambara N, Sakai T, Kishi Y, Kodama K, et al. (2001) The morbidity, time course and predictive factors for persistent post-thoracotomy pain. Eur J Pain 5: 89–96.
37. Katz J, Seltzer Z (2009) Transition from acute to chronic postsurgical pain: risk factors and protective factors. Expert Rev Neurother 9: 723–744.
38. Kalso E, Perttunen K, Kaasinen S (1992) Pain after thoracic surgery. Acta Anaesthesiol Scand 36: 96–100.
39. Tiippana E, Nilsson E, Kalso E (2003) Post-thoracotomy pain after thoracic epidural analgesia: a prospective follow-up study. Acta Anaesthesiol Scand 47: 433–438.
40. Khan IH, McManus KG, McCraith A, McGuigan JA (2000) Muscle sparing thoracotomy: a biomechanical analysis confirms preservation of muscle strength but no improvement in wound discomfort. Eur J Cardiothorac Surg 18: 656–661.
41. American Society of Anesthesiologists Task Force on Acute Pain M (2012) Practice guidelines for acute pain management in the perioperative setting: an updated report by the American Society of Anesthesiologists Task Force on Acute Pain Management. Anesthesiology 116: 248–273.
42. Wildgaard K, Kehlet H (2011) Chronic post-thoracotomy pain—What is new in pathogenic mechanisms and strategies for prevention? Techniques in Regional Anesthesia and Pain Management 15: 83–89.
43. Wildgaard K, Ringsted TK, Ravn J, Werner MU, Kehlet H (2013) Late sensory changes following chest drain insertion during thoracotomy. Acta Anaesthesiol Scand 57: 776–783.
44. Miyazaki T, Sakai T, Yamasaki N, Tsuchiya T, Matsumoto K, et al. (2013) Chest tube insertion is one important factor leading to intercostal nerve impairment in thoracic surgery. Gen Thorac Cardiovasc Surg.
45. Forcella D, Pompeo E, Coniglione F, Gatti A, Mineo TC (2009) A new technique for continuous intercostal-intrapleural analgesia in videothoracoscopic surgery. J Thorac Cardiovasc Surg 137: e48–49.
46. Nakamura H, Taniguchi Y, Miwa K, Adachi Y, Fujioka S, et al. (2009) The use of Blake drains following general thoracic surgery: is it an acceptable option? Interact Cardiovasc Thorac Surg 8: 58–61.

11

The Anti-Diabetic Drug Metformin Protects against Chemotherapy-Induced Peripheral Neuropathy in a Mouse Model

Qi-Liang Mao-Ying[1,2], Annemieke Kavelaars[1], Karen Krukowski[1], Xiao-Jiao Huo[1], Wenjun Zhou[1], Theodore J. Price[3], Charles Cleeland[4], Cobi J. Heijnen[1]*

1 Neuroimmunology Laboratory, Department of Symptom Research, University of Texas M.D. Anderson Cancer Center, Houston, Texas, United States of America, **2** Department of Integrative Medicine and Neurobiology, State Key Laboratory of Medical Neurobiology, School of Basic Medical Sciences, Fudan University, Shanghai, People's Republic of China, **3** School of Behavioral and Brain Sciences, University of Texas at Dallas, Richardson, Texas, United States of America, **4** Department of Symptom Research, University of Texas M.D. Anderson Cancer Center, Houston, Texas, United States of America

Abstract

Chemotherapy-induced peripheral neuropathy (CIPN) characterized by loss of sensory sensitivity and pain in hands and feet is the major dose-limiting toxicity of many chemotherapeutics. At present, there are no FDA-approved treatments for CIPN. The anti-diabetic drug metformin is the most widely used prescription drug in the world and improves glycemic control in diabetes patients. There is some evidence that metformin enhances the efficacy of cancer treatment. The aim of this study was to test the hypothesis that metformin protects against chemotherapy-induced neuropathic pain and sensory deficits. Mice were treated with cisplatin together with metformin or saline. Cisplatin induced increased sensitivity to mechanical stimulation (mechanical allodynia) as measured using the von Frey test. Co-administration of metformin almost completely prevented the cisplatin-induced mechanical allodynia. Co-administration of metformin also prevented paclitaxel-induced mechanical allodynia. The capacity of the mice to detect an adhesive patch on their hind paw was used as a novel indicator of chemotherapy-induced sensory deficits. Co-administration of metformin prevented the cisplatin-induced increase in latency to detect the adhesive patch indicating that metformin prevents sensory deficits as well. Moreover, metformin prevented the reduction in density of intra-epidermal nerve fibers (IENFs) in the paw that develops as a result of cisplatin treatment. We conclude that metformin protects against pain and loss of tactile function in a mouse model of CIPN. The finding that metformin reduces loss of peripheral nerve endings indicates that mechanism underlying the beneficial effects of metformin includes a neuroprotective activity. Because metformin is widely used for treatment of type II diabetes, has a broad safety profile, and is currently being tested as an adjuvant drug in cancer treatment, clinical translation of these findings could be rapidly achieved.

Editor: David D. McKemy, University of South California, United States of America

Funding: This work was supported by National Cancer Institute of the National Institute of Health PO1 CA124787 (CC); National Institute of Neurological Diseases and Stroke of the National Institute of Health RO1 NS073939 (AK), RO1 NS74999 (AK), and RO1 NS065926 (TJP); National Institute of General Medical Sciences of the National Institute of Health RO1 GM102575 (TJP); United States Pain Relief Committee (CJH, CC); and STARS award Universtiy of Texas System (AK). The funders had no role in study design, data collection and analysis, decision to publish, or preparation of the manuscript.

Competing Interests: The authors have declared that no competing interests exist.

* Email: cjheijnen@mdanderson.org

Introduction

Chemotherapy-induced peripheral neuropathy (CIPN), characterized by a glove-and-stocking distribution of sensory changes including dysesthesia, paraesthesia, and pain, occurs on average in 30-40% patients treated for cancer, but the incidence ranges widely among various studies and compounds from 10–100% [1,2]. A deficit in touch detection that ranges from the pain area into the volar skin outside the area of perceived pain or sensory dysfunction has also been reported in patients treated with chemotherapy [2,3]. In patients treated for cancer, the pain, numbness and tingling in hand and feet develop during treatment and frequently continue even after completion of therapy. Moreover, this peripheral neuropathy is a major dose-limiting adverse effect of multiple chemotherapeutic agents, including cisplatin (cis-diamminedichloroplatinmum) and paclitaxel. At present, there are no FDA-approved treatments for chemotherapy-induced neuropathy. Therefore, identification of drugs that provide effective prevention and/or treatment of chemotherapy-induced peripheral neuropathy would be a major step forward in improving treatment adherence and quality of life in patients treated with chemotherapeutics.

Metformin, a classic and widely used anti-diabetic drug, activates adenosine monophosphate-activated protein kinase (AMPK). Recent findings show that metformin reverses established mechanical allodynia in models of neuropathic pain induced by spinal nerve ligation in rats and spared nerve injury in mice [4,5]. Moreover, metformin attenuates hyperexcitability in sensory neurons that develops following exposure to growth factors and cytokines that have previously been linked to chemotherapy-induced neuropathic pain [6]. In addition, metformin has neuroprotective effects in murine models of neurodegenerative disorders including diabetes-associated brain neurodegeneration [7,8], ethanol-induced neuronal apoptosis [9] and experimental stroke [10]. There is evidence that metformin enhances the efficacy of anti-cancer treatment [11,12] an effect that has been widely attributed to the drug's action on AMPK. However, whether metformin protects against cisplatin-induced neuropathy has not been tested.

Intraepidermal nerve fibers (IENFs) are free nerve ending arising from unmyelinated and thinly myelinated sensory neurons within the dermis and are important for transmission of peripheral pain [13]. In humans treated with chemotherapy, the density of epidermal nerve fibers in the fingertip, palm and forearm are either absent or reduced, indicating damage to distal nerves [1]. Similarly, in rats and mice receiving repeated treatment with platinum-based chemotherapeutic agents a significant reduction in IENF density is observed in the foot pad [13,14,15]. In 2011, J. Boyette-Davis et al. reported that minocycline treatment effectively prevented IENF loss as well as mechanical allodynia in oxaliplatin-treated rats [13]. This finding revealed that peripheral nerve damage leading to a reduction in IENFs may be involved in chemotherapy-induced neuropathic pain. In addition, IENFs are known to be important for normal tactile sensation [16,17]. Hence, treatments that protect against chemotherapeutic-induced retraction and/or damage of IENFs may reduce the development of neuropathic pain and alleviate dysesthesias that are common dose limiting complaints in patients.

Here we have tested the hypothesis that metformin may protect against chemotherapy-induced neuropathic pain, dysesthesia and loss of IENFs in the hind paw of mice. This hypothesis is based on the notion that AMPK activation may lead to the production of direct and/or indirect neuroprotective and anti-hyperexcitability effects in the peripheral nervous system that would alleviate multiple facets of chemotherapy-induced sensory symptoms [18]. Our findings show that metformin is broadly effective in a preclinical mouse model suggesting that these findings may rapidly translate into transformative treatment strategies for the alleviation of these dose-limiting side effects.

Materials and Methods

Animals

C57Bl/6J mice at 12 weeks of age at the beginning of the experiment were used in this study. Mice were housed on a 12 h light/dark cycle with free access to food and water. All behaviors were observed during the dark phase of the light cycle with red light. All procedures were consistent with the National Institute of Health Guidelines for the Care and Use of Laboratory Animals and the Ethical Issues of the International Association for the Study of Pain [19] and were approved by the Institutional Animal Care and Use Committee of Texas A&M University (protocol number 12020).

Drug treatments

After repeat exposure to the test environment and baseline measurements of behavior, C57Bl/6J mice were intraperitoneally (i.p.) treated with cisplatin (Sigma-Aldrich, St. Louis MI) daily at a dosage of 2.3 mg/kg for 5 days, followed by 5 days of rest, for two cycles with a total cumulative dose of 23 mg/kg cisplatin [19]. Control mice received an equivalent volume of saline. Metformin hydrochloride (Sigma-Aldrich) was freshly prepared in saline daily. Metformin (200 mg/kg) or saline was given i.p. for seven consecutive days, beginning 24 h prior to the first dose of cisplatin of each cycle or 24 h before the start of the second cisplatin cycle. A separate group of mice was treated with paclitaxel (i.p 10 mg/kg) every other day for two weeks. In this group, metformin (200 mg/kg i.p.) was given daily starting 24 h before the first dose of paclitaxel. On days when both cisplatin or paclitaxel and metformin were administered, metformin was given 30–60 min prior to cisplatin or paclitaxel. Lidocaine hydrochloride (Sigma-Aldrich; 5 µl 4% in saline) or saline was injected into the hind paw of control mice 10 minutes before the adhesive removal test.

Von Frey test for mechanical allodynia

Mechanical allodynia was measured as the hind paw withdrawal response to von Frey hair stimulation using the up-and-down method as we described previously [20]. Mice were placed in a plastic cage ($10\times10\times13$ cm^3) with a mesh floor for 30 min prior to testing. Subsequently, a series of von Frey hairs (0.02, 0.07, 0.16, 0.4, 0.6, 1.0 and 1.4 g) (Stoelting, Wood Dale, IL) were applied perpendicular to the mid-plantar surface of hind paw. A trial began with the application of the 0.16 g hair. A positive response was defined as a clear paw withdrawal or shaking. Whenever a positive response occurred, the next lower hair was applied, and whenever a negative response occurred, the next higher hair was applied. The testing consisted of five more stimuli after the first change in response occurred, and the pattern of response was converted to the 50% withdrawal threshold using the method described previously [21] and specified in the supporting information (File S1).

Rotarod test for motor impairment

To control for the possibility that behavioral changes are due to the motor impairment in cisplatin treated mice, motor function was assessed using the rotarod apparatus (Med Associates INC, Georigia, VE). Briefly, mice were placed individually on the rotating system and trained for three days at 16 rpm with three trials per day. Each trial lasted for three minutes; on the third day all mice completed the 3 minute training session. In the actual motor function test, an accelerated rotarod assay (4–40 rpm over 5 min) was evaluated for three trails and the latency to fall was recorded. For details see supporting information section (File S2).

Adhesive removal test for tactile hyposensitivity behavior

In order to examine the effect of cisplatin on sensory function, we used a modification of the adhesive removal test [22]. Briefly, a round adhesive patch (3/16" Teeny Touch-Spots, USA Scientific INC. Ocalo, FL) was placed on the plantar surface of the hind paws. The animal performance in a testing cage ($20\times20\times13$ cm^3) was recorded in 15 min. The time until the mouse started to shake its paw or bring the paw to the mouth was recorded as a measure of the latency until the mouse noticed the presence of the adhesive patch on the paw. For details see supporting information section (File S1).

Immunostaining for IENFs

For quantification of IENFs, 3×3 mm^2 biopsies were dissected from the central plantar surface of the hind paws. Biopsies were immediately placed in Zamboni's fixative for 24 hrs, and transferred to 20% sucrose for at least 24 hrs, frozen in Optimal Cutting Temperature compound (OCT), and sliced into 25 µm sections. The sections were blocked for 2 hrs at room temperature in 0.1 M PBS containing 5% normal donkey serum/0.3% Triton X-100. The blocking solution was removed and the sections were incubated with an antibody against the pan neuronal marker PGP9.5 (AbD Serotec, Raleigh, NC; Rabbit, 1:2000) along with anti-Collagen IV antibody (Southern Biotech, Birmingham, AL; Goat, 1:100) at 4 °C overnight. Then the sections were washed in wash buffer (3 times one hour), and incubated with Alexa-594-donkey anti-rabbit (Life Technologies, Grand Island, NY 1:500) and Alexa-488-donkey anti-goat (Invitrogen, Grand Island, NY 1:500) at 4 °C overnight. Sections were washed in wash buffer and then three randomly chosen slices from each paw were quantified under a Leica fluorescence microscope. Nerve fibers that crossed the collagen stained dermal/epidermal junction into the epidermis were counted in three fields of each slice using the 40× objective. The length of the epidermis within each field was measured using ImageJ. IENF density was determined as the total number of fibers/length of epidermis (IENFs/mm). For details see supporting information section (File S4). Representative images captured by using In Cell 6000 microscope are shown.

Statistical analysis

Data are expressed as mean ± SEM. Statistical analysis was carried out using repeated measure analysis of variance or dependent t test or one-way ANOVA followed by Bonferroni analysis. $P<0.05$ was considered statistically significant. Methods for calculating 50% withdrawal thresholds are detailed in file S5. Raw data are provided in the supporting information file S6.

Results

Effect of metformin on chemotherapy-induced neuropathic pain

Mice were treated with two rounds of 5 daily i.p. injections with cisplatin with 5 days rest in between (Figure 1a). Figure 1b demonstrates cisplatin induced persistent mechanical allodynia measured at 3 and 5 weeks after the 1st cisplatin injection. Metformin was administered at a dose that is used to treat diabetic mice (200 mg/kg daily) and that is efficacious in surgical nerve injury-induced neuropathic pain [4], for 2 rounds of 7 days, beginning 24 hours prior to the 1st dose of cisplatin of each cycle. Co-administration of metformin treatment completely prevented cisplatin-induced mechanical allodynia (Figure 1b). Metformin treatment alone did not have any effect on mechanical sensitivity (Figure 1b).

To determine whether metformin treatment should be started together with cisplatin or can be delayed, we delayed metformin treatment until the 2nd round of cisplatin treatment. The results in Figure 1c show that this delayed metformin treatment had no effect on mechanical allodynia. These results strongly suggested that concomitant but not delayed treatment with metformin prevents cisplatin-induced mechanical allodynia.

The beneficial effect of metformin was not limited to cisplatin-induced mechanical allodynia; also paclitaxel-induced mechanical allodynia was prevented by administration of metformin starting 24 hours prior to the first dose of paclitaxel (Figure 1d).

Metformin treatment did not affect body weight when given alone and did not have any effect on the transient loss of bodyweight in mice treated with cisplatin (Figure 1e) or paclitaxel (Data not shown).

Cisplatin-induced sensory deficits and metformin treatment

The effect of cisplatin on the time-to-respond to an adhesive patch on the hind paw was recorded as a novel indicator of chemotherapy-induced sensory deficit. In cisplatin-treated mice the time-to-respond to the adhesive patch on the hind paw was significantly prolonged at 3 and 5 weeks after the 1st cisplatin injection when compared to saline-treated mice (Figure 2a). Co-administration of metformin prevented the increase in latency to respond to the adhesive patch on the paw, whereas delayed treatment did not have any effect (Figure 2a, c). The time between the first response to the adhesive patch and subsequent removal of the patch was not affected by cisplatin treatment indicating normal motor function (data not shown). In addition, cisplatin-treated mice showed normal performance on a rotarod indicating that the prolonged time-to-respond to the patch on the hind paw cannot be attributed to potential cisplatin-induced motor function deficits (Figure 2d). As a positive control, the data in Figure 2e show that the time-to-respond to the adhesive patch was also significantly increased in lidocaine-treated mice. Collectively, our findings support the notion that the increase in time-to-respond to the adhesive patch in cisplatin-treated mice is related to a sensory deficit, which is prevented by metformin treatment.

Protective effect of metformin on cisplatin-induced IENF loss

IENF loss had been reported in rat models of chemotherapy-induced neuropathy using cisplatin, oxaliplatin, taxol, paclitaxel and vincristine [13,14,23,24]. We analyzed the effect of metformin treatment on the IENF density in hind and fore paw of cisplatin treated mice at 5 weeks after the first cisplatin treatment. Saline-treated mice showed abundant distribution of nerve fibers entering the epidermis. The IENF density was significantly decreased in response to cisplatin-treatment (Figure 3a–b). Notably, metformin significantly protected against this cisplatin-induced IENF loss (Figure 3c). There were no significant differences between metformin-treated cisplatin mice and saline- treated mice (Figure 3d).

Discussion

The AMP kinase agonist metformin is an anti-diabetic drug that has been safely and widely used for the treatment of type 2 diabetes for decades. This is the first study to show that metformin protects against cisplatin- and paclitaxel-induced mechanical allodynia in a mouse model. Additionally, this is the first study to demonstrate a loss of sensory sensitivity associated with CIPN in a mouse model. We show that cisplatin increases the time to detect an adhesive patch on the hind paw and that metformin prevents development of this sign of sensory impairment or 'numbness' in cisplatin-treated mice. In search for an underlying mechanism, we show that metformin treatment protects against the loss of IENFs that occurs in response to cisplatin treatment. Collectively, these findings indicate that metformin protects against cisplatin-induced peripheral neuropathy by reducing peripheral nerve damage. We propose that these findings represent the discovery of a safe preventive treatment for chemotherapy-induced neuropathy. Because metformin is already widely used, rapid clinical translation of these findings should be possible.

Metformin is the first-line treatment for type II diabetes because of its insulin sensitizing effects [25]. Individuals with obesity or polycystic ovary syndrome are also frequently treated with metformin. In 2012, over 61 million prescriptions for metformin were filed in the United States [26]. There is evidence that metformin treatment of diabetics reduces the risk of cancer in this population. In addition, preclinical and clinical studies indicate that metformin treatment may increase the efficacy of cancer treatment. In a retrospective study in breast cancer patients with diabetes, patients treated with metformin had higher complete pathologic response rates to neoadjuvant therapy than diabetic patients treated with other antidiabetic drugs [27]. Similarly two retrospective cohort studies indicated that metformin treatment of

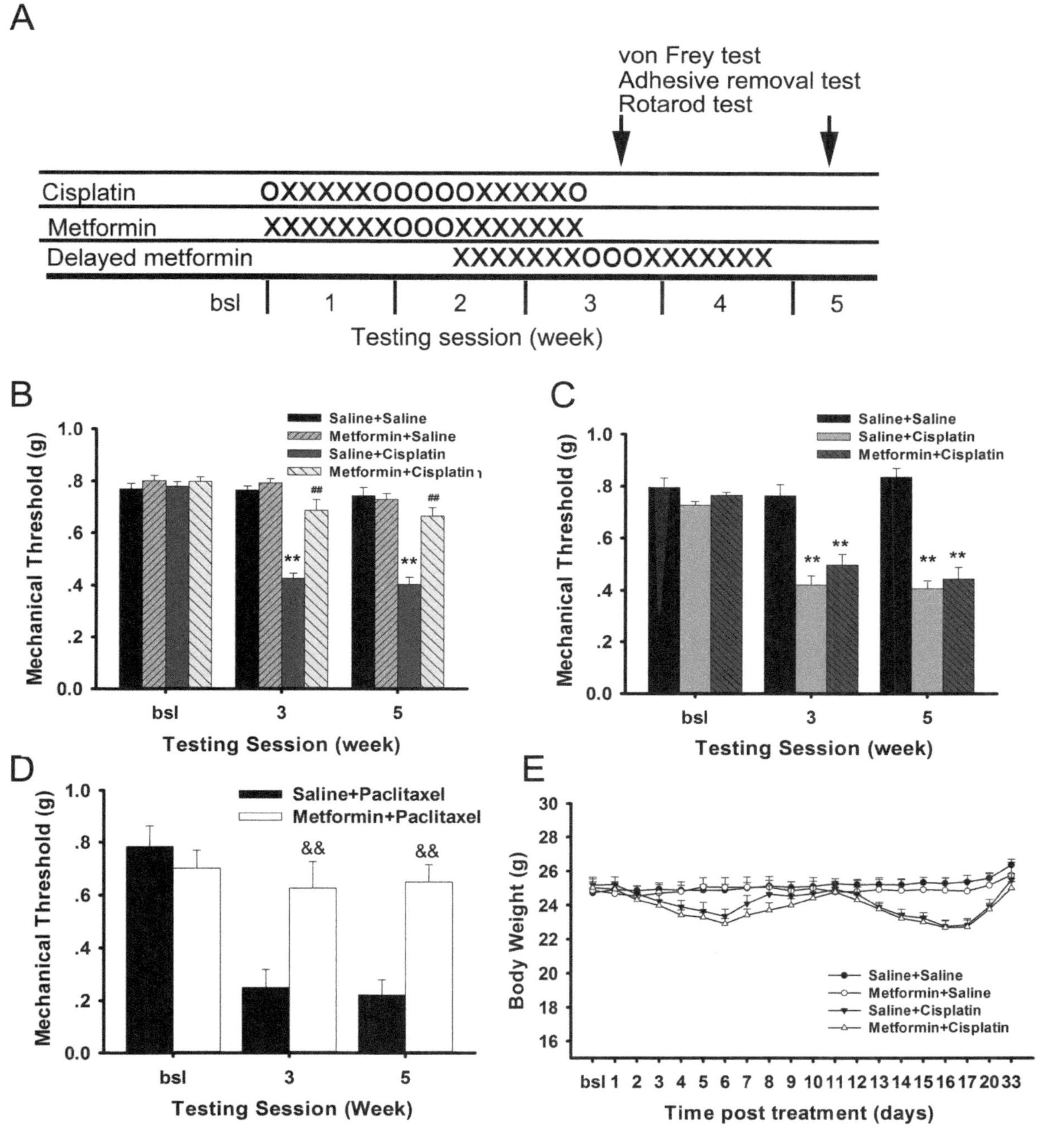

Figure 1. Effect of metformin on cisplatin- or paclitaxel-induced mechanical allodynia in mice. A). Treatment schedule; X: injection; O: no treatment. B) Mice (n = 10–12/group) were treated with cisplatin (cumulative dose 23 mg/kg i.p.) and metformin (200 mg/kg/dose i.p.) as depicted in panel A. Mechanical allodynia was quantified with von Frey hairs using the up and down method. C). Effect of delayed metformin treatment on cisplatin-induced mechanical allodynia. Mice (n = 8/group) received i.p. injections with cisplatin (cumulative dose 23 mg/kg i.p.) and delayed metformin (200 mg/kg/dose i.p.) as depicted in panel A and mechanical allodynia was monitored. D). Mice (n = 4–7/group) were treated with paclitaxel (10 mg/kg/every other day, i.p. for two weeks) and metformin (200 mg/kg i.p. daily from one day before until one day after paclitaxel) and mechanical allodynia was measured. E). Change in body weight after cisplatin and metformin treatment. ** $p<0.01$ vs. Saline+Saline group; ## $p<0.01$ vs. Saline+Cisplatin; && $p<0.01$ vs. Saline+Paclitaxel.

diabetic patients with ovarian cancer may prolong disease specific and progression-free survival [28,29,30]. Preclinical data demonstrate that metformin inhibits cancer cell growth in vitro, enhances anti-tumor effects of chemotherapeutics in vitro, inhibits the inflammatory response associated with cancer and prolongs remission in response to chemotherapy in mouse xenograft models of cancer [31,32,33,34]. Collectively these findings have given rise to an increasing number of clinical trials aimed at examining the efficacy of metformin in cancer treatment. The data we show here identify a potential additional beneficial effect of metformin in

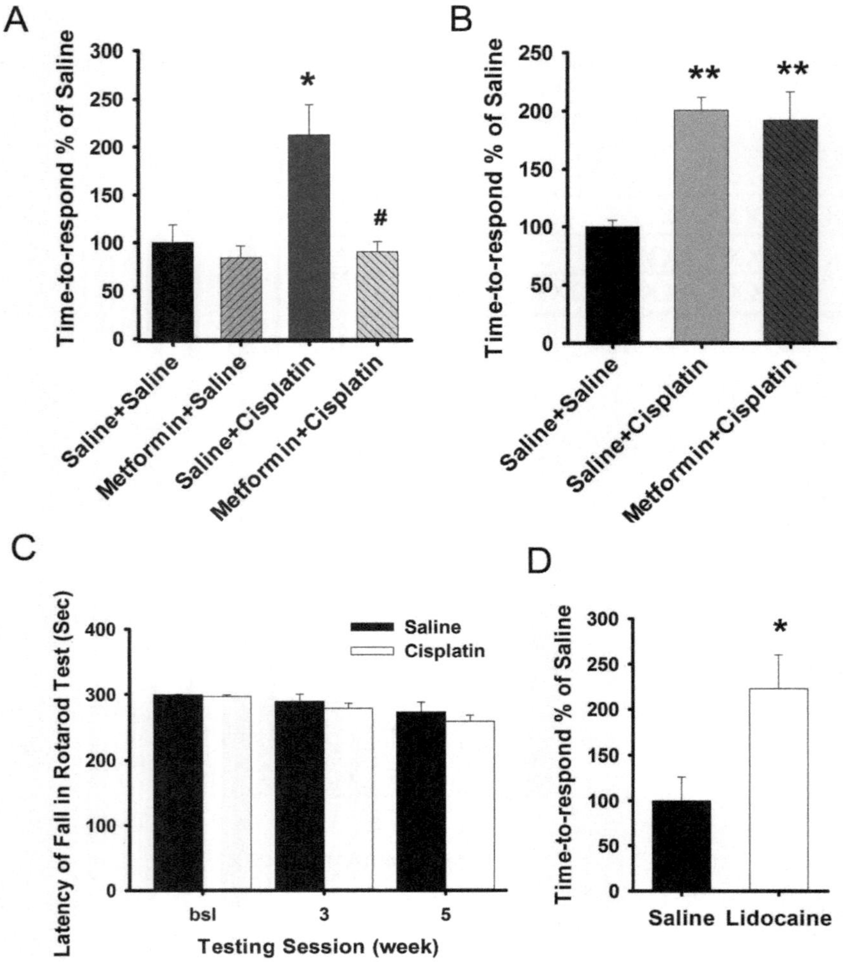

Figure 2. Effect of metformin treatment on cisplatin-induced sensory deficits. A). Mice (n = 6–10/group) were treated with cisplatin and metformin as described in Figure 1. The time to respond to an adhesive patch on the hind paw was monitored. B). Effect of delayed metformin on cisplatin induced sensory deficits (n = 7–8/group). C). Effect of cisplatin treatment on rotarod performance. Mice (n = 6/group) were treated with cisplatin and their performance on the rotarod was monitored as an index of motor coordination. E). Mice (n = 7/group) were treated with lidocaine (5 μL, 4% in saline) or saline and 10 mins. later, the time to respond to an adhesive patch on the hind paw was measured. * $p<0.05$, ** $p<0.01$ vs. Saline+Saline; # $p<0.05$ vs. Saline+Cisplatin.

cancer treatment. Our finding that metformin protects against chemotherapy-induced peripheral neuropathy urges for inclusion of systematic assessment of neuropathy in trials with metformin in cancer patients.

Recent studies have shown that metformin alleviates pain amplification that occurs in response to peripheral nerve injury in mice and rats [4,18]. In these surgical models of neuropathic pain, it was shown that metformin reverses already existing mechanical allodynia. We show here that metformin prevented development of cisplatin- and paclitaxel-induced mechanical allodynia only when treatment was started before start of the administration of these chemotherapeutics. In contrast to what was observed in traumatic models of neuropathy, we did not observe any beneficial effect of metformin when treatment was started after the first round of cisplatin treatment, when mechanical allodynia had already developed. This result is in contrast to previous observations in the spared nerve injury model in mice and spinal nerve ligation injury model in rats where metformin treatment after establishment of neuropathic allodynia effectively reversed this symptom of peripheral nerve injury. While the reasons for this discrepancy between models are not presently clear, there are several possible reasons. First, chemotherapy-induced neuropathy is mechanistically distinct from trauma-induced neuropathy. A therapeutic benefit of AMPK activation in trauma-induced neuropathy is related to decreases in mTOR and MAPK signaling in injured nerves [5,35]. It is not currently known if these signaling pathways are altered in CIPN. On the other hand, CIPN involves clear changes in mitochondrial function that may be an important target for AMPK activation in CIPN [36]. If mitochondria are a relevant target for AMPK activation [37] in CIPN, it may not be possible to reverse this effect once established by the chemotherapeutic treatment. Another possibility is that while the effects of metformin in trauma-induced neuropathy are AMPK-mediated (this hypothesis is supported by similar findings with specific AMPK activating tool compounds), metformin effects in CIPN have a separate mechanism of action. This can be tested with future experiments with AMPK activating tool compounds. One AMPK-independent possibility is metformin-mediated blockade of organic cation transporter 2 [38] which is required for oxaliplatin-induced CIPN [39]. While these mechanism-based studies are

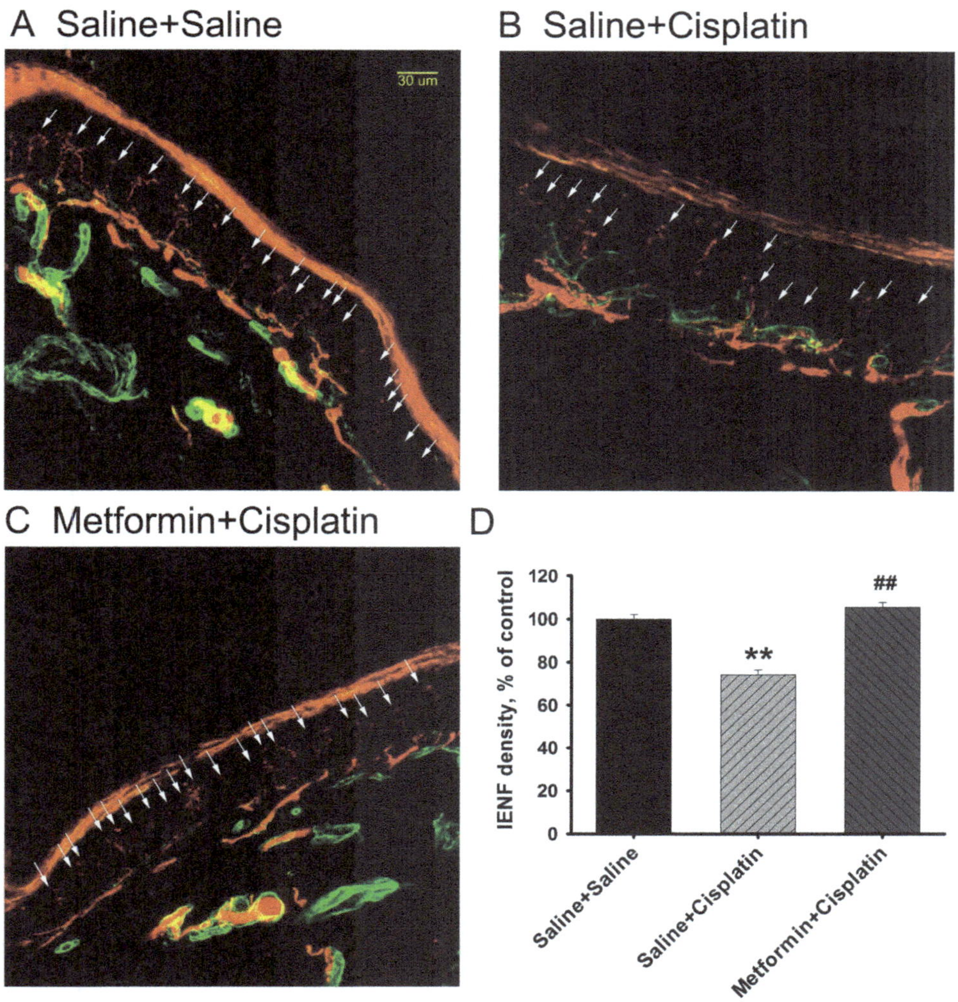

Figure 3. Effect of metformin on loss of intraepidermal nerve fibers induced by cisplatin. Mice (n = 4–6 per group) were treated with cisplatin and metformin as in figure 1. Paw biopsies obtained from the hind paw at 5 weeks after the start of treatment were stained for intraepidermal nerve fibers (PGP9.5; red) and collagen (green). (A) saline/saline; (B) saline/cisplatin; (C) metformin/cisplatin. White arrows indicate the intraepidermal nerve fibers stained by PGP9.5 (in red), which can clearly be seen crossing the basement membrane (in green) and extending as long lines into the epidermis. (D) Quantification of intraepidermal nerve fiber density. ** $p<0.01$ vs. Saline+Saline; ## $p<0.01$ vs. Saline+Cisplatin.

undoubtedly important, the aim of these studies was to assess metformin as a potential treatment for CIPN and our studies give a clear rationale for preventative clinical trials with this drug.

At present, knowledge about the mechanisms underlying chemotherapy-induced sensory deficits remains limited. Although the pain component of CIPN has received the most attention, sensory deficits are often longer lasting and thus debilitating for patients in daily life. One of the aims of this study was to determine whether cisplatin treatment in mice leads to sensory impairment and to assess the effect of metformin on cisplatin-induced sensory impairment. To that end, we used the adhesive removal test, a sensitive method to evaluate both somatosensory and motor function in rats and mice [22]. In this test, an adhesive patch is placed on the plantar surface of the hind paw, and the latency to a behavioral response to the patch as well as latency to removal of the patch is assessed. The data show that the time to display a behavioral response to the adhesive patch placed on the paw is significantly prolonged in mice treated with cisplatin. This sign of cisplatin-induced 'numbness' was present without evidence of functional motor deficits. We also observed significant IENFs loss in mice treated with cisplatin. These findings are in line with earlier studies showing loss of IENFs in rats treated with chemotherapeutic agents such as paclitaxel [24], vincristine [23], oxaliplatin [13] and cisplatin [14]. In humans exposed to chemotherapy, damage to peripheral nerves in the extremities has also been reported [1]. Moreover, IENFs transmit sensations of tactile, cold, thermal and mechanical origin from the skin, and loss of IENFs has been shown to correspond to loss of these sensations in humans [40]. We show here that mice treated with cisplatin display sensory deficits and los of IENFs in the hind paws consistent with results using the adhesive tactile test. Co-administration of metformin prevented both sensory deficits and loss of IENFs in the paws. These results strongly suggest that the cisplatin-induced of loss of IENFs in the paw contributes to chemotherapy-induced sensory deficits. The protective effect of metformin on loss of IENFs is consistent with earlier reported neuroprotective activity of metformin in models of brain damage. Moreover, in a model of peripheral nerve damage-induced neuropathy it has been shown that metformin increases the level of ApoE, a 34 kDa glycoprotein that is a major determinant of lipid transport and metabolism [18]. In addition, ApoE plays an important role in peripheral and central neuroregeneration and remyelination [18,41,42,43]. It remains to be determined whether metformin-induced increases in ApoE also contribute to the protective effect of metformin in our mouse model of chemotherapy-induced peripheral neuropathic pain.

It may seem contradictory that chemotherapy-induced decrease in IENF density is associated with decreased sensory function, but enhanced pain sensitivity. Electrophysiological and biochemical studies in cisplatin-treated rats show that sensitization of sensory neurons, increased spontaneous activity and prolonged after discharges in response to stimulation, plays a key role in pathological pain behaviors following platinum drugs [44]. This hyperresponsiveness of sensory neurons may be due to up-regulation of a variety of channels in DRG neurons and/or changes in signaling leading to enhanced activity in these channels following cisplatin treatment [19]. While the mechanism of action of metformin has not been elucidated in these studies, the present findings are consistent with an AMPK-mediated mechanism of action because activation of this kinase dampens signaling in pathways linked to sensory neuron hyperexcitability and may modulate the expression of channels via transcription and/or translation regulation downstream of AMPK activation [4,5].

In conclusion, this study is the first to demonstrate that metformin protects against chemotherapy-induced neuropathic pain and numbness in a mouse model. The beneficial effect of metformin is associated with a reduction in the loss of plantar IENFs. Whether these neuroprotective effects of metformin treatment in the mouse model of cisplatin-induced peripheral neuropathy are the direct cause of the protective effect of metformin treatment on pain and numbness need to be further investigated. There are no FDA-approved drugs to treat CIPN. As a result of CIPN a significant subset of patients receives sub-optimal doses of anti-cancer treatment. Moreover, CIPN markedly reduces quality of life both during and after completion of treatment.

Because metformin has already been widely used, these findings strongly argue for an immediately available novel treatment to prevent chemotherapy-induced peripheral neuropathy in patients treated for cancer. The ongoing studies on the usefulness of metformin as an add-on therapy in cancer treatment should include analysis of the potential beneficial effect of metformin on chemotherapy-induced neuropathy as an outcome measure.

Supporting Information

File S1 Von Frey test for mechanical allodynia.

File S2 Rotarod test for motor impairment.

File S3 Adhesive Removal Test.

File S4 Protocol Immunohistochemistry of intraepidermal nerve fibers.

File S5 Excell sheet for calculation of 50% withdrawal threshold.

File S6 Raw data.

Acknowledgments

We thank Dr. P.M. Dougherty, Department of Pain Medicine of MD Anderson Cancer Center for his help on IENF analysis. We thank Dr. Jeannie Zhong from Baylor College of Medicine, Houston, TX for her kind support with image capture.

Author Contributions

Conceived and designed the experiments: QLMY AK KK XJH WZ TJP CC CJH. Performed the experiments: QLMY KK XJH WZ. Analyzed the data: QLMY KK. Contributed to the writing of the manuscript: QLMY AK KK XJH WZ TJP CC CJH.

References

1. Pachman DR, Barton DL, Watson JC, Loprinzi CL (2011) Chemotherapy-induced peripheral neuropathy: prevention and treatment. Clinical pharmacology and therapeutics 90: 377–387.
2. Cata JP, Weng HR, Lee BN, Reuben JM, Dougherty PM (2006) Clinical and experimental findings in humans and animals with chemotherapy-induced peripheral neuropathy. Minerva anestesiologica 72: 151–169.
3. Cata JP, Weng HR, Burton AW, Villareal H, Giralt S, et al. (2007) Quantitative sensory findings in patients with bortezomib-induced pain. The journal of pain: official journal of the American Pain Society 8: 296–306.
4. Melemedjian OK, Khoutorsky A, Sorge RE, Yan J, Asiedu MN, et al. (2013) mTORC1 inhibition induces pain via IRS-1-dependent feedback activation of ERK. Pain 154: 1080–1091.
5. Melemedjian OK, Asiedu MN, Tillu DV, Sanoja R, Yan J, et al. (2011) Targeting adenosine monophosphate-activated protein kinase (AMPK) in preclinical models reveals a potential mechanism for the treatment of neuropathic pain. Molecular pain 7: 70.
6. Melemedjian OK, Mejia GL, Lepow TS, Zoph OK, Price TJ (2013) Bidirectional regulation of P body formation mediated by eIF4F complex formation in sensory neurons. Neuroscience letters.
7. Correia S, Carvalho C, Santos MS, Proenca T, Nunes E, et al. (2008) Metformin protects the brain against the oxidative imbalance promoted by type 2 diabetes. Medicinal chemistry 4: 358–364.
8. El-Mir MY, Detaille D, G RV, Delgado-Esteban M, Guigas B, et al. (2008) Neuroprotective role of antidiabetic drug metformin against apoptotic cell death in primary cortical neurons. Journal of molecular neuroscience: MN 34: 77–87.
9. Ullah I, Ullah N, Naseer MI, Lee HY, Kim MO (2012) Neuroprotection with metformin and thymoquinone against ethanol-induced apoptotic neurodegeneration in prenatal rat cortical neurons. BMC neuroscience 13: 11.
10. Li J, Benashski SE, Venna VR, McCullough LD (2010) Effects of metformin in experimental stroke. Stroke; a journal of cerebral circulation 41: 2645–2652.
11. Buac D, Kona FR, Seth AK, Dou QP (2013) Regulation of metformin response by breast cancer associated gene 2. Neoplasia 15: 1379–1390.
12. Garofalo C, Capristo M, Manara MC, Mancarella C, Landuzzi L, et al. (2013) Metformin as an Adjuvant Drug against Pediatric Sarcomas: Hypoxia Limits Therapeutic Effects of the Drug. PloS one 8: e83832.
13. Boyette-Davis J, Dougherty PM (2011) Protection against oxaliplatin-induced mechanical hyperalgesia and intraepidermal nerve fiber loss by minocycline. Experimental neurology 229: 353–357.
14. Lauria G, Lombardi R, Borgna M, Penza P, Bianchi R, et al. (2005) Intraepidermal nerve fiber density in rat foot pad: neuropathologic-neurophysiologic correlation. Journal of the peripheral nervous system: JPNS 10: 202–208.
15. Verdu E, Vilches JJ, Rodriguez FJ, Ceballos D, Valero A, et al. (1999) Physiological and immunohistochemical characterization of cisplatin-induced neuropathy in mice. Muscle & nerve 22: 329–340.
16. Schuning J, Scherens A, Haussleiter IS, Schwenkreis P, Krumova EK, et al. (2009) Sensory changes and loss of intraepidermal nerve fibers in painful unilateral nerve injury. The Clinical journal of pain 25: 683–690.
17. Wu JZ, Dong RG, Rakheja S, Schopper AW, Smutz WP (2004) A structural fingertip model for simulating of the biomechanics of tactile sensation. Medical engineering & physics 26: 165–175.
18. Melemedjian OK, Yassine HN, Shy A, Price TJ (2013) Proteomic and functional annotation analysis of injured peripheral nerves reveals ApoE as a protein upregulated by injury that is modulated by metformin treatment. Molecular pain 9: 14.
19. Ta LE, Bieber AJ, Carlton SM, Loprinzi CL, Low PA, et al. (2010) Transient Receptor Potential Vanilloid 1 is essential for cisplatin-induced heat hyperalgesia in mice. Molecular pain 6: 15.
20. Wang H, Heijnen CJ, Eijkelkamp N, Garza Carbajal A, Schedlowski M, et al. (2011) GRK2 in sensory neurons regulates epinephrine-induced signalling and duration of mechanical hyperalgesia. Pain 152: 1649–1658.

21. Chaplan SR, Bach FW, Pogrel JW, Chung JM, Yaksh TL (1994) Quantitative assessment of tactile allodynia in the rat paw. Journal of neuroscience methods 53: 55–63.
22. Bouet V, Boulouard M, Toutain J, Divoux D, Bernaudin M, et al. (2009) The adhesive removal test: a sensitive method to assess sensorimotor deficits in mice. Nature protocols 4: 1560–1564.
23. Siau C, Xiao W, Bennett GJ (2006) Paclitaxel- and vincristine-evoked painful peripheral neuropathies: loss of epidermal innervation and activation of Langerhans cells. Experimental neurology 201: 507–514.
24. Boyette-Davis J, Xin W, Zhang H, Dougherty PM (2011) Intraepidermal nerve fiber loss corresponds to the development of taxol-induced hyperalgesia and can be prevented by treatment with minocycline. Pain 152: 308–313.
25. Scheen AJ, Lefebvre PJ (1993) Pharmacological treatment of the obese diabetic patient. Diabete & metabolisme 19: 547–559.
26. Informatics IIfH, editors (2013) Declining medicine use and costs: For better or worse? A review of the use of medicines in the United States in 2012: IMS Institute for Healthcare Informatics, Parsippany, NJ.
27. Jiralerspong S, Palla SL, Giordano SH, Meric-Bernstam F, Liedtke C, et al. (2009) Metformin and pathologic complete responses to neoadjuvant chemotherapy in diabetic patients with breast cancer. Journal of clinical oncology: official journal of the American Society of Clinical Oncology 27: 3297–3302.
28. Dilokthornsakul P, Chaiyakunapruk N, Termrungruanglert W, Pratoomsoot C, Saokeaw S, et al. (2013) The effects of metformin on ovarian cancer: a systematic review. International journal of gynecological cancer: official journal of the International Gynecological Cancer Society 23: 1544–1551.
29. Kumar S, Meuter A, Thapa P, Langstraat C, Giri S, et al. (2013) Metformin intake is associated with better survival in ovarian cancer: a case-control study. Cancer 119: 555–562.
30. Romero IL, McCormick A, McEwen KA, Park S, Karrison T, et al. (2012) Relationship of type II diabetes and metformin use to ovarian cancer progression, survival, and chemosensitivity. Obstetrics and gynecology 119: 61–67.
31. Cufi S, Corominas-Faja B, Vazquez-Martin A, Oliveras-Ferraros C, Dorca J, et al. (2012) Metformin-induced preferential killing of breast cancer initiating CD44+CD24-/low cells is sufficient to overcome primary resistance to trastuzumab in HER2+ human breast cancer xenografts. Oncotarget 3: 395–398.
32. Cheong JH, Park ES, Liang J, Dennison JB, Tsavachidou D, et al. (2011) Dual inhibition of tumor energy pathway by 2-deoxyglucose and metformin is effective against a broad spectrum of preclinical cancer models. Molecular cancer therapeutics 10: 2350–2362.
33. Hirsch HA, Iliopoulos D, Struhl K (2013) Metformin inhibits the inflammatory response associated with cellular transformation and cancer stem cell growth. Proceedings of the National Academy of Sciences of the United States of America 110: 972–977.
34. Chen G, Xu S, Renko K, Derwahl M (2012) Metformin inhibits growth of thyroid carcinoma cells, suppresses self-renewal of derived cancer stem cells, and potentiates the effect of chemotherapeutic agents. The Journal of clinical endocrinology and metabolism 97: E510–520.
35. Melemedjian OK, Price TJ (2012) Dendritic spine plasticity as an underlying mechanism of neuropathic pain: commentary on Tan et al. Experimental neurology 233: 740–744.
36. Flatters SJ, Bennett GJ (2006) Studies of peripheral sensory nerves in paclitaxel-induced painful peripheral neuropathy: evidence for mitochondrial dysfunction. Pain 122: 245–257.
37. Hardie DG, Ross FA, Hawley SA (2012) AMPK: a nutrient and energy sensor that maintains energy homeostasis. Nature reviews Molecular cell biology 13: 251–262.
38. Kimura N, Masuda S, Tanihara Y, Ueo H, Okuda M, et al. (2005) Metformin is a superior substrate for renal organic cation transporter OCT2 rather than hepatic OCT1. Drug metabolism and pharmacokinetics 20: 379–386.
39. Sprowl JA, Ciarimboli G, Lancaster CS, Giovinazzo H, Gibson AA, et al. (2013) Oxaliplatin-induced neurotoxicity is dependent on the organic cation transporter OCT2. Proceedings of the National Academy of Sciences of the United States of America 110: 11199–11204.
40. Nolano M, Simone DA, Wendelschafer-Crabb G, Johnson T, Hazen E, et al. (1999) Topical capsaicin in humans: parallel loss of epidermal nerve fibers and pain sensation. Pain 81: 135–145.
41. Ignatius MJ, Gebicke-Harter PJ, Skene JH, Schilling JW, Weisgraber KH, et al. (1986) Expression of apolipoprotein E during nerve degeneration and regeneration. Proceedings of the National Academy of Sciences of the United States of America 83: 1125–1129.
42. Handelmann GE, Boyles JK, Weisgraber KH, Mahley RW, Pitas RE (1992) Effects of apolipoprotein E, beta-very low density lipoproteins, and cholesterol on the extension of neurites by rabbit dorsal root ganglion neurons in vitro. Journal of lipid research 33: 1677–1688.
43. Li FQ, Fowler KA, Neil JE, Colton CA, Vitek MP (2010) An apolipoprotein E-mimetic stimulates axonal regeneration and remyelination after peripheral nerve injury. The Journal of pharmacology and experimental therapeutics 334: 106–115.
44. Cata JP, Weng HR, Dougherty PM (2008) Behavioral and electrophysiological studies in rats with cisplatin-induced chemoneuropathy. Brain research 1230: 91–98.

12

Genetic Variation in Iron Metabolism Is Associated with Neuropathic Pain and Pain Severity in HIV-Infected Patients on Antiretroviral Therapy

Asha R. Kallianpur[1,2]*, Peilin Jia[3], Ronald J. Ellis[4], Zhongming Zhao[3], Cinnamon Bloss[5], Wanqing Wen[6], Christina M. Marra[7], Todd Hulgan[6], David M. Simpson[8], Susan Morgello[8], Justin C. McArthur[9], David B. Clifford[10], Ann C. Collier[11], Benjamin B. Gelman[12], J. Allen McCutchan[13], Donald Franklin[14], David C. Samuels[15], Debralee Rosario[14], Emily Holzinger[15], Deborah G. Murdock[15], Scott Letendre[13], Igor Grant[16], for the CHARTER Study Group

1 Department of Genomic Medicine, Lerner Research Institute, Cleveland Clinic Foundation, Cleveland, Ohio, United States of America, **2** Department of Molecular Medicine, Cleveland Clinic Lerner College of Medicine of Case Western Reserve University, Cleveland, Ohio, United States of America, **3** Department of Biomedical Informatics, Vanderbilt University School of Medicine, Nashville, Tennessee, United States of America, **4** Department of Neurology, University of California San Diego, San Diego, California, United States of America, **5** Scripps Genomic Medicine, Scripps Translational Science Institute, and Scripps Health, La Jolla, California, United States of America, **6** Department of Medicine, Vanderbilt University School of Medicine, Nashville, Tennessee, United States of America, **7** Department of Neurology, University of Washington, Seattle, Washington, United States of America, **8** Department of Neurology, Icahn School of Medicine of Mt. Sinai, New York, New York, United States of America, **9** Department of Neurology, Johns Hopkins University, Baltimore, Maryland, United States of America, **10** Department of Neurology, Washington University, St. Louis, Missouri, United States of America, **11** Department of Medicine, University of Washington, Seattle, Washington, United States of America, **12** Department of Pathology, University of Texas Medical Branch, Galveston, Texas, United States of America, **13** Department of Medicine, University of California San Diego, San Diego, California, United States of America, **14** HIV Neurobehavioral Research Center & CHARTER Center, University of California San Diego, San Diego, California, United States of America, **15** Department of Molecular Physiology and Biophysics and Center for Human Genetics Research, Vanderbilt University School of Medicine, Nashville, Tennessee, United States of America, **16** Department of Psychiatry, University of California San Diego, San Diego, California, United States of America

Abstract

HIV sensory neuropathy and distal neuropathic pain (DNP) are common, disabling complications associated with combination antiretroviral therapy (cART). We previously associated iron-regulatory genetic polymorphisms with a reduced risk of HIV sensory neuropathy during more neurotoxic types of cART. We here evaluated the impact of polymorphisms in 19 iron-regulatory genes on DNP in 560 HIV-infected subjects from a prospective, observational study, who underwent neurological examinations to ascertain peripheral neuropathy and structured interviews to ascertain DNP. Genotype-DNP associations were explored by logistic regression and permutation-based analytical methods. Among 559 evaluable subjects, 331 (59%) developed HIV-SN, and 168 (30%) reported DNP. Fifteen polymorphisms in 8 genes ($p<0.05$) and 5 variants in 4 genes ($p<0.01$) were nominally associated with DNP: polymorphisms in *TF*, *TFRC*, *BMP6*, *ACO1*, *SLC11A2*, and *FXN* conferred reduced risk (adjusted odds ratios [ORs] ranging from 0.2 to 0.7, all $p<0.05$); other variants in *TF*, *CP*, *ACO1*, *BMP6*, and *B2M* conferred increased risk (ORs ranging from 1.3 to 3.1, all $p<0.05$). Risks associated with some variants were statistically significant either in black or white subgroups but were consistent in direction. *ACO1* rs2026739 remained significantly associated with DNP in whites (permutation $p<0.0001$) after correction for multiple tests. Several of the same iron-regulatory-gene polymorphisms, including *ACO1* rs2026739, were also associated with severity of DNP (all $p<0.05$). Common polymorphisms in iron-management genes are associated with DNP and with DNP severity in HIV-infected persons receiving cART. Consistent risk estimates across population subgroups and persistence of the *ACO1* rs2026739 association after adjustment for multiple testing suggest that genetic variation in iron-regulation and transport modulates susceptibility to DNP.

Editor: Kostas Pantopoulos, Lady Davis Institute for Medical Research/McGill University, Canada

Funding: The co-authors of this manuscript have no pertinent financial disclosures. Funding support for this work was provided by the following grants: National Institutes of Health contracts N01 MH22005 and HHSN271201000036C from the National Institutes of Health (to CHARTER PI Igor Grant) and 1R01 MH 095621 (to PIs Asha Kallianpur and Todd Hulgan). The funders had no role in study design, data collection and analysis, decision to publish, or preparation of the manuscript.

Competing Interests: The authors have declared that no competing interests exist.

* Email: kalliaa@ccf.org

Introduction

The success of combination antiretroviral therapy (cART) in human immunodeficiency virus (HIV) infection has focused attention on addressing long-term complications that reduce quality of life, such as peripheral neuropathy [1]. Peripheral neuropathy in HIV infection is a distal symmetric, often painful, sensory polyneuropathy associated with the virus itself and/or to toxic effects of certain antiretroviral drugs, particularly the dideoxy-nucleoside reverse-transcriptase inhibitors (so-called "D-drug" NRTIs) such as didanosine and stavudine [2,3]. Clinically and histopathologically, neuropathy due to HIV infection in the pre-cART era and the neuropathy associated with cART toxicity are usually indistinguishable; both are encompassed by the term "HIV sensory neuropathy" (HIV-SN). HIV-SN may first manifest or worsen upon initiation of cART and is associated with sensory loss, paresthesias, and distal neuropathic pain (DNP) or dysesthesias. The known mitochondrial toxicity of D-drugs and dysregulated inflammation have both been implicated in its pathogenesis, but the pathophysiology of HIV-SN remains incompletely understood [2,4–8].

Development of DNP is particularly disabling [9–11], because the symptoms respond poorly to analgesic medications that are used to treat other types of neuropathic pain [1,12–15]. HIV-SN therefore has an adverse impact on quality of life, social and emotional functioning, and neuropsychological test performance, and DNP in particular contributes to depression, physical deconditioning, and non-adherence to treatment [10,11,16–18]. Although substitution of less toxic antiretroviral drugs lowers the risk of HIV-SN, older D-drugs like stavudine are likely to remain in use in low-resource settings for some time as part of generic, fixed-dose cART regimens, and the study of HIV-SN and DNP remains very relevant [19,20]. Improved understanding of the biological mechanisms underlying painful HIV-SN may lead to better ways of categorizing and therapeutically targeting DNP [21–23].

Iron is a critical micronutrient for metabolically active cells such as neurons, and a carefully controlled supply of iron is essential for mitochondrial function, axonal transport, and myelination [24–26]. Iron transport also plays an important role in regulating macrophage-mediated inflammation via the hepcidin pathway [27–30]. Hepcidin, a peptide hormone which is synthesized in the liver in response to inflammatory stimuli, leads to iron sequestration within the reticuloendothelial cell (macrophage-monocyte) compartment, potentiating macrophage oxidative killing via Fenton chemistry while reducing availability of iron to microorganisms. We previously reported associations between iron-loading, single-nucleotide polymorphisms (SNPs) in the hemochromatosis (*HFE*) gene and reduced risk of HIV-SN in HIV-infected individuals exposed to D-drug-containing cART [31]. While improved cellular and mitochondrial iron delivery might play a protective role in individuals with *HFE* variants, in whom the action of hepcidin is reduced, these associations could also be explained by the known linkage of *HFE* to the HLA Class I locus and thereby to other immunomodulatory haplotypes [31,32]. Studies of non-HLA-linked genetic variants that are prevalent in racially diverse populations, unlike *HFE* gene variants, are needed to determine whether iron-transport is of fundamental importance in susceptibility to HIV-SN and neuropathic symptoms like DNP.

We hypothesized that like *HFE* variants, common variants in other iron-management but non-HLA-Class I-linked genes modulate susceptibility to cART-associated HIV-SN and DNP in HIV-infected individuals, and that these genes impact neuropathy phenotypes independent of race/ethnicity and disease-related factors. This study assessed the role of variants in key iron-transport and iron-regulatory genes (henceforth termed "the ferrome" for brevity) in susceptibility to neuropathy phenotypes in a racially diverse, HIV-infected population, the CNS HIV Antiretroviral Therapy Effects Research (CHARTER) Cohort. CHARTER is the largest U.S.-based prospective study of neurological complications in HIV/AIDS in the cART era [33]. Particular strengths of CHARTER include its clear definition of neurological phenotypes and sensitive and specific methods of ascertaining HIV-SN. This analysis specifically targeted genes that encode components of the nuclear and mitochondrial ferrome, for which SNP genotypes were available from a genomic study conducted previously in CHARTER. In addition to several SNPs that were nominally associated with DNP, a common variant (rs2026739) in the cytoplasmic aconitase gene (*ACO1*) was identified to be statistically associated with DNP after multiple-testing correction.

Patients and Methods

Study population

The CHARTER Study is a prospective, observational study conducted at six outpatient centers within the U.S.: Johns Hopkins University, Baltimore, Maryland; Mount Sinai School of Medicine, New York, NY; the University of California, San Diego, CA; the University of Texas Medical Branch, Galveston, TX; the University of Washington, Seattle, WA; and Washington University, St Louis, MO. Data collection was standardized across centers and employed a protocol of comprehensive neuromedical, neurobehavioral, and laboratory assessments, including: nadir CD4+ T-cell count, cART history, D-drug exposure, history of a major depressive disorder, and demographic information (from structured interviews), as well as current CD4+ T-cell count, HIV plasma viral load, and hepatitis C viral serology (from laboratory data). Further details regarding CHARTER Study eligibility and enrollment procedures have been reported previously [1]. A subset of CHARTER Study subjects ($N = 579$) was recruited between 2003 and 2007 to a cross-sectional genomic sub-study of peripheral neuropathy. Genetic study eligibility criteria included the ability to provide details of cART use and to undergo a structured interview and examination for signs/symptoms of HIV-SN; individuals with active opportunistic infections, uncontrolled psychiatric disorders, or who were unable to cooperate with detailed evaluations over the course of a full day were excluded.

Ethics Statement. The CHARTER Study and this study were approved by the University of California-San Diego Human Research Protections Program (Biomedical Institutional Review Board) and by the Institutional Review Boards (IRBs) of the following participating CHARTER institutions: the Johns Hopkins University School of Medicine IRB, Icahn School of Medicine at Mount Sinai IRB, University of Texas (Medical Branch) IRB, University of Washington School of Medicine IRB, and Washington University -St. Louis School of Medicine IRB. The present study was conducted according to the principles expressed in the Declaration of Helsinki. All study subjects whose data are reported herein provided written informed consent.

Ascertainment of neuropathy and distal neuropathic pain

Standardized, targeted neurological examinations were performed by physicians and nurses trained in neurological AIDS disorders. HIV-SN and DNP were identified using criteria published previously [1,10]. Briefly, participants were queried at baseline and each follow-up visit about symptoms of HIV-SN and DNP, specifically, tingling, or burning, aching, shooting, or stabbing pain in a bilateral, predominantly distal distribution (*e.g.*, in the fingers and toes only, extending to the ankles or wrists, or extending to the knees or elbows). If subjects endorsed tingling in this distribution, they were considered to have paresthesias; if they endorsed any of the pain symptoms in this distribution, they were considered to have a positive self-report of DNP; loss of sensation in the lower extremities was also assessed on examination. HIV-SN cases were defined by the bilateral presence of at least one of the following signs at any visit: diminished vibration sense, reduced sharp-dull discrimination in the feet and toes, reduced ankle reflexes, and DNP cases by the above-mentioned pain symptoms; controls did not have any of these signs or symptoms of peripheral nerve disease. DNP was also classified into the following 5 severity levels by structured survey; none, slight (occasional, fleeting), mild (frequent), moderate (frequent, disabling) or severe (constant, daily, disabling, and requiring treatment with analgesics or other medications).

Genomic DNA isolation and gene selection

Genomic DNA was isolated from whole blood samples using PUREGENE (Gentra Systems Inc., Minneapolis, MN, USA). Samples were subjected to whole-genome nuclear genotyping using the Affymetrix Genome-Wide Human SNP Array 6.0 platform (Affymetrix, Inc., Santa Clara, CA). Among 579 extracted samples, 560 yielded analyzable genotypes that passed quality-control filters using the Platform for the Analysis, Translation, and Organization of large scale data (PLATO) [34]. Sample genotyping efficiency was 95%. Variants with less than 95% genotyping efficiency or minor allele frequencies (MAFs) less than 1% in the study population were excluded from analysis.

Genes reported in the published literature to be associated with iron metabolism and/or neurological phenotypes were searched in the publicly available Online Mendelian Inheritance in Man database (http://www.ncbi.nlm.nih.gov/omim). We then identified 20 genes based on their well-recognized direct or indirect involvement in iron metabolism, transport, storage, or regulation (*e.g.*, the hepcidin pathway). SNPs mapping to the following iron-regulatory and transport genes were selected for this exploratory analysis based on their inclusion in the Affymetrix Genome-Wide Human SNP Array 6.0: *HFE*, *HFE2*, *SLC40A1*, *SLC11A1*, *HAMP*, *TF*, *TFRC*, *TFR2*, *BMP2*, *BMP6*, *CP*, *SLC11A2*, *FXN*, *FTMT*, *FTH1*, *ACO1*, *ACO2*, *B2M* and *ATP13A2*. Nineteen of these genes were covered by the Affymetrix 6.0 chip, and the platform provided evaluable genotypic information for 192 candidate SNPs (Table S1). Many of these iron-related genes/SNPs have also been previously reported to play a role in iron transport within the nervous system, and genes previously linked to neurodegenerative diseases and neural differentiation were included [35]. Based on the common disease-common variant hypothesis, this list was further narrowed to those SNPs with MAFs of at least 5% in one or both of the largest subsets of the CHARTER study population (non-Hispanic blacks or non-Hispanic whites, henceforth referred to as blacks or whites, respectively) [36]. Using a typical analysis strategy that has been applied in numerous previous studies, we used all available genotyped SNPs in those genes, though some of them may be correlated due to LD structure.

Statistical methods

General approach. The role of iron-related genes in susceptibility to cART-associated HIV-SN and DNP was evaluated by both multivariable logistic regression and permutation analysis. Since the SNPs analyzed could not be assumed to be independent, Bonferroni adjustment of statistical tests would almost certainly overcorrect and result in unacceptable Type II error; permutation-based analysis is a complementary statistical method that accounts for multiple statistical tests, gene size, and linkage disequilibrium [37,38]. Specifically, the observed p-value from the real dataset is compared to the distribution of p-values generated from 1000 permutated sample sets which randomly switch case/control labels while maintaining the same case/control ratio [37]. An empirical p-value is generated by the number of permutation sets whose p-values are less than the observed p-value divided by 1000.

Population stratification was also evaluated in our analyses by adjustment for four principal components variables (PCs) representing ancestry-related genetic information, which were generated from genome-wide genotype data in CHARTER and used as covariates in multivariate logistic regression models, in addition to adjustment for self-reported race/ethnicity. Logistic regression models stratified by self-reported race/ethnicity were also explored (black or white; other categories were omitted due to insufficient numbers). The degree of potential overlap between individual PCs was also evaluated by plotting these variables against one another (Figure S1).

The following neuropathy outcomes were analyzed: presence of *at least 1 sign* of HIV-SN, *at least 2 signs* of HIV-SN, and DNP. Each outcome was analyzed as a dichotomous variable. Potential confounders were identified by univariable logistic regression to calculate unadjusted odds ratios (ORs) and by prior published associations of these variables with HIV-SN, neuropathy symptoms (loss of sensation, paresthesias, and/or dysesthesias/DNP), or DNP alone in CHARTER.[1,9,33]. Significant variables were then included in all multivariable logistic models with or without race-stratification. These phenotype-specific covariates were as follows: age (years), cumulative D-drug exposure (months), CD4+ T-cell nadir, $\log_{10}$[plasma HIV RNA], hepatitis C virus (HCV) serologic status (positive/negative), protease inhibitor use (0 or ≥ 1 protease inhibitor), current or prior major depressive disorder (yes/no), self-reported race (in non-stratified models), and the 4 genomic sequence-derived ancestry PC variables in HIV-SN analyses; and age, cumulative D-drug exposure, CD4+ T-cell nadir, $\log_{10}$[plasma HIV RNA], self-reported race (in non-stratified analyses), and the 4 PC variables in analyses of neuropathy symptoms and DNP. In order to account for the effects of diabetes in some subjects who might also be on treatment for this condition, we used a more stringent blood glucose criterion for ascertaining diabetes than is normally used for non-fasting blood glucose levels ($\geq$126 mg/dL, rather than $\geq$200 mg/dL). By this criterion, 66 subjects (11.8%) were coded as diabetic. Since additional adjustment for diabetes by this method did not alter p-values appreciably for any of the studied SNPs, we did not include this covariate in final regression models. (Hemoglobin A1c levels, which would have allowed for more accurate diabetes diagnosis, were available in $<$10% subjects, and blood glucose values were missing in 6 subjects.)

The reported associations of genetic variants with presence or absence of HIV-SN or DNP made no genetic model assumptions regarding dominant or recessive allelic effects (genotypes were coded as 0, 1, or 2, based on the number of minor alleles present); all SNPs in the genes studied were bi-allelic.

For analysis of DNP severity, genotypes were dichotomized (variant alleles present or absent) to optimize power, and p-values were obtained using Pearson's chi-square test or, for those SNPs with fewer than 5 observations per cell, Fisher's exact test.

Multivariable single-SNP analyses. Statistical tests were performed using publicly available R software (http://www.r-project.org/). For each phenotype, logistic regression was used for single-marker association tests, while adjusting for phenotype-specific covariates in addition to race as a categorical covariate and ancestry PCs, as discussed above [1,9]. Additional adjustment for cART-naïve status beyond inclusion of D-drug exposure and HIV viral load did not significantly alter results; hence, this variable was not included in multivariable models. PC variables were computed in advance based on genome-wide genotype data available in all 560 CHARTER study participants. Permutation tests were conducted by randomizing case/control labels in multivariable models while keeping the same numbers of cases and controls as in the original dataset. We generated 1000 permutation datasets. An empirical p-value was computed for each SNP in each phenotype, according to $p_{emp} = \#\{P(\pi) < P(\text{real})/1000$, where $P(\pi)$ is the p-value in the πth permutation [38,39].

Results of association tests for two key genes, *CP* and *ACO1*, with neuropathic pain were depicted using the LocusZoom tool (Figure 1, generated using HapMap Phase II CEU) [40].

The p-values for all statistical tests were two-tailed, and for this exploratory analysis, the value of α (statistical significance) was set at 0.05 to identify SNPs of potential interest in this exploratory study. A Bonferroni correction for multiple statistical tests was also applied by multiplying p-values obtained for each association test by 192, the number of SNPs evaluated to identify more robust associations.

Results

Genotypes from the CHARTER genome study were available for 192 SNPs encompassing 19 iron-regulatory or iron-transport-related (ferrome) genes queried (Table S1): *HFE*, *HJV*, *FPN1*, *SLC11A1*, *HAMP*, *TF*, *TFRC*, *TFR2*, *BMP2*, *BMP6*, *CP*,

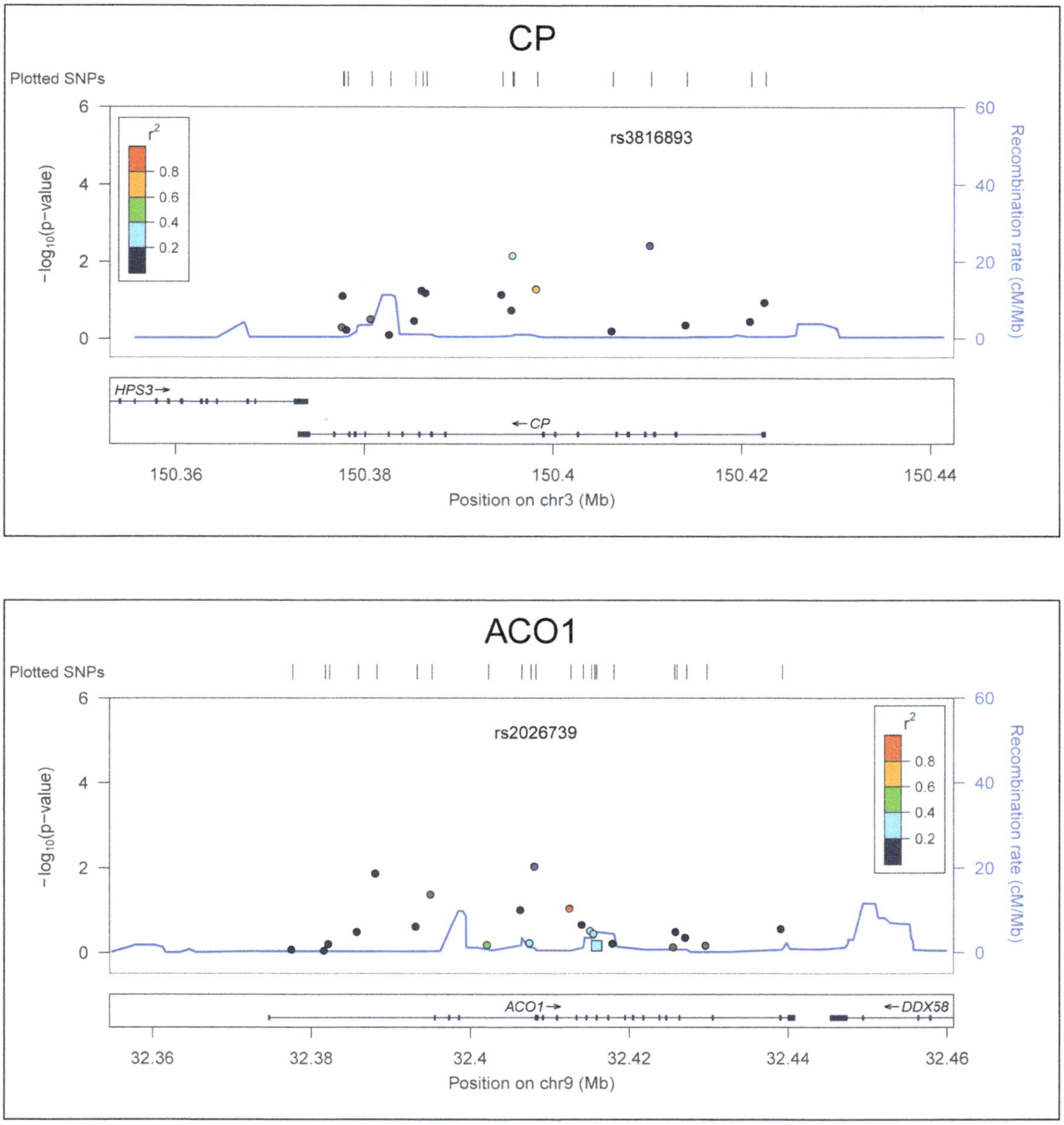

Figure 1. Representative Linkage Disequilibrium (LD) plot. The LD plot for two representative SNPs that were statistically significantly associated with neuropathic pain in the CHARTER cohort is displayed: *CP* rs3816893 and *ACO1* rs2026739. Each plot shows the degree of LD between the SNP of interest (rs number) and all other SNPs analyzed in the same gene, color-coded according to the r^2 value (correlation of frequencies in this sample). The LD is based on HapMap Phase II CEU data. Association p-values are displayed on the y-axis and chromosomal distance (Mb) on the x-axis.

SLC11A2, *FXN*, *FTMT*, *FTH1*, *ACO1*, *ACO2*, *B2M*, and *ATP13A2*. Genotypes at the *HEPH* locus on the X chromosome, which encodes a ceruloplasmin-like, membrane-bound ferroxidase that is important in transmembrane iron transport, and genotypes at the *HFE* C187G locus (previously studied by the authors in HIV-infected subjects) were not covered by the Affymetrix Human SNP Array 6.0 platform. The CHARTER genomic study provided genotypes at all other loci of interest in >99% of subjects; of 559 evaluable individuals, 21% were women, and the mean age of the population was 44 years (range 21–68). Self-reported race/ethnicity was 43% (n = 242) black, 44% (n = 247) white, 11% (n = 58) Hispanic, and 2% Asian or "Other" (n = 11). Due to insufficient power for analyses in subjects of Hispanic, Asian or "Other" ancestry, only analyses performed in non-Hispanic blacks, whites, or the entire CHARTER genetic study population are reported. As shown in Figure S1, the 4 genome-derived PC variables in multivariable models of neuropathic pain accurately represented distinct ancestral strata in this study sample.

Demographic and HIV disease characteristics of subjects with and without HIV-SN are presented in Table 1. Among 559 evaluable subjects, 331 (59%) had at least one sign of HIV-SN, and 160 (29%) exhibited more severe HIV-SN (at least two signs). Fifty percent of the study population (281 subjects) reported at least one neuropathic symptom, including paresthesias, loss of sensation, dysesthesias, and/or DNP in both lower extremities. Ascertainment of dysesthesias correlated so closely with DNP that only results for DNP will be discussed henceforth. A total of 168 subjects (30% of this study sample) experienced DNP of some degree of severity. CHARTER study subjects with HIV-SN (at least one sign) and those who reported neuropathic symptoms and/or DNP were older than subjects without these complications ($p<0.01$). No significant differences were noted with regard to educational level (*data not shown*), self-reported race/ethnicity, or sex, but subjects reporting DNP tended to be female (26% *vs.* 19%, $p = 0.06$). Individuals with HIV-SN of any severity and those who reported neuropathy symptoms other than DNP had a lower CD4 nadir than corresponding controls [median (IQR) for cases *vs.* controls, respectively, were 112 (31, 246) *vs.* 242 (125, 391) cells/µL, $p<0.01$ for at least one HIV-SN sign; 107 (23, 214) *vs.* 200 (70, 350), $p<0.01$ for at least two signs; and 151 (37, 275) *vs.* 198 (60, 348), $p<0.01$ for neuropathy symptoms]. Median viral load was lower among HIV-SN cases than controls [median (IQR) 1.7 (1.7, 3.3) *vs.* 2.6 (1.7, 4.2) $\log_{10}$ (HIV RNA copies/mL), respectively, $p<0.01$] but not statistically different between subjects with or without neuropathy symptoms and DNP. Substantially fewer individuals with HIV-SN and DNP were cART-naïve as compared to controls (6% of cases with at least one sign of HIV-SN *vs.* 29% of controls; 8% of DNP cases *vs.* 19% of controls, $p<0.01$ for both). Cumulative D-drug exposure was also higher among cases than controls in all outcome categories, including DNP [*e.g.*, median (IQR) 14 (0, 53) *vs.* 0 (0, 21) months for DNP]; all p-values<0.01]. HIV-SN of any severity was associated with the use of protease inhibitors (53% current use in subjects with at least one sign *vs.* 31% of controls, $p<0.01$. Co-infection with hepatitis C virus (HCV) was more common among HIV-SN cases (28% of cases with at least one sign *vs.* 19% of controls; 31% of cases with at least two signs *vs.* 22% of controls, $p<0.05$ for both). History of a major depressive disorder was more frequently reported by subjects without HIV-SN (46%) than among HIV-SN cases (36%, $p<0.05$) and was slightly more common among individuals with DNP.

Results of multivariable logistic regression and permutation analyses evaluating associations of selected SNPs with HIV-SN phenotypes, including DNP, are summarized in Table 2, adjusted for potential confounders, including self-reported race and 4 PC variables that captured racial admixture. Twelve SNPs in 8 iron-related genes were associated with at least one sign of HIV-SN ($p<0.05$) by permutation analyses, as compared with 13 SNPs in the same 8 genes analyzed by logistic regression. One variant (rs1049296 in the gene *TF*) was also associated with HIV-SN with a p-value<0.01. One variant in the *HFE* gene was also associated with reduced risk of HIV-SN in this population, replicating a prior association of this gene with reduced risk of HIV-SN [31]. More severe HIV-SN was associated with 10 SNPs in 7 iron-related genes ($p<0.05$) and with 4 SNPs in 4 genes ($p<0.01$) by permutation analysis. Fourteen SNPs in 8 iron-regulatory genes were significantly associated with DNP ($p<0.05$) by logistic regression and 15 SNPs by permutation analysis, including two variants (rs3816893 in the gene *CP* and rs2026739 in the gene *ACO1*). These SNPs were also associated with more severe HIV-SN (at least two signs, *data not shown*). Eighteen SNPs in 6 genes were associated in permutation analysis with the presence of one or a combination of uncomfortable neuropathy symptoms (paresthesias, loss of sensation, or dysesthesias/DNP, $p<0.05$). Four variants in 2 of these genes, including *CP* rs3816893 and *CP* rs13072552, were strongly associated with neuropathy symptoms by logistic regression (all p-values<0.01) as well as by permutation analysis ($p<0.0001$ for both SNPs mentioned), thereby also meeting criteria for significance after correction for multiple testing.

A summary of iron-regulatory gene variants significantly associated in multivariable-adjusted analyses with DNP in CHARTER subjects stratified by self-reported race, with estimated ORs and 95% confidence intervals (CIs), is presented in Table 3. Eight iron-regulatory or iron-transport-related genes, *TF*, *CP*, *TFRC*, *BMP6*, *ACO1*, *FXN*, *SLC11A2*, and *B2M* were associated with DNP. Five SNPs in 4 iron regulatory genes, *TF* rs2718796, *CP* rs13072552 and rs3816893, *ACO1* rs2026739, and *B2M* rs16966334, were associated with increased risk in the combined CHARTER population by both logistic regression and permutation analysis in the entire population, with ORs ranging from 1.5 to 3.1 (all $p<0.01$). Race-stratified analyses revealed, however, that statistically significant associations for some of these SNPs occurred primarily within black or white subgroups. Point estimates for the associations of *CP* rs3816893 and *B2M* rs16966334 with DNP were greater in blacks than in whites and statistically significant only in blacks [OR 2.6 (95% CI 1.3–5.0) and 2.8 (95% CI 1.3–6.0), respectively, both $p<0.01$], while those for *ACO1* rs2026739 and *B2M* rs1901531 were statistically significant among whites only [OR 2.3 (95% CI 1.4–3.7, $p<0.0001$) and OR 2.2 (95% CI 1.3–3.8, $p<0.01$), respectively]. With the exception of *B2M* rs1901531, point estimates for ORs associating SNPs with DNP in this population were consistent in direction and very similar in magnitude across race-stratified analyses (black and white subgroups). Several additional SNPs were nominally associated with DNP by logistic regression as well as permutation-based methods of analysis, including *FXN* rs3793451 (all $p<0.05$). Two variants, *TF* rs8177306 and *ACO1* rs4495514, could not be analyzed in whites due to insufficient numbers of variant alleles.

The strong association of SNP rs2026739 in *ACO1* with DNP in whites by both logistic regression and permutation analysis remained statistically significant after adjustment for multiple testing ($p_{emp}<0.0001$). Notably, no linkage disequilibrium was observed between statistically significant SNPs and other SNPs within the same genes, as exemplified in the LD maps for *CP* and *ACO1* (SNPs rs3816893 and rs2026739), shown in Figure 1.

Table 1. Characteristics of neuropathy cases and controls in the CHARTER genetic study population.

Baseline Characteristic	HIV-SN, ≥1 sign		*p*-value*	HIV-SN, ≥2 signs		*p*-value*	Neuropathy Symptoms†		*p*- value*	Neuropathic Pain		*p*-value*
	Cases N = 331	Controls N = 228		Cases N = 160	Controls N = 399		Cases N = 281	Controls N = 274		Cases N = 168	Controls N = 390	
Age, mean ± SD	46±8	40±8	<0.01	42±8	47±8	<0.01	45±8	42±8	<0.01	46±8	43±9	<0.01
Race/ethnicity, %			0.10			0.80			0.23			0..30
Black	46	40		43	43		40	47		38	46	
White	44	44		46	44		48	40		49	42	
Hispanic	9	13		10	11		10	11		11	10	
Other	1	3		1	2		2	2		2	2	
Sex, % women	19	23	0.23	18	22	0.23	23	18	0.13	26	19	0.06
CD4+ T-cell nadir, cells/uL, median(IQR)	112 (31, 246)	242 (125, 391)	<0.01	107 (23, 214)	200 (70, 350)	<0.01	151 (37, 275)	198 (60, 348)	<0.01	139 (56, 267)	187 (54, 325)	0.09
Log_{10} [HIV RNA copies/mL], median (IQR)	1.7 (1.7, 3.3)	2.6 (1.7, 4.2)	<0.01	1.7 (1.7, 3.0)	2.3 (1.7, 4.1)	<0.01	1.7 (1.7, 3.4)	2.2 (1.7, 4.0)	0.09	1.7 (1.7, 3.6)	2.0 (1.7, 3.9)	0.31
cART-naïve, %	6	29	<0.01	3	20	<0.01	11	20	<0.01	8	19	<0.01
Current PI use, % yes	53	31	<0.01	56	40	<0.01	48	40	0.14	46	44	0.49
Cumulative D-drug use, median mos.,(IQR)	14 (0, 53)	0 (0, 21)	<0.01	17 (0, 48)	0 (0, 36)	<0.01	11 (0, 41)	0 (0, 43)	0.01	12 (0, 48)	0 (0, 36)	<0.01
HCV positive, %	28	19	<0.05	31	22	<0.05	24	25	0.73	24	25	0.78
Current/prior major depression, %	36	46	<0.05	32	43	<0.05	42	39	0.43	43	39	0.39

Abbreviations: SD, standard deviation; *HIV-SN*, HIV sensory neuropathy; *cART*, combination antiretroviral therapy; *PI*, protease inhibitor; *HCV*, hepatitis C virus; *mos.*, months; *IQR*, interquartile range.
†Neuropathy symptoms included bilateral paresthesias, dysesthesias/neuropathic pain, and/or loss of sensation in the lower extremities.
**p*-values<0.05 are statistically significant.

Table 2. Summary of significant results from multivariable analyses of peripheral neuropathy in CHARTER subjects.

Neuropathy Phenotype	**p-values from Logistic regression***		**Empirical p-values from Permutation***	
	No. of Significant genes (SNPs)			
	$p<0.05$	**$p<0.01$**	**$p_{emp}<0.05$**	**$p_{emp}<0.01$**
HIV-SN, ≥1 sign	8 (13)	1 (1)	8 (12)	(0)
HIV-SN, ≥2 signs	7 (12)	4 (4)	7 (10)	4 (4)
Neuropathic pain	8 (14)	4 (5)	8 (15)	4 (5)
≥1 Neuropathy symptom(s)[¥]	7 (18)	2 (4)	6 (18)	2 (4)

*Models shown were adjusted for the following covariates: age, cumulative D-drug exposure, $CD4^+$ T-cell nadir, plasma HIV RNA concentration, self-reported race, protease inhibitor use, HCV status, history of major depression, and 4 ancestry by principal components (for HIV-SN); first five of the same factors plus principal components (for neuropathic pain or neuropathy symptoms).
[¥]Includes presence of paresthesias, loss of sensation, and/or dysesthesias/neuropathic pain.
Analyses were performed with no genetic model assumptions (genotypes at each locus were coded as 0, 1, or 2 minor alleles).
Abbreviations: HIV-SN, HIV-sensory neuropathy.

The prevalence of ferromic variants was compared across three categories of severity of DNP, which was graded as *none* (0); *slight or mild* (1–2); and *moderate to severe* (3–4) in race-stratified analyses (Table 4). Only associations with p-values≤0.05 are presented. Polymorphisms in *ACO1* (rs2026739), *B2M* (rs16966334 and rs1901531), *CP* (rs3816893), *TF* (rs2718796 and rs8177306), and *TFRC* rs480760, most of which are very common among both blacks and whites, showed statistically significant associations with DNP severity in one or both subgroups as well as in the entire study population.

Discussion

This represents the first study to associate key iron-regulatory and iron-transport-pathway genes, which make up the human ferrome and are critical for maintenance of neuronal metabolism and mitochondrial function, with painful neuropathy in HIV-infected subjects. Our results particularly support the concept that iron metabolism plays a role in the pathophysiology of DNP for the following reasons: 1) the same genomic variants showed associations with DNP by conventional regression and by permutation-based analytical methods, which account for the effects of multiple statistical tests, gene size, and linkage disequilibrium; 2) thirteen of the same SNPs (in 7 genes) were also associated with the *severity* of DNP in this population; and 3) point estimates for ORs were consistent in direction and very similar in magnitude in both blacks and whites, as might be anticipated for valid, fundamental biological associations. Furthermore, ACO1 SNP rs2026739 retained its statistically significant association with DNP after adjustment for multiple testing. Our observation that associations of certain SNPs (*e.g.*, in *CP*, *ACO1*, *TF*, and *B2M* genes) with DNP and with DNP severity predominate in either blacks or whites may in part explain reported population differences with regard to pain threshold and pain-related disability, albeit in non-HIV-infected populations [41,42]. Interaction with race-specific genomic and lifestyle factors within these population subgroups is also possible. With the exception of *BMP6*, none of the genes we associated with DNP occurs on chromosome 6*p*, indicating that genomic variation in iron metabolism and transport *per se*, not linkage disequilibrium with HLA Class I-linked haplotypes that modulate inflammation, is likely to be responsible for the observed associations.

Several lines of evidence support a role for iron metabolism in the development of HIV-SN and/or DNP, which remain significant problems even in the era of newer-generation cART [43,44]. Common variants in the iron-loading *HFE* gene were associated with reduced risk of HIV-SN during mitochondrial-toxic cART regimens in AIDS Clinical Trial Group Study 384, and the protective association with *HFE* was replicated in this study [31]. HIV infection itself induces cellular iron dysregulation, possibly via downregulation of macrophage Hfe expression by the viral Nef protein and induction of the pro-inflammatory, iron-regulatory hormone hepcidin [45–47]. Restless legs syndrome (RLS), a disorder characterized by unpleasant sensations in the lower extremities that are relieved by movement, has been reported in some studies to be more prevalent in HIV-infected individuals with painful neuropathy and has been likened to a unique form of neuropathic pain [48,49]. Systemic iron deficiency, brain iron deficiency, and activation of the hypoxia-inducible factor pathway have been linked to the development of RLS, and in a significant subset of patients, iron supplementation alleviates symptoms [50–52]. The biological plausibility of a role for iron metabolism in the pathophysiology of inflammatory peripheral neuropathy and DNP is also suggested by prior experimental studies and growing appreciation within the field of iron metabolism of the importance of iron transport and its tight regulation to maintenance of energy metabolism in highly metabolically active cells such as neurons, and to immune regulation [27,47,53–57]. Iron transport is critical to neuronal energy metabolism and axoplasmic transport [58–60]. Inhibitors of heme oxygenase, which catalyzes the breakdown of heme to iron, biliverdin and carbon monoxide, have been shown to have analgesic effects in some models of inflammatory or neuropathic pain [61]. Genetic variation in iron transport has also been associated with altered inflammatory cytokine levels, which at least in part mediate neuropathic pain [62–66]. Involvement of bone morphogenetic proteins in pain perception and sensitivity has also been reported in rodent models [67].

The *ACO1* and *FXN* genes are important for cellular energy metabolism and mitochondrial iron transport: *ACO1* encodes a bifunctional protein containing an iron-sulfur cluster that reversibly binds to regulatory elements in transferrin receptor (Tfr) and ferritin mRNAs depending on ambient cellular iron levels [55]. This protein functions as a cytoplasmic aconitase under low-iron conditions, upregulating synthesis of Tfr (the major cellular iron importer) by stabilizing Tfr mRNA, while preventing translation of ferritin (the principal iron storage protein in the cell); the reverse occurs when ambient iron levels are high [68]. The *FXN* gene,

Table 3. Genetic variants associated with neuropathic pain.

SNP	Gene	All Subjects (390 Cases/168 Controls)			White (163 Cases/83 Controls)			Black (179 Cases/63 Controls)		
		OR (95% CI)	p	p_{emp}	OR (95% CI)	p	p_{emp}	OR (95% CI)	p	p_{emp}
rs2718796_g	*TF*	3.1 (1.4–7.3)	0.007	0.003	5.0 (1.1–28.1)	0.045	0.026	3.0 (0.7–12.3)	0.118	0.055
rs8177306_g	*TF*	0.4 (0.2–0.9)	0.023	0.017	–	–	–	0.5 (0.2–1.0)	0.060	0.059
rs13072552_t	*CP*	1.6 (1.1–2.4)	0.007	0.008	1.5 (0.7–3.1)	0.292	0.280	1.5 (1.0–2.4)	0.054	0.071
rs13075921_c	*CP*	1.6 (1.0–2.4)	0.048	0.035	1.4 (0.7–2.8)	0.343	0.358	2.1 (1.0–4.0)	0.037	0.049
rs3816893_t	*CP*	1.9 (1.2–3.0)	0.004	0.002	1.6 (0.8–3.3)	0.165	0.151	2.6 (1.3–5.0)	0.005	0.006
rs480760_t	*TFRC*	0.6 (0.4–0.9)	0.042	0.042	0.8 (0.2–2.1)	0.660	0.678	0.7 (0.0–1.1)	0.098	0.094
rs270388_t	*BMP6*	1.3 (1.0–1.8)	0.057	0.049	1.2 (0.7–2.2)	0.430	0.448	1.2 (0.2–1.9)	0.323	0.314
rs267202_a	*BMP6*	0.8 (0.6–1.0)	0.050	0.066	0.8 (0.5–1.3)	0.414	0.424	0.7 (0.5–1.1)	0.162	0.182
rs267206_c	*BMP6*	1.4 (1.0–2.0)	0.029	0.034	1.5 (0.9–2.6)	0.098	0.118	1.4 (0.9–2.2)	0.173	0.196
rs7033149_g	*ACO1*	1.6 (1.1–2.4)	0.013	0.012	1.7 (0.9–3.2)	0.118	0.128	1.7 (1.0–2.9)	0.044	0.046
rs4495514_t	*ACO1*	0.4 (0.2–0.9)	0.040	0.036	–	–	–	0.5 (0.2–1.1)	0.118	0.112
rs2026739_g	*ACO1*	1.5 (1.1–2.0)	0.009	0.007	2.3 (1.4–3.7)	0.001	<0.0001	1.3 (0.8–2.1)	0.233	0.228
rs3793451_t	*FXN*	0.4 (0.2–0.9)	0.046	0.047	0.3 (0.1–0.9)	0.047	0.054	0.6 (0.1–2.1)	0.513	0.526
rs224446_t	*SLC11A2*	0.7 (0.4–1.0)	0.047	0.047	0.7 (0.4–1.2)	0.222	0.233	0.9 (0.4–2.0)	0.899	0.897
rs16966334_g	*B2M*	2.4 (1.3–4.2)	0.003	0.006	1.3 (0.3–4.7)	0.708	0.726	2.8 (1.3–6.0)	0.008	0.004
rs1901531_c	*B2M*	1.6 (1.1–2.5)	0.028	0.023	2.2 (1.3–3.8)	0.004	0.006	0.5 (0.1–1.3)	0.262	0.265

The *p*-values (*p*) shown were obtained by multivariable logistic regression, adjusting for age, total D-drug exposure, $CD4^+$ T-cell nadir, plasma HIV RNA concentration, all 4 principal component ancestry variables, and self-reported race (if not race-stratified) and by permutation analysis (empiric *p*-value, p_{emp}). *Abbreviations: OR*, odds ratio; *95% CI*, 95% Confidence Interval; *TF*, transferrin; *CP*, ceruloplasmin; *TFRC*, transferrin receptor 1; *BMP6*, bone morphogenetic protein 6; *ACO1*, cytoplasmic aconitase; *SLC11A2*, divalent metal transporter 1; *B2M*, beta-2 microglobulin.

Table 4. Iron-transport-related genes associated with severity of distal neuropathic pain in CHARTER.

Gene/SNP	Neuropathic Pain Severity (n,%)[1]			All subjects N = 558	Blacks N = 242	Whites N = 247	Allele Frequency[3] Overall (B/W)
	None	Slight/Mild	Mod/Severe	*p*-value for trend[2]			
ACO1							
rs2026739_g	209 (54)	76 (66)	38 (73)	0.013	0.148	0.002	0.46 (0.54/0.36)
rs7033149_g	133 (34)	52 (44)	24 (46)	0.044	0.089	0.222	0.20 (0.30/0.14)
rs4495514_t	39 (10)	3 (3)	4 (8)	0.027	0.111	---[4]	0.05 (0.11/---)
B2M							
rs16966334_g	37 (10)	20 (17)	7 (13)	0.027	0.009	0.618	0.06 (0.08/0.02)
rs1901531_c	71 (18)	29 (25)	16 (31)	0.009	0.316	0.005	0.12 (0.04/0.21)
BMP6							
rs267202_a	258 (67)	68 (59)	24 (47)	0.008	0.078	0.206	0.57 (0.57/0.50)
rs376308_g	243 (63)	59 (51)	23 (44)	0.014	0.203	0.315	0.49 (0.58/0.35)
CP							
rs9853335_c	38 (10)	16 (15)	10 (20)	0.034	0.758	0.124	0.06 (0.02/0.11)
rs3816893_t	65 (17)	32 (27)	10 (19)	0.024	0.011	0.210	0.10 (0.12/0.10)
FXN							
rs3793451_t	46 (12)	7 (6)	4 (8)	0.051	0.289	0.094	0.06 (0.04/0.04)
TF							
rs2718796_g	14 (3)	5 (4)	9 (17)	0.004	0.154	0.009	0.03 (0.02/0.02)
rs8177306_g	54 (14)	7 (6)	4 (8)	0.009	0.026	---[4]	0.08 (0.18/---)
TFRC							
rs480760_t	110 (28)	22 (19)	8 (15)	0.005	0.038	0.476	0.19 (0.37/0.05)

[1]Numbers of subjects shown are for entire study population, including 10.4% non-Hispanic Black and 2.1% "Other" self-reported race/ethnicity.
[2]*P*-values presented were obtained using a non-parametric test for trend.
[3]Allele frequency in entire CHARTER study population.
[4]Allele not present in whites.
Abbreviations: Mod/Sev, moderate to severe neuropathic pain; B/W, Non-Hispanic Blacks/Whites; *ACO1*, cytoplasmic aconitase (iron-regulatory protein 1); *B2M*, beta-2 microglobulin; *BMP6*, bone morphogenetic protein-6; *CP*, ceruloplasmin; *TF*, transferrin; *TFRC*, transferrin receptor 1.

which is mutated in Friedreich's ataxia, regulates mitochondrial iron utilization and export; a defect in the encoded frataxin molecule in this disease results in progressive mitochondrial iron accumulation and oxidative injury in a variety of tissues with high metabolic demand, including the heart and central nervous system [69–71]. Beta-2 microglobulin is a ubiquitous iron- and Hfe-stabilizing protein which also promotes nerve repair following injury, and it is a marker of disease progression in a variety of diseases, but it has not previously been associated with DNP [72]. The *CP* rs3816893 and rs1302552 SNPs, which were associated with DNP alone in this population, also showed strong associations with the presence of neuropathy symptoms in general, which included paresthesias and loss of sensation. These SNP associations also met multiple-testing criteria for significance after permutation analysis, lending support to a role for *CP* in DNP. Ceruloplasmin is a ferroxidase of critical importance to neuronal copper and iron regulation and in neuronal protection against iron-mediated oxidative injury in the central and peripheral nervous systems [73]. The non-synonymous *CP* SNP rs13072552 has been associated in genome-wide association studies with higher serum ceruloplasmin levels [74]. While serum ceruloplasmin is an acute-phase reactant (levels rise during acute inflammation), serum ceruloplasmin levels may also be a marker of oxidative neuronal injury, as in diabetic neuropathy.[75]. Disturbances in ceruloplasmin homeostasis have been linked to other neurodegenerative diseases, and to neuropathic pain in the constriction injury rat model of neuropathic pain.[76]. Similarly, transferrin levels have been associated with peripheral neuropathy after bariatric surgery, which has been shown to disrupt iron homeostasis [77].

Iron transport in all tissues is intricately balanced with cellular and mitochondrial iron demand; indeed, recent studies including our own suggest that iron levels regulate mitochondrial biogenesis, a determinant of mitochondrial function [78]. (*Kallianpur et al, unpublished data*) Therefore, it should not be surprising if altered iron transport increases susceptibility to HIV-SN and DNP, especially in individuals exposed to mitochondria-toxic forms of cART. Mitochondrial injury, as well as activation of glia in the spinal cord and dorsal root ganglia due to HIV envelope glycoprotein gp120, with consequent release of inflammatory cytokines, may be involved in the pathogenesis of DNP [79]. Finally, others have reported that dysregulated iron transport also alters glutamate metabolism, which is implicated in both drug-induced and non-toxic peripheral neuropathies [80–82].

This study has some acknowledged limitations. The functional effects of these SNPs in iron-related genes are currently unknown. Since regulation of iron metabolism occurs largely at the post-transcriptional level, we speculate that many of these variants alter gene regulation and protein levels rather than protein structure or function. Assay of serum protein levels was not possible as part of this study, but *CP* rs13072552 has been linked to increased ceruloplasmin levels [74], and several of the genes identified here encode measurable serum proteins that may be investigated in future studies. The functional relatedness of the genes we selected in iron metabolism, in addition to tightly coordinated regulation of some of these genes (*e.g.*, *ACO1* and *TFRC*) in order to fine tune cellular iron access, storage, and utilization, argue against reliance on genome-wide levels of significance or stringent multiple-testing corrections in an exploratory study of this type; individual iron-regulatory SNP genotypes are highly unlikely to be independent, as represented in Figure 1. In this situation, correction for the number of genes analyzed may be a more logical approach: with this type of correction, *TF* rs2718796, *CP* rs3816893, and *B2M* rs16966334, as well as *ACO1* rs2026739 in whites, remain statistically significant or nominally significant. (As noted, the *ACO1* SNP also remained significant after Bonferroni correction for multiple tests.) We did not adjust in our analyses for height or alcohol consumption, factors which can influence susceptibility to neuropathy, but not necessarily DNP. However, alcohol consumption was not associated with DNP on univariable analysis. Information about hair color, which has been correlated with neuropathic pain sensitivity, was not available [83]. We also attempted to address the potential effect of diabetes on genetic associations with peripheral neuropathy and DNP in this population. Glycosylated hemoglobin values were not available for analysis on most subjects, but additional adjustment for the possible presence of treated or untreated diabetes, ascertained using a more stringent-than-normal cut-off for non-fasting blood glucose values, did not significantly impact our results. Finally, the purpose of this study was to build on our prior findings of iron-related genetic associations with HIV-SN and to test the hypothesis that iron metabolism, rather than inflammation alone, plays a role in HIV-associated DNP; we intentionally did not study an exhaustive list of iron-regulatory genes. Much of the ferrome therefore remains to be studied. Keltner et al recently reported that HIV-associated DNP is associated in CHARTER subjects with reduced total cortical gray matter volumes on neuroimaging; cortical gray matter volumes have also been linked to R2* relaxation times, a sensitive measure of brain iron content [84,85].

In summary, SNPs in eight iron-related genes selected for analysis showed significant and biologically plausible associations with DNP, independent of known potential confounders; SNPs in 7 of these genes also predicted DNP severity, adding to the biological plausibility argument. Most importantly, the common ACO1 rs2026739 variant remained significantly associated with DNP and DNP severity after stringent correction for multiple tests. Furthermore, associations with DNP were relatively robust, and point estimates for SNP associations were similar in direction and magnitude in blacks and whites, if not statistically significant in both groups. These results support the concept that the ferrome may be involved in the pathogenesis of HIV-SN and DNP in HIV-infected individuals on cART. These new genetic associations will require replication in other population samples as well as further functional characterization to determine underlying biological mechanisms that may be therapeutically targeted.

Supporting Information

Figure S1 Minimal overlap between ancestry principal components (PCs). PCs plotted against one another demonstrate appropriate clustering, with few outliers. *Black dots*: black; *blue dots:* Hispanic; *red dots:* white; *cyan dots:* other.

Table S1 Iron-related genes and variants evaluated in relation to neuropathy in CHARTER.

Acknowledgments

The authors would like to express gratitude to all CHARTER study participants. We also thank all CHARTER investigators and site PIs, who assisted in subject recruitment:

The CNS HIV Antiretroviral Therapy Effects Research (CHARTER) Study is affiliated with the University of California-San Diego, Johns Hopkins University School of Medicine, Mount Sinai School of Medicine, Washington University- Saint Louis, University of Texas- Galveston, and the University of Washington-Seattle and is headquarted at the University of California-San Diego. Members of the CHARTER Study Group include: Director, Igor Grant, M.D.; Co-Directors, Scott Letendre, M.D.,

Ronald Ellis, M.D., Ph.D., Thomas Marcotte, Ph.D.; Center Manager, Donald Franklin, Jr.; Neuromedical component: Ronald Ellis, M.D., Ph.D. (PI); J. Allen McCutchan, M.D., Terry Alexander, R.N.; Laboratory, Pharmacology and Immunology Component: Scott Letendre, M.D. (P.I.), Edmund Capparelli, Pharm.D.; Neurobehavioral Component: Robert K. Heaton, Ph.D. (P.I.), J. Hampton Atkinson, M.D., Steven Paul Woods, Psy.D., Matthew Dawson; Virology Component: Davey M. Smith, M.D. (P.I.), Joseph K. Wong, M.D.; Imaging Component: Christine Fennema-Notestine, Ph.D. (Co-P.I.), Michael J. Taylor, Ph.D. (Co-P.I.), Rebecca Theilmann, Ph.D.; Data Management Component: Anthony C. Gamst, Ph.D. (P.I.), Clint Cushman, Ph.D; Statistics Component: Ian Abramson, Ph.D. (P.I.), Florin Vaida, Ph.D.; Johns Hopkins University Site: Justin McArthur (P.I.), Mary Smith; Mount Sinai School of Medicine Site: Susan Morgello, M.D. (Co-P.I.) and David Simpson, M.D. (Co-P.I.), Letty Mintz, N.P.; University of California, San Diego Site: J. Allen McCutchan, M.D. (P.I.), Will Toperoff, N.P.; University of Washington, Seattle Site: Ann Collier, M.D. (Co-P.I.) and Christina Marra, M.D. (Co-P.I.), Trudy Jones, M.N., A.R.N.P.; University of Texas, Galveston Site: Benjamin Gelman, M.D., Ph.D. (P.I.), Eleanor Head, R.N., B.S.N.; and Washington University, St. Louis Site: David Clifford, M.D. (P.I.), Muhammad Al-Lozi, M.D., Mengesha Teshome, M.D.

The views expressed in this article are those of the authors and do not reflect the official policy or position of the United States Government.

Author Contributions

Analyzed the data: ARK PJ WW ZZ. Contributed reagents/materials/analysis tools: IG SLL RJE ACC CMM DMS DBC SM JCM BBG JAM DF DR CB TH EH. Wrote the paper: ARK PJ. Assisted in interpretation of genotyping results: CB PJ DCS. Participated in discussion of analysis results and commented on the manuscript: PJ RJE ZZ TH CB BBG DGM DCS SLL.

References

1. Ellis RJ, Rosario D, Clifford DB, McArthur JC, Simpson D, et al. (2010) Continued high prevalence and adverse clinical impact of human immunodeficiency virus-associated sensory neuropathy in the era of combination antiretroviral therapy: the CHARTER Study. Arch Neurol 67: 552–558.
2. Kallianpur AR, Hulgan T (2009) Pharmacogenetics of nucleoside reverse-transcriptase inhibitor-associated peripheral neuropathy. Pharmacogenomics 10: 623–637.
3. Hitchcock SA, Meyer HP, Gwyther E (2008) Neuropathic pain in AIDS patients prior to antiretroviral therapy. S Afr Med J 98: 889–892.
4. Apostolova N, Blas-Garcia A, Esplugues JV (2011) Mitochondrial interference by anti-HIV drugs: mechanisms beyond Pol-gamma inhibition. Trends in Pharmacological Sciences 32: 715–725.
5. Hulgan T, Haas DW, Haines JL, Ritchie MD, Robbins GK, et al. (2005) Mitochondrial haplogroups and peripheral neuropathy during antiretroviral therapy: an adult AIDS clinical trials group study. AIDS 19: 1341–1349.
6. Hulgan T, Tebas P, Canter JA, Mulligan K, Haas DW, et al. (2008) Hemochromatosis gene polymorphisms, mitochondrial haplogroups, and peripheral lipoatrophy during antiretroviral therapy. J Infect Dis 197: 858–866.
7. Kamerman PR, Moss PJ, Weber J, Wallace VC, Rice AS, et al. (2012) Pathogenesis of HIV-associated sensory neuropathy: evidence from in vivo and in vitro experimental models. J Peripher Nerv Syst 17: 19–31.
8. Keswani SC, Jack C, Zhou C, Hoke A (2006) Establishment of a rodent model of HIV-associated sensory neuropathy. J Neurosci 26: 10299–10304.
9. Ellis RJ, Marquie-Beck J, Delaney P, Alexander T, Clifford DB, et al. (2008) Human immunodeficiency virus protease inhibitors and risk for peripheral neuropathy. Ann Neurol 64: 566–572.
10. Robinson-Papp J, Morgello S, Vaida F, Fitzsimons C, Simpson DM, et al. (2010) Association of self-reported painful symptoms with clinical and neurophysiologic signs in HIV-associated sensory neuropathy. Pain 151: 732–736.
11. Lucey BP, Clifford DB, Creighton J, Edwards RR, McArthur JC, et al. (2011) Relationship of depression and catastrophizing to pain, disability, and medication adherence in patients with HIV-associated sensory neuropathy. Aids Care-Psychological and Socio-Medical Aspects of Aids/Hiv 23: 921–928.
12. Phillips TJ, Cherry CL, Cox S, Marshall SJ, Rice AS (2010) Pharmacological treatment of painful HIV-associated sensory neuropathy: a systematic review and meta-analysis of randomised controlled trials. PLoS One 5: e14433.
13. Chetty S, Baalbergen E, Bhigjee AI, Kamerman P, Ouma J, et al. (2012) Clinical practice guidelines for management of neuropathic pain: expert panel recommendations for South Africa. Samj South African Medical Journal 102: 312–325.
14. Derry S, Moore RA (2012) Topical capsaicin (low concentration) for chronic neuropathic pain in adults. Cochrane Database Syst Rev 9: CD010111.
15. Evans SR, Simpson DM, Kitch DW, King A, Clifford DB, et al. (2007) A Randomized Trial Evaluating Prosaptide (TM) for HIV-Associated Sensory Neuropathies: Use of an Electronic Diary to Record Neuropathic Pain. PLoS One 2: e551.
16. Keltner JR, Vaida F, Ellis RJ, Moeller-Bertram T, Fitzsimmons C, et al. (2012) Health-related quality of life 'well-being' in HIV distal neuropathic pain is more strongly associated with depression severity than with pain intensity. Psychosomatics 53: 380–386.
17. Fellows RP, Byrd DA, Elliott K, Robinson-Papp J, Mindt MR, et al. (2012) Distal sensory polyneuropathy is associated with neuropsychological test performance among persons with HIV. J Int Neuropsychol Soc 18: 898–907.
18. Davis L, Evans S, Fishman B, Haley A, Spielman LA (2004) Predictors of attrition in HIV-positive subjects with peripheral neuropathic pain. Aids Care-Psychological and Socio-Medical Aspects of Aids/Hiv 16: 395–402.
19. Oshinaike O, Akinbami A, Ojo O, Ogbera A, Okubadejo N, et al. (2012) Influence of Age and Neurotoxic HAART Use on Frequency of HIV Sensory Neuropathy. AIDS Res Treat 2012: 961510.
20. Pahuja M, Grobler A, Glesby MJ, Karim F, Parker G, et al. (2012) Effects of a reduced dose of stavudine on the incidence and severity of peripheral neuropathy in HIV-infected adults in South Africa. Antiviral Therapy 17: 737–743.
21. Backonja M, Woolf CJ (2010) Future directions in neuropathic pain therapy: closing the translational loop. Oncologist 15 Suppl 2: 24–29.
22. Maag R, Baron R (2006) Neuropathic pain: translational research and impact for patient care. Curr Pain Headache Rep 10: 191–198.
23. Max MB, Stewart WF (2008) The molecular epidemiology of pain: a new discipline for drug discovery. Nature Reviews Drug Discovery 7: 647–658.
24. Galy B, Ferring-Appel D, Sauer SW, Kaden S, Lyoumi S, et al. (2010) Iron regulatory proteins secure mitochondrial iron sufficiency and function. Cell Metab 12: 194–201.
25. Millecamps S, Julien JP (2013) Axonal transport deficits and neurodegenerative diseases. Nature Reviews Neuroscience 14: 161–176.
26. Sheftel AD, Lill R (2009) The power plant of the cell is also a smithy: the emerging role of mitochondria in cellular iron homeostasis. Ann Med 41: 82–99.
27. Drakesmith H, Prentice AM (2012) Hepcidin and the Iron-Infection Axis. Science 338: 768–772.
28. Wu X, Yung LM, Cheng WH, Yu PB, Babitt JL, et al. (2012) Hepcidin regulation by BMP signaling in macrophages is lipopolysaccharide dependent. PLoS One 7: e44622.
29. Zhang X, Rovin BH (2013) Beyond anemia: hepcidin, monocytes and inflammation. Biol Chem 394: 231–238.
30. Johnson EE, Sandgren A, Cherayil BJ, Murray M, Wessling-Resnick M (2010) Role of ferroportin in macrophage-mediated immunity. Infect Immun 78: 5099–5106.
31. Kallianpur AR, Hulgan T, Canter JA, Ritchie MD, Haines JL, et al. (2006) Hemochromatosis (HFE) gene mutations and peripheral neuropathy during antiretroviral therapy. AIDS 20: 1503–1513.
32. Bulaj ZJ, Griffen LM, Jorde LB, Edwards CQ, Kushner JP (1996) Clinical and biochemical abnormalities in people heterozygous for hemochromatosis. N Engl J Med 335: 1799–1805.
33. Holzinger ER, Hulgan T, Ellis RJ, Samuels DC, Ritchie MD, et al. (2012) Mitochondrial DNA variation and HIV-associated sensory neuropathy in CHARTER. J Neurovirol 18: 511–520.
34. Grady BJ, Dudek S, Ritchie MD (2009) Finding Unique Filter Sets in PLATO: Preparation for Efficient Interaction Analysis. Genetic Epidemiology 33: 788–788.
35. Kumar KR, Djarmati-Westenberger A, Grunewald A (2011) Genetics of Parkinson's disease. Semin Neurol 31: 433–440.
36. Reich DE, Lander ES (2001) On the allelic spectrum of human disease. Trends Genet 17: 502–510.
37. Purcell S, Neale B, Todd-Brown K, Thomas L, Ferreira MA, et al. (2007) PLINK: a tool set for whole-genome association and population-based linkage analyses. American Journal of Human Genetics 81: 559–575.
38. Jia P, Wang L, Fanous AH, Chen X, Kendler KS, et al. (2012) A bias-reducing pathway enrichment analysis of genome-wide association data confirmed association of the MHC region with schizophrenia. J Med Genet 49: 96–103.
39. Bush WS, Moore JH (2012) Chapter 11: Genome-wide association studies. PLoS Comput Biol 8: e1002822.
40. Pruim RJ, Welch RP, Sanna S, Teslovich TM, Chines PS, et al. (2010) LocusZoom: regional visualization of genome-wide association scan results. Bioinformatics 26: 2336–2337.
41. Cano A, Mayo A, Ventimiglia M (2006) Coping, pain severity, interference, and disability: the potential mediating and moderating roles of race and education. Journal of Pain 7: 459–468.
42. Wandner LD, Scipio CD, Hirsh AT, Torres CA, Robinson ME (2012) The perception of pain in others: how gender, race, and age influence pain expectations. Journal of Pain 13: 220–227.
43. Lorber M, Haddad S (2013) Hypersensitivity and desensitization to darunavir in a case of HIV infection with triple-class drug resistance: case description and review of the literature. J Int Assoc Provid AIDS Care 12: 378–379.

44. Kranick SM, Nath A (2012) Neurologic complications of HIV-1 infection and its treatment in the era of antiretroviral therapy. Continuum (Minneap Minn) 18: 1319–1337.
45. Boelaert JR, Weinberg GA, Weinberg ED (1996) Altered iron metabolism in HIV infection: mechanisms, possible consequences, and proposals for management. Infect Agents Dis 5: 36–46.
46. Drakesmith H, Chen N, Ledermann H, Screaton G, Townsend A, et al. (2005) HIV-1 Nef down-regulates the hemochromatosis protein HFE, manipulating cellular iron homeostasis. Proc Natl Acad Sci U S A 102: 11017–11022.
47. Finberg KE (2013) Regulation of systemic iron homeostasis. Curr Opin Hematol 20: 208–214.
48. Bentley AJ, Rosman KD, Mitchell D (2007) Can the sensory symptoms of restless legs syndrome be assessed using a qualitative pain questionnaire? Clin J Pain 23: 62–66.
49. Gemignani F, Vitetta F, Brindani F, Contini M, Negrotti A (2013) Painful polyneuropathy associated with restless legs syndrome. Clinical features and sensory profile. Sleep Med 14: 79–84.
50. Connor JR, Ponnuru P, Wang XS, Patton SM, Allen RP, et al. (2011) Profile of altered brain iron acquisition in restless legs syndrome. Brain 134: 959–968.
51. Patton SM, Ponnuru P, Snyder AM, Podskalny GD, Connor JR (2011) Hypoxia-inducible factor pathway activation in restless legs syndrome patients. Eur J Neurol 18: 1329–1335.
52. Hare D, Ayton S, Bush A, Lei P (2013) A delicate balance: Iron metabolism and diseases of the brain. Front Aging Neurosci 5: 34.
53. Dowling P, Klinker F, Amaya F, Paulus W, Liebetanz D (2009) Iron-deficiency sensitizes mice to acute pain stimuli and formalin-induced nociception. J Nutr 139: 2087–2092.
54. Dubovy P (2011) Wallerian degeneration and peripheral nerve conditions for both axonal regeneration and neuropathic pain induction. Ann Anat 193: 267–275.
55. Gille G, Reichmann H (2011) Iron-dependent functions of mitochondria–relation to neurodegeneration. J Neural Transm 118: 349–359.
56. Joseph EK, Levine JD (2006) Mitochondrial electron transport in models of neuropathic and inflammatory pain. Pain 121: 105–114.
57. Richardson DR, Lane DJ, Becker EM, Huang ML, Whitnall M, et al. (2010) Mitochondrial iron trafficking and the integration of iron metabolism between the mitochondrion and cytosol. Proc Natl Acad Sci U S A 107: 10775–10782.
58. Carlson ES, Tkac I, Magid R, O'Connor MB, Andrews NC, et al. (2009) Iron is essential for neuron development and memory function in mouse hippocampus. J Nutr 139: 672–679.
59. Moos T, Rosengren Nielsen T (2006) Ferroportin in the postnatal rat brain: implications for axonal transport and neuronal export of iron. Seminars in Pediatric Neurology 13: 149–157.
60. Moos T, Bernth N, Courtois Y, Morgan EH (2011) Developmental iron uptake and axonal transport in the retina of the rat. Mol Cell Neurosci 46: 607–613.
61. Li X, Clark JD (2003) Heme oxygenase type 2 participates in the development of chronic inflammatory and neuropathic pain. Journal of Pain 4: 101–107.
62. Mitchell RM, Lee SY, Randazzo WT, Simmons Z, Connor JR (2009) Influence of HFE variants and cellular iron on monocyte chemoattractant protein-1. J Neuroinflammation 6: 6.
63. Lawless MW, White M, Mankan AK, O'Dwyer MJ, Norris S (2007) Elevated MCP-1 serum levels are associated with the H63D mutation and not the C282Y mutation in hereditary hemochromatosis. Tissue Antigens 70: 294–300.
64. Uceyler N, Rogausch JP, Toyka KV, Sommer C (2007) Differential expression of cytokines in painful and painless neuropathies. Neurology 69: 42–49.
65. Leung L, Cahill CM (2010) TNF-alpha and neuropathic pain - a review. Journal of Neuroinflammation 7: 27.
66. Foulkes T, Wood JN (2008) Pain Genes. Plos Genetics 4: e1000086
67. Tramullas M, Lantero A, Diaz A, Morchon N, Merino D, et al. (2010) BAMBI (bone morphogenetic protein and activin membrane-bound inhibitor) reveals the involvement of the transforming growth factor-beta family in pain modulation. J Neurosci 30: 1502–1511.
68. Wang J, Pantopoulos K (2011) Regulation of cellular iron metabolism. Biochem J 434: 365–381.
69. Calabrese V, Lodi R, Tonon C, D'Agata V, Sapienza M, et al. (2005) Oxidative stress, mitochondrial dysfunction and cellular stress response in Friedreich's ataxia. J Neurol Sci 233: 145–162.
70. Stemmler TL, Lesuisse E, Pain D, Dancis A (2010) Frataxin and mitochondrial FeS cluster biogenesis. J Biol Chem 285: 26737–26743.
71. Ye H, Rouault TA (2010) Human iron-sulfur cluster assembly, cellular iron homeostasis, and disease. Biochemistry 49: 4945–4956.
72. Staats KA, Schonefeldt S, Van Rillaer M, Van Hoecke A, Van Damme P, et al. (2013) Beta-2 microglobulin is important for disease progression in a murine model for amyotrophic lateral sclerosis. Front Cell Neurosci 7: 249.
73. Ayton S, Zhang M, Roberts BR, Lam LQ, Lind M, et al. (2014) Ceruloplasmin and beta-amyloid precursor protein confer neuroprotection in traumatic brain injury and lower neuronal iron. Free Radic Biol Med. Feb 7 (Epub ahead of print).
74. Tang WH, Wu Y, Hartiala J, Fan Y, Stewart AF, et al. (2012) Clinical and genetic association of serum ceruloplasmin with cardiovascular risk. Arterioscler Thromb Vasc Biol 32: 516–522.
75. El Boghdady NA, Badr GA (2012) Evaluation of oxidative stress markers and vascular risk factors in patients with diabetic peripheral neuropathy. Cell Biochem Funct 30: 328–334.
76. Tan EC, Bahrami S, Kozlov AV, Kurvers HA, Ter Laak HJ, et al. (2009) The oxidative response in the chronic constriction injury model of neuropathic pain. J Surg Res 152: 84–88.
77. Thaisetthawatkul P, Collazo-Clavell ML, Sarr MG, Norell JE, Dyck PJ (2004) A controlled study of peripheral neuropathy after bariatric surgery. Neurology 63: 1462–1470.
78. Rensvold JW, Ong SE, Jeevananthan A, Carr SA, Mootha VK, et al. (2013) Complementary RNA and Protein Profiling Identifies Iron as a Key Regulator of Mitochondrial Biogenesis. Cell Rep 3: 237–245.
79. Hao S (2013) The Molecular and Pharmacological Mechanisms of HIV-Related Neuropathic Pain. Curr Neuropharmacol 11: 499–512.
80. Li JY, Wang X, Ji PT, Li XF, Guan GH, et al. (2012) Peripheral nerve injury decreases the expression of metabolic glutamate receptor 7 in dorsal root ganglion neurons. Neurosci Lett 531: 52–56.
81. Yan X, Jiang E, Gao M, Weng HR (2013) Endogenous activation of presynaptic NMDA receptors enhances glutamate release from the primary afferents in the spinal dorsal horn in a rat model of neuropathic pain. J Physiol 591: 2001–2019.
82. Mitchell RM, Lee SY, Simmons Z, Connor JR (2011) HFE polymorphisms affect cellular glutamate regulation. Neurobiol Aging 32: 1114–1123.
83. Belfer I, Dai F (2010) Phenotyping and Genotyping Neuropathic Pain. Curr Pain Headache Rep 14: 203–212.
84. Keltner JR, Fennema-Notestine C, Vaida F, Wang D, Franklin DR, et al; for the CHARTER Group (2014) HIV-associated distal neuropathic pain is associated with smaller total cerebral cortical gray matter. J Neurovirol Feb 19 (Epub ahead of print).
85. Ropele S, Wattjes MP, Langkammer C, Kilsdonk ID, de Graaf WL, et al. (2013) Multicenter R2* mapping in the healthy brain. Magn Reson Med May 8 (Epub ahead of print).

Curcumin Alleviates Neuropathic Pain by Inhibiting p300/CBP Histone Acetyltransferase Activity-Regulated Expression of BDNF and Cox-2 in a Rat Model

Xiaoyan Zhu[1], Qian Li[1], Ruimin Chang[2], Dong Yang[3], Zongbing Song[1], Qulian Guo[1], Changsheng Huang[1]*

1 Department of Anesthesiology, Xiangya Hospital of Central South University, Changsha, China, **2** Liver Cancer Laboratory, Xiangya Hospital of Central South University, Changsha, China, **3** Department of Anesthesiology, Union Hospital, Tongji Medical College, Huazhong University of Science and Technology, Wuhan, China

Abstract

The management of neuropathic pain is still a major challenge because of its unresponsiveness to most common treatments. Curcumin has been reported to play an active role in the treatment of various neurological disorders, such as neuropathic pain. Curcumin has long been recognized as a p300/CREB-binding protein (CBP) inhibitor of histone acetyltransferase (HAT) activity. However, this mechanism has never been investigated for the treatment of neuropathic pain with curcumin. The aim of the present study was to investigate the anti-nociceptive role of curcumin in the chronic constriction injury (CCI) rat model of neuropathic pain. Furthermore, with this model we investigated the effect of curcumin on P300/CBP HAT activity-regulated release of the pro-nociceptive molecules, brain-derived neurotrophic factor (BDNF) and cyclooxygenase-2 (Cox-2). Treatment with 40 and 60 mg/kg body weight curcumin for 7 consecutive days significantly attenuated CCI-induced thermal hyperalgesia and mechanical allodynia, whereas 20 mg/kg curcumin showed no significant analgesic effect. Chromatin immunoprecipitation analysis revealed that curcumin dose-dependently reduced the recruitment of p300/CBP and acetyl-Histone H3/acetyl-Histone H4 to the promoter of BDNF and Cox-2 genes. A similar dose-dependent decrease of BDNF and Cox-2 in the spinal cord was also observed after curcumin treatment. These results indicated that curcumin exerted a therapeutic role in neuropathic pain by down-regulating p300/CBP HAT activity-mediated gene expression of BDNF and Cox-2.

Editor: Daqing Ma, Imperial College London, Chelsea & Westminster Hospital, United Kingdom

Funding: This project was supported by National Natural Science Foundation of China (81000478, 81171053) and Science and Technology Planning Project of Hunan Province, China (2012WK3019). The funders had no role in study design, data collection and analysis, decision to publish, or preparation of the manuscript.

Competing Interests: The authors have declared that no competing interests exist.

* E-mail: docthuang2005@hotmail.com

Introduction

Neuropathic pain is caused by a lesion or disease affecting the nervous systems, and is generally manifested as spontaneous pain, hyperalgesia, and allodynia [1,2]. Treatment of neuropathic pain is still a major challenge because of its unresponsiveness to most available pharmacotherapy [3]. Even opioid drugs, which are commonly used analgesics, are often considered to not have an effect on neuropathic pain [4,5]. Therefore, the search for novel drug molecules has become one of the most important strategies for the management of neuropathic pain.

Curcuma longa (tumeric) is a rhizomatous herbaceous perennial plant of the ginger family. It is commonly found in traditional Chinese medicine, such as in Xiaoyao-san, and is used to treat symptoms of mental stress, hypochondriac pain, and mania. 1, 7-bis (4-hydroxy-3-methoxyphenyl)-1, 6-heptadiene-3, 5-dione (curcumin) is the main ingredient of curcuma longa, and has a variety of effects, such as anti-oxidative, anti-inflammatory, immunomodulatory, and neuro-protective [6,7]. Curcumin has neuroprotective effects in various neurological disorders, such as Alzheimer's disease [8], tardive dyskinesia [9], major depression [10], and diabetic neuropathy [11,12]. Recently, several studies have demonstrated an anti-nociceptive effect of curcumin in neuropathic pain [13,14]. However, its mechanism of action is not clearly understood.

Curcumin plays a major role as a p300/CREB-binding protein (CBP) inhibitor of histone acetyltransferase (HAT) activity [15,16,17]. p300 and CBP are two distinct but functionally-related proteins that belong to the HAT family, which is involved in the regulation of gene expression in eukaryotes [18,19]. Dysfunction of p300/CBP HAT activity contributes to various disorders in the central nervous system [20,21,22]. One of our previous studies has demonstrated that the manifestation of neuropathic pain induced by chronic constriction injury (CCI) is related to increased expression of P300/CBP in the rat spinal dorsal horn [23]. Furthermore, we have shown that inhibition of p300 HAT activity downregulates a pain-related downstream gene and is accompanied by an alleviation of neuropathic pain [24]. These results raise the question of whether curcumin exerts its anti-nociceptive effects by inhibiting the activity of p300/CBP HAT.

Therefore, the aim of this study was to determine the anti-nociceptive role of curcumin and its effect on the release of pro-nociceptive molecules, brain-derived neurotrophic factor (BDNF) and cyclooxygenase-2 (Cox-2) in a chronic constriction injury (CCI) rat model of neuropathic pain. The expression of BDNF and Cox-2 has been shown to be regulated by HAT activity of p300/CBP [25,26,27]. We investigated the co-expression of these pro-nociceptive molecules with P300/CBP in the rat spinal dorsal horn after CCI and curcumin treatment. We then determined the changes in the recruitment of P300/CBP and histone H3 acetylation at lysine 9 (H3K9ac)/histone H4 acetylation at lysine 5 (H4K5ac) to the promoter region of these genes. The changes in the expression of these molecules were consequently examined. Our study demonstrated for the first time that curcumin inhibited the activity of p300/CBP HAT, which subsequently enabled the management of neuropathic pain.

Materials and Methods

Animals

A total of 60 male Sprague-Dawley rats (220–250 g) were provided by the animal experimental center of Central South University of China. Rats were housed in plastic cages in a climate-controlled room under a 12:12-h light-dark cycle, with free access to food and water. All procedures were approved by the Animal Care Committee of Central South University of China, and conformed with the United States Public Health Service Policy on Humane Care and Use of Laboratory Animals and the Guide for the Care and Use of Laboratory Animals (1996). All efforts were made to minimize animal suffering and the number of animals used.

CCI Model

Rats were anesthetized with 10% chloral hydrate (300–350 mg/kg, intraperitoneally [i.p.]). CCI was then established, as previously described [28]. In brief, the left common sciatic nerve was exposed and freed from the surrounding loose connective tissue. Four snug ligatures (4-0 chromic gut) with about 1 mm spacing were placed around the nerve proximal to the trifurcation. All nerve ligations were performed by the same member of our team to avoid variation. In the sham group, the nerve was exposed but not ligated. Rats that had undergone CCI surgery and demonstrated vigorous mechanical and thermal hypersensitivity of nerve injury were used for further experiments.

Drug Treatments

Curcumin (Sigma-Aldrich, Santa Clara, CA, USA) was dissolved in 20% dimethyl sulfoxide (DMSO) with 80% normal saline solution, as performed in previous studies [29,30]. Curcumin was administered to CCI rats at 20, 40 or 60 mg/kg body weight (i.p.) (n = 10 per group). The vehicle (20% DMSO with 80% normal saline solution) was given (i.p.) to sham-operated rats (n = 10) and CCI rats (n = 20) as controls. Drug delivery was not performed until 7 days after CCI surgery to ensure the establishment of neuropathic pain. Drugs were then administered once a day until 14 days after the CCI or sham operation.

Behavioral Measurements

The thermal withdrawal latency and mechanical withdrawal threshold of all rats were measured before CCI surgery, and 3, 5, 7, 10, 12, and 14 days after CCI. All the measurements were performed by the same observer who was blind to the animal treatments.

The Hargreaves test [31] was used to evaluate the thermal withdraw latency by a plantar algesimeter (Tes7370, Ugo Basile, Comerio, Italy). Rats were placed in clear plastic cages on an elevated glass plate. A constant intensity radiant heat source was focused underneath the glass and aimed at the plantar surface of the ipsilateral hindpaw. A digital timer automatically read the duration between the start of stimuli and paw withdrawal. Measurements were repeated three times at intervals of 5 min, and the mean value of the three measurements was taken as the latency. A cutoff time of 25 s of irradiation was used to avoid any tissue damage.

The mechanical withdraw threshold of the ipsilateral hindpaw was measured by an electronic von Frey anesthesiometer (2390 series; IITC Instruments, Woodland Hills, USA), as described previously [32]. Briefly, the rats were placed in a plastic cage on a metal mesh floor and were allowed to adapt to this set-up prior to testing. A hand-held force transducer fitted with a 0.7 mm^2 polypropylene tip was applied to the plantar surface of the ipsilateral hindpaw. Measurements were repeated three times at intervals of 5 min, and the mechanical threshold was defined as the force (g) initiating a withdrawal response averaged from the three measurements.

Tissue Preparation

The spinal cord tissue was processed, as described in our previous study [33]. Rats were sacrificed at the completion of behavioral measurements (i.e. 14 days after CCI). L4-L5 segments of lumbar spinal cords were quickly removed and stored at −80°C. Ten Rats from the vehicle-treated CCI group were used for immunohistological observation. These rats were anesthetized and perfused with 400 ml normal saline followed by 40 0 ml 4% paraformaldehyde, and L4-L5 segments of lumbar spinal cords were then removed and post-fixed with 4% paraformaldehyde for 8 h at 4°C.

Double-labeling Immunofluorescence

Tissues were fixed with 4% paraformaldehyde for 8 h and then dehydrated and embedded in paraffin. They were cut at a thickness of 5 μm. The sections were dewaxed and treated with 0.01 M citrate buffer at 80°C for 20 min for antigen retrieval, and then blocked with 10% horse serum for 1 h. Sections were then incubated for 24 h at 4°C with anti-CBP antibody (1:200; Santa Cruz) or anti-p300 antibody (1:200; Santa Cruz), and then incubated with biotinylated anti-mouse IgG (1:200; Santa Cruz) for 2 h, followed by red dihydroxyfluorane (1:100; Jackson) incubation for 2 h. Sections were then blocked with 3% goat serum for 1 h, incubated with anti-Cox-2 antibody (1:200; Abcam) or anti-BDNF antibody (1:200; Santa Cruz) overnight at 4°C, followed by biotinylated anti-rabbit IgG (1:500; Santa Cruz) for 2 h and green dihydroxyfluorane (1:200; Jackson) incubation for 2 h. Sections without primary antibody served as the negative controls. Sections were then scanned with a Leica confocal laser scanning microscope (TCS SP5, Mannheim, Germany).

Chromatin Immunoprecipitation (ChIP) Assay and Quantitative Real-time Polymerase Chain Reaction (qRT-PCR)

ChIP assays were performed using the ChIP assay kit (Upstate Biotechnology, USA). The lumber spinal cord segments were cut into 1 mm slices and crossed-linked with 1.5% formaldehyde for 10 minutes. After neutralization in glycine and homogenization in PBS, the cell suspension was centrifuged at 12,000 g for 10 minutes, and sodium dodecyl sulfate (SDS) lysis buffer was added to the pellets. One third of the lysate was used as the DNA input control. The remaining two thirds of the lysate was diluted 10-fold followed by incubation with antibodies against p300, CBP, H3K9ac, H4K5ac, or non-immune IgG, overnight at 4°C. The immunoprecipitated protein-DNA complexes were collected using protein A agarose beads (Upstate Biotechnology, USA). The precipitates were washed extensively and incubated in the elution buffer (25 mM Tris-HCl, 10 mM EDTA, 0.5% SDS, pH 8) at 60°C for 15 min. The input tissue and protein-DNA complexes were subjected to reverse cross-linking, proteinase K digestion, and purification. Real-time PCR amplification then followed, using specific promoter primers containing the putative p300/CBP binding sites for BDNF: forward 5′-TCTCCCTGCCTCATCCCT-3′, reverse 5′-CA-GAGTCTTCCTTTGCCTAC-3′; for Cox-2: forward 5′-AC-CTCTGCGATGCTCTTCCG-3′, reverse 5′-GCTCAGGCGCTTTGCCAATA-3′. All the specific promoter primers were designed as previously described [33]. qRT-PCR was performed by the ABI Prism 7900 Sequence Detection System (Applied Biosystems, Foster City, USA) with the following conditions: 95°C for 5 min, followed by 40 cycles at 94°C for 20 s, 56°C or 59°C for BDNF or Cox-2, respectively for 20 s, and 72°C for 20 s. Each PCR reaction was done in triplicate. A standard curve for absolute quantification was generated with the standard DNA for each PCR product. The absolute copy numbers of the target genes was normalized against those of β-actin, which served as an internal control gene [34].

Western Immunoblot Analysis

Proteins were extracted and subjected to SDS-polyacrylamide gel electrophoresis on 10% polyacrylamide gels, then electrophoretically transferred to polyvinylidene difluoride membranes (Millipore, Massachusetts, USA). After membranes were blocked with 5% nonfat milk in Tris-buffered saline (TBS) (pH 7.5) plus 0.05% Tween 20 for 1 h, they were probed (overnight at 4°C) with rabbit polyclonal anti-BDNF (1:300; Santa Cruz) or anti-Cox-2 (1:800; Abcam). Mouse monoclonal anti-β-actin (1:5000; Abcam) served as the internal control protein. Antibodies were diluted in TBS containing 5% nonfat milk. Horseradish peroxidase-conjugated goat anti-rabbit and anti-mouse antibodies (both 1:500; Santa Cruz) were used as the secondary antibody respectively. Protein brands were visualized by enhanced chemiluminescence (ECL) using an ECL kit (Pierce, USA). Quantity One software (Bio-Rad) was used for densitometric analysis. The results were normalized to β-actin levels.

Statistical Analysis

All data are expressed as the mean ± SEM. A two-way repeated-measure analysis of variance (ANOVA) followed by the Tukey's post hoc multiple comparisons test was used to examine the behavioral data at different time-points and across all groups. Data of protein and gene levels from each independent group were compared using an one-way ANOVA followed by the Tukey's post hoc multiple comparisons test was used to examine protein and gene levels from each independent group. Significance was reached at values of $p<0.05$ or $p<0.01$.

Results

Curcumin attenuated thermal hyperalgesia and mechanical allodynia in CCI rats Neuropathic pain in rats can be examined by measuring the paw withdrawal latency or threshold to thermal or mechanical stimulation, respectively [24,35]. Thermal withdrawal latency represents thermal hyperalgesia, and mechanical withdrawal threshold reflects mechanical allodynia. Time-course changes of thermal withdrawal latency and mechanical withdrawal threshold occurred (Fig. 1 A and B, respectively) in the ipsilateral hindpaw of rats with or without curcumin injection. CCI rats from each group demonstrated a significant ($p<0.05$) reduction of thermal latency and mechanical threshold prior to curcumin treatment compared with sham-operated rats. Thermal latency and mechanical threshold were low in rats treated with vehicle until 14 days after CCI, indicating that CCI-induced thermal hyperalgesia and mechanical allodynia were sustained. Thermal latency and mechanical threshold were significantly ($p<0.05$) increased with 40 and 60 mg/kg curcumin for 7 days in a dose-dependent manner. Compared with vehicle-treated rats, thermal latency increased by 58.2% and 70.6% for 40 mg/kg and 60 mg/kg, respectively. Mechanical threshold increased by 49.3% and 54% for 40 mg/kg and 60 mg/kg, respectively compared with vehicle-treated rats. Thermal latency and mechanical threshold were significantly ($p<0.05$) increased in rats as early as 5 days after 60 mg/kg curcumin. Neither thermal latency nor mechanical threshold was significantly altered at any time point in rats receiving 20 mg/kg curcumin.

BDNF and Cox-2 Co-localized with p300/CBP Immunoreactive Cells

Molecular changes in the dorsal horn contribute to the central sensitization of neuropathic pain. BDNF and Cox-2 are recognized as pro-nociceptive factors, which are peripherally and centrally up-regulated in response to peripheral nerve injury. After CCI, Cox-2 is increased in the lumbar spinal cord between laminae I–IV of the dorsal horn ipsilateral to injury [36]. CCI also increased BDNF in the superficial (I and II) and deeper laminae (IV and V) of ipsilateral dorsal horn [37]. In the present study we used double immunofluorescence to investigate whether the presence of spinal BDNF and Cox-2 induced by CCI is regulated by P300/CBP protein. P300/CBP-immunoreactivity was observed throughout the dorsal horn and was localized in the nuclei. These results are in line with those from [38]. Intense immunoreactivity for BDNF (Fig. 2) and Cox-2 (Fig. 3) was found in laminae I–IV of the ipsilateral lumbar dorsal horn. Immunoreactivity for BDNF and Cox-2 was mainly localized in the cytoplasm and cell membranes surrounding immunoreactive P300/CBP cells, suggesting that the transcription of BDNF and Cox-2 occurred in nuclei in which P300/CBP was present. These co-localizations suggested that P300/CBP regulated the spinal expression of BDNF and Cox-2 in response to CCI.

Curcumin Reduced p300/CBP-mediated Hyper-acetylation of Histone at BDNF and Cox-2 Promoters

Histone hyper-acetylation at promoter region generally raises gene transcription [39,40]. Gene transcription of BDNF and Cox-2 are known to be regulated by p300/CBP-mediated histone acetylation at their promoters. The promoter region of Cox-2 examined in this study has been previously shown by our group to be regulated by P300 protein [33]. BDNF has multiple promoters with each of them regulating an individual transcript [41], thus exerting a distinct role in different pathophysiological conditions. Among the different transcripts of BDNF, the pain promoter transcript has been recognized to be regulated by promoter I [42]. In the present study, P300/CBP-mediated histone acetylation was examined at promoter I of BDNF.

ChIP analysis was introduced to detect the changes of p300/CBP and H3K9ac/H4K5ac protein at the promoter of BDNF and Cox-2, respectively. Binding of p300, CBP, and H3K9ac, but not H4K5ac, to BDNF promoter significantly ($p<0.05$ for p300 and CBP; $p<0.01$ for H3K9ac) increased in vehicle-treated CCI rats compared with sham-operated rats. Curcumin treatment differentially down-regulated the recruitments of the above proteins to

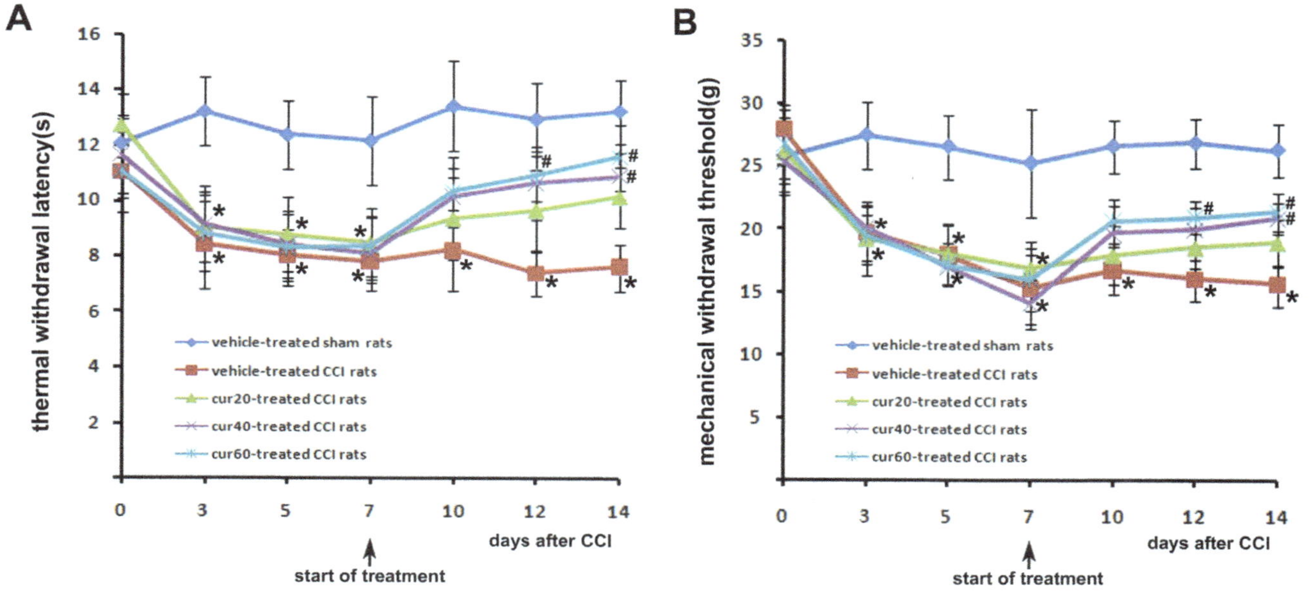

Figure 1. Time-course changes of thermal withdrawal latency (A) and mechanical withdrawal threshold (B) in the ipsilateral hindpaw of rats. Treatment with vehicle or curcumin started 7 days after CCI and was given once daily until 14 days after CCI. *$p<0.05$, CCI versus sham; #$p<0.05$ curcumin versus vehicle (n = 10 per group). cur20: curcumin 20 mg/kg; cur40: curcumin 40 mg/kg; cur60: curcumin 60 mg/kg.

the BDNF promoter in a dose-dependently manner. At 20 mg/kg, a significant ($p<0.05$) decrease in binding of only CBP at the BDNF promoter was observed. At 40 mg/kg, a significant reduction in binding of P300/CBP ($p<0.05$ for p300; $p<0.01$ for CBP), and not H3K9ac/H4K5ac, at the BDNF promoter was observed. At 60 mg/kg, all four proteins were significantly (p300, CBP and H3K9ac: $p<0.01$ for p300, CBP, and H3k9ac; $p<0.05$ for H4K5ac) reduced at the BDNF promoter (Fig. 4 A). P300/CBP and H3K9ac/H4K5ac were all markedly ($p<0.01$ for p300; $p<0.05$ for CBP, H3K9ac, and H4K5ac) up-regulated in the promoter region of the Cox-2 gene in response to CCI. In addition, protein binding at the Cox-2 promoter was altered by

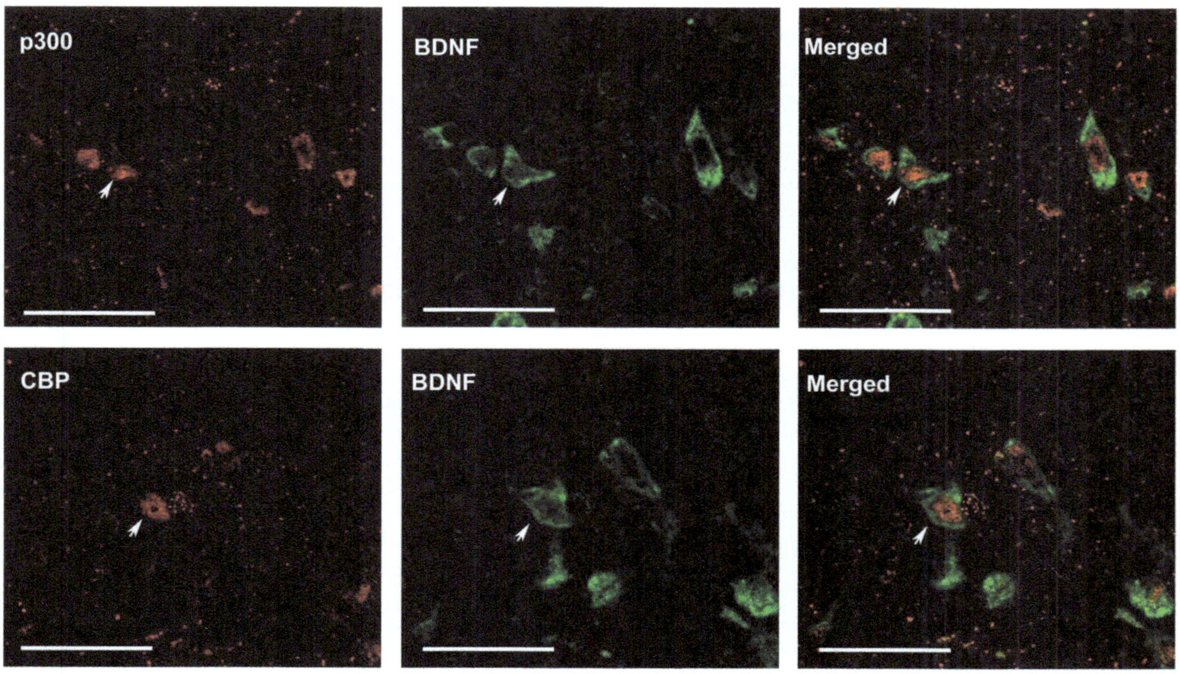

Figure 2. Double immunofluorescence staining of p300/CREB binding protein (CBP) and brain derived neurotrophic factor (BDNF) in the ipsilateral spinal dorsal horn (laminae I–IV) of vehicle-treated CCI rats. Immunoreactivity of BDNF is localized in the cytoplasm and cell membranes surrounding immunoreactive p300 or CBP nuclei. Arrows indicate the co-localization of BDNF and p300 or CBP. Scale bar = 45 μm.

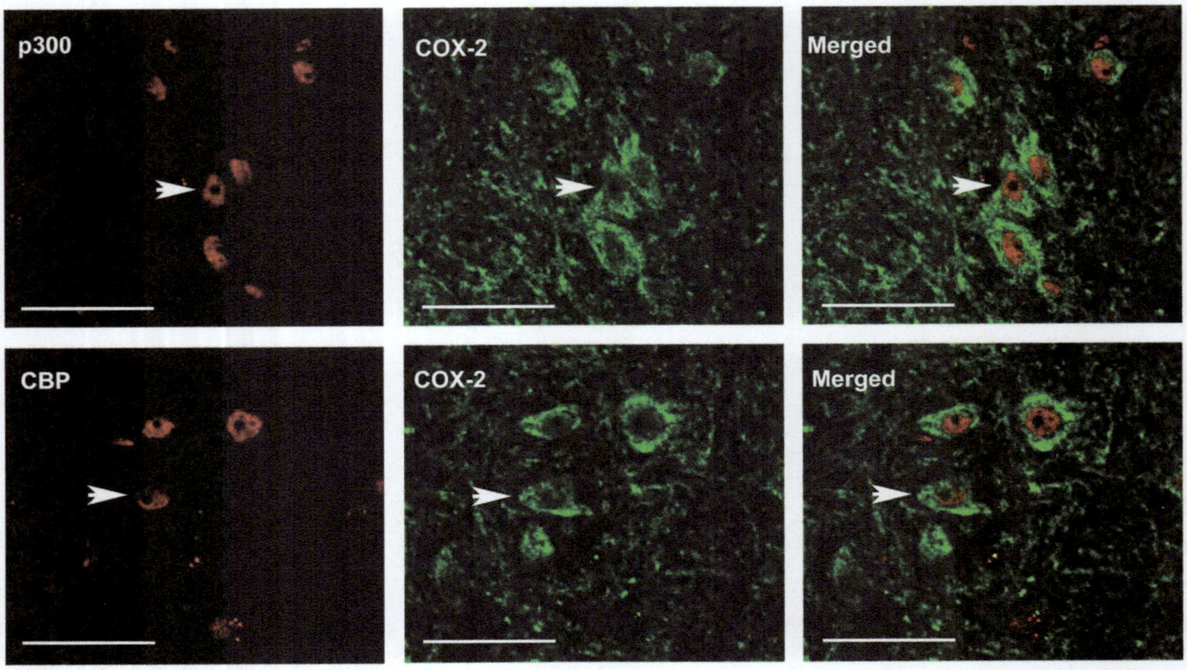

Figure 3. Double immunofluorescence staining of p300/CBP and cyclooxygenase-2 (Cox-2) in the ipsilateral spinal dorsal horn (laminae I–IV) of vehicle-treated CCI rats. Cox-2 is localized in the cytoplasm and cell membranes surrounding immunoreactive P300 or CBP nuclei. Arrows indicate the co-localization of Cox-2 and p300 or CBP. Scale bar = 45 μm.

curcumin treatment in the pattern similar to the changes at the BDNF promoter. However, the reduction of P300 binding occurred at 20 mg/kg and the binding of H3K9ac occurred at 40 mg/kg treatment (Fig. 4 B).

Curcumin Reduced the Spinal Gene Expression of BDNF and Cox-2

qRT-PCR was employed to determine the mRNA expression of BDNF and Cox-2 to investigate whether curcumin-induced transcriptional modification leads to the expressional changes of these two pro-nociceptive molecules. mRNA expression of BDNF and Cox-2 increased 2.05 and 2.38 fold ($p<0.01$) 14 days after CCI (Fig. 5). Consistent with the results from the ChIP assay, curcumin dose-dependently reduced the expression of BDNF and Cox-2. BDNF gene expression was significantly ($p<0.01$) reduced after a 7-day treatment of 40 mg/kg or 60 mg/kg curcumin (Fig. 5A). However, 20 mg/kg curcumin did not affect BDNF gene expression. Similarly, Cox-2 gene expression was significantly ($p<0.05$) reduced after the treatment of 60 mg/kg curcumin (Fig. 5B). Although not significant, 20 mg/kg and 40 mg/kg curcumin tended to decrease the gene expression of Cox-2 compared with rats treated with vehicle.

These results were confirmed at the post-transcription level, in which western immunoblotting analysis revealed that CCI increased BDNF and Cox-2 protein (Fig. 6). Furthermore, the change in protein expression levels of BDNF and Cox-2 in protein level after curcumin treatment was consistent with that of mRNA expression. BDNF was significantly ($p<0.05$) decreased after the treatment with 40 or 60 mg/kg curcumin (Fig. 6, A and B). Similarly, a significant ($p<0.05$) reduction of Cox-2 protein was observed after the treatment of 60 mg/kg, but not 20 or 40 mg/kg, curcumin (Fig. 6, C and D).

Discussion

Findings of the present study indicated that the anti-nociceptive effect of curcumin on neuropathic pain resulted from peripheral nerve injury. These results are in agreement with previous studies [13,14]. Our results showed that curcumin attenuated thermal hyperalgesia and mechanical allodynia in a dose-dependent manner. Thermal hyperalgesia and mechanical allodynia were attenuated with the treatment of 40 and 60 mg/kg curcumin. However, 20 mg/kg curcumin exerted no significant analgesic effect. This finding is similar to [30], in which 25 mg/kg curcumin failed to ameliorate formalin-induced orofacial pain in rats. The time course of thermal latency and mechanical threshold in the present study demonstrated that even at the highest dose, a significant anti-nociceptive effect of curcumin occurred at least 5 days after the commencement of daily treatment. This result is in accordance with a previous finding which showed that chronic, but not acute curcumin treatment is effective in controlling neuropathic nociception [13].

Peripheral nerve injury induces long-lasting changes of pain-related molecules in the spinal cord [43,44], and thus mainly account for the central mechanisms underlying neuropathic pain. BDNF [45,46,47,48,49,50] and Cox-2 [51,52,53,54,55,56] are well-documented pro-nociceptive molecules that are expressed in the spinal dorsal horn after peripheral nerve injury. The present results of immunofluoresence staining showed that increased BDNF and Cox-2 were co-localized in p300/CBP-positive cells, indicating a potential relationship between these molecules and P300/CBP proteins. The ChIP assay further verified that CCI increased the binding of P300/CBP proteins to the promoter of both BDNF and Cox-2 genes. Therefore, the recruitment of P300/CBP to the gene promoter may promote transcription of the target gene. For example, N-methyl-D-aspartic acid receptor-mediated activation of BDNF has been associated with the

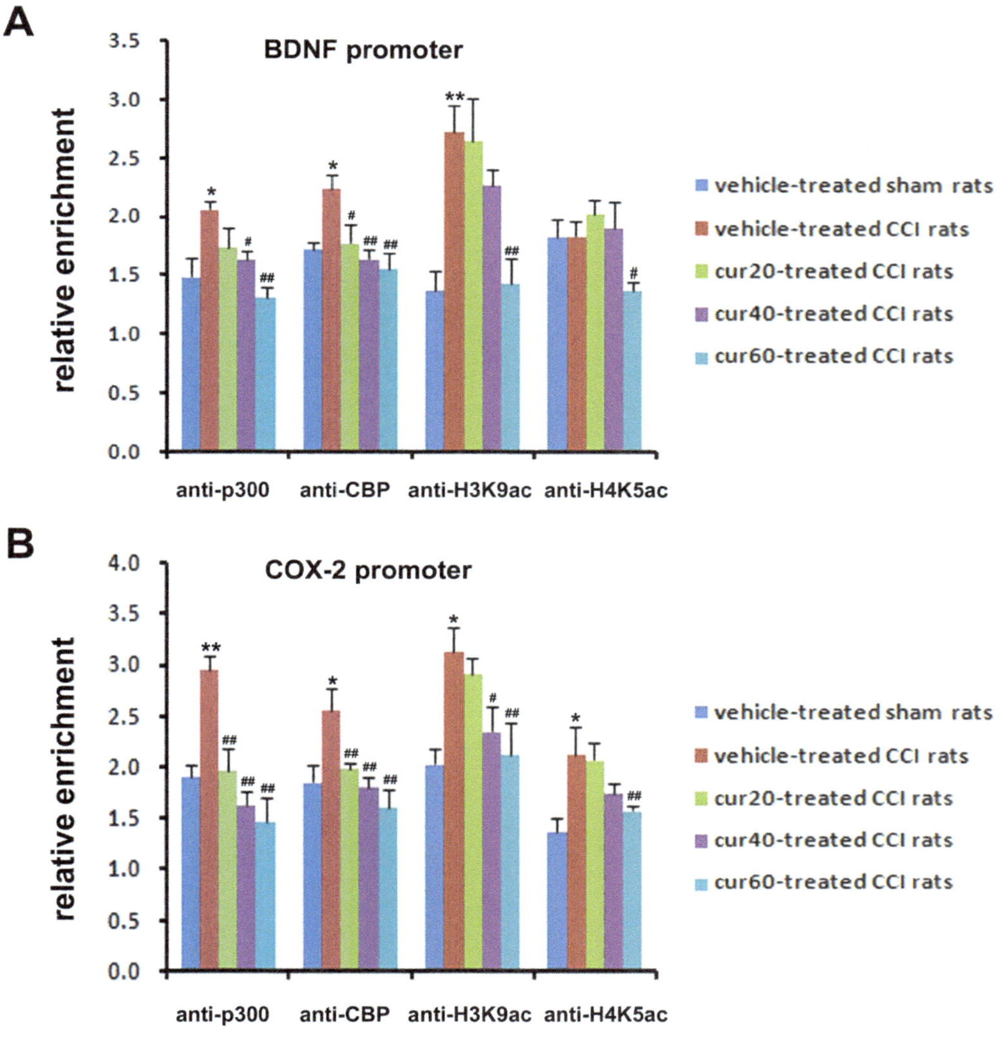

Figure 4. Binding of p300/CBP and H3K9ac/H4K5ac to the promoter of BDNF and Cox-2 gene. The chromatin immunoprecipitation assay was performed with antibodies against p300, CBP, H3K9ac, H4K5ac or non-immune rabbit IgG, after 7 days of treatment with DMSO or curcumin at 20, 40, and 60 mg/kg body weight. Binding of p300/CBP and H3K9ac/H4K5ac to the BDNF promoter (A). Binding of p300/CBP and H3K9ac/H4K5ac to the Cox-2 promoter (B). *$p<0.05$, CCI versus sham; **$p<0.01$, CCI versus sham; $^{\#}p<0.05$ curcumin versus vehicle; $^{\#\#}p<0.01$ curcumin versus vehicle ($n=10$ per group). cur20: curcumin 20 mg/kg; cur40: curcumin 40 mg/kg; cur60: curcumin 60 mg/kg.

enrichment of CBP at the BDNF gene promoter I [26]. In addition, pro-inflammatory mediators enhance the binding of P300 to the Cox-2 promoter, and this effect is essential for transcriptional activation of Cox-2 [27].

P300/CBP at the gene promoter have two main functions. Firstly, they serve as a platform for integrating other required transcriptional components, such as transcription factors [57,58]. Secondly, they exhibit HAT activity, by which an acetyl group is transferred to a lysine residue of histone. The acetylation level of histone has been established to be a key mechanism in regulating transcription [59,60]. Moreover, acetylation at specific sites of histone accounts for the transcription of different genes. In the present study, the expression of H3K9ac, but not H4K5ac, was increased at the BDNF promoter I after CCI. This finding is in agreement with that of Schmidt et al. [61], who demonstrated an association between increased BDNF transcription with increased H3K9ac at BDNF promoter I. In contrast, H3K9ac and H4K5ac have been shown to increase at the Cox-2 promoter after CCI, indicating acetylation at multiple lysine residues involved in the transcription regulation of the Cox-2 gene [62,63,64]. Because H3K9 and H4K5 are targets of P300/CBP HAT [65,66,67], the increased binding of P300/CBP and the consequent hyper-acetylation of histone at the promoter of BDNF and Cox-2 may have contributed to CCI-induced up-regulation of these molecules in the present study.

Curcumin has been reported to repress p300/CBP HAT activity-dependent transcriptional activation [15,16,17]. In the present study, the ChIP assay demonstrated that curcumin dose-dependently inhibited the binding of P300/CBP and H3K9ac/H4K5ac to the promoter of BDNF and Cox-2. Because curcumin has little effect on histone acetylation mediated by other HATs, such as PCAF or GCN5 [15,68], reduced histone acetylation in this study may have been attributed to suppressed HAT activity of P300/CBP. In parallel with the ChIP results, reduced gene and protein expression of BDNF and Cox-2 was revealed, suggesting that curcumin treatment reduced the transcriptional followed by

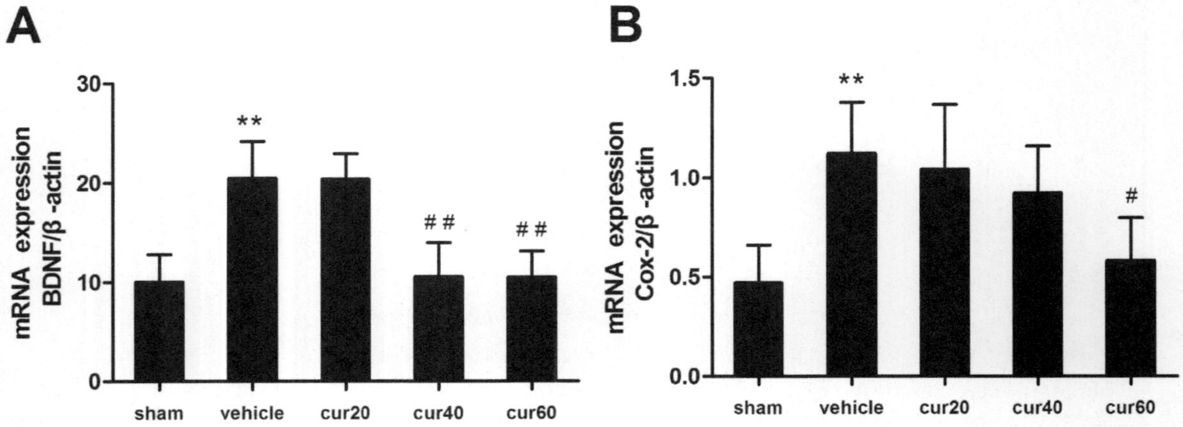

Figure 5. mRNA expression of BDNF and Cox-2. Quantitative real time polymerase chain reaction was performed 7 days after treatment with vehicle or 20, 40 and 60 mg/kg body weight curcumin. Relative amount of BDNF gene (A). Relative amount of Cox-2 gene (B). Data were normalized to the β-actin gene. **$p<0.01$, CCI versus sham; $^{\#}p<0.05$ curcumin versus vehicle; $^{\#\#}p<0.01$ curcumin versus vehicle (n = 10 per group). sham: vehicle-treated sham rats; vehicle: vehicle-treated CCI rats; cur20: curcumin 20 mg/kg-treated CCI rats; cur40: curcumin 40 mg/kg-treated CCI rats; cur60: curcumin 60 mg/kg-treated CCI rats.

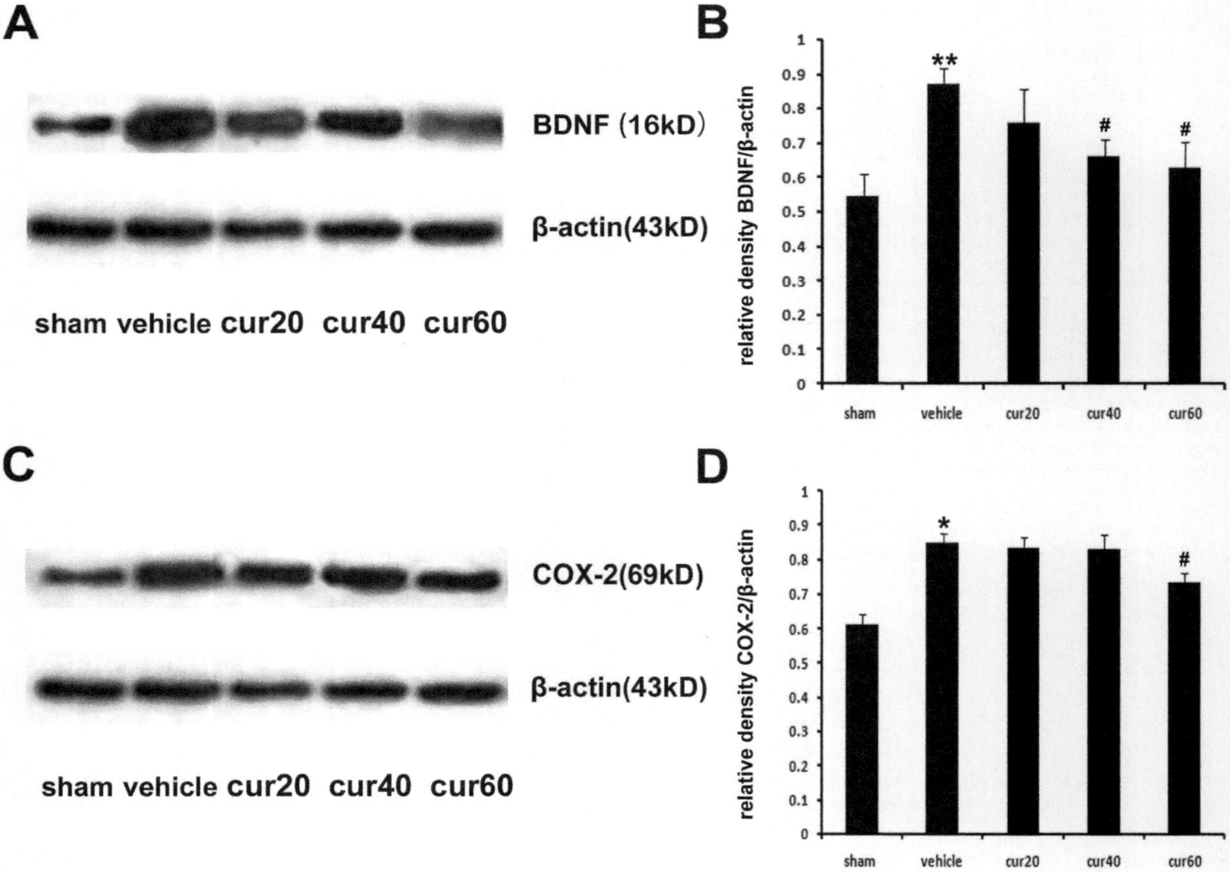

Figure 6. Protein expression of BDNF and Cox-2 protein. Western immunoblotting analysis was performed 7 days after treatment with vehicle or 20, 40 and 60 mg/kg body curcumin. β-actin was used as an internal control. Representative images of BDNF expression (A). Relative amount of BDNF protein (B). Representative images of Cox-2 expression (C). Relative amount of Cox-2 protein (D). *$p<0.05$, CCI versus sham; **$p<0.01$, CCI versus sham; $^{\#}p<0.05$ curcumin versus vehicle (n = 10 per group). Sham: vehicle-treated sham rats; vehicle: vehicle-treated CCI rats; cur20: curcumin 20 mg/kg-treated CCI rats; cur40: curcumin 40 mg/kg-treated CCI rats; cur60: curcumin 60 mg/kg-treated CCI rats.

post-transcriptional level of BDNF and Cox-2 by inhibiting HAT activity of P300/CBP proteins.

Recently, 141 patients suffering from neuropathic pain were treated with a formula containing curcumin as one of the major ingredients to test the safety and efficacy of this compound in the management of neuropathic pain [69]. However, a better understanding of the mechanisms of curcumin is necessary before its development as a therapeutic strategy for the treatment of neuropathic pain. Several possible mechanisms for its anti-nociceptive effect have been indicated, such as anti-oxidative [70] and anti-inflammatory [71,72]. The present study showed for the first time that as a P300/CBP HAT inhibitor, curcumin alleviated neuropathic pain by down-regulating P300/CBP HAT-regulated gene expression.

Author Contributions

Conceived and designed the experiments: CH QG. Performed the experiments: XZ QL RC DY ZS. Analyzed the data: XZ QL ZS. Contributed reagents/materials/analysis tools: QL RC. Wrote the paper: CH QG.

References

1. Haanpää M, Attal N, Backonja M, Baron R, Bennett M, et al. (2011) NeuPSIG guidelines on neuropathic pain assessment. Pain 152: 14–27.
2. Treede RD, Jensen TS, Campbell JN, Cruccu G, Dostrovsky JO, et al. (2008) Neuropathic pain: Redefinition and a grading system for clinical and research purposes. Neurology 70: 1630–1635.
3. Dworkin RH, O'Connor AB, Audette J, Baron R, Gourlay GK, et al. (2010) Recommendations for the pharmacological management of neuropathic pain: an overview and literature update. Mayo Clin Proc 85: S3–14.
4. Ossipov MH, Lopez Y, Nichols ML, Bian D, Porreca F (1995) Inhibition by spinal morphine of the tail-flick response is attenuated in rats with nerve ligation injury. Neurosci Lett 199: 83–86.
5. Idanpaan-Heikkila JJ, Guilbaud G, Kayser V (1997) Prevention of tolerance to the antinociceptive effects of systemic morphine by a selective cholecystokinin-B receptor antagonist in a rat model of peripheral neuropathy. J Pharmacol Exp Ther 282: 1366–1372.
6. Yadav VS, Mishra KP, Singh DP, Mehrotra S, Singh VK (2005) Immunomodulatory effects of curcumin. Immunopharmacol Immunotoxicol 27: 485–497.
7. Reeta KH, Mehla J, Gupta YK (2010) Curcumin ameliorates cognitive dysfunction and oxidative damage in phenobarbitone and carbamazepine administered rats. Eur J Pharmacol 644: 106–112.
8. Mishra S, Palanivelu K (2008) The effect of curcumin (turmeric) on Alzheimer's disease: An overview. Ann Indian Acad Neurol 11: 13–19.
9. Bishnoi M, Chopra K, Kulkarni SK (2008) Protective effect of Curcumin, the active principle of turmeric (Curcuma longa) in haloperidol-induced orofacial dyskinesia and associated behavioural, biochemical and neurochemical changes in rat brain. Pharmacol Biochem Behav 88: 511–522.
10. Kulkarni SK, Bhutani MK, Bishnoi M (2008) Antidepressant activity of curcumin: involvement of serotonin and dopamine system. Psychopharmacology (Berl) 201: 435–442.
11. Sharma S, Chopra K, Kulkarni SK (2007) Effect of insulin and its combination with resveratrol or curcumin in attenuation of diabetic neuropathic pain: participation of nitric oxide and TNF-alpha. Phytother Res 21: 278–283.
12. Sharma S, Kulkarni SK, Agrewala JN, Chopra K (2006) Curcumin attenuates thermal hyperalgesia in a diabetic mouse model of neuropathic pain. Eur J Pharmacol 536: 256–261.
13. Zhao X, Xu Y, Zhao Q, Chen CR, Liu AM, et al. (2012) Curcumin exerts antinociceptive effects in a mouse model of neuropathic pain: descending monoamine system and opioid receptors are differentially involved. Neuropharmacology 62: 843–854.
14. Ji FT, Liang JJ, Liu L, Cao MH, Li F (2013) Curcumin exerts antinociceptive effects by inhibiting the activation of astrocytes in spinal dorsal horn and the intracellular extracellular signal-regulated kinase signaling pathway in rat model of chronic constriction injury. Chin Med J (Engl) 126: 1125–1131.
15. Balasubramanyam K, Varier RA, Altaf M, Swaminathan V, Siddappa NB, et al. (2004) Curcumin, a novel p300/CREB-binding protein-specific inhibitor of acetyltransferase, represses the acetylation of histone/nonhistone proteins and histone acetyltransferase-dependent chromatin transcription. J Biol Chem 279: 51163–51171.
16. Puglia C, Frasca G, Musumeci T, Rizza L, Puglisi G, et al. (2012) Curcumin loaded NLC induces histone hypoacetylation in the CNS after intraperitoneal administration in mice. Eur J Pharm Biopharm 81: 288–293.
17. Morimoto T, Sunagawa Y, Kawamura T, Takaya T, Wada H, et al. (2008) The dietary compound curcumin inhibits p300 histone acetyltransferase activity and prevents heart failure in rats. J Clin Invest 118: 868–878.
18. Chan HM, La Thangue NB (2001) p300/CBP proteins: HATs for transcriptional bridges and scaffolds. J Cell Sci 114: 2363–2373.
19. Liu X, Wang L, Zhao K, Thompson PR, Hwang Y, et al. (2008) The structural basis of protein acetylation by the p300/CBP transcriptional coactivator. Nature 451: 846–850.
20. Min SW, Cho SH, Zhou Y, Schroeder S, Haroutunian V, et al. (2010) Acetylation of tau inhibits its degradation and contributes to tauopathy. Neuron 67: 953–966.
21. Valor LM, Viosca J, Lopez-Atalaya JP, Barco A (2013) Lysine Acetyltransferases CBP and p300 as Therapeutic Targets in Cognitive and Neurodegenerative Disorders. Curr Pharm Des 19: 5051–5064.
22. Renthal W, Nestler EJ (2009) Histone acetylation in drug addiction. Semin Cell Dev Biol 20: 387–394.
23. Zhu XY, Huang CS, Li Q, Guo QL, Wang Y, et al. (2012) Temporal Distribution of p300/CBP Immunoreactivity in the Adult Rat Spinal Dorsal Horn Following Chronic Constriction Injury (CCI). Cell Mol Neurobiol 33: 197–204.
24. Zhu XY, Huang CS, Li Q, Chang RM, Song ZB, et al. (2012) p300 exerts an epigenetic role in chronic neuropathic pain through its acetyltransferase activity in rats following chronic constriction injury (CCI). Mol Pain 8: 84.
25. Caccamo A, Maldonado MA, Bokov AF, Majumder S, Oddo S (2010) CBP gene transfer increases BDNF levels and ameliorates learning and memory deficits in a mouse model of Alzheimer's disease. Proc Natl Acad Sci U S A 107: 22687–22692.
26. Tian F, Hu XZ, Wu X, Jiang H, Pan H, et al. (2009) Dynamic chromatin remodeling events in hippocampal neurons are associated with NMDA receptor-mediated activation of Bdnf gene promoter 1. J Neurochem 109: 1375–1388.
27. Deng WG, Zhu Y, Wu KK (2004) Role of p300 and PCAF in regulating cyclooxygenase-2 promoter activation by inflammatory mediators. Blood 103: 2135–2142.
28. Bennett GJ, Xie YK (1988) A peripheral mononeuropathy in rat that produces disorders of pain sensation like those seen in man. Pain 33: 87–107.
29. Yeon KY, Kim SA, Kim YH, Lee MK, Ahn DK, et al. (2010) Curcumin produces an antihyperalgesic effect via antagonism of TRPV1. J Dent Res 89: 170–174.
30. Mittal N, Joshi R, Hota D, Chakrabarti A (2009) Evaluation of antihyperalgesic effect of curcumin on formalin-induced orofacial pain in rat. Phytother Res 23: 507–512.
31. Hargreaves K, Dubner R, Brown F, Flores C, Joris J (1988) A new and sensitive method for measuring thermal nociception in cutaneous hyperalgesia. Pain 32: 77–88.
32. Vivancos GG, Verri WA Jr, Cunha TM, Schivo IR, Parada CA, et al. (2004) An electronic pressure-meter nociception paw test for rats. Braz J Med Biol Res 37: 391–399.
33. Zhu XY, Huang CS, Li Q, Chang RM, Song ZB, et al. (2012) p300 exerts an epigenetic role in chronic neuropathic pain through its acetyltransferase activity in rats following chronic constriction injury (CCI). Mol Pain 8: 84.
34. Piller N, Decosterd I, Suter MR (2013) Reverse transcription quantitative real-time polymerase chain reaction reference genes in the spared nerve injury model of neuropathic pain: validation and literature search. BMC Res Notes 6: 266.
35. Huang C, Zou W, Lee K, Wang E, Zhu X, et al. (2012) Different symptoms of neuropathic pain can be induced by different degrees of compressive force on the C7 dorsal root of rats. Spine J 12: 1154–1160.
36. Jean YH, Chen WF, Sung CS, Duh CY, Huang SY, et al. (2009) Capnellene, a natural marine compound derived from soft coral, attenuates chronic constriction injury-induced neuropathic pain in rats. Br J Pharmacol 158: 713–725.
37. Ha SO, Kim JK, Hong HS, Kim DS, Cho HJ (2001) Expression of brain-derived neurotrophic factor in rat dorsal root ganglia, spinal cord and gracile nuclei in experimental models of neuropathic pain. Neuroscience 107: 301–309.
38. Zhu XY, Huang CS, Li Q, Guo QL, Wang Y, et al. (2013) Temporal distribution of p300/CBP immunoreactivity in the adult rat spinal dorsal horn following chronic constriction injury (CCI). Cell Mol Neurobiol 33: 197–204.
39. Mutskov V, Gerber D, Angelov D, Ausio J, Workman J, et al. (1998) Persistent interactions of core histone tails with nucleosomal DNA following acetylation and transcription factor binding. Mol Cell Biol 18: 6293–6304.
40. Ura K, Kurumizaka H, Dimitrov S, Almouzni G, Wolffe AP (1997) Histone acetylation: influence on transcription, nucleosome mobility and positioning, and linker histone-dependent transcriptional repression. Embo J 16: 2096–2107.
41. Timmusk T, Palm K, Metsis M, Reintam T, Paalme V, et al. (1993) Multiple promoters direct tissue-specific expression of the rat BDNF gene. Neuron 10: 475–489.
42. Kobayashi H, Yokoyama M, Matsuoka Y, Omori M, Itano Y, et al. (2008) Expression changes of multiple brain-derived neurotrophic factor transcripts in selective spinal nerve ligation model and complete Freund's adjuvant model. Brain Res 1206: 13–19.

43. Woolf CJ (2010) Central sensitization: implications for the diagnosis and treatment of pain. Pain 152: S2–15.
44. Wall PD, McMahon SB, Koltzenburg M (2006) Wall and Melzack's textbook of pain. In: McMahon SB, Koltzenburg M, editors. Central consequences of peripheral nerve damage. Oxford: Churchill Livingstone. 947–959.
45. Quintao NL, Santos AR, Campos MM, Calixto JB (2008) The role of neurotrophic factors in genesis and maintenance of mechanical hypernociception after brachial plexus avulsion in mice. Pain 136: 125–133.
46. Yajima Y, Narita M, Usui A, Kaneko C, Miyatake M, et al. (2005) Direct evidence for the involvement of brain-derived neurotrophic factor in the development of a neuropathic pain-like state in mice. J Neurochem 93: 584–594.
47. Wang X, Ratnam J, Zou B, England PM, Basbaum AI (2009) TrkB signaling is required for both the induction and maintenance of tissue and nerve injury-induced persistent pain. J Neurosci 29: 5508–5515.
48. Guo W, Robbins MT, Wei F, Zou S, Dubner R, et al. (2006) Supraspinal brain-derived neurotrophic factor signaling: a novel mechanism for descending pain facilitation. J Neurosci 26: 126–137.
49. Geng SJ, Liao FF, Dang WH, Ding X, Liu XD, et al. (2010) Contribution of the spinal cord BDNF to the development of neuropathic pain by activation of the NR2B-containing NMDA receptors in rats with spinal nerve ligation. Exp Neurol 222: 256–266.
50. Constandil L, Aguilera R, Goich M, Hernandez A, Alvarez P, et al. (2008) Involvement of spinal cord BDNF in the generation and maintenance of chronic neuropathic pain in rats. Brain Res Bull 86: 454–459.
51. Ma W, Du W, Eisenach JC (2002) Role for both spinal cord COX-1 and COX-2 in maintenance of mechanical hypersensitivity following peripheral nerve injury. Brain Res 937: 94–99.
52. Seybold VS, Jia Y-P, Abrahams LG (2003) Cyclo-oxygenase-2 contributes to central sensitization in rats with peripheral inflammation. Pain 105: 47–55.
53. Zhao Z CS, Eisenach JC, Busija DW, Pan HL (2000) Spinal cyclooxygenase-2 is involved in development of allodynia after nerve injury in rats. Neuroscience 97: 743–748.
54. Zhao FY, Spanswick D, Martindale JC, Reeve AJ, Chessell IP (2007) GW406381, a novel COX-2 inhibitor, attenuates spontaneous ectopic discharge in sural nerves of rats following chronic constriction injury. Pain 128: 78–87.
55. Durrenberger PF, Facer P, Casula MA, Yiangou Y, Gray RA, et al. (2006) Prostanoid receptor EP1 and Cox-2 in injured human nerves and a rat model of nerve injury: a time-course study. BMC Neurol 6: 1.
56. Ohtori S, Takahashi K, Aoki Y, Doya H, Ozawa T, et al. (2004) Spinal neural cyclooxygenase-2 mediates pain caused in a rat model of lumbar disk herniation. J Pain 5: 385–391.
57. Shiama N (1997) The p300/CBP family: integrating signals with transcription factors and chromatin. Trends Cell Biol 7: 230–236.
58. Goodman RH, Smolik S (2000) CBP/p300 in cell growth, transformation, and development. Genes Dev 14: 1553–1577.
59. Brownell JE, Allis CD (1996) Special HATs for special occasions: linking histone acetylation to chromatin assembly and gene activation. Curr Opin Genet Dev 6: 176–184.
60. Wade PA, Pruss D, Wolffe AP (1997) Histone acetylation: chromatin in action. Trends Biochem Sci 22: 128–132.
61. Schmidt HD, Sangrey GR, Darnell SB, Schassburger RL, Cha JH, et al. (2012) Increased brain-derived neurotrophic factor (BDNF) expression in the ventral tegmental area during cocaine abstinence is associated with increased histone acetylation at BDNF exon I-containing promoters. J Neurochem 120: 202–209.
62. Soliman ML, Ohm JE, Rosenberger TA (2013) Acetate Reduces PGE2 Release and Modulates Phospholipase and Cyclooxygenase Levels in Neuroglia Stimulated with Lipopolysaccharide. Lipids 48: 651–662.
63. Miao F, Gonzalo IG, Lanting L, Natarajan R (2004) In vivo chromatin remodeling events leading to inflammatory gene transcription under diabetic conditions. J Biol Chem 279: 18091–18097.
64. Martin TA, Jayanthi S, McCoy MT, Brannock C, Ladenheim B, et al. (2012) Methamphetamine causes differential alterations in gene expression and patterns of histone acetylation/hypoacetylation in the rat nucleus accumbens. PLoS One 7: e34236.
65. Wang D, Xia X, Weiss RE, Refetoff S, Yen PM (2010) Distinct and histone-specific modifications mediate positive versus negative transcriptional regulation of TSHalpha promoter. PLoS One 5: e9853.
66. Crump NT, Hazzalin CA, Bowers EM, Alani RM, Cole PA, et al. (2011) Dynamic acetylation of all lysine-4 trimethylated histone H3 is evolutionarily conserved and mediated by p300/CBP. Proc Natl Acad Sci U S A 108: 7814–7819.
67. Yuan H, Reddy MA, Sun G, Lanting L, Wang M, et al. (2012) Involvement of p300/CBP and epigenetic histone acetylation in TGF-beta1-mediated gene transcription in mesangial cells. Am J Physiol Renal Physiol 304: F601–613.
68. Marcu MG, Jung YJ, Lee S, Chung EJ, Lee MJ, et al. (2006) Curcumin is an inhibitor of p300 histone acetylatransferase. Med Chem 2: 169–174.
69. Di Pierro F, Settembre R (2013) Safety and efficacy of an add-on therapy with curcumin phytosome and piperine and/or lipoic acid in subjects with a diagnosis of peripheral neuropathy treated with dexibuprofen. J Pain Res 6: 497–503.
70. Al Moundhri MS, Al-Salam S, Al Mahrouqee A, Beegam S, Ali BH (2013) The effect of curcumin on oxaliplatin and cisplatin neurotoxicity in rats: some behavioral, biochemical, and histopathological studies. J Med Toxicol 9: 25–33.
71. Li Y, Zhang Y, Liu DB, Liu HY, Hou WG, et al. (2013) Curcumin attenuates diabetic neuropathic pain by downregulating TNF-alpha in a rat model. Int J Med Sci 10: 377–381.
72. Joshi RP, Negi G, Kumar A, Pawar YB, Munjal B, et al. (2013) SNEDDS curcumin formulation leads to enhanced protection from pain and functional deficits associated with diabetic neuropathy: An insight into its mechanism for neuroprotection. Nanomedicine 9: 776–785.

Full Inhibition of Spinal FAAH Leads to TRPV1-Mediated Analgesic Effects in Neuropathic Rats and Possible Lipoxygenase-Mediated Remodeling of Anandamide Metabolism

Katarzyna Starowicz[1], Wioletta Makuch[1], Michal Korostynski[2], Natalia Malek[1], Michal Slezak[2], Magdalena Zychowska[1], Stefania Petrosino[3], Luciano De Petrocellis[4], Luigia Cristino[4], Barbara Przewlocka[1]*, Vincenzo Di Marzo[3]*

1 Dept. of Pain Pharmacology, Institute of Pharmacology, Polish Academy of Sciences, Smetna, Krakow, Poland, **2** Dept. of Molecular Neuropharmacology, Institute of Pharmacology, Polish Academy of Sciences, Smetna, Krakow, Poland, **3** Endocannabinoid Research Group, Istituto di Chimica Biomolecolare, CNR, Pozzuoli (Naples), Italy, **4** Endocannabinoid Research Group, Istituto di Cibernetica, CNR, Pozzuoli (Naples), Italy

Abstract

Neuropathic pain elevates spinal anandamide (AEA) levels in a way further increased when URB597, an inhibitor of AEA hydrolysis by fatty acid amide hydrolase (FAAH), is injected intrathecally. Spinal AEA reduces neuropathic pain by acting at both cannabinoid CB1 receptors and transient receptor potential vanilloid-1 (TRPV1) channels. Yet, intrathecal URB597 is only partially effective at counteracting neuropathic pain. We investigated the effect of high doses of intrathecal URB597 on allodynia and hyperalgesia in rats with chronic constriction injury (CCI) of the sciatic nerve. Among those tested, the 200 μg/rat dose of URB597 was the only one that elevated the levels of the FAAH non-endocannabinoid and anti-inflammatory substrates, oleoylethanolamide (OEA) and palmitoylethanolamide (PEA), and of the endocannabinoid FAAH substrate, 2-arachidonoylglycerol, and fully inhibited thermal and tactile nociception, although in a manner blocked almost uniquely by TRPV1 antagonism. Surprisingly, this dose of URB597 decreased spinal AEA levels. RT-qPCR and western blot analyses demonstrated altered spinal expression of lipoxygenases (LOX), and baicalein, an inhibitor of 12/15-LOX, significantly reduced URB597 analgesic effects, suggesting the occurrence of alternative pathways of AEA metabolism. Using immunofluorescence techniques, FAAH, 15-LOX and TRPV1 were found to co-localize in dorsal spinal horn neurons of CCI rats. Finally, 15-hydroxy-AEA, a 15-LOX derivative of AEA, potently and efficaciously activated the rat recombinant TRPV1 channel. We suggest that intrathecally injected URB597 at full analgesic efficacy unmasks a secondary route of AEA metabolism via 15-LOX with possible formation of 15-hydroxy-AEA, which, together with OEA and PEA, may contribute at producing TRPV1-mediated analgesia in CCI rats.

Editor: Bernard Le Foll, Centre for Addiction and Mental Health, Canada

Funding: This work was supported by Dept.'s of Pain Pharmacology statutory funds and by a grant (N N401 015235), both of which were from Ministry of Science and Higher Education, Warsaw, Poland. Dr. V. Di Marzo is grateful to the National Institutes of Health for partly funding this study (grant nr. DA009789). The funders had no role in study design, data collection and analysis, decision to publish, or preparation of the manuscript.

Competing Interests: The authors have declared that no competing interests exist.

* E-mail: przebar@if-pan.krakow.pl (BP); vdimarzo@icmib.na.cnr.it (VDM)

Introduction

The endocannabinoid system includes the cannabinoid CB_1 and CB_2 receptors (two G-protein-coupled receptors activated also by the main psychotropic component of *Cannabis sativa*, Δ^9-tetrahydrocannabinol [1]), and the endogenous agonists at these receptors, i.e. the endocannabinoids anandamide (AEA) and 2-arachidonoyl glycerol (2-AG)]. AEA also activates the transient receptor potential vanilloid-1 (TRPV1) channel [2], which transduces the pronociceptive and heat-like effects of another plant natural product, the pungent component of hot peppers, capsaicin [3,4,5,6]. TRPV1 usually, but not always, plays in pain transmission a role opposite to cannabinoid receptors [7,8] and, therefore, the possible effects on pain of the activation of this channel by AEA have been thoroughly studied [9,10,11].

Enzymes for endocannabinoid catabolism have been characterized. Fatty acid amide hydrolase (FAAH) catalyzes the hydrolysis of AEA and its two congeners, the acylethanolamides oleoylethanolamide (OEA) and palmitoylethanolamide (PEA), which occur in higher tissue concentrations than AEA and produce their effects in a mostly cannabinoid receptor-independent manner. FAAH catalyzes also the hydrolysis of 2-AG [12,13], which, however, is usually degraded in vivo by monoacylglycerol lipase [14]. Additionally, lipoxygenase (LOX)- and cyclooxygenase (COX)-2- catalyzed oxygenation of endocannabinoids generate several bioactive compounds [15,16]. Whilst COX-2 derivatives are inactive at cannabinoid receptors and TRPV1 [16], LOX products of AEA are still able to activate these targets [17,18].

TRPV1 and CB_1 co-localization in the spinal cord and dorsal root ganglia opens interesting possibilities for the development of

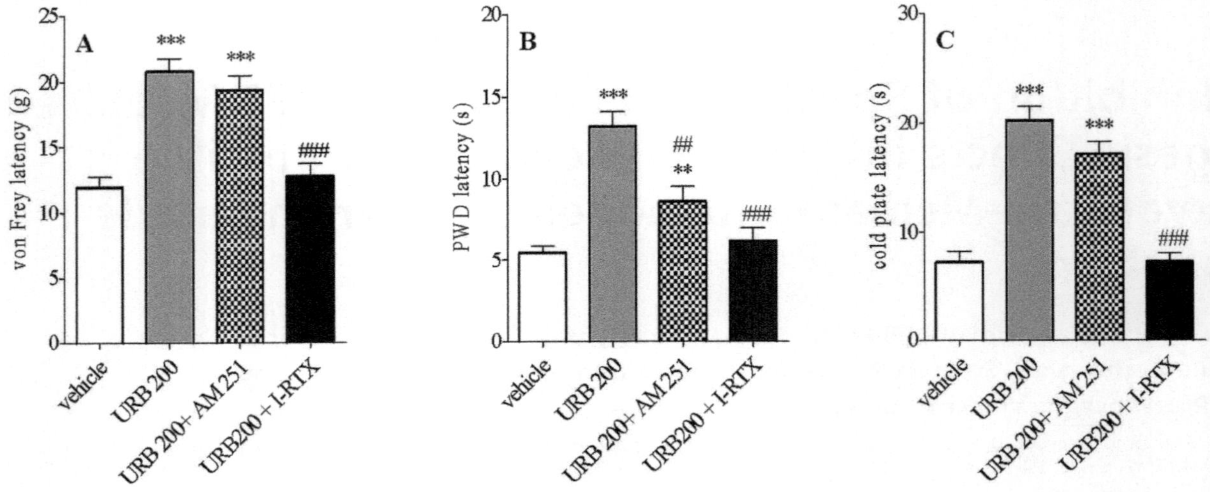

Figure 1. Effect of URB597 (a selective inhibitor of the enzyme fatty acid amide hydrolase, FAAH) at the dose of 200 μg, on mechanical allodynia (A), thermal hyperalgesia (B) and cold allodynia (C) in CCI rats. Experiments were conducted 7 days after the CCI. Antagonists (I-RTX or AM251) were administered 15 min before URB597 and behavioral evaluations were made 30 min after the last administration. The doses of I-RTX and AM251 used for antagonism of URB597 effects had no effect on allodynia and hyperalgesia *per se* (for details, please refer to [23]). All drugs were given i.t. in a volume of 10 μl. Data represents mean values ± SEM (n = 8). Statistical analyses were performed with one-way ANOVA with Bonferroni as post test. **p<0.01; ***p<0.001 versus vehicle-treated rats (veh); ##p<0.01 and ###p<0.001 versus URB597-treated rats.

novel therapeutics against neuropathic pain. Administration of FAAH inhibitors, like URB597 [19], to rodents enhances the levels of AEA, PEA, OEA and/or 2-AG in various tissues involved in pain perception [20,21,22]. Depending on the dose of URB597, or the time after its injection in the periaqueductal grey, either a suppression or an increase in thermal nociception via TRPV1 or CB_1 receptors, respectively, was observed [21]. Intrathecal injection of URB597 elevates AEA levels and produces antihyperalgesic and anti-allodynic effects in neuropathic rats via CB_1 or TRPV1-mediated mechanisms depending on the dose used [23]. Therefore, local injection of FAAH inhibitors offers the opportunity to investigate the role of FAAH substrates and their molecular targets in pain control. Yet, the possibility that full FAAH inhibition unmasks other pathways for AEA metabolism, with likely consequences on nociception, has been poorly investigated (see [24] for a rare example). Therefore, the present study aimed at elucidating the mechanism of action of a fully effective analgesic dose of URB597 in rats with chronic constriction injury (CCI) of the sciatic nerve, by establishing how it modifies endocannabinoid and acylethanolamide levels in the spinal cord and determining the contribution of CB_1, TRPV1 and LOX to its effects.

Results

Anti-allodynic and Anti-hyperalgesic Effects of Intrathecal Administration of the FAAH Inhibitor, URB597 in CCI Rats

We assessed the selective FAAH inhibitor, URB597, on signs of neuropathic pain in rats subjected to CCI. URB597 at doses of 10 and 100 μg was effective at reducing mechanical allodynia ($p<0.001$) and thermal hyperalgesia ($p<0.001$) as well as cold allodynia ($p<0.001$) ([23] and data not shown). However, URB597 was maximally effective at exerting these effects at the dose of 200 μg, when monitoring mechanical allodynia (Fig. 1A, $p<0.001$, 174% over vehicle), thermal hyperalgesia (Fig. 1B, $p<0.001$, 242% over vehicle) and cold allodynia (Fig. 1C, $p<0.001$, 281% over vehicle) (Fig. 1). The analgesic effects observed with this high dose of URB597 were significantly attenuated by pretreatment with the selective TRPV1 antagonist, 5'-iodoresiniferatoxin (I-RTX), starting at 15 min after i.t. injection and still present at 60 min (data not shown). I-RTX significantly reduced URB597-mediated tactile allodynia, thermal hyperalgesia and cold allodynia. Pretreatment with the CB_1 receptor antagonist, AM251, affected URB597 (200 μg)–mediated analgesia in Hargreaves test only at 30 min after i.t. injection (Fig. 1B). All remaining values from rats pretreated with AM251 did not differ significantly from those treated with URB597 (200 μg) alone (Fig. 1 A–C).

Both types of treatment (URB597 200 μg alone or preceeded by I-RTX or AM251) and time after injection yielded statistically different effects. Data analysis were as follows: for tactile allodynia (drug injected: $F_{3,112} = 29.67$; time: $F_{3,112} = 13.36$; parameters mutually $p<0.001$); for Hargreaves test (drug: $F_{3,112} = 17.29$; time: $F_{3,112} = 7.05$; parameters $p<0.0001$ and $p<0.0002$, respectively); for cold plate test (drug: $F_{3,112} = 29.27$; time: $F_{3,112} = 13.33$; parameters mutually $p<0.0001$). Neither I-RTX nor AM251 had effect on allodynia *per se* at the doses used (for details see also: [23]).

Effect of FAAH Inhibition on the Levels of Endogenous AEA, Related Fatty Acid Amides and 2-AG in the Spinal Cord of CCI Rats

In separate experiments, we assessed the levels of AEA, 2-AG, PEA and OEA in the lumbar spinal cord of sham-operated and CCI rats treated with URB597 vs. vehicle (Fig. 2). Seven days after CCI, AEA levels were increased both in the ipsi- and contralateral side (Fig. 1A, 60.6% and 95% elevation *vs.* sham-operated rats, $p<0.05$ and $p<0.001$, respectively). By contrast, administration of URB597 at the dose of 200 μg resulted in a significant decrease in spinal AEA levels (ipsilateral: 45.5% reduction vs. sham-vehicle rats, $p<0.05$ and 66% reduction vs. CCI-vehicle rats, $p<0.001$; contralateral: 20% reduction vs. sham-vehicle rats, $p>0.05$ and 59% reduction vs. CCI- vehicle rats, $p<0.05$).

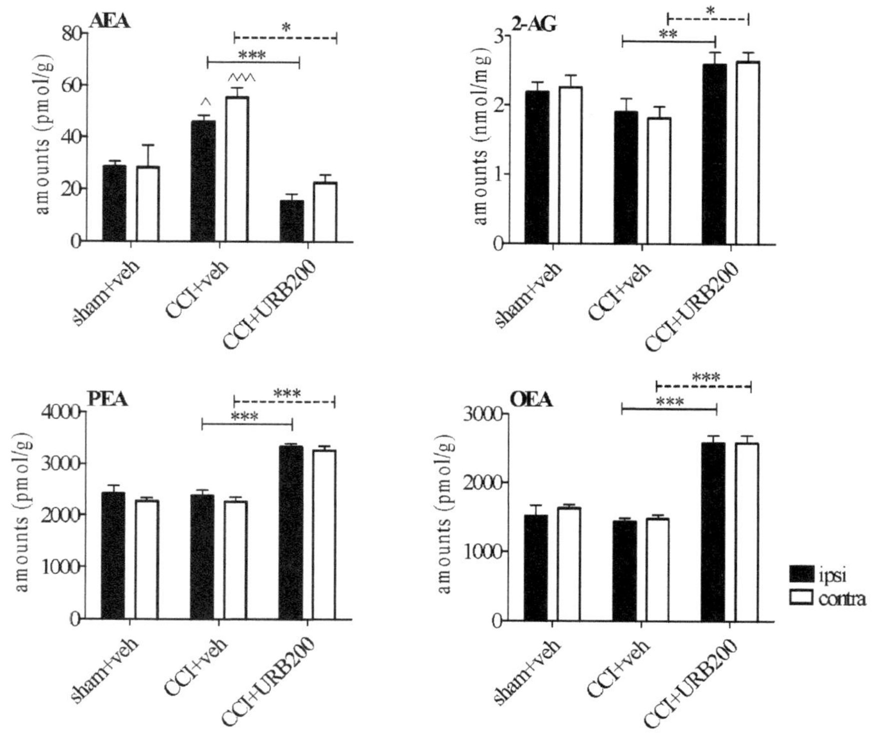

Figure 2. LC-MS analysis of anandamide (AEA),2-arachidonoylglycerol(2-AG), palmitoylethanolamide (PEA) and oleoylethanolamide (OEA) in the ipsilateral (black bars) and contralateral (open bars) parts of the lumbar spinal cords of sham-operated and CCI rats in response to pharmacological modulation of its endogenous levels evoked by URB597 (200 µg) administration. Experiments were conducted 7 days after the CCI.URB597 was given i.t. in a volume of 10 µl. Data are means ± SEM of n = 6 rats. Means were compared by two-way ANOVA with side and treatment as a variable factors with Bonferroni as post test. ^$p<0.05$; ^^^$p<0.001$ versus sham-operated, vehicle (veh) injected group, *$p<0.05$; **$p<0.01$ and ***$p<0.001$ versus CCI, veh injected rats.

Intrathecal delivery of URB597 (200 µg) resulted in a significant increase of 2-AG levels, both ipsi- and contralateral (36.8% ($p<0.05$) and 45.5% ($p<0.01$)) *vs.* CCI-vehicle rats (Fig. 2B). Likewise, we observed a significant increase in PEA levels by 40% at the ipsilateral side ($p<0.001$) and 44% at the contralateral side ($p<0.001$) *vs.* CCI-vehicle rats (Fig. 2C). URB597 treatment (200 µg) caused a significant elevation also of OEA by 80% and 75% *vs.* CCI-vehicle rats (Fig. 2D, $p<0.001$ mutually).

Two-way analysis of variance resulted in the general conclusion that only the treatment procedure, but not side of the injury (ipsi- *vs.* contralateral), affected the presented results in a significant manner.

Gene Expression Level of the Major Lipoxygenases in CCI Rats

Quantitative PCR (qPCR) analysis revealed that the abundance levels of *Alox15* (15-LOX) transcript were highly elevated (20-fold change versus control, $p<0.05$) seven days after CCI (Fig. 3C). The effects were observed in the lumbar spinal cord, both ipsi- and contralateral to the injury. The mRNA levels of *Alox5* (5-LOX, Fig. 3A) and *Alox12* (12-LOX, Fig. 3B) did not significantly change between the experimental groups.

15-LOX Protein Expression in the Rat Dorsal Horn

To determine whether up-regulation of 15-LOX transcript in the lumbar dorsal horn (DH) was accompanied by corresponding changes in its protein levels, Western blot analysis was performed at 7 days after CCI, i.e. at the same time as mRNA measurements. In the control DH, 15-LOX proteins of 73 kDa were found. No significant differences from control animals were observed between ipsi and contralateral DH of naïve and sham-vehicle animals. A significant elevation of 15-LOX protein was observed exclusively on the ipsilateral side (249% vs. CCI contralateral; 247% vs. naïve and sham) (Fig. 4).

Effect of Baicalein, an Inhibitor of LOX Activity, on the Analgesic Effects of URB597 in CCI Rats

The 12/15-LOX inhibitor, baicalein (1.5 µg), produced no effects in the absence of URB597 following CCI (Fig. 5A–C). Intrathecal injection of baicalein (1.5 µg) 15 min before URB597 (200 µg) injection highly and significantly reduced its anti-analgesic and anti allodynic actions (Fig. 5A–C, $p<0.001$ for von Frey $F_{(3,31)}$ 95.7, Hargreaves $F_{(3,31)}$ 54.3 and cold plate tests $F_{(3,31)}$ 40.5). However, all drug combinations were still active at attenuating neuropathic pain signs in rats ($p<0.001$ for von Frey test and $p<0.01$ for Hargreaves and cold plate tests).

FAAH, TRPV1 and 15-LOX are Highly Colocalized in the Lumbar Spinal Cord of CCI Rats

Immunohistochemical localization of TRPV1 receptor, FAAH and, in view of the results of the q-PCR analyses, 15-LOX, was measured in the DH of CCI and sham operated rats by means of immunofluorescence (Fig. 6). In the lumbar DH lamina II/III, both in the sham and controlateral side to CCI spinal cord we observed relatively few TRPV1-positive (15.5±3.4%) or 15-LOX-positive (18.4±2.6%) neurons, whereas FAAH was more abun-

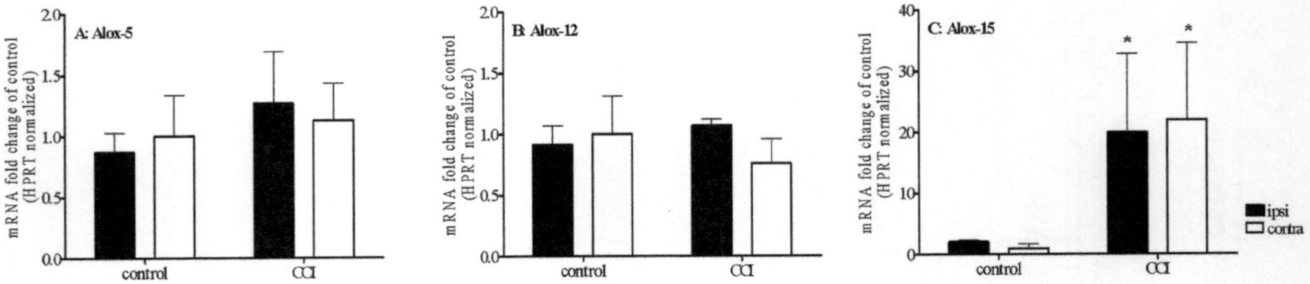

Figure 3. The results of qPCR analyses of LOX-15, LOX-12 and LOX-5 gene expression levels in the dorsal part of the lumbar (L5–L6) spinal cord of neuropathic rats. Tissue was dissected 7 days after the CCI. The data are presented as means251658240±251658240SEM, which represent normalized averages derived from 4–6 samples per each group. Statistical analysis was performed using a two-way ANOVA followed by Bonferroni post-test (*$p<0.05$).

dant, especially in the fibers and scattered puncta in the lamina II. Noteworthy, no significant double or triple immunoexpression was found in the controlateral CCI or sham lumbar spinal cord. In the ispilateral side to CCI we found a significant increase of both TRPV1 and 15-LOX immunoreactivity in the lumbar spinal cord. A density of 78.3±8.5% TRPV1-positive and 65.5±10.5% 15-LOX positive neurons were observed within lamina II/III of the DH, with main localization of 15-LOX neurons in lamina II. TRPV1 was co-localized with 15-LOX in 86.8±14.5% of the cell bodies of lamina II. Among these cell bodies, 50.5±8.7% showed 15-LOX/FAAH/TRPV1 co-localization (Fig. 6), thus demonstrating that TRPV1-ir neurons in the DH of rats with CCI might metabolize AEA via both 15-LOX and FAAH. FAAH staining was also observed in fibres (Fig. 6).

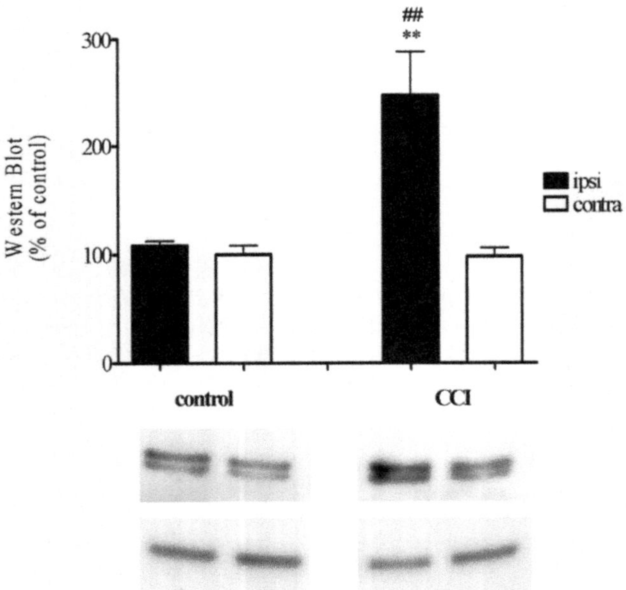

Figure 4. Western blot analysis of LOX-15 protein levels measured in the lumbar dorsal horn (L5–L6) of the spinal cord on day 7 of control (sham) and CCI in rats. The data are presented as means ± SEM, which represent GAPDH (lower line) normalized averages derived from 6 samples per each group Results are presented as a % of control densitometry analysis of all sections. Statistical analyses were performed with one-way ANOVA with Bonferroni as post-hoc test. **$p<0.01$ ipsilateral versus contralateral of CCI-exposed rats and ## $p<0.01$ CCI ipsilateral versus control (naïve and sham) rats.

The 15-LOX Derivative of AEA, 15(S)-hydroxy-AEA, Stimulates Intracellular Calcium Elevation via TRPV1

The addition of 15(*S*)-hydroxy-AEA activates to HEK-293 cells stably transfected with the rat recombinant TRPV1 caused intracellular Ca^{2+} elevation with an efficacy that was 37.3±0.8% of that of 4 μM ionomycin, and a potency (EC_{50}) of 11.3±0.9 μM (Fig. 7A). Under the same conditions, AEA exhibited higher efficacy (49.5±0.9%) and potency (0.24±0.03 μM). To further characterise the specificity of TRPV1 agonism of 15(*S*)-hydroxy-AEA, we evaluated the effect on $[Ca^{2+}]_i$ either in wild type HEK293 (i.e. not transfected with the TRPV1 construct, WT) or after pre-treatment with the TRPV1 antagonist I-RTX [25]. In both cases, 15(*S*)-hydroxy-AEA exhibited much lower efficacy, if any. Finally, 15(*S*)-hydroxy-AEA was also able to desensitise TRPV1-mediated elevation of $[Ca^{2+}]_i$ induced by capsaicin (0.1 μM), with an $IC_{50} = 16.0 \pm 0.5$ μM. Again, AEA was more potent at desensitizing TRPV1 to the effect of capsaicin (Fig. 7B).

Discussion

In the present study, the spinal administration of a high dose of the FAAH inhibitor, URB597, caused anti-allodynic and anti-hyperalgesic effects in neuropathic rats. The effects of URB597 were blocked by a selective TRPV1 receptor antagonist (I-RTX) and significantly attenuated by a 12/15-LOX inhibitor (baicalein). CCI was accompanied by increased levels of AEA and increased co-localization of TRPV1 with AEA catabolic enzymes: 15-LOX and FAAH in the lumbar spinal cord. The analgesic effects of URB597 (200 μg) were accompanied by increased spinal levels of PEA, OEA and 2-AG and, surprisingly, decreased levels of AEA as compared with matched vehicle-treated CCI controls. Our pharmacological and molecular data support the possibility that the full inactivation of FAAH, together with CCI-induced over-expression of TRPV1 and 15-LOX in the DH of the spinal cord, trigger: 1) an alternative pathway of AEA metabolism leading to15-LOX-derived metabolites that inhibit nociception via TRPV1 desensitization; and 2) elevation of the levels of AEA-related acylethanolamides with possibly similar TRPV1-mediated analgesic actions, i.e. PEA and OEA. Our findings, together with our previous investigation of the effects of lower intrathecal doses of URB597, or of varying doses of AEA [23], suggest that elevation of spinal AEA levels with increasing doses of a locally injected FAAH inhibitor, produce anti-hyperalgesic and anti-allodynic actions via mechanisms that progressively involve TRPV1 channel desensitization rather than CB_1 receptor activation (CB_2 receptors are not a likely target for cannabinoid-mediated antinociception in CCI model and AEA is only a partial

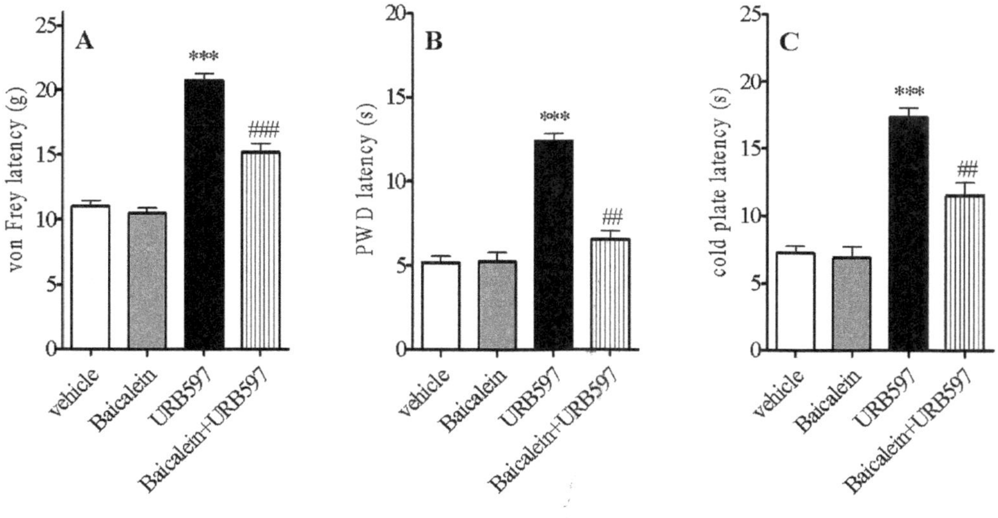

Figure 5. Effect of baicalein, an antioxidant 12/15-lipoxygenase inhibitor, on the behavioral effects of URB597 (200 μg) on mechanical allodynia (A), thermal hyperalgesia (B) and cold allodynia (C) in CCI rats. Experiments were conducted 7 days after the CCI. Baicalein was administered 15 min before URB597 and behavioral evaluations were made 30 min after the last administration. The dose of baicalein used for antagonism of URB597 had no effect on allodynia and hyperalgesia *per se*. Drugs were given i.t. in a volume of 10 μl. Data represents mean values ± SEM (n = 8). Statistical analyses were performed with one-way ANOVA with Bonferroni as post test. **p<0.01; ***p<0.001 versus vehicle-treated rats (veh); ##p<0.01 and ###p<0.001 versus URB597-treated rats.

agonist at CB2 receptors [26,27,28]). FAAH inhibition would result first in elevation of AEA levels to an extent that is high enough to activate/desensitize this channel [23], and then in the elevation of the levels of other TRPV1-active acylethanolamides and in the activation of AEA catabolic pathways leading to other TRPV1-active metabolites (present data). Thus, potent inhibition of FAAH may cause fully effective analgesic actions against neuropathic pain as a result of a complex readaptation of endocannabinoid metabolism and signaling, involving AEA-lipoxygenation, PEA and OEA.

It should be emphasized that the concentrations required for AEA to stimulate TRPV1 are usually higher than those necessary for CB_1 stimulation [29], and that other acylethanolamides that are substrates for FAAH are less potent than AEA at activating these channels [30]. On the other hand, the substrate concentration requirements for several enzymes to efficiently catalyze the oxygenation of AEA are higher than those required for this endocannabinoid/endovanilloid to be hydrolyzed by FAAH [15,17], suggesting that such enzymes may play a role in AEA inactivation only when FAAH is fully inhibited and AEA levels increased beyond a certain threshold. As a consequence, the doses of URB597 used to inhibit FAAH, and the subsequent extent of elevation of AEA levels, become an important issue to investigate. We tested, here and previously, URB597 at two different concentrations, 10 μg and 100 μg, and observed that spinal AEA reduces neuropathic pain via CB_1 or TRPV1, depending on its local concentration, bioavailability, tissue level elevation and subcellular distribution [23]. Furthermore, a previous study [21] showed that, depending on the dose used for site injections into the periaqueductal gray (PAG), or on the interval of time since its administration, URB597 either suppresses or increases thermal nociception in healthy rats *via* TRPV1 or CB_1 receptors, respectively (please refer to [21],[31] for detailed mechanism description). In the present study, the anti-allodynic and anti-hyperalgesic actions of URB597 at the 200 μg dose were antagonized almost uniquely by I-RTX. It was, therefore, surprising to find that, following this treatment, the spinal levels of endogenous AEA were decreased, rather than being further increased. On the other hand, a significant augmentation of 2-AG, PEA and OEA concentrations was detected instead. The concomitant increase of 2-AG levels, an endocannabinoid FAAH substrate already reported to be up-regulated following local injections of URB597 (see [21] and [32] for review), would explain why CB_1 antagonism with AM251 still tended to reduce at 15 and 60 min, and significantly attenuated at 30 min, URB597-mediated analgesia in the Hargreaves test, thus suggesting the presence of a transitory involvement of CB_1 receptors in some of URB597 effects in this test. Indeed, the increase of brain and spinal cord 2-AG levels obtained by the administration of inhibitors of 2-AG inactivation by monoacylglycerol lipase was previously shown to reduce mechanical and cold allodynia in the CCI model [33,34]. On the other hand, the increase by URB597 of the levels of OEA and PEA, which are also substrates for FAAH, would explain why the effects of the high dose of the FAAH inhibitor were antagonized by I-RTX. In fact, a role for OEA in inflammatory pain has been demonstrated [35], and it has been proposed that this compound acts not only *via* nuclear peroxisome proliferator-activated receptor (PPAR)-α and-γ, but also TRPV1 ([30,36,37] for review). Also PEA exhibits anti-allodynic and anti-hyperalgesic effects in a murine model of neuropathic pain *via* multiple mechanisms [38]. PEA can act as an allosteric enhancer of AEA actions at TRPV1 [39] or activate and desensitize this channel, in part directly and in part via PPAR-α activation [40]. Thermal hyperalgesia and mechanical allodynia in CCI mice were relieved by repeated administration of PEA [38], and for this reason this compound is thought to be involved in the endogenous protective mechanisms that are activated in the body as a result of different types of tissue damage and hence also in neuropathic pain [41].

To explain the decrease in AEA levels induced by the highest dose of URB597, we hypothesized that, following full inactivation of FAAH, alternative pathways of AEA metabolism might come into play to form AEA metabolites that inhibit nociception. Because of its arachidonate-containing chemical structure, AEA is not only subjected to hydrolysis but can also be metabolized by

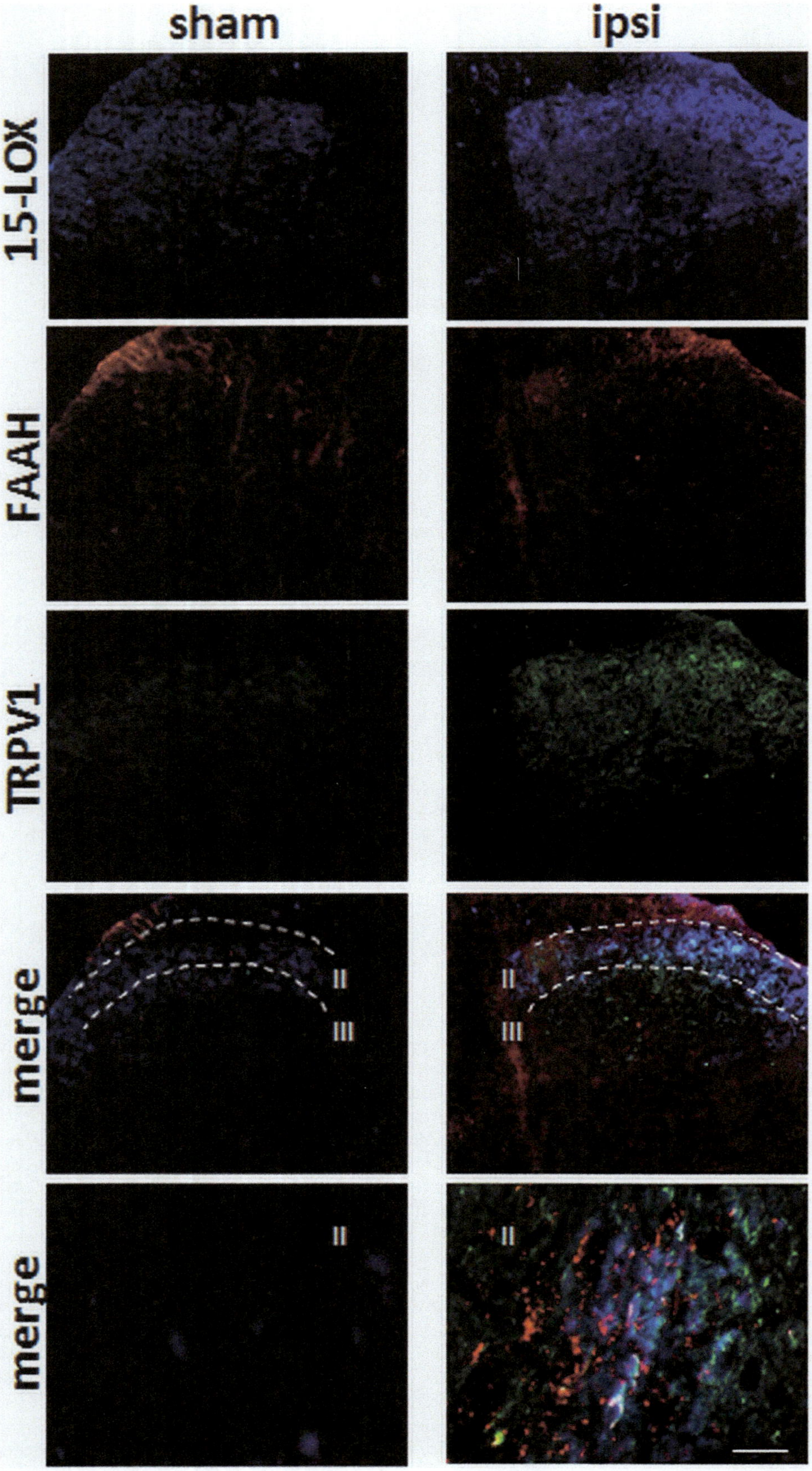
sham
ipsi
15-LOX
FAAH
TRPV1
merge
II
III
II
III
merge
II
II

Figure 6. Effect of sciatic nerve CCI on 15-LOX, FAAH and TRPV1 immunoreactivities in sham operated and ipsilateral lumbar dorsal horn of the spinal cord. After sciatic nerve-CCI, a significant increase of 15-LOX/TRPV1 immunoexpression is observed especially in lamina II. FAAH immunoreactivity is located both in fibers and puncta in the cytoplasm of 15-LOX/TRPV1 neurons. Scale bar = 100 μm, and 30 μm in merged images.

several of the same enzymes that are responsible for arachidonic acid oxidation, including COX-2 and lipoxygenases [42]. COX-2 is responsible for catalyzing the oxidation of AEA and 2-AG into various prostamides and prostaglandin-glycerol esters, respectively [43]. A major COX-2 metabolite of AEA, prostamide $F_{2\alpha}$, was recently identified in the spinal cord of mice with knee inflammation. However, this compound was found to contribute to analgesia rather than counteracting it, in a way mediated by specific receptors [24]. Previous data had shown that prostamide $F_{2\alpha}$ is inactive at TRPV1 channels [16], and therefore COX-2 inhibitors were not tested in the present study. Oxidative metabolism of AEA by 12-LOX and 15-LOX, instead, results in the formation of 12- and 15-hydroperoxy-AEA, respectively

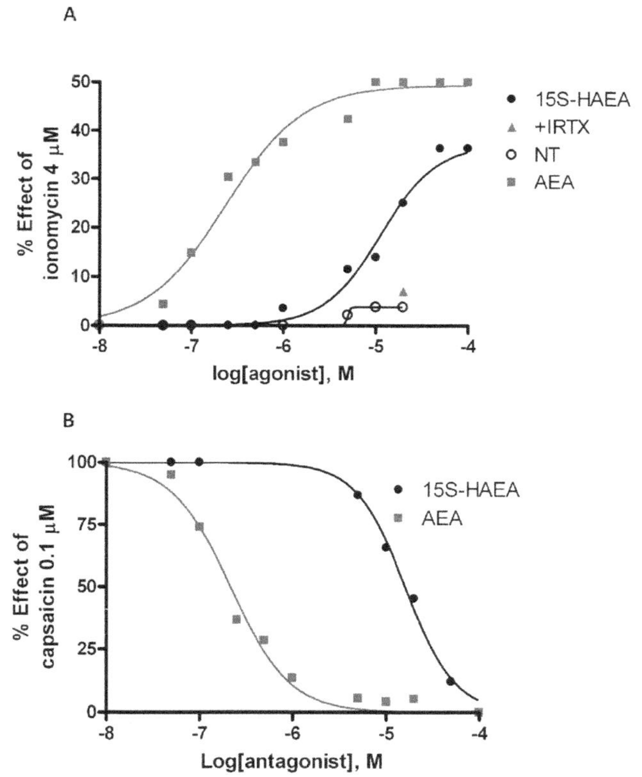

Figure 7. Effect of anandamide (squares) and 15(*S*)-hydroxy-anandamide (15S-HAEA) (filled circles) on intracellular Ca^{2+} elevation in HEK-293 cells overexpressing the rat recombinant TRPV1 channel (A). The effect of 5 min pre-incubation with the TRPV1 antagonist iodo-resiniferatoxin (I-RTX) (triangle), tested against 2 μM 15S-HAEA, and the effect of 15S-HAEA in wild-type HEK293 (i.e. not transfected with the TRPV1 construct, NT) are also shown. Desensitization, by 5 min pre-incubation with anandamide (squares) or15(S)-hydroxy-anandamide (15S-HAEA) (filled circles), of capsaicin (0.1 μM)-induced Ca^{2+} elevation in HEK-293 cells overexpressing the rat recombinant TRPV1 channel (B). In (A) data are expressed as % of the effect of ionomycin (4 μM, 'maximal response'), and in (B) as % of the effect of capsaicin (0.1 μM). Data are means of n = 3 separate determinations. Standard error bars are not shown for the safe of clarity and were never higher than 10% of the means.

[17,44], which exert their biological activities via established receptors, including the cannabinoid receptors, PPAR-α and TRPV1 [17,18,42,45]. Indeed, the TRPV1-mediated contractile action of AEA on guinea-pig isolated bronchi was attenuated by LOX inhibitors [18]. Thus, AEA lipoxygenation, together with the increase in OEA and PEA levels, might also have contributed to the TRPV1-mediated effects of the high dose of URB597. Accordingly, we observed here that CCI induced the up-regulation of spinal 15-LOX mRNA, and thus we investigated the expression of this enzyme in the DH of spinal cord of CCI rats. Using western blot analyses, we found that spinal 15-LOX protein levels were significantly up-regulated. Furthermore, using immunofluorescence techniques, we observed a very high degree of co-localization among FAAH, TRPV1 and 15-LOX in more than 50% of the cell bodies in lamina II, which was instead nearly absent in sham rats. We suggest that the activity of 15-LOX may be controlled at two different molecular levels: 1) regulation of gene expression, which occurs on both sides of the DH; and 2) regulation of mRNA translation to the active protein, only on the injured side.

Based on these data, we hypothesize that, when FAAH is fully inhibited in certain spinal neurons, AEA levels can reach threshold levels to be recognized by 15-LOX in the same neurons and produce 15(*S*)-hydroxy-AEA, which is capable of acting at TRPV1 in the same cells, desensitize it and produce analgesic effects. Accordingly, when baicalein was co-administered with URB597, the analgesic effect was partly lost, which also suggests that, when both FAAH and LOX enzymes are inactivated, AEA can still be metabolized to yet other compounds that might: 1) either have no antinociceptive action and represent a new mechanism for the termination of AEA signaling [46]; or 2) even exacerbate pain, as in the case of prostamide$F_{2\alpha}$ [24]. In agreement with the hypothesis that 15-LOX metabolizes AEA to TRPV1 agonists, we report here that 15(*S*)-hydroxy-AEA is relatively potent and quite efficacious at stimulating intracellular calcium elevation in a TRPV1-mediated manner in HEK-293 cells overexpressing the rat recombinant TRPV1, but not in wild-type HEK-293 cells, and equally potent at desensitizing TRPV1 to the action of capsaicin. This finding is in agreement with a previous study indicating that 15(*S*)-hydroxy-AEA can displace the specific binding of [^{3}H]-resiniferatoxin (a high affinity TRPV1 ligand) to mouse brain membranes [47]. Interestingly, in this previous study, the authors also reported that 15(*S*)-hydroxy-AEA stimulates the activity of an acylethanolamide-biosynthesizing enzyme, and inhibits FAAH as well as the activity of a 2-AG-biosynthesizing enzyme [47]. Thus, the formation of 15(*S*)-hydroxy-AEA might reinforce further and prolong the inhibition of FAAH, contribute to elevate the levels of TRPV1-active acylethanolamides by both inhibiting their degradation and stimulating their biosynthesis, sustain its own biosynthesis from AEA, and counteract CB_1 activation by 2-AG, thereby leading, together with OEA and PEA, to an overall prolonged activation/desensitization of TRPV1 signaling, with subsequent anti-hyperalgesic and anti-allodynic effects in neuropathic rats. Notably, also 15(*S*)-HETE, a major arachidonic acid metabolite from the 15-lipoxygenase pathway, was shown to have anti-inflammatory roles [48]. Furthermore, varying expression patterns of the two major 15-LOX isoforms may underlie different production patterns of downstream lipid mediators (e.g., 15-

HETE and 13-HODE) in different tissues [49], thus contributing in different, or even opposing ways, to pain signaling or its modulation.

In conclusion, we have provided here a new example of the complex network surrounding AEA signaling and of the potential complications of the pharmacological manipulation of the levels of this endocannabinoid/endovanilloid mediator, which may result in the readaptation of this network, whilst still leading, at least in neuropathic rats, to the counteraction of hyperalgesia and allodynia. Our findings support the use of high doses of intrathecal FAAH inhibitors as analgesic drugs for chronic pain.

Summary

Following full inhibition of its hydrolysis, AEA might be metabolized to 15(*S*)-hydroxy-AEA, which, together with OEA and PEA, may produce TRPV1-mediated anti-hyperalgesic and anti-allodynic effects in neuropathic rats.

Materials and Methods

Animals

Male Wistar rats (Charles River, Hamburg, Germany), initially weighing between 250–275 g, were used for all experiments. Animals were housed individually, under a 12:12 h light/dark cycle and free access to food and water. All experiments were carried out between 9:00 am and 12:0 am. All animals were allowed to acclimatize to their holding cages for 3–4 days before any behavioral, or surgical procedures were carried out. Experimental procedures followed the guidelines of the IASP [50] and were approved by the Local Bioethics Committee of the Institute of Pharmacology (Cracow, Poland). Care was taken to reduce both number of animals used and suffering during the experiments.

Intrathecal Catheterization

Rats were chronically implanted with intrathecal (i.t.) catheters according to [51] under pentobarbital anesthesia (60 mg/kg; i.p.). The catheter (PE 10,Clay Adams) sterilized by immersion in 70% ethanol, and flushed with sterile water prior to insertion was carefully introduced through atlanto-occipital membrane to the subarachnoid space at the rostral level of the spinal cord lumbar enlargement (L4–L6). Rats exhibiting postoperative neurological deficits (approximately 5–10%) were excluded from the study.

Sciatic Nerve Surgery

Peripheral neuropathy was induced by chronic constriction injury (CCI) to the sciatic nerve, as described by [52]. The sciatic nerve injury was performed under sodium pentobarbital anesthesia (60 mg/kg, i.p.)7 days after implantation of the i.t. catheter. The biceps femoris and the gluteus superficialis were separated, and the right sciatic nerve was exposed. Proximal to the sciatic trifurcation, about 7 mm of nerve was freed of adhering tissue and the injury was produced by tying four loose ligatures (4/0 silk, 1 mm spacing) around the sciatic nerve. The twitch of muscles during ligation prevented us from applying it too strongly. The total length of nerve affected was 4–5 mm. In sham-operated rats, the sciatic nerve was visualized and left intact.

Nociceptive Testing

On the day of the experiment, behavioral testing was carried out over 30 min before, then over a 1 h period (15, 30 and 60 min) after i.t. drug administration. All experiments were conducted at day 7 after the sciatic nerve ligation in order to avoid the inflammatory component of pain, which could appear in initial state after injury.

Tactile allodynia (von Frey test). For the assessment of tactile allodynia, rats were tested for their foot withdrawal threshold in response to automatic von Frey apparatus (Dynamic Plantar Aesthesiometer Cat. No.37400, Ugo Basile Italy). Rats were placed in plastic cages with wire net floor 5 min before the experiment. The von Frey filament was applied to the midplantar surface of the ipsilateral hind paw and the measurements of applied mechanical force were taken automatically. Hind paws were tested two times in 3-min intervals, and the response mean value was calculated. The strength of the von Frey stimuli in our experiments ranged from 0.5 to 26 g.

Thermal hyperalgesia (Hargreaves test). For the assessment of paw withdrawal latency (PWD) to a noxious thermal stimulus the Analgesia Meter (mod 33, IITC INC., Landing, NJ) was used [53]. On the day of experiment, each animal was placed in a plastic cage with a heated glass floor. After 5 min of habituation, a noxious thermal stimulus - light beam was focused onto the plantar aspect of a hindpaw until the animal lifted a paw away from the heat source. The paw withdrawal latency was automatically displayed to the nearest 0.1 s. A cut-off latency of 20 s was used to avoid tissue damage. The latency of nociceptive reaction was measured in seconds under basal condition and after i.t. treatment with drugs.

Cold hyperalgesia. The hyperalgesia was assessed using the cold plate test (Cold/Hot Plate Analgesia Meter No.05044 Columbus Instruments, USA). The temperature of the cold plate was kept at 5°C, the cut-off latency was 30 s. The rats were placed on the cold plate and the time until lifting of the hind paw was recorded, the injured paw exhibiting a lower reaction latency.

Drugs

Anandamide (AEA), AM251, 5'-Iodoresiniferatoxin (I-RTX) and baicalein were purchased from Tocris (Bristol, UK) and URB597 from Sigma-Aldrich (Poznan, Poland). 15(*S*)-hydroxy-AEA and capaicin were purchased from Cayman Chemical (Ann Arbor, MI, USA). URB597 and AM251 were made up in a vehicle solution comprising (v/v%) 18% dimethyl sulphoxide (DMSO), 1% ethanol, 1% Tween-80 and 80% saline. Stock solution of AEA and I-RTX were prepared in ethanol and furtherdiluted with saline. URB597 was used at the dose of 200 μg (58 mM); 1.5 μg of baicalein (555 μM), 5 μg of I-RTX (0.66 mM); 30 μg of AM251 (5.4 mM). Each dose was injected intrathecally in volume of 10 μl.

Experimental Design

Groups of 8 animals per treatment were used, with each animal used for one treatment only. In behavioral experiments vehicle-treated (i.t.) CCI animals formed the control group. We did not observe changes in their response values throughout the testing period (0–60 min). Additionally, in all testing procedures we measured also the contralateral paw response for all tested drugs. These values were not altered by the treatment applied (data not shown).

The first series of experiments was performed to characterize the effect of pharmacological elevation of endogenous spinal AEA levels and, to examine whether TRPV1 or CB_1 receptor antagonists would block the behavioral effects caused by the FAAH inhibitor. To this end, rats were injected with URB597 alone, or i.t. administration of TRPV1 or CB_1 antagonists (I-RTX or AM251) was followed by URB597 15 min later.

In the second series of experiments we assessed the possible influence of lipoxygenation products on the behavioral effects elicited by URB597 and again assessed the involvement of TRPV1 or cannabinoid CB_1 receptors in the observed effects, by blocking these receptors with theirs specific antagonists.

All behavioral paradigms included time-course testing, ranging from 0 to 60 min after i.t. drug administration. For the clarity of graphs, most representative data relate to 30 min after i.t. administration.

The doses of I-RTX and AM251 tested for antagonism of AEA and/or URB597 effects were selected in order not to have any effect on allodynia and hyperalgesia *per se* (for details see [23]).

Tissue Collection, RNA Preparation and Quantitative Real-time PCR

Seven days after CCI rats were decapitated,spinal cords were dissected rapidly. The samples were placed in individual tubes with the tissue storage reagent RNA later (Qiagen Inc., Valencia, CA, USA), frozen on dry ice, and stored at −70°C until RNA isolation. Samples were thawed at room temperature and homogenized in 1 ml Trizol reagent (Invitrogen, Carlsbad, CA, USA). RNA isolation was performed according to the manufacturer's protocol. The total RNA concentration was measured using a NanoDrop ND-1000 Spectrometer (NanoDrop Technologies Inc., Montchanin, DE, USA). RNA quality was determined by chip-based capillary electrophoresis using an RNA 6000 Nano LabChip Kit and Agilent Bioanalyzer 2100 (Agilent, Palo Alto, CA, USA). Total RNA from ipsilateral lumbar (L4–L6) dorsal part of the spinal cord of two animals was pooled.

Reverse transcription was performed with Omniscript Reverse Transcriptase enzyme (Qiagen) at 37°C for 60 minutes. The reaction was carried out in the presence of the RNase inhibitor rRNAsin (Promega, Madison, WI, USA), and an oligo(dT_{16}) primer (Qiagen) was used to selectively amplify mRNA. qPCR reactions were performed using Assay-On-Demand TaqMan (Applied Biosystems, Foster City, CA, USA). The following assays were used Rn00563172_m1 (*Alox5*), Rn01461082_m1 (*Alox12*), Rn00696151_m1 (*Alox15*) and Rn01527838_m1 (*Hprt*). Reactions were run on a Real-Time PCR iCycler device (BioRad, Hercules, CA, USA) with the 3.0 a software version. Threshold cycle values were calculated automatically with default parameters. The amplification efficiency for each assay was determined by running a standard dilution curve. Expression of the *Hprt1* transcript with stable level between the control and CCI groups was quantified to control for variation in cDNA amounts. The threshold cycle (CT) value for each gene was normalized with the CT value of *Hprt*. The abundance of RNA was calculated as $2^{-(\text{normalized threshold cycle})}$.

Western Blot

The lumbar (L5–L6) region of the spinal cord was removed and divided into ipsilateral and contralateral parts with respect to the side of injury or left and right in the case of naive mice. Tissue samples were homogenized in RIPA buffer with proteases and phospatases inhibitors (Sigma-Aldrich) and cleared by centrifugation (10,000 ×g, 4°C, 30 min). The protein concentration in the supernatant was determined using the BCA Protein Assay Kit (Sigma-Aldrich). Samples containing 30 µg of protein were heated for 8 min at 99°C in loading buffer (50 mMTris–HCl, 2% SDS, 2% β-mercaptoethanol, 8% glycerol and 0.1% bromophenol blue) and resolved by SDS-PAGE on 10% polyacrylamide gels. After gel electrophoresis, proteins were electrophoretically transferred to PVDF membranes (Trans-Blot; Bio-Rad). The blots were blocked using 5% blocking buffer (2.5% albumin +2.5% non-fat drymilk)in TBST (Tris-buffered saline with 0.1% Tween 20) for 1 h. Blots were incubated with rabbit polyclonal anti-LOX15 at 0,5 ug/ml concentration (Aviva Systems Biology Corp.). Blots were incubated overnight at 4°C with primary antibodies and then incubated with a peroxidase-conjugated secondary antibody (goat anti-rabbit/mouse IgG, Bio-Rad) at a dilution of 1:1000 for 1 h at room temperature. After three 10 min washes in TBST, immunocomplexes were detected using a Immuno-Star HPR kit (Bio-Rad) and visualized using a Fujifilm LAS-1000 fluorimager system. The blots were stripped and reprobed with a mouse polyclonal anti-GAPDH antibody (1:1000 dilution) (Millipore) as loading control. Relative levels of immunoreactivity were quantified using the Fujifilm Image Gauge software.

Measurement of Anandamide and Other Spinal Fatty Acid Amides by *liquid chromatography*–mass Spectrometry (LC-MS)

A sham operation of the sciatic nerve (nerve was exposed, but not touched) formed a control group for all LC-MS experiments. Sham animals did not produce neuropathic symptoms, i.e. no changes in withdrawal repose to mechanical and thermal stimulation were observed.Seven days after the induction of the CCI ipsilateral and contralateral lumbar sections of the spinal cord (n = 6) were sectioned and homogenized in 5 vol of chloroform:-methanol:Tris-HCl 50 mM (2:1:1) containing 10 pmol of d8-AEA, d4-palmitoylethanolamide (PEA), d5–2-arachidonoylglycerol (2-AG), d4palmitoylethanolamide (PEA) and d4–oleoylethanolamide (OEA). Homogenates were centrifuged at 13000×g for 16 min (4°C), the aqueous phase plus debris were collected and extracted again twice with 1 vol of chloroform. The organic phases from the three extractions were pooled and the organic solvents evaporated in a rotating evaporator.

Lyophilized extracts were resuspended in chloroform:methanol (99:1, v v–1). The solutions were then purified by open bed chromatography on silica as previously described [54]. Fractions eluted with chloroform:methanol (9:1, v v−1) and containing AEA, PEA, 2-AG and OEA, were collected and the excess solvent evaporated with a rotating evaporator, and aliquots analysed by isotope dilution-liquid chromatography/atmospheric pressure chemical ionization/mass spectrometry (MS) carried out under conditions described previously [54] and allowing the separations of 2-AG, PEA, AEA and OEA. Results are expressed as nmol per g of wet tissue, or pmol per mg in the case of 2-AG.

Immunofluorescence Microscopy

Animals (n = 3 CCI and n = 3 sham operated rats) were deeply anaesthetized with pentobarbital and perfused transcardially with saline followed by ice-cold 4% paraformaldehyde in 0.1 M phosphate buffer (PB), pH 7.4. Spinal cords were removed, post-fixed for 2 h and then washed. Tissues to be cut at cryostat were cryoprotected overnight in PB containing 30% (w/v) sucrose at 4°C. Serial cryostat sections were cut at 14 mm and mounted onto gelatine-coated slides (Mezel, Germany). For double immunofluorescence, serial sections were incubated for 1 h in 10% normal donkey serum (NDS, Jackson Immunoresearch Laboratories, West Grove, PA) in PB containing 0.3% Triton X-100 (block solution). Subsequently the sections were incubated for 2 days at 4°C in a humid chamber with the respective polyclonal antibodies (all diluted in block solution). All sections were processed for guinea pig anti-TRPV1 receptor immunostaining (1:400, Novus Biologicals, Cambridge, UK) as well as goat anti-FAAH (1:200, Santa Cruz, Heidelberg, Germany) and rabbit anti-15-LOX (1:200, Abcam, Cambridge, UK) immunostaining. After three washes in PB, triple immunofluorescence was revealed by incubation for 2 h in the appropriate fluorochrome-conjugated secondary antibody: Alexa Fluor488 donkey anti-guinea pig, Alexa Fluor546 donkey anti-goat and Alexa Fluor350 donkey anti-rabbit all diluted

1:200 in NDS. Thereafter, sections were washed with PB and coverslipped with Aquatex mounting medium (Merck, Darmstadt, Germany).

Controls of immunostaining included: (1) preabsorption of diluted antibodies with their respective immunizing peptides, and (2) omission of either the primary antisera or the secondary antibodies. These control experiments did not show notable staining. The sections processed for immunofluorescence were studied with an epifluorescence microscope (Leica DMI6000). Images were acquired using the digital camera Leica DFC 320 connected to the microscope and the image analysis software Leica IM500, which allows both single and merged pictures acquisitions. Digital images were processed in Adobe Photoshop, with brightness and contrast being the only adjustments made.

Quantification of immunoreactivity.Quantification of the mean percentage value of the number of neurons TRPV1/FAAH, TRPV1/15-LOX, 15-LOX/FAAH and TRPV1/15-LOX/FAAH labeled was performed, by an observer blinded to the experimental protocols. The total number of neurons was counted bycresyl violet in the lamina II/III of DH of adjacent immunolabelled sections and only in the cells whose nucleus, unstained or lightly stained, was in the focal plane. The level of section evaluated for immunohistochemistry study covered, bi-laterally, the entire extension of lumbar DH on a total of 20 sections per animal (3 animals per group).

Intracellular Calcium Assays

HEK-293 (human embryonic kidney) wild type and stably transfected cells overexpressing the rat TRPV1-cDNA cells were grown as monolayers in EMEM supplemented with nonessential amino acids, 10% fetal bovine serum, and 2 mM glutamine, maintained under 5% CO2 at 37°C plated on 100-mm diameter Petri dishes. On the day of the experiment, the cells were loaded for 1 h at 25°C with the methyl ester Fluo-4-AM (Invitrogen), 4 μM in DMSO containing 0.02% Pluronic F-127 (Invitrogen). After loading, cells were washed twice in Tyrode's buffer (145 mMNaCl, 2.5 mMKCl, 1.5 mM $CaCl_2$, 1.2 mM $MgCl_2$, 10 mM D-glucose, and 10 mM HEPES, pH 7.4), resuspended in the same buffer, and transferred to the quartz cuvette of the spectrofluorimeter (Perkin-Elmer LS50B) under continuous stirring. $[Ca^{2+}]_i$ was determined before and after the addition of various concentrations of test compound by measuring cell fluorescence (λ_{EX} = 488 nm, λ_{EM} = 516 nm). Curve fitting (sigmoidal dose-response variable slope) and parameter estimation were performed with GraphPad Prism® (GraphPad Software Inc., San Diego, CA). Potency was expressed as the concentration of test substance exerting a half-maximal agonist effect (i.e. half-maximal increases in $[Ca^{2+}]_i$) (EC_{50}). The efficacy of TRPV1 agonists was first determined by normalizing their effect to the maximum Ca^{2+} influx effect on $[Ca^{2+}]_i$ observed with application of 4 μM ionomycin. Desensitizing behaviour was evaluated against capsaicin (0.1 μM) by adding the test compound in the quartz cuvette 5 min before stimulation of cells with agonists. Data are expressed as the concentration exerting a half-maximal inhibition of agonist-induced $[Ca^{2+}]_i$ elevation (IC_{50}), which was calculated again using GraphPad Prism® software. The effect on $[Ca^{2+}]_i$ exerted by agonist alone was taken as 100%. Dose response curves were fitted by a sigmoidal regression with variable slope. All determinations were performed at least in triplicate.

Statistical Analyses

All data are reported as mean ± SEM and were analyzed using one-way analysis of variance (ANOVA) in the case of behavioral experiments and two-way analysis of variance in the case of qPCR, western blot and LC-MS analyses, with follow-up comparisons using Bonferroni post-hoc test. Results with $p<0.05$ were considered significant.

Author Contributions

Conceived and designed the experiments: KS BP VDM. Performed the experiments: KS WM MK NM MS MZ SP LDP LC. Analyzed the data: KS MK NM LDP LC. Contributed reagents/materials/analysis tools: KS BP LDP LC VDM. Wrote the paper: KS BP VDM.

References

1. Di Marzo V, De Petrocellis L (2012) Why do cannabinoid receptors have more than one endogenous ligand? Philos Trans R Soc Lond B Biol Sci 367: 3216–28.
2. Zygmunt PM, Petersson J, Andersson DA, Chuang H, Sørgård M, et al. (1999) Vanilloid receptors on sensory nerves mediate the vasodilator action of anandamide. Nature 400: 452–457.
3. Cortright DN, Szallasi A (2009) TRP channels and pain. Curr Pharm Des 15: 1736–49. Review.
4. Chung MK, Jung SJ, Oh SB (2011) Role of TRP channels in pain sensation. Adv Exp Med Biol 704: 615–36. Review.
5. Starowicz K, Nigam S, Di Marzo V (2007) Biochemistry and pharmacology of endovanilloids.Pharmacol Ther 114: 13–33.
6. Starowicz K, Maione S, Cristino L, Palazzo E, Marabese I, et al. (2007) Tonic endovanilloid facilitation of glutamate release in brainstem descending antinocice-ptive pathways. J Neurosci 27: 13739–749.
7. Alawi K, Keeble J (2010) The paradoxical role of the transient receptor potential vanilloid 1 receptor in inflammation. Pharmacol Ther 125: 181–95.
8. Talwar R, Potluri VK (2011) Cannabinoid 1 (CB1) receptor–pharmacology, role in pain and recent developments in emerging CB1 agonists. CNS Neurol Disord Drug Targets 10: 536–44.
9. Ross RA, Gibson TM, Brockie HC, Leslie M, Pashmi G, et al. (2001) Structure – activity relationship for the endogenous cannabinoid, anandamide, and certain of its analogues at vanilloid receptors in transfected cells and vas deferens. Br J Pharmacol 132: 631–40.
10. Di Marzo V, Blumberg PM, Szallasi A (2002) Endovanilloid signaling in pain. Curr Opin Neurobiol 12: 372–79.
11. Rice ASC, Farquhar-Smith WP, Nagi I (2002) Endocannabinoids and pain: spinal and peripheral analgesia in inflammation and neuropathy. Prostaglandins Leukot Essent Fatty Acids 66: 243−56.
12. Goparaju SK, Ueda N, Yamaguchi H, Yamamoto S (1998) Anandamide amidohydrolase reacting with 2-arachidonoylglycerol, another cannabinoid receptor ligand. FEBS Lett 422: 69–73.
13. Lang W, Qin C, Lin S, Khanolkar AD, Goutopoulos A, et al. (1999) Substrate specificity and stereoselectivity of rat brain microsomal anandamide amidohydrolase. J Med Chem 42: 896–902.
14. Dinh TP, Freund TF, Piomelli D (2002) A role for monoglyceride lipase in 2-arachidonoylglycerol inactivation. Chem Phys Lipids 121: 149–58.
15. Kozak KR, Gupta RA, Moody JS, Ji C, Boeglin WE, et al (2002) 15-Lipoxygenase metabolism of 2-arachidonoylglycerol. Generation of a peroxisome proliferator-activated receptor α agonist. J Biol Chem 277: 23278–286.
16. Matias I, Chen J, De Petrocellis L, Bisogno T, Ligresti A, et al. (2004) Prostaglandin ethanolamides (prostamides): in vitro pharmacology and metabolism,J Pharmacol Exp Ther 309: 745–57.
17. Edgemond WS, Hillard CJ, Falck JR, Kearn CS, Campbell WB (1998) Human platelets and polymorphonuclear leukocytes synthesize oxygenated derivatives of arachidonylethanolamide (anandamide): their affinities for cannabinoid receptors and pathways of inactivation. Mol Pharmacol 54: 180–88.
18. Craib SJ, Ellington HC, Pertwee RG, Ross RA (2001) A possible role of lipoxygenase in the activation of vanilloid receptors by anandamide in the guinea-pig bronchus. Br J Pharmacol 134: 30–37.
19. Tarzia G, Duranti A, Tontini A, Piersanti G, Mor M, et al (2003) Design, synthesis, and structure-activity relationships of alkylcarbamic acid aryl esters, a new class of fatty acid amide hydrolase inhibitors. J Med Chem. 46: 2352–60.
20. de Lago E, Petrosino S, Valenti M, Morera E, Ortega-Gutierrez S, et al. (2005) Effect of repeated systemic administration of selective inhibitors of endocannabinoid inactivation on rat brain endocannabinoid levels. Biochem Pharmacol 70: 446–52.
21. Maione S, Bisogno T, de Novellis V, Palazzo E, Cristino L, et al. (2006) Elevation of endocannabinoid levels in the ventrolateral periaqueductal grey through inhibition of fatty acid amide hydrolase affects descending nociceptive pathways via both cannabinoid receptor type 1 and transient receptor potential vanilloid type-1 receptors. J Pharmacol Exp Ther 16: 969–82.

22. Petrosino S, Palazzo E, de Novellis V, Bisogno T, Rossi F, et al. (2007) Changes in spinal and supraspinal endocannabinoid levels in neuropathic rats. Neuropharmacology 52: 415–22.
23. Starowicz K, Makuch W, Osikowicz M, Piscitelli F, Petrosino S, et al. (2012) Spinal anandamide produces analgesia in neuropathic rats: possible CB(1)- and TRPV1-mediated mechanisms. Neuropharmacology 62: 1746–55.
24. Gatta L, Piscitelli F, Giordano C, Boccella S, Lichtman A, et al. (2012) Discovery of prostamide f(2α) and its role in inflammatory pain and dorsal horn nociceptive neuron hyperexcitability. PLoS One 7: e31111.
25. Wahl P, Foged C, Tullin S, Thomsen C (2001) Iodo-resiniferatoxin, a new potent vanilloid receptor antagonist. Mol Pharmacol 59: 9–15.
26. Gonsiorek W, Lunn C, Fan X, Narula S, Lundell D, et al. (2000) Endocannabinoid 2-arachidonyl glycerol is a full agonist through human type 2 cannabinoid receptor: antagonism by anandamide. Mol. Pharmacol. 57: 1045–1050.
27. Sugiura T, Kondo S, Kishimoto S, Miyashita T, Nakane S, et al. (2000) Evidence that 2-arachidonoylglycerol but not N-palmitoylethanolamine or anandamide is the physiological ligand for the cannabinoid CB2 receptor. Comparison of the agonistic activities of various cannabinoid receptor ligands in HL-60 cells. J. Biol. Chem. 275: 605–612.
28. Brownjohn PW, Ashton JC (2012) Spinal cannabinoid CB2 receptors as a target for neuropathic pain: an investigation using chronic constriction injury. Neuroscience 203: 180–193.
29. Ross RA (2003) Anandamide and vanilloid TRPV1 receptors. Br J Pharmacol 140: 790–801.
30. Movahed P, Jonsson BA, Birnir B, Wingstrand JA, Jorgensen TD, et al. (2005) Endogenous unsaturated C18 N-acylethanolamines are vanilloid receptor (TRPV1) agonists. J Biol Chem280: 38496–504.
31. Starowicz K, Cristino L, Di Marzo V (2008) TRPV1 receptors in the central nervous system: potential for previously unforeseen therapeutic applications. Curr Pharm Des 14: 42–54.
32. Di Marzo V, Maccarrone M (2008) FAAH and anandamide: is 2-AG really the odd one out? Trends Pharmacol Sci 29: 229–33.
33. Kinsey SG, Long JZ, O'Neal ST, Abdullah RA, Poklis JL, et al. (2009) Blockade of endocannabinoid-degrading enzymes attenuates neuropathic pain. J. Pharmacol. Exp. Ther. 330: 902–910.
34. Kinsey SG, Long JZ, Cravatt BF, Lichtman AH (2010) Fatty acid amide hydrolase and monoacylglycerol lipase inhibitors produce anti-allodynic effects in mice through distinct cannabinoid receptor mechanisms. J Pain 11: 1420–1428.
35. Suardíaz M, Estivill-Torrús G, Goicoechea C, Bilbao A, Rodríguez de Fonseca F (2007) Analgesic properties of oleoylethanolamide (OEA) in visceral and inflammatory pain. Pain 133: 99–110.
36. Wang X, Miyares RL, Ahern GP (2005) Oleoylethanolamide excites vagal sensory neurones, induces visceral pain and reduces short-term food intake in mice via capsaicin receptor TRPV1. J Physiol 564: 541–7.
37. Re G, Barbero R, Miolo A, Di Marzo V (2007) Palmitoylethanolamide, endocannabinoids and related cannabimimetic compounds in protection against tissue inflammation and pain: potential use in companion animals.Vet J 173: 21–30.
38. Costa B, Comelli F, Bettoni I, Colleoni M, Giagnoni G (2008) The endogenous fatty acid amide, palmitoylethanolamide, has anti-allodynic and anti-hyperalgesic effects in a murine model of neuropathic pain: involvement of CB(1), TRPV1 and PPARgamma receptors and neurotrophic factors. Pain 139: 541–50.
39. De Petrocellis L, Bisogno T, Maccarrone M, Davis JB, Finazzi-Agro A, et al. (2001) The activity of anandamide at vanilloid VR1 receptors requires facilitated transport across the cell membrane and is limited by intracellular metabolism. J Biol Chem 276: 12856–63.
40. Ambrosino P, Soldovieri M, Russo C, Taglialatela M (2013) Activation and Desensitization of Trpv1 Channels in Sensory Neurons by the Peroxisome Proliferator-Activated Receptor α Agonist Palmitoylethanolamide. Br J Pharmacol 168: 1430–1434.
41. Re G, Barbero R, Miolo A, Di Marzo V (2007) Palmitoylethanolamide, endocannabinoids and related cannabimimetic compounds in protection against tissue inflammation and pain: potential use in companion animals. Vet. J. 173: 21–30.
42. Di Marzo V (2006) Endocannabinoids: synthesis and degradation. In: Amara SG, Bamberg E, Fleischmann BK, Gudermann TH, Hebert SC, et al., editors. Review of Physiology Biochemistry and Pharmacology. Berlin: Springer. 1–24.
43. Woodward DF, Carling RW, Cornell CL, Fliri HG, Martos JL, et al. (2008) The pharmacology and therapeutic relevance of endocannabinoid derived cyclo-oxygenase (COX)-2 products. Pharmacol Ther 120: 71–80.
44. Veldhuis WB, van der Stelt M, Wadman MW, van Zadelhoff G, Maccarrone M, et al. (2003) Neuroprotection by the endogenous cannabinoid anandamide and arvanil against in vivo excitotoxicity in the rat: role of vanilloid receptors and lipoxygenases. J Neurosci 23: 4127–33.
45. Kozak KR, Gupta RA, Moody JS, Ji C, Boeglin WE, et al. (2002) 15-Lipoxygenase metabolism of 2-arachidonoylglycerol. Generation of a peroxisome proliferator-activated receptor α agonist. J Biol Chem 277: 23278–286.
46. Forsell PK, Brunnström A, Johannesson M, Claesson HE (2012) Metabolism of anandamide into eoxamides by 15-lipoxygenase-1 and glutathione transferases. Lipids 47: 781–91.
47. Amadio D, Fezza F, Catanzaro G, Incani O, van Zadelhoff G, et al. (2010) Methylation and acetylation of 15-hydroxyanandamide modulate its interaction with the endocannabinoid system.Biochimie 92: 378–87.
48. Mabalirajan U, Agrawal A, Ghosh B (2012) 15-Lipoxygenase eicosanoids are the putative ligands for vanilloid receptors and peroxisome proliferator-activated receptors (PPARs). Proc Natl Acad Sci U S A 109: E1.
49. Umar A (2012) Is 15-LOX-1 a tumor suppressor? J Natl Cancer Inst. 104: 645–7.
50. Zimmermann M (1983) Ethical guidelines for investigations of experimental pain in conscious animals. Pain 16: 109–110.
51. Yaksh TL, Rudy TA (1976) Chronic catheterization of the spinal subarachnoid space. Physiol Behav 17: 1031–36.
52. Bennett GJ, Xie YK (1988) A peripheral mononeuropathy in rat that produces disorders of pain sensation like those seen in man. Pain 1: 87–107.
53. Hargreaves K, Dubner R, Brown F, Flores C, Joris J (1988) A new and sensitive method for measuring thermal nociception in cutaneous hyperalgesia. Pain 32: 77–88.
54. Bisogno T, Sepe N, Melck D, Maurelli S, De Petrocellis L, et al. (1997) Biosynthesis, release and degradation of the novel endogenous cannabimimetic metabolite 2-arachidonoylglycerol in mouse neuroblastoma cells.Biochem J. 322: 671–677.

Adherence of French GPs to Chronic Neuropathic Pain Clinical Guidelines: Results of a Cross-Sectional, Randomized, "e" Case-Vignette Survey

Valéria Martinez[1,2]*, Nadine Attal[2,3], Bertrand Vanzo[4], Eric Vicaut[5], Jean Michel Gautier[6], Didier Bouhassira[2,3], Michel Lantéri-Minet[7,8]

1 Anesthésiologie-Réanimation, Hôpital Raymond-Poincaré, Garches, France, **2** INSERM U-987, Centre d'Evaluation et de Traitement de la Douleur, CHU Ambroise Paré, Boulogne-Billancourt, France, **3** Université Versailles-Saint-Quentin, Versailles, France, **4** General Practitioner, Athis Mons, France, **5** Unité de Recherche Clinique - Hôpital Fernand Widal, Paris, France, **6** Réseau InterCLUD Languedoc Roussillon, CHRU Montpellier, Montpellier, France, **7** CHU de Nice, Centre d'Evaluation et Traitement de la Douleur, Nice, France, **8** INSERM/UdA, U1107, Neuro-Dol, Université de Clermont-Ferrand, Clermont-Ferrand, France

Abstract

Background and aims: The French Pain Society published guidelines for neuropathic pain management in 2010. Our aim was to evaluate the compliance of GPs with these guidelines three years later.

Methods: We used "e" case vignette methodology for this non interventional study. A national panel of randomly selected GPs was included. We used eight "e" case-vignettes relating to chronic pain, differing in terms of the type of pain (neuropathic/non neuropathic), etiology (cancer, postoperative pain, low back pain with or without radicular pain, diabetes) and symptoms. GPs received two randomly selected consecutive "e" case vignettes (with/without neuropathic pain). We analyzed their ability to recognize neuropathic pain and to prescribe appropriate first-line treatment.

Results: From the 1265 GPs in the database, we recruited 443 (35.0%), 334 of whom logged onto the web site (26.4%) and 319 (25.2%) of whom completed the survey. Among these GPs, 170 (53.3%) were aware of the guidelines, 136 (42.6%) were able to follow them, and 110 (34.5%) used the DN4 diagnostic tool. Sensitivity for neuropathic pain recognition was 87.8% (CI: 84.2%; 91.4%). However, postoperative neuropathic pain was less well diagnosed (77.9%; CI: 69.6%; 86.2%) than diabetic pain (95.2%; CI: 90.0%; 100.0%), cancer pain (90.6%; CI: 83.5%; 97.8%) and typical radicular pain (90.7%; CI: 84.9%; 96.5%). When neuropathic pain was correctly recognized, the likelihood of appropriate first-line treatment prescription was 90.6% (CI: 87.4%; 93.8%). The treatments proposed were pregabaline (71.8%), gabapentine (43.9%), amiptriptylline (23.2%) and duloxetine (18.2%). However, ibuprofen (11%), acetaminophen-codeine (29.5%) and clonazepam (10%) were still prescribed.

Conclusions: The compliance of GPs with clinical practice guidelines appeared to be satisfactory, but differed between etiologies.

Editor: Laxmaiah Manchikanti, University of Louisville, United States of America

Funding: This study was supported by Pfizer. The sponsor financed the data collection and statistical analysis of the data, which was performed by an independent clinical research organization (ITEC, Bordeaux, France). The funders had no role in the study design and analysis, decision to publish or preparation of the manuscript.

Competing Interests: The authors received honoraria from Pfizer for their participation in the scientific committee of the study.

* E-mail: valeria.martinez.aphp@gmail.com

Introduction

Neuropathic pain constitutes a significant burden for society in terms of impaired quality of life, comorbidities and cost [1–3]. Classical causes of neuropathic pain include diabetes, shingles, spinal cord injury, stroke, multiple sclerosis, cancer and HIV infection, but also more common conditions, such as radicular pain related to radiculopathy, and traumatic or postsurgical nerve injuries [4].

Several large epidemiological surveys have highlighted the under-treatment of neuropathic pain in France in either the general population [5] or in specialist settings [6]. Screening tools have been developed to increase the awareness and recognition of neuropathic pain, particularly by non-specialists [7–9]. The use of these tools may also contribute to reduce false positive diagnoses, which are probably also common in clinical practice.

Evidence-based recommendations for the assessment and management of neuropathic pain have also been developed in recent years [10–13]. In France, the French Pain Society (*Société Française d'Etude et Traitement de la Douleur*/SFETD), in particular, has proposed and disseminated evidence-based recommendations targeting all health professionals, with the aim of facilitating neuropathic pain recognition and management in the ambulatory care setting [14]. These recommendations emphasize the importance of screening tools (particularly the DN4, which was developed in France [7]) as a first step in the diagnosis of neuropathic pain, and propose first- and second-line drug treatments for neuropathic pain, regardless of its etiology, akin to European or international recommendations.

However, very few studies have investigated the real-life impact of evidence-based recommendations on physicians' practices. In the USA, a study by Dworkin and colleagues [15] suggested that the drug treatment of post-herpetic neuralgia by primary care physicians was roughly consistent with the US recommendations issued some years before. However, this study was retrospective and restricted to post-herpetic neuralgia, a condition that is easier for non-specialists to diagnose than many other neurological pain conditions.

Our aim in this study was to describe chronic neuropathic pain management practices among general practitioners (GPs), focusing on the criteria used in decision-making processes and compliance with current French recommendations. We used "case vignettes", a valid and reliable method that is gaining widespread acceptance for quality-of-care assessments in current clinical practice [16–20]. This method provides an effective evaluation of the behavior of physicians in the setting of diagnosis or treatment decisions, and of their compliance with recommendations. It therefore appeared an appropriate method in the context of the objectives of this study.

Materials and Methods

Ethics statement

This study was conducted in accordance with French regulatory requirements. The protocol and all administrative documents, including the financial agreement, with investigators paid for their participation, were approved by the National Medical Council (*Conseil National de l'Ordre des Médecins*; CNOM). The database was declared to the National Data Protection Authority (*Commission Nationale de l'Informatique et des Libertés*; CNIL). Submission to an ethics committee was not required under French law.

Selection of participants

We calculated that a sample of 300 GPs would be required to estimate any percentage with a maximum 95% CI of ±6.5%, taking into account a design effect related to the non-independence of observations made by the same physician. The rate of participation in e-CRF studies is generally about 30%, with 75% of participants being highly active. We therefore decided to select a representative random sample of 1,332 GPs for this study. To this end, we sent a questionnaire, by mail, to the 84,832 GPs practicing in mainland France (listed in the CEGEDIM database), on January 2nd, 2012, asking them whether they would be interested in participating in a non-interventional study. We selected a random sample of 1,332 physicians from the 4,299 GPs who expressed interest in participating in this study between January and July 2012. Contact information was incorrect for 67 GPs, so 1,265 GPs were finally included in our database. In October 2012, we sent these GPs a proposal for participation in this survey. Any physician who did not respond to this mailing was contacted by telephone two weeks later, and attempts at contact were continued until the planned number of participants was reached. In total, 465 GPs agreed to take part in this survey, of whom 443 signed a contract for participation and were issued with a center number. The flow chart for GP selection is summarized in Figure 1.

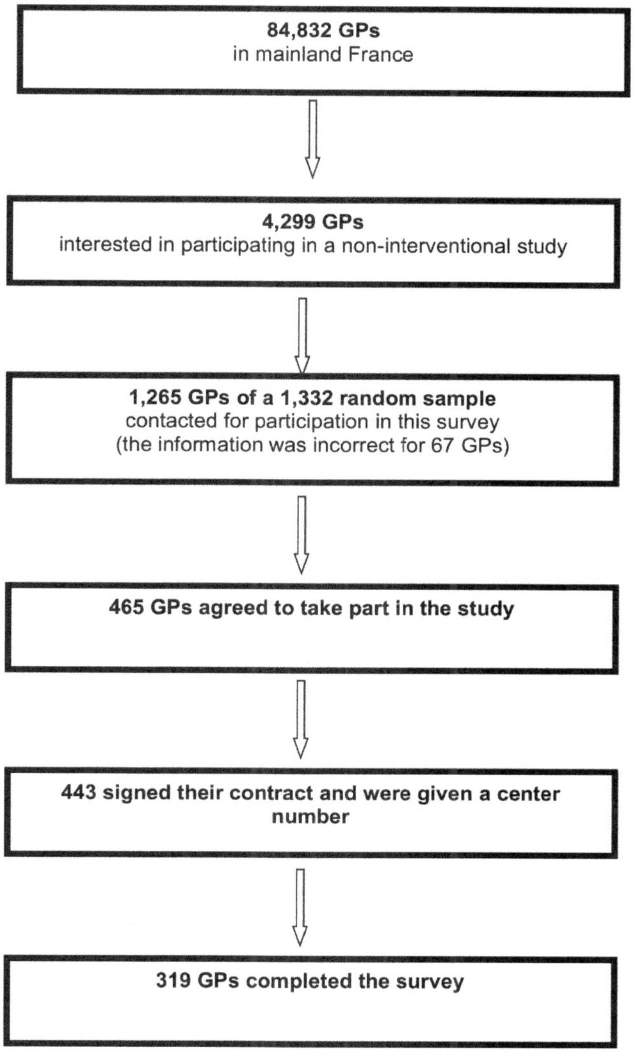

Figure 1. Flow chart of the study.

Construction of case-vignettes

Case vignettes were developed by a multidisciplinary panel of experts (authors of this paper) in the field of neuropathic pain, practicing as GPs, clinicians or nurses in neurology or anesthesiology. The description of clinical cases was based on epidemiological and descriptive data characterizing neuropathic pain [21]. Each clinical case was designed to be realistic and concrete, matching as closely as possible the cases observed in clinical practice. We focused on four etiologies of peripheral neuropathic pain frequently encountered in general medical practice: painful diabetic polyneuropathy, cancer chemotherapy-induced peripheral neuropathy [22], typical radicular pain [23] and post-operative neuropathic pain [24–26]. In assessments of performance for the identification of neuropathic pain, we considered two types of chronic pain for each etiology: nociceptive chronic pain and peripheral neuropathic pain. Based on these conditions, we constructed eight case-vignettes, each with a different scenario. The eight case-vignettes are given in File S1.

The scenario needed to be simple, brief (length <15 lines-200 words), with no potential pitfalls. Each case-vignette was constructed in the same way: age, sex, patient's history, chronic pain history, reason for consultation, clinical symptoms, data from clinical examination, with or without results from additional investigations.

Scenarios differed in terms of both symptoms (e.g. burning pain *vs* aching pain) and elements of clinical examination (e.g. allodynia *vs* pain triggered by joint mobilization). The symptoms and clinical examination findings leading to the diagnosis of neuropathic pain were chosen from among the most discriminative, although none of them is specific [7,11,27] and were consistent with those used in validated screening tools, such as the DN4 (*Douleur neuropathique en 4 questions*) [7]. Clinical cases of neuropathic pain included at least six discriminative neuropathic elements, whereas non-neuropathic cases presented fewer than two neuropathic characteristics (see cases n°7 and 8 in File S1).

Non-discriminative clinical elements of neuropathic pain were systematically included in the description of all clinical cases: high pain intensity on a numerical rating scale (>7/10) and comorbid conditions (anxiety, depression).

Construction of the case-vignette questionnaire

The proposed questions and their corresponding items dealt with the different elements for the diagnosis and management of neuropathic pain set out in SFETD recommendations (see Key points in File S1). The construction of this closed-ended questionnaire superimposed over the recommendations made it possible to carry out a relevant assessment of knowledge and facilitated the analysis of responses. The number of questions and items was the same for each case. The knowledge of the GPs was assessed through four multiple-choice questions: i) diagnostic elements, four items, ii) elements from the patient's clinical history guiding diagnosis, four items, iii) elements from clinical examination guiding diagnosis, three items, iv) drugs proposed for first-line treatment, seven items.

The case-vignette questionnaire is shown in in File S1. The list of first-line drugs includes duloxetine, which is authorized only for the treatment of painful diabetic peripheral neuropathy in France.

Procedure

Eight case-vignettes were constructed, corresponding to four neuropathic cases and four non-neuropathic cases (Table 1). By combining these vignettes two-by-two (one neuropathic case and one non-neuropathic case), we obtained 12 possible combinations, which we tested on 20 GPs, to evaluate their comprehensibility. This testing step identified two combinations as too similar to each other (diabetic polyneuropathy and cancer chemotherapy-induced polyneuropathy), and these combinations were therefore removed. Each GP had to provide a response for a set of two case-vignettes randomly selected from the 10 remaining combinations. GPs were blind to the mode of case distribution.

The case-vignettes were stored in a database on a dedicated server for this survey (a web-based application). GPs could access their two assigned case-vignettes at any time, *via* a personal online account protected by a specific and confidential login and password assigned to them after validation of the financial agreement. Once all fields of the case-vignette questionnaire had been completed, the questionnaire was saved automatically on the administrator's account, preventing any further modification.

Table 1. The eight case-vignettes.

	Neuropathic pain	Non-neuropathic pain
Diabetes	Case 1	Case 2
Cancer	Case 3	Case 4
Low back pain	Case 5	Case 6
Postoperative pain	Case 7	Case 8

In the event of an incorrect diagnosis after the response to the first three questions, GPs were given the correct diagnosis so that they could answer the question relating to therapeutic strategy with the correct diagnosis in mind.

Before completing the case-vignette questionnaires, the participants provided the following information: their age, sex, duration of practice, practice in an urban/rural area, number of chronic pain patients seen per week (and the percentage of these patients with neuropathic pain). After validation of the responses, they were also asked the following questions: *"Are you aware of the SFETD recommendations? Do you implement them? Are you aware of the DN4 tool* (Douleur Neuropathique en 4 questions)? *Do you use it?"*

Statistical analysis

For continuous variables, we determined the mean and standard deviation. For categorical variables, the number and percentage of subjects in each category are summarized. We used Student's t test to assess differences for continuous variables. Chi^2 tests of association were used to test for sequence order differences for categorical variables. The threshold for significance was set at $p = 0.05$.

We determined the percentage of cases correctly diagnosed, with its 95% confidence interval (CI). A similar analysis was performed for each of the eight case-vignettes, according to the type of pain (neuropathic or non-neuropathic) and the underlying disease. The percentages of GPs making 0, 1 and 2 corrected diagnoses were determined.

The elements of the patient's history and clinical examination used to reach the diagnosis were described separately for each of the eight case-vignettes, according to the type of pain (neuropathic or non-neuropathic) and the disease, and for the following subgroups: correct diagnosis/misdiagnosis, knowledge of recommendations (YES/NO) and their implementation (YES/NO), knowledge of the DN4 tool (YES/NO) and its use (YES/NO). The results obtained were compared with the expected responses.

Prescriptions of analgesic treatments were described separately for each of the eight case-vignettes and according to: the type of pain (neuropathic or non-neuropathic), knowledge of the recommendations (YES/NO) and their implementation (YES/NO).

We aimed to evaluate compliance with SFETD guidelines. Thus, for each question on the case-vignette questionnaire, we analyzed the number of correct answers and the number of answers containing at least one element of the correct answer, without any element wrongly ticked.

Analyses were performed with SAS version 9.3 (SAS Institute, Cary, NC).

Results

In total, 443 GPs signed a contract and received a center number, but only the 319 duly completing the e-CRF were included in the analysis. We thus evaluated responses for a total of 638 case-vignettes.

Characteristics of connections

An analysis of connection times showed that the participants remained connected for a median of 17 minutes and that the minimum connection time was four minutes. A few extreme values were obtained, probably due to participants forgetting to sign out.

Table 2. GPs' characteristics.

	Statistics	N=319
Sex		
Male	*n(%)*	254 (79.6%)
Female	*n(%)*	65 (20.4%)
Pattern of medical practice		
Alone	*n(%)*	125 (40.1%)
Group practice	*n(%)*	187 (59.9%)
	Missing (n - %)	7 (2.2%)
Urban/Rural		
Rural	*n(%)*	191 (59.9%)
Urban	*n(%)*	128 (40.1%)
Age (years)	*MeanSD*	52.3
	Median	8.4
	Q1;Q3	53.0
	[Min; Max]	[47.0;59.0]
		[31.0;69.0]
Duration of practice		
<10 years	*n(%)*	33 (10.3%)
>=10 years	*n(%)*	286 (89.7%)
Number of chronic pain patients per month	*Mean*	52.8
	SD	46.7
	Median	45.0
	Q1;Q3	[20.0;70.0]
	[Min; Max]	[2.0;400.0]
Number of chronic pain patients with neuropathic pain per month	*Mean*	8.6
	SD	10.8
	Median	5.0
	Q1;Q3	[2.5;10.0]
	[Min; Max]	[0.1;100.0]

SD, standard deviation; Q1–Q3, first and third quartiles; min, minimum; max, maximum.

Characteristics of the participants

The demographic features of the 319 GPs completing the questionnaires for both the clinical cases assigned to them are reported in Table 2.

This sample of physicians was representative of the general population of GPs in terms of their nationwide distribution (with a slight underrepresentation of Ile-de-France) and mean age. Men were overrepresented (79.6% *vs* the expected 59%, based on GP numbers) as frequently reported in studies of this type. Representativeness was assessed on the basis of the French atlas of medical demography (Atlas National CNOM 2012).

Of the 319 GPs completing the questionnaires for both case-vignettes, 53.3% (170/319) were aware of guidelines and 42.6% (136/319) said that they implemented them. The principal reason for not following the recommendations was insufficient knowledge of these recommendations. For the DN4 diagnostic tool, 60.8% of the GPs (194/319) stated that they were aware of it and 34.5% (110/319) reported using it. The main reason for not using this tool was a lack of memorized knowledge.

Evaluation of case-vignettes: diagnosis and therapeutic strategy

Global results. ***Of the 319 GPs***, 58.9% made the correct diagnosis for both the allocated case vignettes. The proportion of GPs giving two correct diagnoses did not between the sexes (58.7% men *vs* 60.0% women; $p = 0.845$) or between types of practice are (56.0% rural *vs* 63.3% urban; $p = 0.434$). The number of accurate diagnoses did not depend on whether the doctors were aware of or implemented the recommendations; similar results were obtained concerning knowledge and use of the DN4 tool. Several case combinations were identified less well than others. The proportions of GPs giving the correct diagnosis for both case vignettes was lowest (Figure 2) when one of the allocated vignettes was a case of cancer with non-neuropathic pain (case no. 4, with case no. 7: 22.6%, or with case no. 5: 34.4%). Postoperative neuropathic pain (case no. 7) also appeared to be difficult to identify, as shown for its combination with case no. 6 (43.8%) or case no. 2 (46.9%).

For the 638 vignettes examined, the correct diagnosis was made in 77.3% of cases. The percentage of correct diagnoses differed considerably between etiologies and was lowest for cancer cases ($p = 0.0002$; Figure 3).

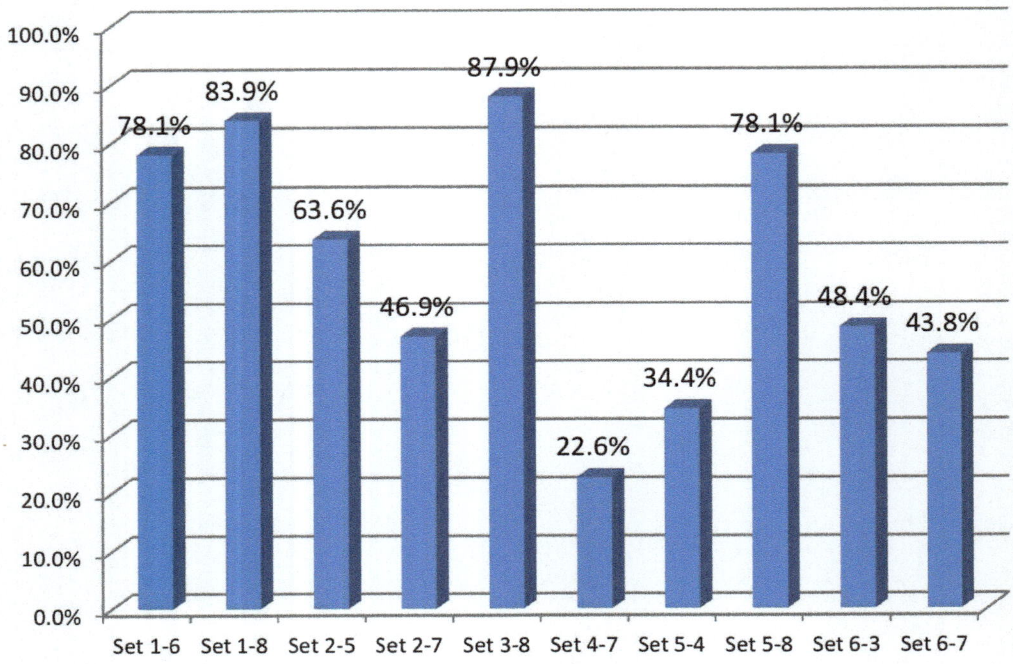

Figure 2. Proportion of investigators (*N* = 319) with 2 correct diagnoses.

Neuropathic pain was well diagnosed in 87.8% (95%CI: 84.2%; 91.4%) of cases (Figure 4), but the frequency of correct diagnosis differed between etiologies (Figure 5). The probability of correct diagnosis seemed to be lower for postoperative neuropathic pain (case no. 7) (77.9%; 95%CI [69.6%; 86.2%]) than for other etiologies (92.0%; 95%CI [88.4%; 95.5%]). Thus, misdiagnosis was 2.8 times more frequent for postoperative neuropathic pain than for other etiologies (22.1% *vs* 8.0%; $p = 0.0005$).

Our analysis of the criteria on which GPs based their diagnosis of neuropathic pain indicated that all items from the patient's history and all items from the clinical examination characterizing this type of pain were recognized in 53.9% and 51.8% of cases, respectively (Table 3). For the 280 GPs making the correct diagnosis, 112 (40%) had ticked at least four correct answers among the seven items proposed; this percentage was significantly lower among the GPs giving the wrong diagnosis (9 of 39 GPs i.e. 23.1%; $p = 0.041$). A case-by-case analysis of the results highlighted differences in the identification of key diagnostic elements as a function of etiology. Indeed, for diabetic neuropathic pain (case no. 1), diagnosis was based mostly on the patient's history rather than clinical examination, whereas, for postoperative neuropathic pain (case no. 7) the key diagnostic elements were more easily identified from clinical examination than from the patient's history. These results are summarized in Table 4.

We found that 53.6% GPs faced with a case of neuropathic pain of any etiology prescribed at least one first-line treatment

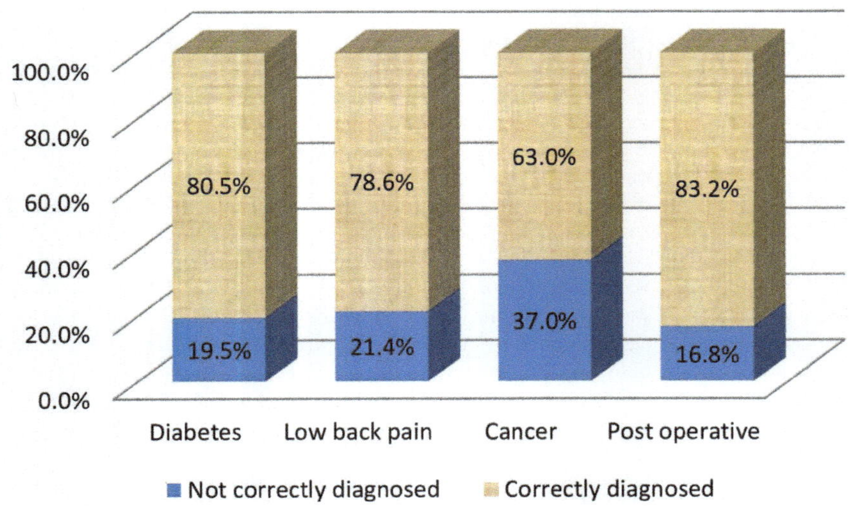

Figure 3. Frequency of correct/incorrect diagnoses by etiology (*N* = 638).

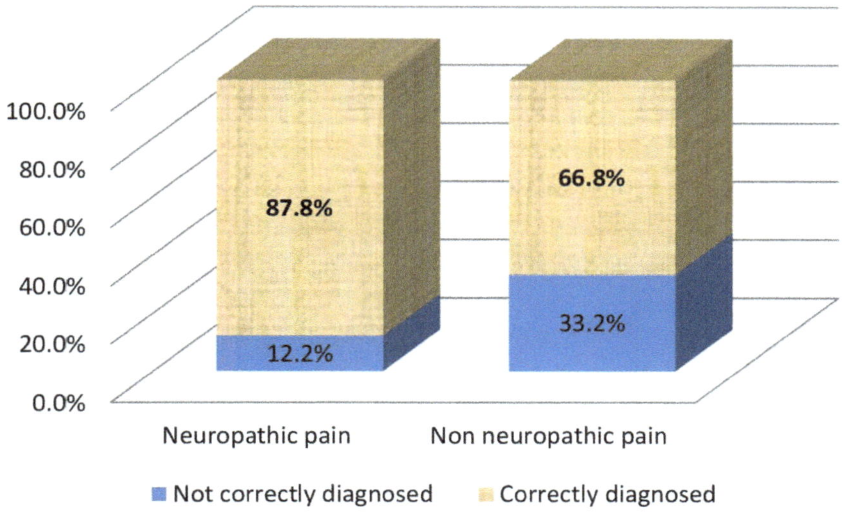

Figure 4. Frequency of correct/incorrect diagnoses by type of pain (*N*=638).

recommended for this type of pain. Significant differences in prescriptions were observed as a function of etiology. Indeed, a first-line treatment was prescribed for 73.0% of diabetes cases but only 48.8% cases of neuropathic pain of other etiologies ($p=0.0006$). Only 4.7% of the GPs identified all the drugs that could be used as first-line treatments for neuropathic pain. A significant disparity in drug prescriptions was observed, with pregabalin prescribed in 71.8% of cases, gabapentin in 43.9% and amitriptyline in 23.2%. The orders of the prescription rates for these three drugs did not depend on etiology. However, for diabetic polyneuropathy, duloxetine replaced amitriptyline as the third most frequently prescribed drug. The questions relating to therapeutic approaches also revealed that many doctors would prescribe inappropriate drugs, such as acetaminophen/codeine, ibuprofen and clonazepam, which were prescribed in 29.5%, 11% and 10% of cases, respectively. Data on drug prescriptions in neuropathic pain are presented in Table 4 and Table 5.

Non-neuropathic pain was well diagnosed in 66.8% of cases. Postoperative pain (case no. 8) was the easiest to identify and cancer pain (case no. 4) proved to be the most difficult. An overdiagnosis of neuropathic pain was observed, with 33.2% of the 319 cases of non-neuropathic pain incorrectly diagnosed as neuropathic pain and a clear predominance of incorrect diagnoses for cancer pain (65.1%). These results are presented in Figures 4 and 5.

Correct diagnosis, with all the correct items ticked for history or clinical examination, was observed in 50.7% and 66.2% of cases, respectively. Other than for postoperative pain, the key elements for a correct diagnosis were more frequently obtained from clinical examination than from history (Table 6).

In terms of therapeutic strategy, regardless of the etiology of non-neuropathic pain, about one third of GPs (36.7%) prescribed both appropriate drugs — ibuprofen and acetaminophen/codeine — and about two thirds (63.6%) prescribed at least one of these

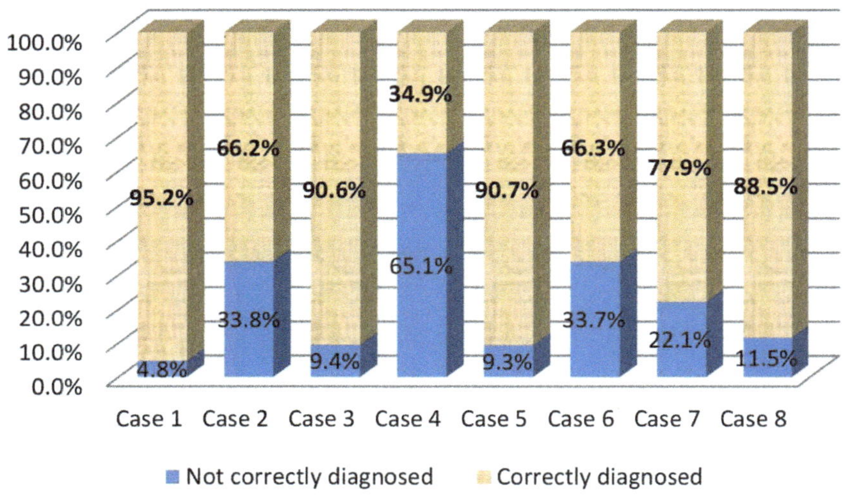

Figure 5. Frequency of correct/incorrect diagnoses for each case-vignette (*N*=638).

Table 3. Key elements for the correct diagnosis of neuropathic pain.

Etiology	Elements from history-exact response rate-	Elements from clinical examination-exact response rate-	p(Mc Nemar)
Diabetes	66.7% (40/60)	35.0% (21/60)	0.0009
Cancer	55.2% (32/58)	56.9% (33/58)	0.8273
Low back pain	54.5% (48/88)	46.6% (41/88)	0.2967
Postoperative pain	41.9% (31/74)	67.6% (50/74)	0.0038
All cases of neuropathic pain	53.9% (151/280)	51.8% (145/280)	0.6146

two drugs. Correct prescription rates were similar whether or not the recommendations were applied (Table 7).

For both neuropathic and non-neuropathic pain, knowledge and implementation of the recommendations, and knowledge and use of the DN4 tool, did not appear to affect the likelihood of recognizing key elements from the patient's history or clinical examination for accurate diagnosis.

Case-by-case results. ***Painful diabetic polyneuropathy*** (case no. 1) was well diagnosed in most cases (95.2%), with 66.7% and 35.0% exact answers for the patient's history and clinical examination, respectively. In terms of therapeutic strategy, the complete list of recommended first-line treatments was rarely given (7.9%), but one of the drugs from this list was proposed in about three in four cases (73.0%). The drug most frequently proposed was pregabalin (73.0% of cases).

Non-neuropathic pain in diabetic patients (case no. 2) was correctly diagnosed in 66.2% of cases, with 46.5% and 97.7% exact answers for the patient's history and clinical examination, respectively. If we considered cases with only one element of the exact answer but with no incorrectly ticked elements, these percentages were 72.1% and 97.7%, respectively. In cases of incorrect diagnosis, no exact answer was obtained for either history or clinical examination. For therapeutic strategy, the two recommended first-line drugs (ibuprofen and acetaminophen/codeine) were proposed together in less than half the cases (41.5%), but one of these drugs was cited in 70.8% of cases. Acetaminophen/codeine was the most frequently proposed drug (80.0% of cases).

Cancer chemotherapy-induced peripheral neuropathy (case no. 3) was well diagnosed in 90.6% of cases, with 55.2% and 56.9% exact answers for the patient's history and clinical examination, respectively. If we considered answers with at least one correct element, these percentages were 58.6% and 70.7%, respectively. For therapeutic management, very few GPs (3.1%) identified all three recommended first-line drugs, but half (51.6%) proposed one of these drugs. The drug most frequently identified was pregabalin (75.0% of cases).

Non-neuropathic pain in cancer (case no. 4) was diagnosed in only 34.9% of cases, with 45.5% and 81.8% exact answers for the patient's history and clinical examination, respectively. Similar results were obtained if we considered responses with at least one correct element. In cases of incorrect diagnosis, no exact answer was obtained for either the patient's history or for clinical examination. The two recommended first-line drugs (ibuprofen and acetaminophen/codeine) were both proposed in 30.2% of cases, but at least one of these two drugs was cited in 65.1% of

Table 4. Key elements leading to correct diagnosis and choice of therapeutic strategy for each of the 8 case-vignettes.

	Case-vignette							
	1	2	3	4	5	6	7	8
	n = 63	*n* = 65	*n* = 64	*n* = 63	*n* = 97	*n* = 95	*n* = 95	*n* = 96
ELEMENTS FROM HISTORY								
Exact answer* (%)	66.7%	46.5%	55.2%	45.5%	54.5%	42.9%	41.9%	60.0%
Correct answer** (%)	71.7%	72.1%	58.6%	45.5%	56.8%	55.6%	45.9%	64.7%
ELEMENTS FROM CLINICAL EXAMINATION								
Exact answer* (%)	35.0%	97.7%	56.9%	81.8%	46.6%	61.9%	67.6%	49.4%
Correct answer (%)	100%***	97.7%	70.7%	81.8%	100%***	61.9%	100%***	77.6%
CORRECT PRESCRIPTIONS								
All first-line drugs proposed	7.9%	41.5%	3.1%	30.0%	5.2%	36.8%	6.3%	37.5%
At least one first-line drug proposed	73.0%	70.8%	51.6%	65.1%	44.3%	62.1%	51.6%	59.4%

* an answer strictly corresponding to the expected answer (the exact answer required all items to be ticked).
** an answer with at least one element of the exact answer, without any element wrongly ticked.

Table 5. Correct prescription rates for neuropathic pain.

Drugs	$N = 319$
Pregabalin/amitryptyline/gabapentin*	15 (4.7%)
Pregabalin	229 (71.8%)
Amitryptyline	74 (23.2%)
Gabapentin	140 (43.9%)
At least one recommended drug**	171 (53.6%)

*all three first-line recommended drugs.
** and no incorrect treatment.

cases. Acetaminophen/codeine was the most frequently proposed drug (79.4% of cases).

Typical radicular pain (case no. 5) was correctly identified in 90.7% of cases, with 54.5% and 46.6% exact answers for the patient's history and clinical examination, respectively. Very few GPs (5.2%) identified all three recommended first-line drugs, and only 44.3% proposed one of these drugs. The most frequently cited drug was pregabalin (64.9% of cases).

Non-neuropathic low back pain (case no. 6) was correctly diagnosed in 66.3% of cases, with 42.9% and 61.9% exact answers for the patient's history and clinical examination, respectively. If we considered answers with at least one correct element, these percentages were 55.6% and 61.9%, respectively. In cases of incorrect diagnosis, exact answers for history and clinical examination were observed in only 9.4% and 3.1% of cases, respectively. The two recommended first-line drugs (ibuprofen and acetaminophen/codeine) were both proposed by 36.8% of GPs, and one of these drugs was proposed by 62.1% of GPs. Acetaminophen/codeine was the most frequently proposed drug (83.2% of cases).

Postoperative neuropathic pain (case no. 7) was well diagnosed in 77.9% of cases, with 41.9% and 67.6% exact answers for the patient's history and clinical examination, respectively. In cases of incorrect diagnosis, exact answers from the patient's history and clinical examination were obtained in 33.3% and 28.6% of cases, respectively. For therapeutic strategy, all three recommended first line treatments was rarely ticked together (6.3%), but one of these drugs was proposed in about half the cases (51.6%). The most frequently cited drug was pregabalin (75.8% of cases).

Postoperative non-neuropathic pain (case no. 8) was diagnosed in 88.5% of cases, with 60.0% and 49.4% exact answers for the patient's history and clinical examination, respectively. If we considered answers with at least one correct element, these percentages were 64.7% and 77.6%, respectively.

Table 7. Correct prescription rates for non-neuropathic pain.

Drugs	$N = 319$
Ibuprofen/acetaminophen-codeine*	117 (36.7%)
Ibuprofen	200 (62.7%)
Acetaminophen-codeine	248 (77.7%)
At least one recommended drug**	203 (63.6%)

* the two first-line recommended drugs.
** and no incorrect treatment.

In cases of wrong diagnosis, no exact answer was given for either history or clinical examination. The two recommended first-line drugs (ibuprofen and acetaminophen/codeine) were both proposed by 37.5% of GPs, and one of these drugs was proposed by 59.4% of GPs.

Discussion

This study is the first to address the issue of the compliance of French general practitioners with current recommendations for the diagnosis and first-line treatment of neuropathic pain [14]. Three years after the publication of French recommendations on neuropathic pain, this study found that only 58.9% of GPs made the correct diagnosis for both the allocated case vignettes. Neuropathic pain was well diagnosed in 87.8% of cases, but only 53.6% of GPs proposed an appropriate first-line treatment. Based on these figures, less than one in two patients (47.1%) consulting for neuropathic pain would receive appropriate treatment.

Diagnosis of neuropathic pain

Accurate diagnosis is the crucial first step toward the successful management of neuropathic pain. We were surprised by the high percentage of correct diagnoses of neuropathic pain obtained in this study (87.8%), given the difficulties encountered in the recognition of this type of pain real life [28,29]. However, the clinical cases submitted to the GPs in this study were simple and somewhat caricatured. Our cases of neuropathic pain included at least seven characteristic features of such pain, whereas four elements are sufficient for the diagnosis of NP with the DN4 tool [7]. Moreover, it has been shown that the use of closed-ended questionnaires with cued items leads to an overestimate of the performance of physicians [30]. The sponsorship of this study by a laboratory heavily involved in research on neuropathic pain may also have resulted in a higher proportion of GPs making the correct diagnosis for neuropathic pain. Thus, although the overall figures appear to be highly satisfactory, further analyses of diagnostic failures can provide us with useful information. Indeed,

Table 6. Key elements for the correct diagnosis of non-neuropathic pain.

Etiology	Elements from history-exact response rate-	Elements from clinical examination-exact response rate-	p(Mc Nemar)
Diabetes	46.5% (20/43)	97.7% (42/43)	<0.0001
Cancer	45.5% (10/22)	81.8% (18/22)	0.0047
Low back pain	42.9% (27/63)	61.9% (39/63)	0.0233
Postoperative pain	60.0% (51/85)	49.4% (42/85)	0.1797
All cases of neuropathic pain	50.7% (108/213)	66.2% (145/213)	0.0011

this detailed analysis identified certain diagnostic difficulties in particular conditions.

Firstly, the large range of answers obtained, depending on the set of two case-vignettes assigned to the GPs, suggested that diagnosis was not always easy. Some cases, such as painful diabetic polyneuropathy, seemed to be much better diagnosed than others, such as postoperative neuropathic pain. We also observed an overdiagnosis of neuropathic pain in cancer patients. Only one in five GPs recognized both non-neuropathic cancer pain and postoperative neuropathic pain. The overdiagnosis of neuropathic pain in some etiologies and its underdiagnosis in others may reflect GPs continuing to think that the nature of pain depends on either its context or its etiology. Parsons *et al.* recently showed that mean time from the onset of postoperative neuropathic pain symptoms to diagnosis was 9.7 months [29]. Indeed, postoperative pain had long been considered purely, until the widespread recognition about 10 years ago of the neuropathic origin of some postoperative pains [31]. By contrast, diabetic neuropathy has been the subject of extensive academic, scientific communication and marketing, potentially accounting for the high frequency of correct diagnosis (92.2%). GPs overdiagnosed neuropathic pain in cancer patients, probably because they were influenced by the background of previous chemotherapy and the presence of two neuropathic elements (e.g. tingling and hypoesthesia) without taking into account clinical presentation (e.g. location of pain away from nerve damage symptoms).

Overall, these results suggest that limited use is made of the findings of clinical examinations in the diagnosis of neuropathic pain. This hypothesis was confirmed by the analysis of answers relating to the elements of the patient's history and clinical examination leading to the diagnosis of neuropathic pain, which provided us with new insight into the decision-making processes of physicians. Indeed, our results indicate that the elements used to arrive at the correct diagnosis differed between etiologies. In diabetic patients, pain descriptors were used for the identification of neuropathic pain, whereas, in postoperative pain, correct diagnoses were based largely on clinical examination. This is a key point, highlighting the essential nature of clinical examination for the diagnosis of neuropathic pain in general practice. This finding closes the debate about whether clinical examinations should be counted among the screening tools helping non-specialists to identify patients with possible neuropathic pain.

Therapeutic management

The management of patients with chronic neuropathic pain is challenging, despite attempts to develop a more rational therapeutic approach [32]. In our study, only one in two GPs proposed at least one of the recommended first-line treatments when faced with a case of confirmed neuropathic pain. This poor result applied to neuropathic pain of all etiologies. Indeed, when multiplied with the probability of prescription of one appropriate first-line treatment, only 69.5%, 46.7%, 40.2% and 40.2% of patients with diabetes, cancer, radicular pain and postoperative pain, respectively, would receive appropriate medical care. These low rates highlight the large proportion of patients that would not have been correctly treated despite the caricatured description of neuropathic pain in the vignettes, its high intensity (7/10 on VAS) and association with sleep disorders and anxiety in all the case-vignettes assigned to the GPs. These findings suggest that the corresponding figures may be even worse in "real life". As for diagnosis, we observed differences according to etiology with neuropathic pain in diabetic patients much better managed than that in patients presenting with low back pain or postoperative pain.

Another key finding of our results is the lack of knowledge of evidence-based therapy, with less than 5% of GPs being able to list all the first-line drugs recommended for the treatment of neuropathic pain. This suggests that physicians have a very superficial knowledge of recommendations, such that patients with contraindications or treatment failure might not necessarily receive appropriate treatment. It is probably easier for GPs to remember one drug per disease, even if further inquiries must subsequently be made, rather than remembering algorithms of various complexities. Pregabalin was by far the most frequently cited drug, regardless of etiology, followed by gabapentin and amitriptyline. This finding may be accounted for by the risk-benefit profile of pregabalin, which is better tolerated and requires fewer precautions for use than amitriptyline [14]. Finally, this study revealed the persistence of non-recommended drug prescriptions, such as acetaminophen/codeine, ibuprofen or clonazepam. Clonazepam, which belongs to the benzodiazepine class, has been misused and abused and has been subject to prescription limitations imposed by the French authorities since January 2012 [33]. The other drugs in this non-recommended list are very often wrongly prescribed, to one inthree patients for ibuprofen and one in five patients for acetaminophen/codeine. Nevertheless, non-recommended drug prescriptions were less frequent than reported in a recent study investigating the treatment of neuropathic pain in the UK general population [34]. An opioid, or a combination of opioid and non-opioid analgesics, was prescribed as a first-line treatment for 25.4% of patients with diabetic neuropathy and 64.0% of patients with neuropathic back pain. By contrast, no benzodiazepine was prescribed. Our results highlight specific issues that should be addressed in the future to optimize the therapeutic management of neuropathic pain in general practice.

Knowledge of SFETD recommendations

In our study, one in two GPs declared that they knew the recommendations for neuropathic pain. This proportion is similar to published findings from surveys carried out in general practice to assess knowledge about recommendations for six common diseases. However, the percentage of GPs stating that they applied recommendations (42%) was much higher in our study than reported for other diseases (17%) [35]. This led us to question the veracity of the GPs' statements, particularly because we were unable to detect any impact on the recognition of neuropathic pain and its therapeutic management. The remuneration of participation by a pharmaceutical company with considerable involvement in pain management might have favored complaisant responses. We therefore considered the reported implementation of the recommendations by GPs to be too dubious for a relevant assessment of the impact of recommendations on medical practice. Other methodological approaches, such as the assessment of practices before/after the publication of recommendations, or before/after training, would be more appropriate for such an analysis.

Strengths and limitations of case-vignettes

Case-vignettes have been used for years to evaluate of the behavior of physicians in the setting of diagnostic testing or treatment decisions. We chose to use this method for our study as it has been shown to be an accurate, valid, feasible and inexpensive tool for measuring the quality of health care [16,17,19,36,37]. Previous studies have demonstrated the utility of case-vignettes for assessing compliance with recommendations, for measuring physicians' practice performance, particularly for comparisons of different groups of physicians, for identifying deviations from guidelines and physicians with non-ideal approaches to patients due to a lack of knowledge, and for defining areas in which scientific knowledge could be strengthened [19,38,39].

This study had several methodological strengths. Case-vignette design was based on epidemiological and descriptive data for neuropathic pain, which we used to create an initial scenario matching current clinical practice in ambulatory care as closely as possible. Case-vignettes were constructed by an expert panel with six members and were further refined after successful testing on a sample of 20 GPs. The assessment criterion was the recognition of neuropathic pain, and the various items proposed in the questionnaire corresponded to the different diagnostic and therapeutic elements addressed in the French recommendations (pain description, clinical examination, first-line medication).

However, our study also had a number of limitations. Men were overrepresented, introducing a selection bias. Nevertheless, the likelihood of recognizing or correctly managing neuropathic pain is unlikely to differ between the sexes, and no significant difference according to sex was identified in this study. This research was sponsored by Pfizer, and we cannot rule out the possibility that this influenced GPs' answers, particularly given the overdiagnosis of neuropathic pain observed.

We selected case-vignettes relating to only four etiologies of chronic pain. The inclusion of a broader range of etiologies would have increased the difficulty of diagnosis and might have generated different results. We presented cases of pure chronic pain that was either neuropathic or nociceptive. The introduction of mixed pain would probably have increased the percentage of misdiagnoses, given the greater complexity of the possible choices.

Despite the great care that we took to ensure that case-vignettes were similar in terms of difficulty (particularly as concerns the number and quality of neuropathic descriptors included in the cases of neuropathic pain), we cannot rule out the possibility that other difficulties influenced the results. For example, case no. 4, "non-neuropathic cancer pain", which was one of the worst diagnosed cases, had specific features. It was the only case among the four cases of non-neuropathic pain presenting two neuropathic elements. Moreover, these elements appeared ahead of all the other items proposed whereas, in other cases, they were presented at the end of the list of items. These various aspects highlight the difficulties involved in drawing up case-vignettes. Thus, case-vignettes seem to be a tool that is more useful for highlighting weaknesses on which communication efforts should focus, rather than providing figures concerning medical practice. As previously reported, it is not possible with the case-vignette method to ensure that the responses obtain reflect the way that the GPs would behave in everyday patient care, even if the design and wording of the vignettes are kept as close as possible to real conditions [40]. Indeed, this method does not take into account either doctor-patient interactions or the relational aspects involved in real life.

Conclusions

The complexity of neuropathic chronic pain poses challenges for both management and diagnosis for primary care physicians. Taking into account our findings and the limitations outlined above, this study highlights to poor adoption of SFETD recommendations, with difficulties recognizing neuropathic pain for certain etiologies, insufficient consideration of clinical examination findings, and the paucity of appropriate first-line drugs recalled by GPs. These results may facilitate the design of specific educational programs and interventions aiming to improve the management of neuropathic pain by GPs in France.

Supporting Information

File S1

Author Contributions

Conceived and designed the experiments: VM NA BV EV JMG DB MLM. Analyzed the data: VM NA BV EV JMG DB MLM. Wrote the paper: VM NA BV EV JMG DB MLM.

References

1. Treede RD, Jensen TS, Campbell JN, Cruccu G, Dostrovsky JO, et al. (2008) Redefinition of neuropathic pain and a grading system for clinical use: consensus statement on clinical and research diagnostic criteria. Neurology 70: 1630–1635.
2. Haanpää ML, Backonja MM, Bennett MI, Bouhassira D, Cruccu G, et al. (2009) Assessment of neuropathic pain in primary care. Am J Med 122 (10 Suppl): S13–21.
3. Radat F, Margot-Duclot A, Attal N (2013) Psychiatric co-morbidities in patients with chronic peripheral neuropathic pain: A multicentre cohort study. Eur J Pain 17: 1547–1557.
4. Attal N, Fermanian C, Fermanian J, Lanteri-Minet M, Alchaar H, et al. (2008) Neuropathic pain: are there distinct subtypes depending on the aetiology or anatomical lesion? Pain 138: 343–353.
5. Attal N, Lanteri-Minet M, Laurent B, Fermanian J, Bouhassira D (2011) The specific disease burden of neuropathic pain: results of a French nationwide survey. Pain 152: 2836–2843.
6. Bouhassira D, Letanoux M, Hartemann A (2013) Chronic pain with neuropathic characteristics in diabetic patients: a French cross-sectional study. PLoS One 8: e74195.
7. Bouhassira D, Attal N, Alchaar H, Boureau F, Brochet B, et al. (2005) Comparison of pain syndromes associated with nervous or somatic lesions and development of a new neuropathic pain diagnostic questionnaire (DN4). Pain 114: 29–36.
8. Bennett MI, Attal N, Backonja MM, Baron R, Bouhassira D, et al. (2007) Using screening tools to identify neuropathic pain. Pain 127: 199–203.
9. Bouhassira D, Attal N (2011) Diagnosis and assessment of neuropathic pain: the saga of clinical tools. Pain 152(3 Suppl): S74–83.
10. Finnerup NB, Otto M, McQuay HJ, Jensen TS, Sindrup SH (2005) Algorithm for neuropathic pain treatment: an evidence based proposal. Pain 118: 289–305.
11. Dworkin RH, O'Connor AB, Backonja M, Farrar JT, Finnerup NB, et al. (2007) Pharmacologic management of neuropathic pain: Evidence-based recommendations. Pain 132: 237–251.
12. Centre for Clinical Practice at NICE (UK) (2010) Neuropathic pain: the pharmacological management of neuropathic pain in adults in non-specialist settings. London: National Institute for Health and Clinical Excellence (UK).
13. Attal N, Cruccu G, Baron R, Haanpaa M, Hansson P, et al. (2010) European Federation of Neurological Societies: EFNS guidelines on the pharmacological treatment of neuropathic pain: 2010 revision. Eur J Neurol 17: e1113–e1188.
14. Martinez V, Attal N, Bouhassira D, Lantéri-Minet M for the French Society for the Study and Treatment of Pain (2010) Chronic neuropathic pain: diagnosis, evaluation and treatment in outpatient services. Guidelines for clinical practice of the French Society for the Study and Treatment of Pain. Douleur analg 23: 51–66.
15. Dworkin RH, Panarites CJ, Armstrong EP, Malone DC, Pham SV (2012) Is treatment of postherpetic neuralgia in the community consistent with evidence-based recommendations? Pain 153: 869–875.
16. Peabody JW, Luck J, Glassman P, Dersselhaus TR, Lee M (2000) Comparison of vignettes, standardized patients, and chart abstraction: a prospective validation study of 3 methods for measuring quality. JAMA 283: 1715–1722.
17. Peabody JW, Luck J, Glassman P, Jain S, Hansen J, et al. (2004) Measuring the quality of physician practice by using clinical vignettes: a prospective validation study. Ann Intern Med 141: 771–780.
18. Peabody JW, Tozija F, Munoz JA, Nordyke RJ, Luck J (2004) Using vignettes to compare the quality of clinical care variation in economically divergent countries. Health Serv Res 39: 1951–1970.
19. Veloski J, Tai S, Evans AS, Nash DB (2005) Clinical vignette-based surveys: a tool for assessing physician practice variation. Am J Med Qual 20: 151–157.
20. Bachmann LM, Muehleisen A, Bock A, ter Riet G, Held U, et al. (2008) Vignette studies of medical choice and judgement to study caregivers' medical decision behaviour: systematic review. BMC Med Res Methodol 8: 50.
21. Bouhassira D, Attal N (2012) Douleurs neuropathiques, Collection: Références en douleur et analgésie, Arnette Editors.

22. Bennett MI, Rayment C, Hjermstad M, Aass N, Caraceni A, et al. (2012) Prevalence and aetiology of neuropathic pain in cancer patients: a systematic review. Pain 153: 359–365.
23. Freynhagen R, Baron R, Gockel U, Tölle TR (2006) painDETECT: a new screening questionnaire to identify neuropathic components in patients with back pain. Curr Med Res Opin 22: 1911–1920.
24. Martinez V, Baudic S, Fletcher D (2013) Chronic postsurgical pain. Ann Fr Anesth Reanim 32: 422–435.
25. Perkins FM, Kehlet H (2000) Chronic pain as an outcome of surgery. A review of predictive factors. Anesthesiology 93: 1123–1133.
26. Johansen A, Romundstad L, Nielsen CS, Schirmer H, Stubhaug A (2012) Persistent postsurgical pain in a general population: prevalence and predictors in the Tromso study. Pain 153: 1390–1396.
27. Woolf CJ, Mannion RJ (1999) Neuropathic pain: aetiology, symptoms, mechanisms, and management. Lancet 353 (9168): 1959–1964.
28. Torrance N, Ferguson JA, Afolabi E, Bennett MI, Serpell MG, et al. (2013) Neuropathic pain in the community: more under-treated than refractory? Pain 154: 690–699.
29. Parsons B, Schaefer C, Mann R, Sadosky A, Daniel S, et al. (2013) Economic and humanistic burden of post-trauma and post-surgical neuropathic pain among adults in the United States. J Pain Res 6: 459–469.
30. Pham T, Roy C, Mariette X, Lioté F, Durieux P, et al. (2009) Effect of response format for clinical vignettes on reporting quality of physician practice BMC Health Serv Res 9: 128.
31. Kehlet H, Jensen TS, WJ (2006) Persistent postsurgical pain: risk factors and prevention. Lancet 367: 1618–1625.
32. Finnerup NB, Sindrup SH, Jensen TS (2010) The evidence for pharmacological treatment of neuropathic pain. Pain 150 (3): 573–581.
33. AFFSAPS (2011) Modification des modalités de prescription et de délivrance du Rivotril. Communiqué de presse.
34. Hall GC, Morant SV, Carroll D, Gabriel ZL, McQuay HJ (2013) An observational descriptive study of the epidemiology and treatment of neuropathic pain in a UK general population. BMC Fam Pract 14: 28.
35. Clerc I, Ventelou B, Guerville MA, Paraponaris A, Verger P (2011) General practitioners and clinical practice guidelines: a reexamination. Med Care Res Rev 68:504–518.
36. Veloski JJ, Fields SK, Boex JR, Blank LL (2005) Measuring professionalism: a review of studies with instruments reported in the literature between 1982 and 2002. Acad Med 80: 366–370.
37. Peabody JW, Liu A (2007) A cross-national comparison of the quality of clinical care using vignettes. Health Policy Plan 22: 294–302.
38. Norcini J (2004) Back to the future: clinical vignettes and the measurement of physician performance. Ann Intern Med 141: 813–814.
39. Dresselhaus TR, Peabody JW, Lee M, Wang MM, Luck J (2000) Measuring compliance with preventive care guidelines: standardized patients, clinical vignettes, and the medical record. J Gen Intern Med 15: 782–788.
40. Dumesnil H, Cortaredona S, Verdoux H, Sebbah R, Paraponaris A, et al. (2012) General practitioners' choices and their determinants when starting treatment for major depression: a cross-sectional, randomized case-vignette survey. PLoS One 7 (12): e52429.

Perineural Mast Cells Are Specifically Enriched in Pancreatic Neuritis and Neuropathic Pain in Pancreatic Cancer and Chronic Pancreatitis

Ihsan Ekin Demir[1]*, Stephan Schorn[1], Elisabeth Schremmer-Danninger[1], Kun Wang[2], Timo Kehl[1], Nathalia A. Giese[4], Hana Algül[3], Helmut Friess[1], Güralp O. Ceyhan[1]

1 Department of Surgery, Klinikum rechts der Isar, Technische Universität München, Munich, Germany, **2** Key laboratory of Carcinogenesis and Translational Research (Ministry of Education), Department of Hepatic, Biliary and Pancreatic Surgery, Peking University School of Oncology, Beijing Cancer Hospital and Institute, Beijing, China, **3** Department of Internal Medicine II, Klinikum rechts der Isar, Technische Universität München, Munich, Germany, **4** Department of General Surgery, University of Heidelberg, Heidelberg, Germany

Abstract

Background: Pancreatic neuritis is a histopathological hallmark of pancreatic neuropathy and correlates to abdominal neuropathic pain sensation in pancreatic adenocarcinoma (PCa) and chronic pancreatitis (CP). However, inflammatory cell subtypes that compose pancreatic neuritis and their correlation to the neuropathic pain syndrome in PCa and CP are yet unknown.

Methods: Inflammatory cells within pancreatic neuritis lesions of patients with PCa (n = 20) and CP (n = 20) were immunolabeled and colorimetrically quantified with the pan-leukocyte marker CD45, with CD68 (macrophages), CD8 (cytotoxic T-lymphocytes), CD4 (T-helper cells), CD20 (B-lymphocytes), NCL-PC (plasma cells), neutrophil elastase, PRG2 (eosinophils), anti-mast cell (MC) tryptase and correlated to pain sensation. Perineural mast cell subtypes were analyzed by double immunolabeling with MC chymase. Expression and neural immunoreactivity of protease-activated receptor type 1 (PAR-1) and type 2 (PAR-2) were analyzed in PCa and CP and correlated to pain status of the patients.

Results: In PCa and CP, nerves were predominantly infiltrated by cytotoxic T-lymphocytes (PCa: 35% of all perineural inflammatory cells, CP: 33%), macrophages (PCa: 39%, CP: 33%) and MC (PCa: 21%, CP: 27%). In both entities, neuropathic pain sensation was associated with a specific increase of perineural MC (PCa without pain: 14% vs. PCa with pain: 31%; CP without pain: 19% vs. CP with pain: 34%), not affecting the frequency of other inflammatory cell subtypes. The vast majority of these MC contained MC chymase. PAR-1 and PAR-2 expression did not correlate to the pain sensation of PCa and CP patients.

Conclusion: Pancreatic neuritis in PC and CP is composed of cytotoxic T-lymphocytes, macrophages and MC. The specific enrichment of MC around intrapancreatic nerves in neuropathic pain due to PCa and CP suggests the presence of MC-induced visceral hypersensitivity in the pancreas. Therefore, pancreatic and enteric neuropathies seem to share a similar type of neuro-immune interaction in the generation of visceral pain.

Editor: Anthony W.I. Lo, The Chinese University of Hong Kong, Hong Kong

Funding: These authors have no support or funding to report.

Competing Interests: The authors have declared that no competing interests exist.

* E-mail: ekin.demir@tum.de

These authors contributed equally to this work.

Introduction

Inflammation and cancer are intertwined in the generation, course and outcome of human malignancies. A specific and unique subtype of cancer-related inflammation is encountered around nerves in pancreatic tumours, especially in pancreatic cancer (PCa) and in the inflammatory pancreatic head tumour associated with chronic pancreatitis (CP). Indeed, both of these tumours frequently contain focal inflammatory cell clusters around intrapancreatic nerves [1,2]. In his seminal electron-microscopic study on nerves in CP, Dale Bockman reported on the presence of severe damage in such nerves which were specifically infiltrated by inflammatory cells [3]. Later studies made the deciding contribution related to the importance of this targeted neural immune cell infiltration termed *pancreatic neuritis* in PCa and CP patients: Increasing frequency and severity of pancreatic neuritis have been shown to bear a major correlation to the severity of abdominal pain sensation and neuroplastic alterations in PCa and CP patients [1,4,5].

Mechanisms of pancreatic neuritis remain to be elucidated. Regarding the inflammatory mediators involved in pancreatic neuritis, interleukin-8 (IL-8), the neuronal chemokine fractalkine

Table 1. Primary antibodies.

Antibody	Species	Type	Dilution	Source
Anti - PGP 9.5	Mouse	Monoclonal	1: 1000	DAKO, Hamburg, Germany
Anti – CD45	Rabbit	Polyclonal	1: 500	Antibodies Online, Aachen, Germany
Anti – CD8	Rabbit	Polyclonal	1: 60	Diagnostic BioSystems, CA, USA
Anti – CD4	Rabbit	Polyclonal	1: 60	Monosan, Uden, Netherlands
Anti – CD68	Mouse	Monoclonal	1: 60	Diagnostic BioSystems, CA, USA
Anti-neutrophil elastase (NE)	Rabbit	Polyclonal	1: 2000	Abcam, Cambridge, UK
Anti-CD20	Mouse	Monoclonal	1:500	Novocastra/Leica, Wetzlar, Germany
Anti-PRG2	Rabbit	Polyclonal	1:500	Sigma-Aldrich, Munich, Germany
Anti-NCL-PC	Mouse	Monoclonal	1:16000	Novocastra/Leica, Wetzlar, Germany
Anti-Mast cell tryptase	Rabbit	Monoclonal	1:800	Abcam, Cambridge, UK
Anti-Mast-cell-chymase	Goat	Polyclonal	1:200	Acris Antibodies, Herford, Germany
Anti-PAR-1	Mouse	monoclonal	1:100	Santa Cruz Biotech., Germany
Anti-PAR-2	Rabbit	Polyclonal	1:4000	LifeSpan/Biozol, Eching, Germany

and its receptor CX3CR1 have been shown to be overexpressed in nerves in CP tissue, and increased endoneural fractalkine presence was detected to correlate to the severity of pancreatic neuritis, tissue macrophage infiltration and pain sensation [6–8].

The exact subtypes and characteristics of the immune cells infiltrating pancreatic nerves are yet unknown. In the only study related to this question, Keith et al. demonstrated in a semi-quantitative fashion the increased presence of eosinophils around nerves in CP and the association between pain sensation and the extent of perineural eosinophilic infiltration [9].

A better understanding of characteristics of the perineural inflammatory cell infiltrate in PCa and CP is likely to allow a deep insight into the mechanisms of pancreatic neuritis. Therefore, in the present study, we aimed at providing a systematic quantitative characterization of pancreatic neuritis-associated inflammatory cell clusters in PCa and CP. For this purpose, we quantified peri- and endoneural leukocytes in normal human pancreas (NP), PCa and CP. Furthermore, we investigated the quantitative distribution of a large panel of leukocyte subset markers in PCa and CP tissue, including CD68 (macrophages), CD8 (cytotoxic T-lymphocytes), CD4 (T-helper cells), CD20 (B-lymphocytes), NCL-PC (plasma cells), neutrophil elastase, proteogylcan 2 / PRG2 (eosinophils) and anti-mast cell (MC) tryptase and chymase within neural inflammatory clusters. Finally, we correlated the amount of these neural inflammatory cell subsets, and the expression of two potential receptors (protease-activated-receptor/PAR-1 and PAR-2) for MC-derived proteases to the neuropathic pain sensation of PCa and CP patients.

Materials and Methods

Ethics statement

The study was approved by the ethics committees of the Technische Universität München, Munich, Germany and the University of Heidelberg, Germany.

Patients and tissues

Pancreatic tissue samples for immunohistochemistry were collected from patients following pancreatic head resection for pancreatic cancer (PCa, n = 20; male/female = 8/12, median age = 66 years) and chronic pancreatitis (CP, n = 20; male/female = 13/7, median age = 51 years). All patients were informed, and written consent was obtained for tissue collection. According to the international classification of the UICC (2009), all patients had stage IIb pancreatic cancer. The etiology of CP was alcoholic in all patients. Due to frequently observed concomitant inflammatory process at the resection margins of pancreatic tissue specimens, normal pancreatic tissue samples were obtained from healthy organ donors (NP, n = 10; male/female = 6/4, median age = 38 years) whenever there was no suitable recipient for transplantation available. The tissue collection was approved by the ethics committees of the Technische Universität München, Munich and University of Heidelberg, Germany. The resected pancreatic tissue samples were divided into parts which were immediately fixed in 4% paraformaldehyde followed by paraffin-embedding, as described previously [1,10].

Abdominal pain

In all PCa and CP patients, the individual pain status (Pain vs. No Pain) and the individual pain score (pain intensity and frequency) were prospectively registered prior to the operation, as described previously [2]. Pain intensity was graded by using a short scale: 0 = none, 1 = mild, 2 = moderate and 3 = strong pain. Pain frequency was graded as 3 = daily, 2 = weekly and 1 = monthly. To calculate the severity of pain, pain intensity and pain frequency of each individual were multiplied. According to the final pain score, the patients were divided into three subgroups: Pain I (0) representing the group of patients without pain, Pain II (1–3) patients who suffered from mild pain and Pain III (4–9), with moderate to severe pain.

Immunohistochemistry & double immunofluorescence labeling

Consecutive 3 μm sections from paraffin-embedded NP, PCa and CP samples were analyzed for the pan-neuronal marker Protein Gene Product 9.5 (PGP 9.5) and for inflammatory cell surface markers including cluster of differentiation 45 (CD45) as pan-leukocyte marker, CD8 as marker of cytotoxic T lymphocytes, CD4 to label T helper lymphocytes, CD68 as marker of macrophages, neutrophil elastase (NE) for neutrophilic granulocytes, CD20 for B-lymphocytes, NCL-PC for plasma cells, PRG2 for eosinophils and anti-mast cell (MC) tryptase and anti-MC chymase to identify mast cells. The protease-activated receptor type 1 (PAR-1) and type 2 (PAR-2) were immunolabeled in additional consecutive sections. The sections were incubated with the primary antibodies at the indicated dilutions overnight in a humid chamber at 4°C (Table 1). The negative controls were incubated with the same IgG or IgM subclass non-immunized antibodies. Primary antibody dilutions were performed with normal goat serum. All antigens were detected through the DAKO Envision System-HRP (Hamburg, Germany) or by Alexa Fluor® 488 and 594 antibodies (Invitrogen, Germany) for the matching species. DAB was used as chromogen. Digital imaging was performed with the Keyence Biorevo BZ-9000 system (Keyence, Neu-Isenburg, Germany).

Quantitative analysis of inflammatory cell distribution around nerves

In order to determine the amount of inflammatory cell subtypes around intrapancreatic nerves, the immunostained area occupied by each cell subtype within neural inflammatory cell clusters was measured via the ImageJ software (ImageJ 1.36b, Wayne Rasband). For this purpose, from each section of a patient, between three to five nerves demonstrating pancreatic neuritis were first identified and subsequently photographed with the help of a consecutive PGP9.5-stained section and a consecutive hematoxylin-eosin-stained section. Pancreatic neuritis was histologically defined and identified as "a cluster of neural inflammatory cells which is in contact with the perineurium and/or endoneurium and can clearly be delineated from the remaining general tissue inflammatory cell infiltrate". After conversion of the RGB image to an 8-bit image, threshold function was used to define a phase with the help of a pre-set threshold which solely labels the area occupied by the immunostained neural inflammatory cells, and the software automatically determined the absolute and per cent area of this phase on each image, as also described previously [10]. The absolute areas measured on each image for the immunoreactivity of CD8, CD4, CD68, CD20, NCL-PC, PRG2, NE, anti-MC-tryptase and -chymase were then related to that for CD45 as the pan-leukocyte marker to determine the distribution of inflammatory cell subsets in the pancreatic neuritis cell

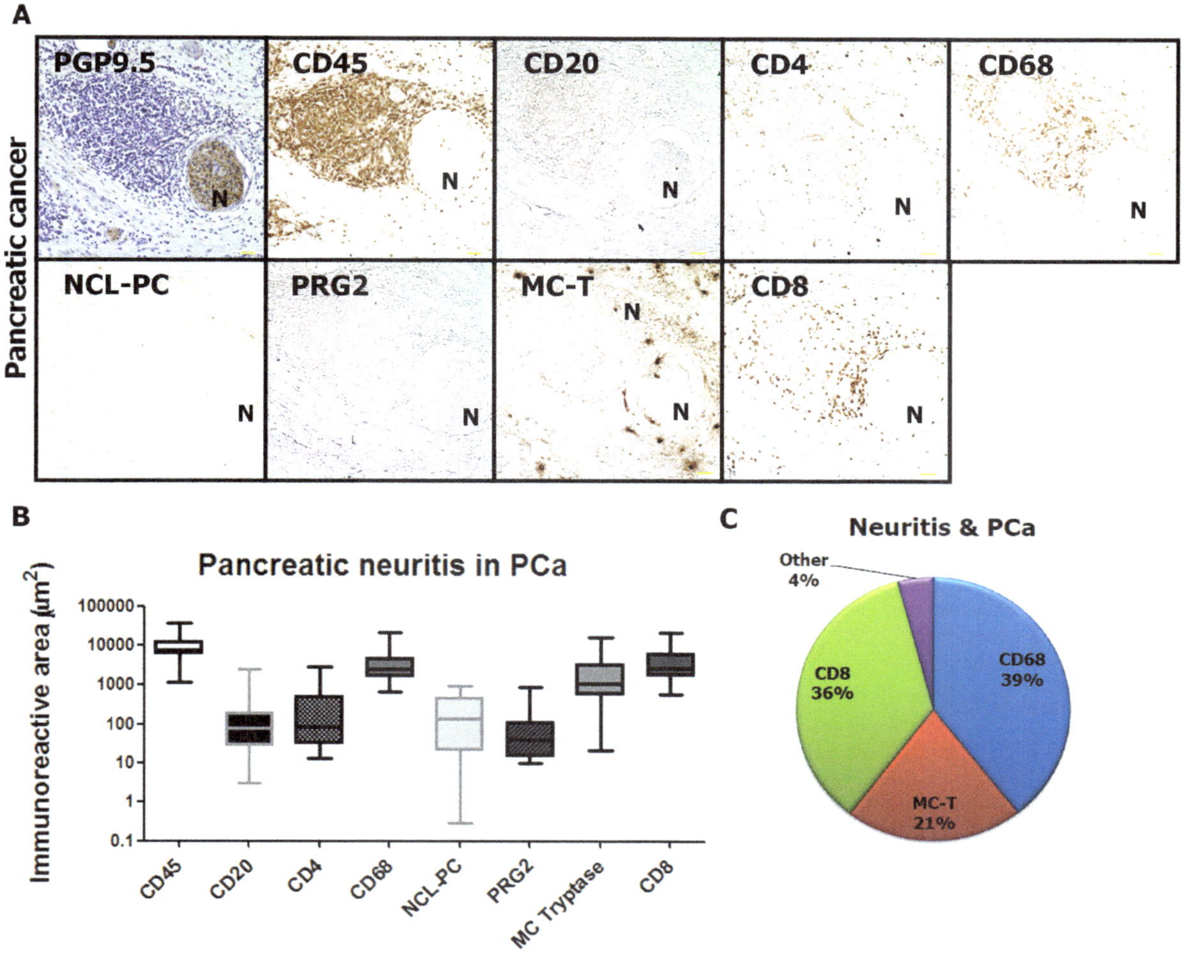

Figure 1. Inflammatory cell subsets composing pancreatic neuritis in pancreatic adenocarcinoma (PCa). (A) Pancreatic neuritis was identified by means of a hematoxylin-counterstained section which was immunolabeled with the pan-neuronal marker PGP9.5 or by means of a hematoyxlin-eosin (H&E)-stained section. Inflammatory cells composing pancreatic neuritis were identified by means of immunolabeling with the pan-leukocyte marker CD45, with CD68 (macrophages), CD8 (cytotoxic T-lymphocytes), CD4 (T-helper cells), CD20 (B-lymphocytes), NCL-PC (plasma cells), neutrophil elastase, PRG2 (eosinophils), anti-mast cell tryptase (MC-T) and correlated to pain sensation. (B–C) In PCa, CD68+ macrophages, $CD8^+$ cytotoxic T lymphocytes and mast cells (MC) dominate the neural inflammatory cell population. "N" stands for the identified nerve. Between three to five nerves with pancreatic neuritis were analyzed from each patient. All images at 200x magnification. Scale bars indicate 50 μm.

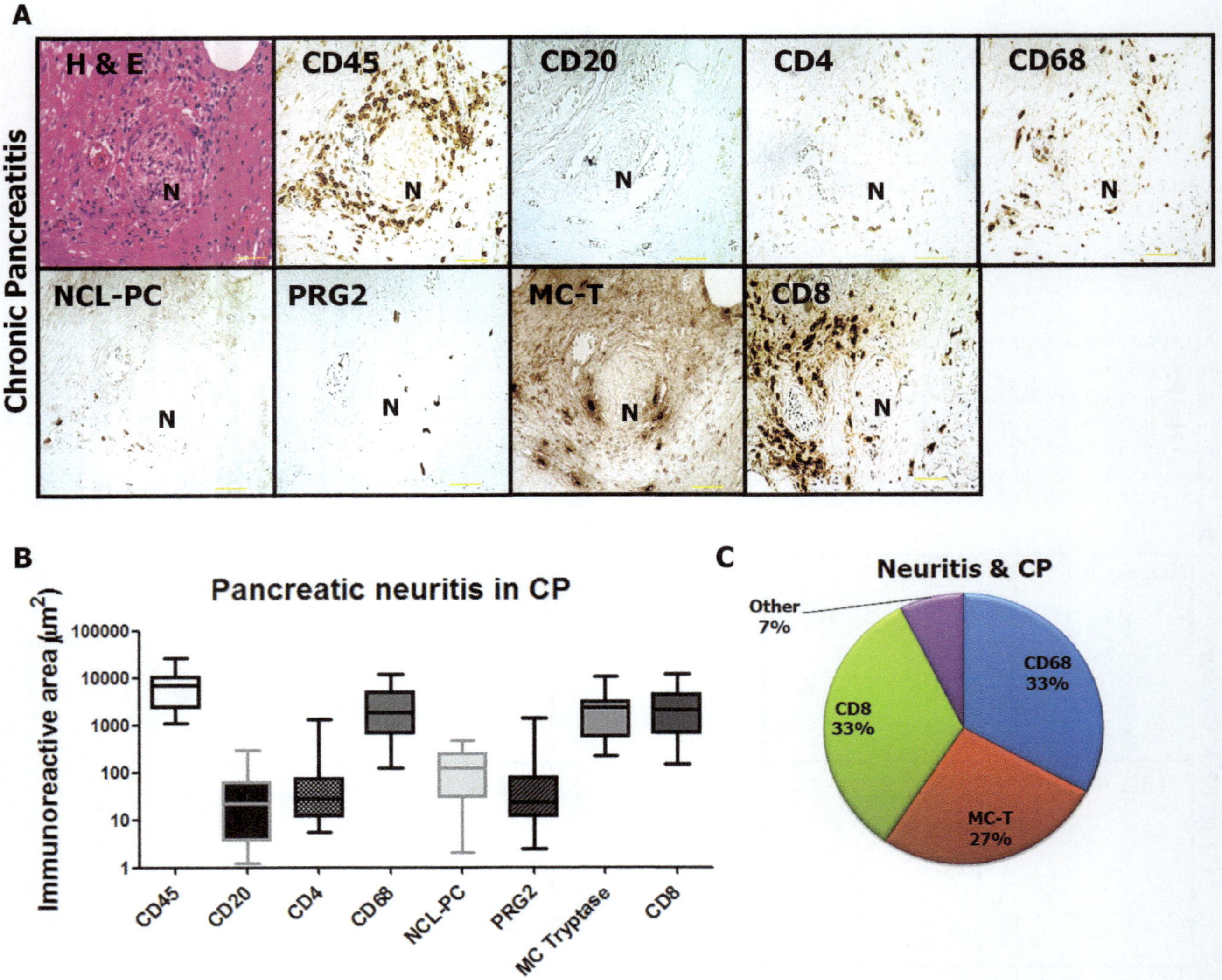

Figure 2. Inflammatory cell subsets composing pancreatic neuritis in chronic pancreatitis (CP). In chronic pancreatitis, pancreatic neuritis showed a similar composition to pancreatic cancer, comprising CD68+ macrophages, $CD8^+$ cytotoxic T lymphocytes and mast cells (MC). "N" stands for the identified nerve. Between three to five nerves with pancreatic neuritis were analyzed from each patient. All images at 200x magnification. Scale bars indicate 50 µm.

population. The photographing and subsequent quantitative analysis were performed by three observers (SS, IED and ESD) blinded to clinical and immunohistochemical data, as described previously [1].

Real-time Light Cycler® Quantitative-Polymerase-Chain-Reaction (QRT-PCR)

Extraction of mRNA from pancreatic tissue was prepared by using TissueLyser II and the RNeasy plus kit (Qiagen/Hilden) according to the manufacturer's instructions. Subsequently, RNA quantity and purity was determined using Nanodrop ND1000 (Peqlab/Erlangen). First-strand cDNA synthesis was performed with the Transcriptor-First-Strand cDNA Synthesis kit (Roche/Mannheim) according to the manufacturer's instructions. Expression of protease-activated-receptor type 1 (PAR-1, GeneBank, GeneID:2149), protease-activated-receptor type 2 (PAR-2, GeneBank, GeneID:2150) and of the reference housekeeping gene cyclophilin-B (CypB, GeneBank, GeneID:5479) were measured with the Roche LightCycler-480 Real-Time PCR System and LightCycler-480 SYBR Green I Master kit. In accordance with the Pfaffl method [11], relative expression was based on the mean crossing-point deviation between the 3 samples normalized to the mean crossing-point deviation for the reference gene, after efficiency correction of the PCR reactions. The relative expression of PAR-1 and PAR-2 in samples was then normalized to the level in normal human pancreas (NP). All primers were obtained from Sigma-Aldrich.

Quantification of neural immunoreactivity for PAR-1 and PAR-2

On each section, the mean neural immunoreactivity for PAR-1 and PAR-2 was determined via ImageJ-based colorimetry, as also shown previously [10]. Briefly, immunolabeled nerves with pancreatic neuritis from each section with PCa or CP were photomicrographed and subjected to the threshold function of the software after conversion into an 8-bit image. The per cent immunostained area in each nerve was determined by the software

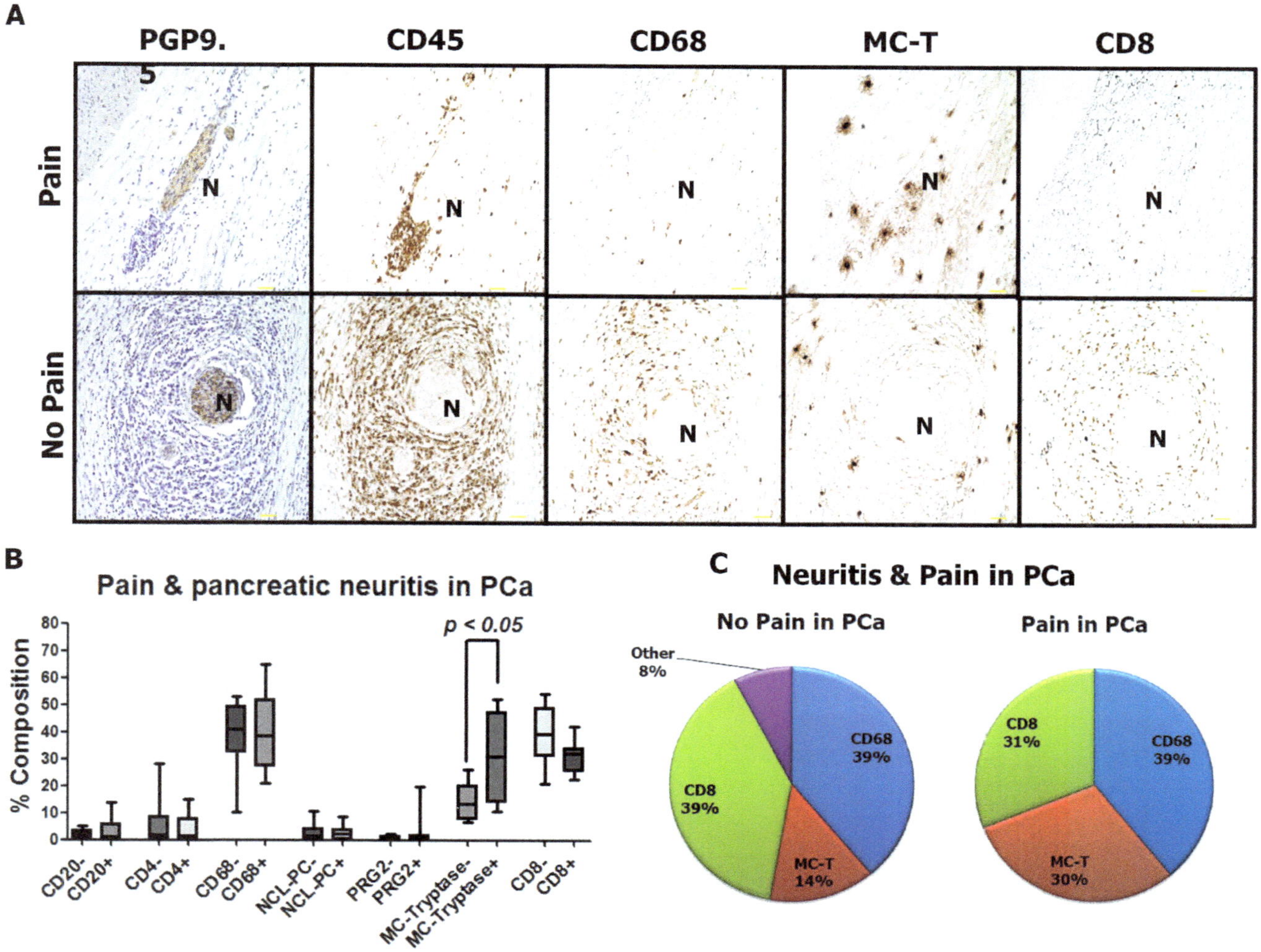

Figure 3. Impact of neuropathic pain upon the composition of pancreatic neuritis in pancreatic adenocarcinoma (PCa). Pain status of PCa patients did not affect the relative distribution of the majority of perineural inflammatory cell subsets in PCa, but it was only mast cells which were specifically enriched around intrapancreatic nerves of PCa patients with pain when compared to patients with no pain. "N" stands for the identified nerve. Between three to five nerves with pancreatic neuritis were analyzed from each patient. All images at 200x magnification. Scale bars indicate 50 μm.

after setting a defined threshold in nerves as regions of interest for each staining (i.e. PAR-1 and PAR-2) and corresponded to neural immunoreactivity. The mean immunoreactivity of each patient was calculated by determining the average neural immunoreactivitiy of all nerves with pancreatic neuritis in each patient.

Statistical analysis

Statistical analysis was performed using the GraphPad Prism 5 Software (La Jolla, CA, USA). For multiple comparisons and due to the interdependence of the measured cell subset areas and percentages within a given neuritis population, Friedman's test followed by Dunn's post hoc test was used. In particular, this test was applied for the comparison of the immunoreactive areas of inflammatory cell subsets, and also for the comparison of their relative (per cent) portion in each neuritis population. For the analysis of PAR-1 and PAR-2 expression between NP, PCa and CP, and for the correlation of neural invasion with perineural mast cell infiltration, Kruskal-Wallis-Test in conjunction with Dunn's post hoc test was used. For comparison of immunoreactivities of each inflammatory cell subtype, and of PAR-1 and PAR-2 neuroimmunoreactivities and expression levels between patients with pain and patients without pain, Mann-Whitney U Test was applied. For these two-group pain analyses, the unpaired t-test was additionally used to confirm the observed differences. For the mast cell subset analysis involving tryptase-chymase co-localization frequency, Fisher's exact test was used. Results are expressed as median (Minimum; Maximum) except for the mRNA expression data which were presented as mean ± standard error of the mean (SEM). Two-sided p-values were always computed, and an effect was considered statistically significant at a p-value ≤ 0.05.

Results

Intrapancreatic nerves in PCa and CP are predominantly infiltrated by cytotoxic T lymphocytes, macrophages and mast cells

As the main aim of the present study, we quantified the amount of leukocytes and leukocyte subpopulations in pancreatic neuritis.

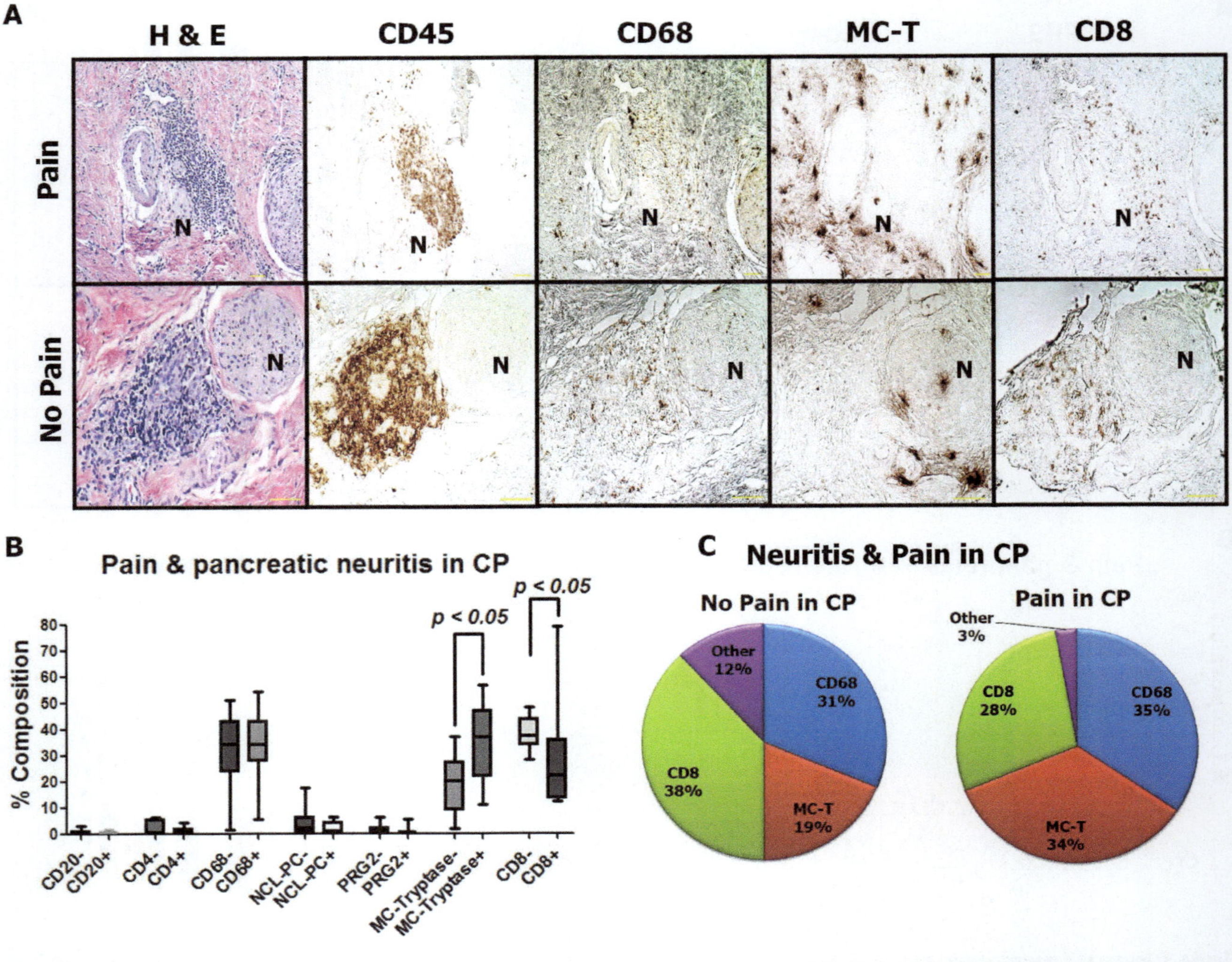

Figure 4. Impact of neuropathic pain upon the composition of pancreatic neuritis in chronic pancreatitis (CP). Similar to PCa, also in CP, patients with pain demonstrated a greater relative amount of mast cells (MC) around intrapancreatic nerves than patients without pain. Furthermore, this increase in the amount of perineural MC was paralleled by decreased amounts of cytotoxic $CD8^+$ T lymphocytes around intrapancreatic nerves. "N" stands for the identified nerve. Between three to five nerves with pancreatic neuritis were analyzed from each patient. All images at 200x magnification. Scale bars indicate 50 μm.

For this purpose, the area occupied by each leukocyte subtype was quantified via colorimetric analysis and expressed in μm^2. In PCa, the pancreatic neuritis immune cell population was mainly composed of $CD68^+$ macrophages [39.87% (10.15; 64.88) of all perineural inflammatory cells, 2545 μm^2 (665.9; 22012)], followed by $CD8^+$ cytotoxic T lymphocytes [33.20% (21.06; 54.11), 2623 μm^2 (586.5; 21092)] and mast cells [MC, 14.46% (0.28; 52.10), 1106 μm^2 (21.51; 16090), Figure 1A–C]. Importantly, all other major inflammatory cell populations were present in hardly detectable amounts [$CD20^+$ B lymphocytes: 0.79% (0.10; 13.84) and 76.84 μm^2 (3.06; 2598); $CD4^+$ T helper cells: 1.61% (0.39; 28.45) and 83.03 μm^2 (13.55; 2962); $NCL\text{-}PC^+$ plasma cells: 1.87% (0.01; 10.54) and 140.9 μm^2 (0.31; 986.9); $PRG2^+$ eosinophils: 0.49% (0.10; 19.77) and 38.71 μm^2 (9.93; 888.8); Figure 1A–C)]. The per cent distribution of leukocyte subpopulations in pancreatic neuritis in PCa is depicted in Figure 1C.

In CP, the distribution of perineural inflammatory cell subtypes strongly resembled that in PCa. Also here, $CD8^+$ cytotoxic T lymphocytes [34.17% (12.27; 78.97) and 2064 μm^2 (142.7; 11334)], $CD68^+$ macrophages [34.40% (1.562; 54.22) and 1852 μm^2 (126.9; 11667)] and mast cells [24.16% (1.78; 56.63) and 2339 μm^2 (221.1; 10155)] were most prevalent in pancreatic neuritis lesions (Figure 2A–C). The remaining inflammatory cell subtypes were only occasionally detected around intrapancreatic nerves [$CD20^+$ B lymphocytes: 0.57% (0.07; 3.19) and 21.93 μm^2 (1.27; 293.9); $CD4^+$ T helper cells: 0.56% (0.16; 6.22) and 27.77 μm^2 (5.38; 1325); $NCL\text{-}PC^+$ plasma cells: 1.20% (0.05; 17.44)and 121.3 μm^2 (2.08; 474.3); $PRG2^+$ eosinophils: 0.61% (0.13; 6.24) and 23.33 μm^2 (2.41; 1384); Figure 2A–C]. The per cent distribution of leukocyte subpopulations in pancreatic neuritis in CP is depicted in Figure 2C.

Neuropathic pain in PCa is associated with specifically increased mast cell infiltration around intrapancreatic nerves

One of the major aims of this study was to compare the distribution of the above-mentioned leukocyte subpopulations

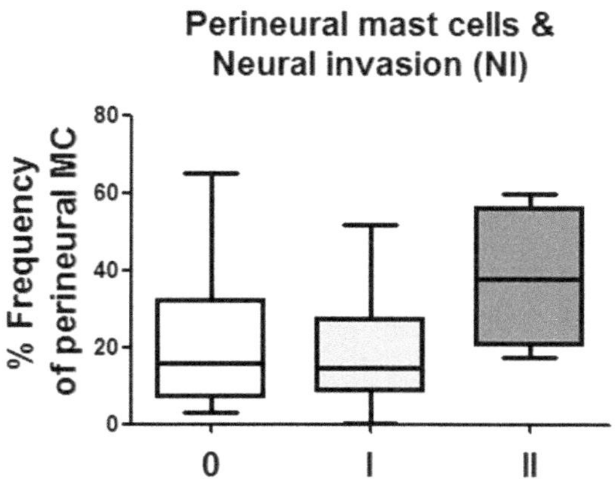

Figure 5. Neural invasion in pancreatic cancer (PCa) and perineural mast cell infiltration. Intrapancreatic nerves in PCa tissues were evaluated for the presence of neural invasion (NI) and classified into the NI degrees "0 / no invasion", "1 / peri-neural invasion" and "2 / endo-neural invasion). In our cohort, the relative perineural mast cell amounts did not differ between the varying degrees of NI in human PCa. Results are presented as median (minimum; maximum).

among PCa patients with and without abdominal pain. Looking at the whole amount of leukocytes in the neural inflammatory cell infiltrates, PCa patients with pain did not demonstrate any difference in the size of the inflammatory cell population per nerve [7574 μm^2 (3121; 36358)] when compared to PCa patients without pain [7320 μm^2 (1155; 33793)]. The analysis of inflammatory cell subtypes revealed that there was a shift in the distribution of only a single inflammatory cell subset among PCa patients with pain: The amount of perineural mast cells was specifically increased among PCa patients with pain [PCaP, 30.96% (10.75; 52.10) and 3081 μm^2 (21.51; 16090)] than among patients without pain [PCaN, 13.41% (6.64; 26.29) and 777.6 μm^2 (69.93; 3228), $p < 0.05$ Figure 3A–C]. All other inflammatory cell subtypes did not demonstrate any significant variation with the pain status of PCa patients [CD8$^+$ cytotoxic T lymphocytes in PCaP: 32.22% (22.62; 42.07) and 2802 μm^2 (116; 10933) vs. 39.57% (21.06; 54.11) and 2208 μm^2 (586.5; 21092) in PCaN; CD68$^+$ macrophages: 38.74% (21.21; 64.88) and 2628 μm^2 (1214; 22012) in PCaP vs. 40.99% (10.15; 53.00) and 2486 μm^2 (665.9; 8097) in PCaN; CD20$^+$ B lymphocytes: 0.77% (0.23; 5.11) and 70.64 μm^2 (3.36; 2598) in PCaP vs. 1.1% (0.10; 13.84) and 83.04 μm^2 (3.06; 418.8) in PCaN; CD4$^+$ T helper cells: 1.42% (0.39; 15.13) and 82.62 μm^2 (30.62; 562.9) in PCaP vs. 1.79% (0.41; 28.45) and 83.03 μm^2 (13.55; 2962) in PCaN; NCL-PC$^+$ plasma cells: 2.08% (0.01; 8.61) and 245.4 μm^2 (0.31; 986.9) in PCaP vs. 1.46% (0.20; 10.54) and 69.83 μm^2 (9.50; 597.9) in PCaN; PRG2$^+$ eosinophils: 0.50% (0.14; 19.77) and 48.98 μm^2 (10.75; 888.8) in PCaP and 0.53% (0.10; 2.44) and 26.99 μm^2 (9.93; 156.6) in PCaN; Figure 3A–C). The per cent distribution of leukocyte subpopulations in pancreatic neuritis among PCa patients with versus without pain is depicted in Figure 3C.

Neuropathic pain in CP is characterized by increased perineural mast cell infiltration and suppression of perineural cytotoxic T lymphocytes in pancreatic neuritis

Although pancreatic neuritis was first described in CP by some pioneering studies [5,9], the influence of pain upon the distribution of inflammatory cell subsets in CP-associated pancreatic neuritis are widely unknown. When we compared the amount of leukocytes around intrapancreatic nerves in CP patients with vs. without pain, there were interestingly smaller amounts of perineural inflammatory cells among CP patients with pain [(CPP, median perineural CD45-immunoreactive area: 4333 μm^2 (1118; 10375)] than among CP patients without pain [(CPN, median perineural CD45-immunoreactive area: 9831 μm^2 (1687; 25685)]. This shrinkage of the perineural inflammatory cell infiltrate in CPP was accompanied by a specific increase in the relative proportion of mast cells in this inflammatory cell proportion [CPP: 36.93% (10.92; 56.63) vs. CPN: 20.25% (1.78; 37.22)], but not in the absolute amounts of perineural mast cells [CPP: 1546 μm^2 (455.8; 3129) vs. CPN: 2833 μm^2 (221.1; 7396)]. Furthermore, both the absolute and the relative amount of CD8$^+$ T lymphocytes were diminished in painful CP [CPP: 22.35% (12.27; 78.97) and 768.6 μm^2 (142.7; 11334) vs. CPN: 37.32% (28.31; 48.09) and 3628 μm^2 (653.0; 7365)]. There were no further major alterations in the relative or absolute amounts of other inflammatory cell subtypes among CP patients with pain [CD68$^+$ macrophages: 34.40% (5.57; 54.22) and 1409 μm^2 (546.8; 4811) in CPP vs. 34.29% (1.56; 51.03) and 3129 μm^2 (126.9; 6613) in CPN; CD20$^+$ B lymphocytes: 0.50% (0.07; 1.65) and 7.07 μm^2 (1.27; 40.86) in CPP vs. 0.76% (0.08; 3.19) and 61.42 μm^2 (2.57; 293.9) in CPN; CD4$^+$ T helper cells: 0.50% (0.16; 4.10) and 14.47 μm^2 (5.38; 208.3) in CPP vs. 0.87% (0.28; 6.22) and 46.73 μm^2 (21.97; 351.2) in CPN; NCL-PC$^+$ plasma cells: 1.06% (0.05; 6.32) and 49.05 μm^2 (2.08; 264.0) in CPP vs. 2.38% (0.45; 17.44) and 151.5 μm^2 (8.58; 474.3) in CPN; PRG2$^+$ eosinophils: 0.42% (0.15; 5.48) and 16.22 μm^2 (2.41; 174.1) in CPP and 0.94% (0.13; 6.24) and 39.42 μm^2 (3.34; 1384) in CPN; Figure 4A–C)]. The per cent distribution of leukocyte subpopulations in pancreatic neuritis among CP patients with versus without pain is depicted in Figure 4C.

Perineural mast cell infiltration does not correlate to neural invasion in pancreatic cancer

Neural invasion (NI) is one of the histopathological hallmarks of PCa and is encountered in up to 100% of PCa specimens [12]. As we observed a specific increase in the amount of perineural MC in painful PCa, one major question which arose at this point was whether perineural MC infiltration also correlates to enhanced tumor invasion of nerves. For this purpose, we classified the severity of NI in PCa specimens into three categories ("0/no invasion", "I/peri-neural invasion" and "II/endo-neural invasion"[1]) and correlated the NI severity to the relative amount of perineural MC. Here, there was no correlation between perineural MC infiltration and increasing severity of NI in PCa [no invasion/ Grade 0: 15.73% (3.08; 65.16), peri-neural invasion/Grade I: 14.79% (0.34; 51.71) and endo-neural invasion/Grade II: 37.67% (17.65; 60.05), $p = 0.08$, Figure 5].

Expression and neural immunoreactivity of PAR-1 and PAR-2 in PCa and CP

Neurons can become sensitized by the action of thrombin upon the protease-activated receptor type 1 (PAR-1) or of MC-derived proteases (such as tryptase) upon protease-activated receptor type 2 (PAR-2) [13]. As we observed significantly elevated mast cell amounts around intrapancreatic nerves in PCa and CP, we also quantified the levels of PAR-1 and PAR-2 in these tissues and additionally in intrapancreatic nerves. Here, the comparison of mRNA expression for PAR-1 and PAR-2 in NP, PCa and CP did not show any major difference in the levels of these receptors (Figure 6A). Similarly, when PCa and CP patients were stratified into the "No Pain" and "Pain" groups, the mRNA levels of these

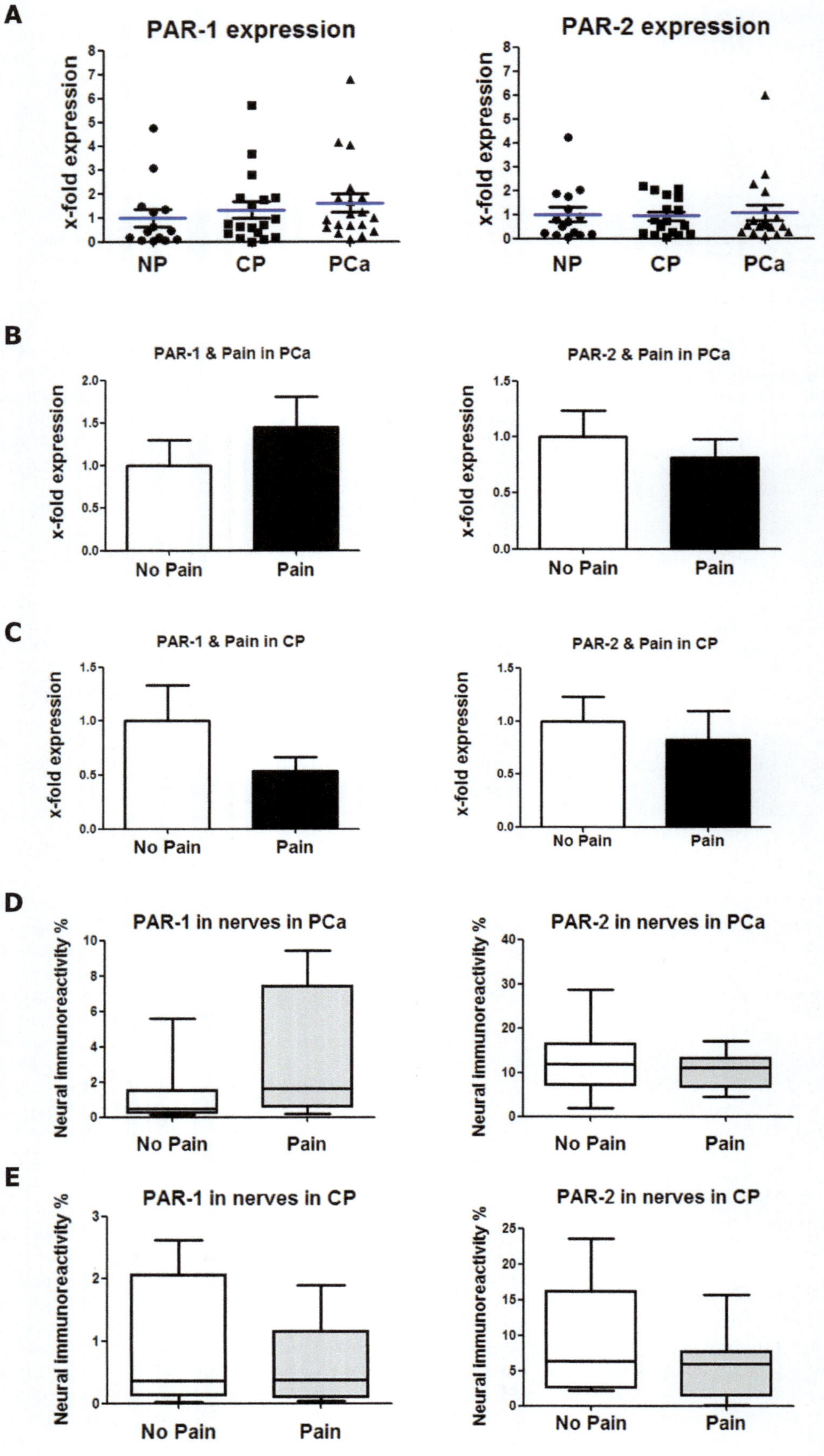
A
PAR-1 expression
PAR-2 expression
x-fold expression
NP
CP
PCa
B
PAR-1 & Pain in PCa
PAR-2 & Pain in PCa
x-fold expression
No Pain
Pain
C
PAR-1 & Pain in CP
PAR-2 & Pain in CP
x-fold expression
No Pain
Pain
D
PAR-1 in nerves in PCa
PAR-2 in nerves in PCa
Neural immunoreactivity %
No Pain
Pain
E
PAR-1 in nerves in CP
PAR-2 in nerves in CP
Neural immunoreactivity %
No Pain
Pain

Figure 6. Protease-activated-receptor (PAR) type 1 (PAR-1) and type 2 (PAR-2) in human pancreatic cancer (PCa) and chronic pancreatitis (CP). (A) Expression of PAR-1 and PAR-2 was compared between normal human pancreas (NP), CP and PCa tissues via qRT-PCR and did not differ between these three entities. Expression was normalized first to the housekeeping gene cyclophilin B and then to NP. (B) In PCa, the tissue levels of PAR-1 and PAR-2 did not differ between patients with pain versus patients without pain. (C) Similarly, also in CP, there was no difference in the tissue mRNA levels of PAR-1 and PAR-2 in patients with no pain versus with pain. (D) Intrapancreatic nerves in PCa were analyzed for the immunoreactivity for PAR-1 and PAR-2 and correlated to the pain status of patients. Here, pain sensation was not associated with differences in the immunoreactivity of intrapancreatic nerves for PAR-1 or PAR-2. (E) In analogy with PCa, also in CP, patients with pain exhibited similar immunoreactivities in nerves for PAR-1 and PAR-2 as patients without pain.

receptors were not different between these groups (Figure 6B–C). When the neural immunoreactivities of these receptors were compared between patients with and without pain, PCa patients with pain tended to exhibit a slightly greater immunoreactivity for PAR-1 [3.272% (0.20;9.44)] than those without pain [1.22% (0.14;5.57), Figure 6D]. However, there was no difference in the PAR-2 immunoreactivity in PCa patients with pain [11.06% (4.45; 17.23)] versus without pain [11.90% (1.843; 28.64), (Figure 6D)]. Similarly, the pain status of CP patients had no influence on the neural immunoreactivity for PAR-1 or PAR-2 in our cohort (Figure 6E).

Neuropathic pain-associated perineural mast cells in PCa and CP are MC_{TC}–type mast cells

In humans, MC can be classified based on their mediator content into two categories: MC_T-type mast cells which contain heparin and tryptase, and MC_{TC}-type mast cells which additionally contain the proteolytic enzyme "chymase" [14]. To determine the prevalent mast cell phenotype in PCa, CP and NP, we performed double-immunofluoresence labelling in pancreatic tissues against mast cell tryptase and mast cell chymase. In NP, mast cells were nearly not detectable at all around intrapancreatic nerves. In all NP patients who were included in the analysis, we could only find three nerves which showed a close spatial association with inflammatory cells. The double immunolabeling of these mast cells showed that all of these cells contained both tryptase and chymase [100% (100;100)], thus classifying them as MC_{TC}-type mast cells (Figure 7A). On the other hand, both in PCa and CP, MC_{TC} type mast cells were again the predominant perineural mast cell phenotype (81.7 ± 4.9% and 77.0 ± 4.0%, respectively), but both disease entities additionally contained perineural MC_T type (tryptase-only) mast cells (18.3 ± 4.9% and 23.7 ± 4.0%, respectively). The subgroup analysis considering the pain status of the patients showed a similar distribution of perineural MC_{TC} and MC_T type mast cells in PCa patients with pain (MC_{TC}: 85.6 ± 6.4% and MC_T: 14.4 ± 6.4%) versus those without pain (MC_{TC}: 77.4 ± 7.4% and MC_T: 22.6 ± 7.4%, Figure 6A). In contrast, CP patients with pain exhibited significantly greater proportions of perineural MC_{TC}-type mast cells (MC_{TC}: 86.9 ± 4.4% and MC_T: 13.1 ± 4.3%, $p<0.0001$) than CP patients without pain (MC_{TC}: 62.9 ± 6.4% and MC_T: 37.1 ± 6.4%; Figure 6A).

Due this observed predominance of chymase-containing perineural mast cells in PCa and CP, we used mast cell chymase as additional marker to verify the specific increase of perineural mast cells in painful PCa and CP. Similar to our observations with mast cell tryptase labeling, pain in PCa and CP was associated with greater relative amounts of chymase-immunoreactive perineural mast cells [PCaP:8.73% (2.53; 16.82) and CPP: 3.70% (0.10; 41.26)] than pain-free PCa and CP [PCaN:0.75% (0.04; 8.71) and CPN: 0.65% (0.01; 7.87), $p<0.05$, Figure 6B].

Discussion

The present study was designed to characterize the cellular subtypes within inflammatory cell infiltrates comprising pancreatic neuritis in human pancreatic cancer (PCa) and chronic pancreatitis (CP). It could demonstrate that cytotoxic T lymphocytes, macrophages and MC are the dominant cell populations in pancreatic neuritis in PCa and CP. Most importantly, out of all cells comprising pancreatic neuritis, it was only perineural MC which were uniquely increased in number around intrapancreatic nerves in PCa and CP patients with neuropathic abdominal pain sensation. The phenotype analysis of these MC revealed their predominant phenotype as chymase-containing MC_{TC} cells.

The presence of pancreatic neuritis is known to correlate to the severity of abdominal pain sensation of PCa and CP patients [1,5]. Furthermore, its degree also bears an association with neuroplastic alterations in PCa and CP, including increased neural density and neural hypertrophy [1]. Moreover, pancreatic neuritis represents the pancreatic counterpart of visceral neuro-inflammation, which is encountered in numerous gastrointestinal (GI) disorders including inflammatory bowel disease (IBD) [15], irritable bowel syndrome (IBS) [16] and appendicitis [17]. In all these disorders, visceral neuro-inflammation is closely related to the generation of pain and organ dysfunction [15]. Therefore, the implications of our findings could be understood in the light of these important aspects of visceral neuro-inflammation.

The generation of pancreatic pain is still only incompletely understood [18,19]. So far, it has become clear that sensitization of nociceptors and neuroplastic alterations at the periphery (i.e. in the pancreas) are closely related to the severity of pain of PCa and CP patients [20]. For CP, it has further been shown that concomitant plasticity in viscero-sensory areas of the central nervous system is present among CP patients with severe pain sensation [19]. The major question which arises at this point is whether perineural intrapancreatic MC can be responsible for the induction of peripheral nociceptive sensitization and peripheral neuroplasticity with consequent central hypersensitivity.

Indeed, there is a considerable number of visceral painful disorders in which MC have been shown to be specifically enriched around intra-organ nerve fibers and correlate to the extent of pain sensation [21]. MC are resident immune cells in the GI tract, skin, lung, brain and other tissues and are classically known as mediators of type I hypersensitivity reactions to allergens or anaphylactic agents by releasing a large set of MC-derived degranulation products like histamine, serotonin, cytokines, prostaglandins, etc. [22]. Moreover, they exhibit a very close spatial association with intra-organ nerves (found sometimes as close as 20 nm away from nerve endings[23]) and a bi-directional mast-cell-neuron-communication [22]. Particularly, mast cells are found in close association with peptidergic nerve fibers containing substance P (SP), calcitonin-gene-related-peptide (CGRP) [24] or those containing nerve growth factor (NGF) which can all bind to their specific receptors on MC and entail MC activation and degranulation [25–27]. Conversely, activated degranulating MC release neuron-activating molecules like histamine, serotonin,

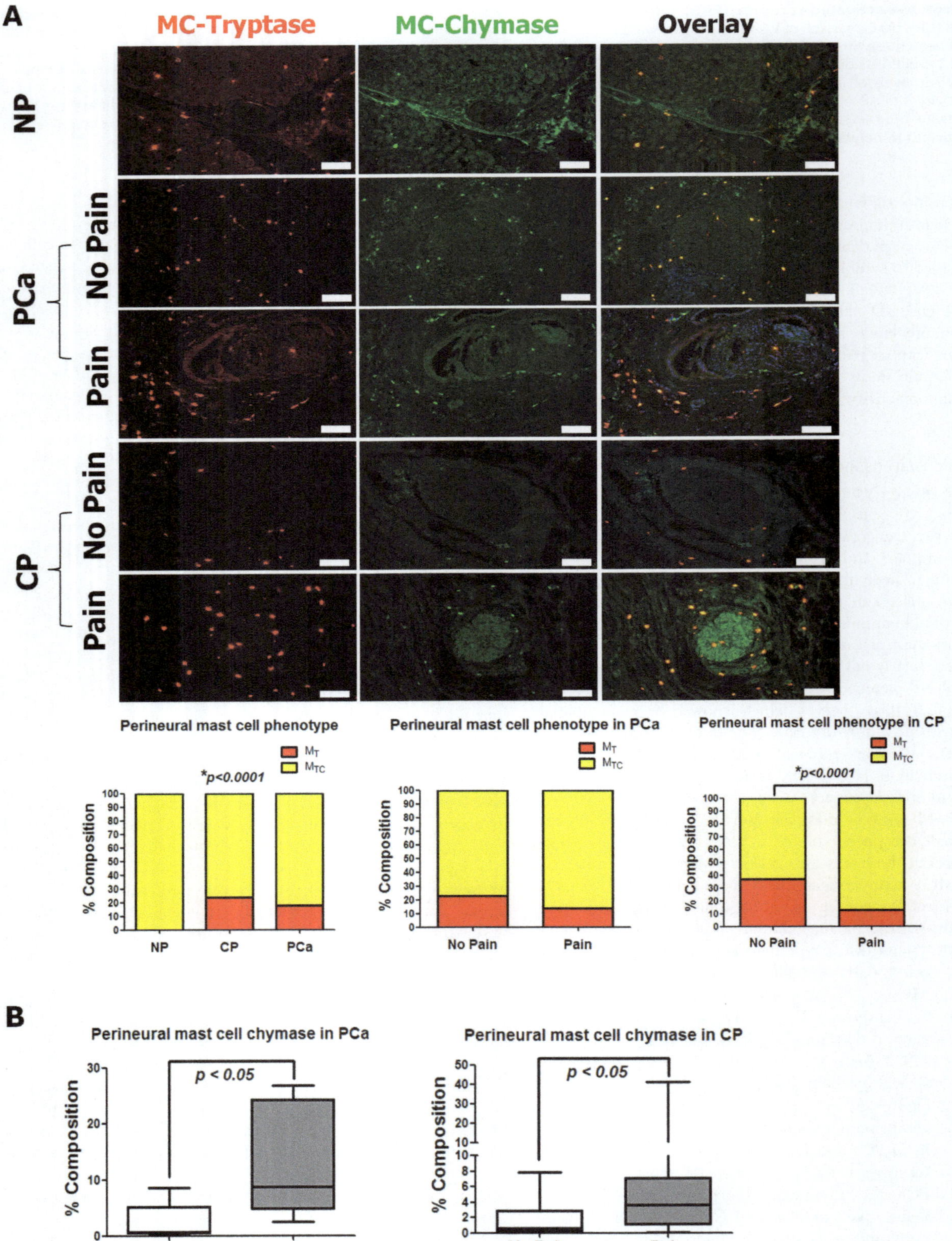

Figure 7. Analysis of mast cell (MC) phenotype in NP, PCa and CP. (A) Human pancreatic tissue samples from NP, PCa and CP were double-immunolabeled for perineural MC-tryptase (red) and MC-chymase (green). In all three entities, the vast majority of perineural MC demonstrated double immunoreactivity (yellow in overlay) for MC-tryptase and -chymase. In CP, there were significantly greater relative amounts of double-immunoreactive MC among patients with pain than among those without pain. The white scale bars indicate 100 μm. (B) In accordance with

increased perineural MC-tryptase in painful PCa and CP, the perineural MC chymase immunoreactivity was significantly greater among PCa and CP patients with pain than in patients without pain. Results are expressed as median (Minimum; Maximum).

NGF, proteases including MC tryptase which can also activate and sensitize peripheral neurons via their corresponding receptors (H1-4, 5HT-3, tyrosine-kinase-receptor A/TrkA, protease-activated-receptor-1/PAR-1) causing pain and dysregulation of neuronal function [28]. Accordingly, neuron-MC-interactions are intensively investigated to understand the pathogenesis of pain in several disorders including migraine, interstitial cystitis, ulcerative colitis, etc.[16,29,30]. In IBS, administration of the MC stabilizing agent ketotifen was recently shown to relieve abdominal pain of IBS patients [31]. Ketotifen is a MC-stabilizing and antihistaminic agent and can inhibit the release of neuron-activating MC-mediators like histamine and tryptase from MC [32]. Based on our results and previous observations on IBS, we believe that administration of such MC-stabilizing agents may reduce the action of these neuron-activating MC-derived factors and can have similar analgesic effects in human PCa and CP.

Neuroplasticity in PCa and CP is characterized by increased presence of neurotrophic factors like NGF, artemin, neurturin and their receptors in intrapancreatic nerves [33,34]. Furthermore, in CP, increased expression of the neuropeptides SP and CGRP has been reported to correlate to the pain sensation of CP patients [35]. Anti-NGF-antibody administration was shown to decrease pancreatic nociceptor excitability in a rat model of CP [36]. Furthermore, in the course of neurogenic inflammation, protease-activated receptors (PAR) are crucially involved in the generation of pancreatic pain [37,38]. Therefore, current literature contains a large series of studies which could demonstrate the overexpression and the involvement of numerous key mediators in the generation of pancreatic pain, and all these molecules are actually known to be crucially involved in the bi-directional communication between MC and nociceptive neurons. Based on our analysis of PAR-1 and PAR-2 in PCa and CP, it seems that these receptors are not differentially regulated in these diseases. However, their presence in intrapancreatic nerves suggests that they may still serve as the receptors for MC-derived proteases.

Intratumoral MC infiltration is a well characterized factor promoting PCa cell invasiveness. Indeed, MC-conditioned media were previously reported to increase the invasiveness, proliferation and migration of PCa cells in vitro [39]. Furthermore, MC infiltration was reported to correlate to higher tumor grade and diminished survival in PCa [39]. However, in our study, there was no correlation between perineural MC infiltration and increasing severity of neural invasion in PCa. Therefore, looking at our results, we assume that perineural mast cell infiltration is primarily related to neuropathic pain and less to the extent of tumor invasion in PCa.

Interestingly, there was a single study which ascribed a role to MC in pancreatic nociception [40]. Here, Hoogerwerf et al. reported increased MC counts in the *whole* pancreatic tissue of CP patients and could also demonstrate decreased abdominal tactile sensitivity of MC-deficient mice with CP [40]. However, the study did not investigate the role of perineural MC which are known to be the actual interacting partner for neurons [23]. Furthermore, there are no other studies in the literature which addressed the potential role of MC in pancreatic neuropathic pain in human PCa.

In summary, the present study elucidated for the first time the major subtypes of inflammatory cells involved in pancreatic neuritis in PCa and CP. Pancreatic neuritis lesions in PCa and CP are mainly composed of cytotoxic T-lymphocytes, macrophages and MC. However, in both disease entities, it is only MC which are uniquely increased in number around intrapancreatic nerves of patients with concomitant abdominal neuropathic pain sensation.

In conclusion, due to the well-established role of MC in numerous painful disorders including enteric neuropathies, MC may be the key inflammatory cell subtype in the generation of pancreatic nociceptor hyperexcitabilty in PCa and CP. Therefore, future studies shall investigate the impact of MC-modulation or MC-stabilization upon pain sensation in experimental and clinical PCa and CP.

Acknowledgments

The authors are grateful to Mr. Bernhard Haller (Institute of Medical Statistics and Epidemiology at Technische Universität München) for the statistical review of the manuscript. The authors also thank Ms. Ulrike Bourquain for her outstanding technical assistance.

Author Contributions

Supervised the experiments: HF IED TK HA GOC. Conceived and designed the experiments: HF GOC HA IED. Performed the experiments: SS ESD IED KW. Analyzed the data: IED SS ESD NAG TK. Wrote the paper: IED SS ESD KW TK HA HF GOC.

References

1. Ceyhan GO, Bergmann F, Kadihasanoglu M, Altintas B, Demir IE, et al. (2009) Pancreatic neuropathy and neuropathic pain--a comprehensive pathomorphological study of 546 cases. Gastroenterology 136: 177-186 e171.
2. Ceyhan GO, Bergmann F, Kadihasanoglu M, Erkan M, Park W, et al. (2007) The neurotrophic factor artemin influences the extent of neural damage and growth in chronic pancreatitis. Gut 56: 534-544.
3. Bockman DE, Buchler M, Malfertheiner P, Beger HG (1988) Analysis of nerves in chronic pancreatitis. Gastroenterology 94: 1459-1469.
4. Ceyhan GO, Demir IE, Maak M, Friess H (2010) Fate of nerves in chronic pancreatitis: Neural remodeling and pancreatic neuropathy. Best Pract Res Clin Gastroenterol 24: 311-322.
5. Di Sebastiano P, Fink T, Weihe E, Friess H, Innocenti P, et al. (1997) Immune cell infiltration and growth-associated protein 43 expression correlate with pain in chronic pancreatitis. Gastroenterology 112: 1648-1655.
6. Ceyhan GO, Deucker S, Demir IE, Erkan M, Schmelz M, et al. (2009) Neural fractalkine expression is closely linked to pain and pancreatic neuritis in human chronic pancreatitis. Lab Invest 89: 347-361.
7. Di Sebastiano P, di Mola FF, Di Febbo C, Baccante G, Porreca E, et al. (2000) Expression of interleukin 8 (IL-8) and substance P in human chronic pancreatitis. Gut 47: 423-428.
8. D'Haese JG, Demir IE, Friess H, Ceyhan GO (2010) Fractalkine/CX3CR1: why a single chemokine-receptor duo bears a major and unique therapeutic potential. Expert Opin Ther Targets 14: 207-219.
9. Keith RG, Keshavjee SH, Kerenyi NR (1985) Neuropathology of chronic pancreatitis in humans. Can J Surg 28: 207-211.
10. Ceyhan GO, Demir IE, Rauch U, Bergmann F, Muller MW, et al. (2009) Pancreatic neuropathy results in "neural remodeling" and altered pancreatic innervation in chronic pancreatitis and pancreatic cancer. Am J Gastroenterol 104: 2555-2565.
11. Pfaffl MW (2001) A new mathematical model for relative quantification in real-time RT-PCR. Nucleic Acids Res 29: e45.
12. Demir IE, Ceyhan GO, Liebl F, D'Haese JG, Maak M, et al. (2010) Neural Invasion in Pancreatic Cancer: The Past, Present and Future. Cancers 2: 1513-1527.
13. Corvera CU, Dery O, McConalogue K, Gamp P, Thoma M, et al. (1999) Thrombin and mast cell tryptase regulate guinea-pig myenteric neurons through proteinase-activated receptors-1 and -2. J Physiol 517 (Pt 3): 741-756.
14. Galli SJ, Borregaard N, Wynn TA (2011) Phenotypic and functional plasticity of cells of innate immunity: macrophages, mast cells and neutrophils. Nat Immunol 12: 1035-1044.

15. Vasina V, Barbara G, Talamonti L, Stanghellini V, Corinaldesi R, et al. (2006) Enteric neuroplasticity evoked by inflammation. Auton Neurosci 126-127: 264-272.
16. Barbara G, Stanghellini V, De Giorgio R, Cremon C, Cottrell GS, et al. (2004) Activated mast cells in proximity to colonic nerves correlate with abdominal pain in irritable bowel syndrome. Gastroenterology 126: 693-702.
17. Di Sebastiano P, Fink T, di Mola FF, Weihe E, Innocenti P, et al. (1999) Neuroimmune appendicitis. Lancet 354: 461-466.
18. Demir IE, Tieftrunk E, Maak M, Friess H, Ceyhan GO (2011) Pain mechanisms in chronic pancreatitis: of a master and his fire. Langenbecks Arch Surg 396: 151-160.
19. Drewes AM, Krarup AL, Detlefsen S, Malmstrom ML, Dimcevski G, et al. (2008) Pain in chronic pancreatitis: the role of neuropathic pain mechanisms. Gut 57: 1616-1627.
20. Ceyhan GO, Michalski CW, Demir IE, Muller MW, Friess H (2008) Pancreatic pain. Best Pract Res Clin Gastroenterol 22: 31-44.
21. Wood JD (2011) Visceral pain: spinal afferents, enteric mast cells, enteric nervous system and stress. Curr Pharm Des 17: 1573-1575.
22. Bauer O, Razin E (2000) Mast Cell-Nerve Interactions. News Physiol Sci 15: 213-218.
23. Stead RH, Dixon MF, Bramwell NH, Riddell RH, Bienenstock J (1989) Mast cells are closely apposed to nerves in the human gastrointestinal mucosa. Gastroenterology 97: 575-585.
24. Stead RH, Tomioka M, Quinonez G, Simon GT, Felten SY, et al. (1987) Intestinal mucosal mast cells in normal and nematode-infected rat intestines are in intimate contact with peptidergic nerves. Proc Natl Acad Sci U S A 84: 2975-2979.
25. Jippo T, Ushio H, Hirota S, Mizuno H, Yamatodani A, et al. (1994) Poor response of cultured mast cells derived from mi/mi mutant mice to nerve growth factor. Blood 84: 2977-2983.
26. De Jonge F, De Laet A, Van Nassauw L, Brown JK, Miller HR, et al. (2004) In vitro activation of murine DRG neurons by CGRP-mediated mucosal mast cell degranulation. Am J Physiol Gastrointest Liver Physiol 287: G178-191.
27. Krumins SA, Broomfield CA (1993) C-terminal substance P fragments elicit histamine release from a murine mast cell line. Neuropeptides 24: 5-10.
28. Buhner S, Schemann M (2012) Mast cell-nerve axis with a focus on the human gut. Biochim Biophys Acta 1822: 85-92.
29. Hagiyama M, Furuno T, Hosokawa Y, Iino T, Ito T, et al. (2011) Enhanced nerve-mast cell interaction by a neuronal short isoform of cell adhesion molecule-1. J Immunol 186: 5983-5992.
30. Levy D, Kainz V, Burstein R, Strassman AM (2012) Mast cell degranulation distinctly activates trigemino-cervical and lumbosacral pain pathways and elicits widespread tactile pain hypersensitivity. Brain Behav Immun 26: 311-317.
31. Klooker TK, Braak B, Koopman KE, Welting O, Wouters MM, et al. (2010) The mast cell stabiliser ketotifen decreases visceral hypersensitivity and improves intestinal symptoms in patients with irritable bowel syndrome. Gut 59: 1213-1221.
32. Franzius D, Hoth M, Penner R (1994) Non-specific effects of calcium entry antagonists in mast cells. Pflugers Arch 428: 433-438.
33. Ceyhan GO, Schafer KH, Kerscher AG, Rauch U, Demir IE, et al. (2010) Nerve growth factor and artemin are paracrine mediators of pancreatic neuropathy in pancreatic adenocarcinoma. Ann Surg 251: 923-931.
34. Demir IE, Wang K, Tieftrunk E, Giese NA, Xing B, et al. (2012) Neuronal plasticity in chronic pancreatitis is mediated via the neurturin/GFRalpha2 axis. Am J Physiol Gastrointest Liver Physiol 303: G1017-1028.
35. Buchler M, Weihe E, Friess H, Malfertheiner P, Bockman E, et al. (1992) Changes in peptidergic innervation in chronic pancreatitis. Pancreas 7: 183-192.
36. Zhu Y, Mehta K, Li C, Xu GY, Liu L, et al. (2012) Systemic administration of anti-NGF increases A-type potassium currents and decreases pancreatic nociceptor excitability in a rat model of chronic pancreatitis. Am J Physiol Gastrointest Liver Physiol 302: G176-181.
37. Liddle RA, Nathan JD (2004) Neurogenic inflammation and pancreatitis. Pancreatology 4: 551-559; discussion 559-560.
38. Hoogerwerf WA, Shenoy M, Winston JH, Xiao SY, He Z, et al. (2004) Trypsin mediates nociception via the proteinase-activated receptor 2: a potentially novel role in pancreatic pain. Gastroenterology 127: 883-891.
39. Strouch MJ, Cheon EC, Salabat MR, Krantz SB, Gounaris E, et al. (2010) Crosstalk between mast cells and pancreatic cancer cells contributes to pancreatic tumor progression. Clin Cancer Res 16: 2257-2265.
40. Hoogerwerf WA, Gondesen K, Xiao SY, Winston JH, Willis WD, et al. (2005) The role of mast cells in the pathogenesis of pain in chronic pancreatitis. BMC Gastroenterol 5: 8.

17

Delta-Opioid Receptor Analgesia Is Independent of Microglial Activation in a Rat Model of Neuropathic Pain

Joanna Mika*⁹, Katarzyna Popiolek-Barczyk⁹, Ewelina Rojewska, Wioletta Makuch, Katarzyna Starowicz, Barbara Przewlocka*

Department of Pain Pharmacology, Institute of Pharmacology, Polish Academy of Sciences, Krakow, Poland

Abstract

The analgesic effect of delta-opioid receptor (DOR) ligands in neuropathic pain is not diminished in contrast to other opioid receptor ligands, which lose their effectiveness as analgesics. In this study, we examine whether this effect is related to nerve injury-induced microglial activation. We therefore investigated the influence of minocycline-induced inhibition of microglial activation on the analgesic effects of opioid receptor agonists: morphine, DAMGO, U50,488H, DPDPE, Deltorphin II and SNC80 after chronic constriction injury (CCI) to the sciatic nerve in rats. Pre-emptive and repeated administration of minocycline (30 mg/kg, i.p.) over 7 days significantly reduced allodynia and hyperalgesia as measured on day 7 after CCI. The antiallodynic and antihyperalgesic effects of intrathecally (i.t.) administered morphine (10–20 μg), DAMGO (1–2 μg) and U50,488H (25–50 μg) were significantly potentiated in rats after minocycline, but no such changes were observed after DPDPE (10–20 μg), deltorphin II (1.5–15 μg) and SNC80 (10–20 μg) administration. Additionally, nerve injury-induced down-regulation of all types of opioid receptors in the spinal cord and dorsal root ganglia was not influenced by minocycline, which indicates that the effects of opioid ligands are dependent on other changes, presumably neuroimmune interactions. Our study of rat primary microglial cell culture using qRT-PCR, Western blotting and immunocytochemistry confirmed the presence of mu-opioid receptors (MOR) and kappa-opioid receptors (KOR), further we provide the first evidence for the lack of DOR on microglial cells. In summary, DOR analgesia is different from analgesia induced by MOR and KOR receptors because it does not dependent on injury-induced microglial activation. DOR agonists appear to be the best candidates for new drugs to treat neuropathic pain.

Editor: Bradley Taylor, University of Kentucky Medical Center, United States of America

Funding: This work was supported by MNiSzW/NCN grant NN405375937, grant OPUS NCN 2011/03/B/NZ4/00042, grant PRELUDIUM NCN 2012/07/N/NZ3/00379, grant MAESTRO NCN 2012/06/A/NZ4/00028 and statutory funds. Katarzyna Popiolek-Barczyk is a Ph.D. student and has a scholarship from the KNOW sponsored by the Ministry of Science and Higher Education, Republic of Poland. The funders had no role in study design, data collection and analysis, decision to publish, or preparation of the manuscript.

Competing Interests: The authors have declared that no competing interests exist.

* Email: przebar@if-pan.krakow.pl (BP); joamika@if-pan.krakow.pl (JM)

⁹ These authors contributed equally to this work.

Introduction

Neuropathic pain has been shown in clinical and animal studies to be resistant to alleviation by morphine [1,2,3,4,5], but the mechanism of this effect is unclear. The classical opioid system modulates nociception through three G-protein-coupled receptors: delta-opioid receptors (DOR) [6,7] kappa-opioid receptors (KOR) [8,9] and mu-opioid receptors (MOR) [8]. Opioid receptors do not necessarily function independently and can exist as heterodimers that modulate their pharmacology [10,11,12]. Several experimental studies have emphasised that the effects of DOR agonists are distinctively more potent than those of MOR and KOR receptors [13,14,15] in neuropathic pain. The field of DOR analgesia has been widely studied [16,17,18] and the DOR agonists seems to be a good drugs that would be effective in neuropathic pain, but still some of the aspects of DOR ligands interactions have to be clarified.

Reduction of morphine antinociceptive potency has been postulated to be a consequence of changes in the activity of opioid systems or opioid-specific signalling [3,19]. Although a reduction in the number of receptors may be a major factor in the reduced efficacy of opioids, it has become clear that many other factors affect the efficacy of morphine. Such factors include heterologous desensitisation between opioid and proinflammatory chemokine receptors via shared G-protein-coupled systems [20], down-regulation of glutamate transporters in glial cells [21] or release of such substances as NO, ATP, excitatory amino acids, prostaglandins, and proinflammatory cytokines from activated glia [22,23,24,25,26,27]. In a previous study, we used minocycline, which is a tetracycline derivative with pleiotropic biological effects, to clarify whether the analgesic opioid effect is associated with the activation of microglia. Minocycline is a potent inhibitor of the microglial activation [22,28,29,30] that impairs microglial viability and migration [31,32]. Minocycline also up-regulates a tissue inhibitors of matrix metalloproteinases (TIMPs) [33], inhibits MMP-9 [34] and has been shown in many studies to have neuroprotective effects [35,36]. Some authors have suggested that minocycline may also reduce pain by inhibiting Ca^{2+} and Na^{+} currents in sensory neurons in DRG [35,37]. It was shown that pain after nerve injury depended on activation of the p38 MAPK signalling pathway in the spinal cord and p38 MAPK was co-localized with activated microglia [38,39]. It was shown [40,41,42] that the level of phospho-p38 MAPK in microglia was reduced after minocycline treatment, which suggests that this kinase is a minocycline target. Little is known about its influence on neurons, but some authors suggest its neuroprotective effects in dopaminergic and glutamatergic neurons [43,44]. We demonstrated in our previous study that chronic administration of minocycline attenuated the development of neuropathic pain and enhanced morphine analgesia [45,46,47]. Filipovic and Zecevic [48] demonstrated in *in vitro* studies that minocycline protects neurons from LPS-induced inflammation by inhibiting the activation of microglia. Activated microglia may weaken morphine analgesia by releasing pronociceptive factors, and the administration of minocycline antagonises this weakening [23,46,47].

The aim of the present study was to determine the extent to which the activation of microglia induced by injury to the sciatic nerve (by chronic constriction injury, CCI) in rats changes the analgesic effect of opioid receptors agonists. Minocycline, a well characterized drug for inhibiting microglial activity [49], was intraperitoneally (i.p.) administered pre-emptively and repeatedly to CCI-exposed rats, subsequently its influence on allodynia and hyperalgesia was measured. On day 7 after CCI, vehicle-treated and minocycline-treated rats received the opioid receptor agonists morphine, DAMGO, U50,488H, DPDPE, deltorphin II and SNC80 intrathecally. We conducted behavioural experiments and simultaneously analysed molecular changes in the transcription of *MOR*, *KOR*, and *DOR* mRNA in the dorsal horn of the lumbar spinal cord and in DRG (L4–L6) at day 7 after injury in CCI-exposed rats after minocycline or vehicle administration. We also analysed the presence of MOR, KOR and DOR in rat primary microglial cell cultures by using qRT-PCR, Western blotting and immunocytochemistry.

Methods

Animals

Male Wistar rats (200–350 g) were housed in cages that were lined with sawdust under a standard 12/12 h light/dark cycle (lights on at 08:00 h), with food and water available *ad lib*. Care was taken to reduce the number of animals used, and all experiments were performed according to the recommendations of IASP [50] and the NIH Guide for the Care and Use of Laboratory Animals and were approved by the II Local Bioethics Committee branch of the National Ethics Committee for Experiments on Animals based at the Institute of Pharmacology, Polish Academy of Sciences (Cracow, Poland).

Surgical preparations

Chronic constriction injury (CCI) was produced in rats by tying four ligatures around the sciatic nerve under sodium pentobarbital anaesthesia (60 mg/kg; i.p.). The *biceps femoris* and the *gluteus superficialis* were separated, and the right sciatic nerve was exposed. The ligatures (4/0 silk) were tied loosely around the nerve distal to the sciatic notch with 1-mm spacing until they elicited a brief twitch in the respective hind limb. The procedure has been described in detail by Bennett and Xie, [51]. After the surgery, all rats developed long-lasting neuropathic pain symptoms such as allodynia and hyperalgesia. Because we have shown in earlier studies that there are no differences between the nociceptive responses of naïve and sham rats [52], we used naïve animals for the behavioural experiments in the present study.

Intrathecal (i.t.) injection

Rats were prepared for intrathecal (i.t.) injection by implanting catheters under pentobarbital anaesthesia (60 mg/kg i.p.). The intrathecal catheter consisted of polyethylene tubing that was 12 cm long (PE 10, Intramedic; Clay Adams, Parsippany, NJ) with an outside diameter of 0.4 mm and a dead space of 10 µl that had been sterilised by immersion in 70% (v/v) ethanol and fully flushed with sterile water before insertion. Rats were placed on a stereotaxic table (David Kopf Instruments, Tujunga, CA), and an incision was made in the atlanto-occipital membrane. The catheter (7.8 cm of its length) was carefully introduced into the subarachnoid space at the rostral level of the spinal cord lumbar enlargement (L4–L5) according to the method of Yaksh and Rudy [53]. After the implantation, the first injection of 10 µl of water was performed slowly and the catheter was tightened. One day after catheter implantation, the rats were monitored for physical impairments. Those showing motor deficits were excluded from further study. Animals were allowed a minimum 1 week of recovery after the surgery before the experiment began. Water for injection or respective drugs were delivered slowly (1–2 min) in a volume of 5 µl through the i.t. catheter and were followed by 10 µl of water for injection, which flushed the catheter.

Behavioural tests

Tactile allodynia (von Frey test). Allodynia was measured in rats subjected to CCI by the use of an automatic von Frey apparatus (Dynamic Plantar Aesthesiometer Cat. No. 37400, Ugo Basile Italy). Rats were placed in plastic cages with a wire net floor 5 min before the experiment. The von Frey filament was applied to the midplantar surface of the hind foot, and measurements were taken automatically [23]. The strength of the von Frey stimuli ranged from 0.5 to 26 g in rats.

Cold hyperalgesia (cold plate test). Hyperalgesia was assessed using the cold plate test (Cold/Hot Plate Analgesia Meter No. 05044 Columbus Instruments, USA) as has been described previously [23,45]. The temperature of the cold plate was maintained at 5°C, and the cut-off latency was 30 s. The rats were placed on the cold plate, and the time until lifting of the hind foot was recorded. The injured foot was the first to react in every case.

Drug administration

The chemicals used in this study and their sources were as follows: morphine hydrochloride – Polfa (Kutno, Poland); DAMGO (Sigma-Aldrich, USA), Deltorphin II (Sigma-Aldrich, USA), DPDPE (Sigma-Aldrich, USA), U50,488H (Tocris, UK), SNC80 (Sigma-Aldrich, USA) and minocycline hydrochloride (Sigma-Aldrich, USA). Minocycline (MC; 30 mg/kg; i.p.) was dissolved in sterile water and pre-emptively administered intraperitoneally 16 h and 1 h before CCI and then twice daily for 7 days. This method of minocycline administration was used throughout the work and is referred to in the text as "repeated administration". The control groups received a vehicle (water for injection) according to the same schedule. One hour after the last morning of minocycline or vehicle administration on day 7 after CCI, morphine (M; 20; 40 µg; 62.3 nM; 124.6 nM), DAMGO (MOR selective ligand; 1; 2 µg; 1.94 nM; 3.9 nM), U50,488H (KOR selective ligand; 25; 50 µg; 61.6 nM; 123.2 nM), DPDPE (DOR I selective ligand; 10; 20 µg; 15.48 nM; 30.96 nM), deltorphin II (del II; DOR II selective ligand; 1.5; 15 µg; 1.9 nM; 19 nM), SNC80 (10; 20 µg; 22.24 nM; 44.48 nM) or a vehicle was intrathecally injected. The von Frey test (25 and 45 min later) and cold plate tests (30 and 50 min later) were

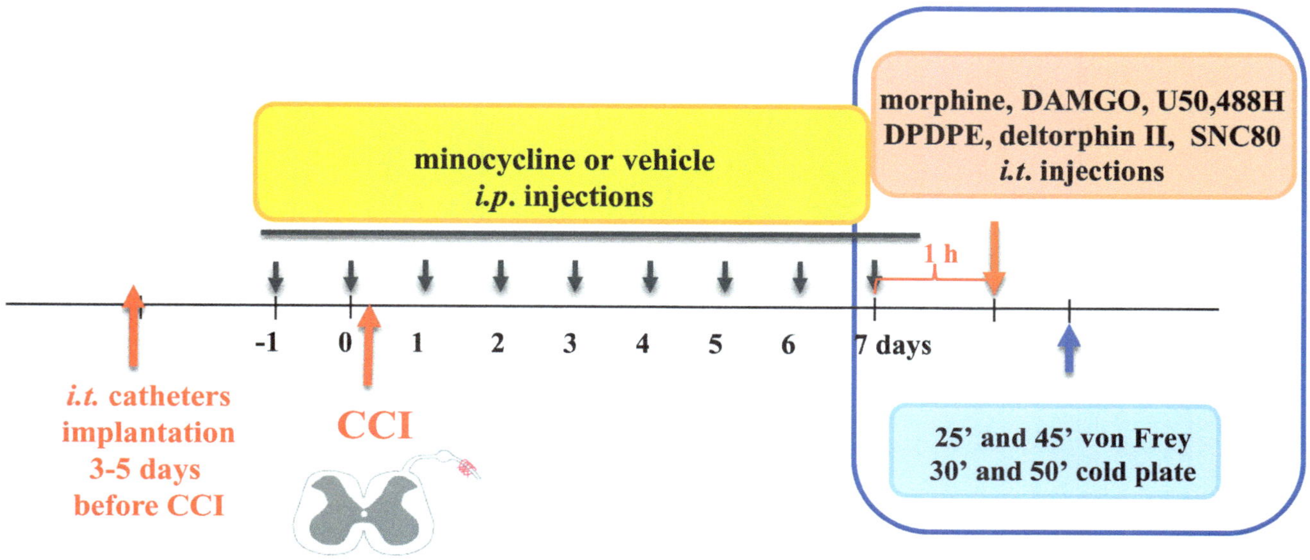

Figure 1. Drug administration.

carried out after vehicle or opioid agonist administration (Figure 1).

Microglial cell cultures and treatments

Primary cultures of microglial cells were prepared from 1-day-old Wistar rat pups as has been previously described [54] Briefly, cells were isolated from the rats' cerebral cortices and were plated at a density of 3×10^5 cells/cm^2 in a culture medium that consisted of DMEM/Glutamax/high glucose (Gibco, USA) supplemented with heat-inactivated 10% foetal bovine serum (Gibco, USA), 100 U/ml penicillin, and 0.1 mg/ml streptomycin (Gibco, USA) on poly-L-lysine coated 75 cm^2 culture flasks and were maintained at 37°C and 5% CO_2. The culture medium was changed after 4 days. The loosely adherent microglial cells were recovered after 9 days by mild shaking and centrifugation. Microglial cells were suspended in a culture medium and plated at a final density of 2×10^5 cells onto 24 well plates and 1.2×10^6 cells onto 6 well plates. Adherent cells were incubated for 48 h in a culture medium before being used for the analyses. Cell specificity was determined using an antibody to OX-42 (microglial marker) in cultures of primary microglia. Levels of mRNA for *C1q* (a microglial marker) and *GFAP* (an astroglial marker) were also investigated. Cultured primary microglia were more than 95% positive for OX-42 and C1q.

We have also analyzed the level of MOR, DOR and KOR mRNA level after LPS-stimulation (data not shown). Cells were prepared as described above and then incubated for 6 h with LPS [100 ng/ml] [55] or vehicle (PBS). We have not observed any significant changes in expression of MOR and KOR transcripts in comparison with vehicle-treated cells. In the LPS-stimulated microglial cells the presence of *DOR* mRNA also haven't been detected. Lipopolysaccharides from *Escherichia coli* 0111:B4 (Sigma-Aldrich, USA).

qRT-PCR analysis of gene expression

Total RNA was extracted according to the method Chomczynski and Sacchi [56] using the TRIzol reagent (Invitrogen) as previously described [57]. The RNA concentration was measured using a NanoDrop ND-1000 Spectrometer (NanoDrop Technologies). Reverse transcription was performed on 500 ng (from cell cultures) or 1000 ng (from tissue) of total RNA using Omniscript reverse transcriptase (Qiagen Inc.) at 37°C for 60 min. cDNA was diluted 1:10 with H_2O. qRT-PCR was performed using Assay-On-Demand TaqMan probes according to the manufacturer's protocol (Applied Biosystems) and run on a Real-Time PCR iCycler device (BioRad, Hercules, CA, USA). Rn00561699_m1 (*Oprd1*), Rn01430371_m1 (*Oprm1*), and Rn00567737_m1 (*Oprk1*) were used as TaqMan primers and probes. The expression of HPRT (a housekeeping gene) was quantified to control for variation in cDNA amounts. Cycle threshold values were calculated automatically by iCycler IQ 3.0 software with default parameters. Abundance of RNA was calculated as $2^{-(\text{threshold cycle})}$.

Western blot analysis

Cell lysates were collected in a RIPA buffer with a protease inhibitor cocktail and cleared by centrifugation (14000×g for 30 min, 4°C). Samples containing 20 µg of protein were heated in a loading buffer (50 mM Tris–HCl, 2% SDS, 2% β-mercaptoethanol, 4% glycerol and 0.1% bromophenol blue) for 5 min at 70°C and resolved by SDS–PAGE on 12% polyacrylamide gels. Following gel electrophoresis, the proteins were electrophoretically transferred to Immune-Blot PVDF membranes (Bio-Rad). The blots were blocked for 30 min using 5% non-fat dry milk (Bio-Rad) in Tris-buffered saline with 0.1% Tween 20 (TBST). The blots were incubated with primary antibodies (rabbit polyclonal anti-MOR, 1:500 [58]; rabbit polyclonal anti-DOR, 1:500 [59]; rabbit polyclonal anti-KOR 1:500, Abcam [58] that had been diluted in a SignalBoost Immunoreaction Enhancer Kit (Merck Millipore) for 24 h at 4°C and then incubated with a goat polyclonal antibody that had been conjugated to horseradish peroxidase (goat anti-rabbit IgG, BioRad) at a dilution of 1:1000 for 1 h at room temperature. After four 5-minute washes in TBST, immunocomplexes were detected using a Lumi-Light Western Blotting Kit and visualised using a Fujifilm LAS-4000 fluorimager system. The blots were washed 4 times for 5 minutes each in TBST and reprobed with a mouse antibody against GAPDH (1:5000, Millipore) as a loading control. The relative levels of immunoreactivity were quantified using Fujifilm Image Gauge software.

Immunocytochemical analysis

We used commercially available specific anti-MOR, anti-KOR and anti-OX/42 antibodies. Cells were fixed for 20 minutes in 4% paraformaldehyde in a 0.1 M phosphate buffer (pH 7.4) and incubated with primary antibodies (rabbit anti-MOR, 1:400 [60], rabbit anti-KOR, 1:400 [61], rabbit anti-DOR, 1:400, [62] Neuromics; mouse anti-OX/42, 1:500, Serotec) for 2 days at 4°C. After three washes in PB, double immunofluorescence was revealed by incubation for 2 h in the appropriate fluorochrome-conjugated secondary antibody, Alexa Fluor546 donkey anti-rabbit and Alexa Fluor488 donkey anti-mouse, diluted 1:500 in 5% NDS. Sections were then washed with PB and coverslipped with an Aquatex mounting medium (Merck, Darmstadt, Germany). Sections without primary antibodies were used as negative controls.

Data analysis

The behavioural data are presented as the mean ± S.E.M of 8–16 rats per group. The results of the experiments were statistically evaluated using one-way analysis of variance (ANOVA). All of the differences between the treatment groups were further analysed with Bonferroni's post-hoc tests. Significant differences in comparisons with vehicle-treated CCI-exposed rats are indicated by $^{*}P$ (<0.05), $^{**}P$ (<0.01) and $^{***}P$ (<0.001). Significant differences between vehicle-treated CCI-exposed rats that had received a single dose of opioid receptor ligands and minocycline-treated CCI-exposed rats that had received a single dose of opioid receptor ligands are indicated by $^{\#}P$ (<0.05), $^{\#\#}P$ (<0.01) and $^{\#\#\#}P$ (<0.001).

The qRT-PCR analyses were performed in three groups: naïve, CCI-exposed and minocycline-treated CCI-exposed rats. The results are presented as fold changes compared with the naïve rats in the ipsilateral dorsal lumbar spinal cord and DRG. The qRT-PCR data are presented as the mean ± S.E.M and represent the normalised averages that were derived from the threshold qRT-PCR cycles from four to eight samples for each group. Intergroup differences were analysed using ANOVAs followed by Bonferroni's multiple comparison tests. Significant differences resulting from comparison with naïve rats are indicated by $^{*}P$ (<0.05), $^{**}P$ (<0.01) and $^{***}P$ (<0.001). The data from 3 to 10 cell cultures are presented.

Results

Repeated administration of minocycline significantly diminished allodynia and hyperalgesia in neuropathic pain in rats

All vehicle-treated CCI rats exhibited neuropathic pain symptoms in the behavioral tests. The rats exhibited strong allodynia on the seventh day after ligation as measured by the von Frey test (11.6 g±0.6 vs. 25.8 g±0.2 for naïve rats) (Fig. 2A,C,E; 3A,C,E) and potent hyperalgesia as measured by the cold plate test (7.6 s±0.9 vs. 29.7 s±0.3 for naïve rats) (Fig. 2B,D,F; 3B,D,F). Repeated administration of minocycline (MC; 30 mg/kg; i.p.) attenuated allodynia (17.4 g±0.5 vs. 11.6 g±0.6 for the vehicle-treated CCI rats) (Fig. 2A,C,E; 3A,C,E) and also hyperalgesia (12.1 s±0.9 vs. 7.6 s±0.9 for the vehicle-treated CCI rats) (Fig. 2B,D,F; 3B,D,F) to a similar extent at both time points.

Repeated administration of minocycline significantly influenced the effects of morphine in neuropathic pain in rats

The doses of morphine effective in neuropathic pain (M; 20 and 40 µg; i.t.) were used. Morphine was injected one hour after the last morning dose of minocycline (30 mg/kg; i.p. repeatedly) or vehicle, and allodynia and hyperalgesia were measured (see Figure 1). Morphine at a dose of 20 µg significantly diminished allodynia 25 and 45 minutes after injection compared with vehicle-treated animals (18.60 g±0.4 vs. 11.6 g±0.6 and 17.57 g±0.39 vs. 11.9 g±0.5, respectively; Fig. 2A). In minocycline-treated animals, the antiallodynic effect of morphine at a dose of 20 µg was potentiated by minocycline at both times as shown in the von Frey test (25 minutes: 22.04 g±0.52 vs. 18.60 g±0.4 for morphine-treated rats, 45 minutes: 22.3 g±0.34 vs. 17.57 g±0.39 for morphine-treated rats; Fig. 2A). Morphine at a dose of 20 µg did not influence thermal hyperalgesia but in the group which was injected repeatedly with minocycline, the antihyperalgesic effect of morphine was demonstrated (30 minutes: 18.30 s±1.6 vs. 11.3 g±0.8 for morphine-treated rats, 50 minutes: 22.5 s±1.7 vs. 13.5 s±1.5 for morphine-treated rats; Fig. 2B). A higher dose of morphine (40 µg) was effective in reducing mechanical allodynia 25 and 45 minutes after injection compared with vehicle-treated animals (25 minutes: 21.1 g±0.48 vs. 11.6 g±0.6, 45 minutes: 23.9 g±0.6 vs. 11.9 g±0.5; Fig. 2A). In minocycline-treated rats, the antiallodynic effect of morphine at a dose of 40 µg was potentiated at both times (25 minutes: 24.84 g±0.27 vs. 21.1 g±0.48, 45 minutes: 23.98 g±0.51 vs. 20.25 g±0.6; Fig. 2A). In opposite to the lower dose, morphine at a dose of 40 µg showed antihyperalgesic effect at both time points (30 minutes: 16.5 s±1.9 vs. 7.6 s±0.9, 50 minutes: 19.1 s±2.2 vs. 8.2 s±0.8; Fig. 2B). The increased effect of morphine at a dose of 40 µg in minocycline-treated group was observed at both time points, however, this effect was more significant after 50 minutes (25.8 s±1.0 vs. 19.1 s±2.2; Fig. 2B).

Repeated administration of minocycline significantly influenced the effects of MOR (DAMGO) and KOR (U50,488H) agonists in neuropathic pain in rats

DAMGO at a dose of 1 µg significantly diminished allodynia 25 and 45 minutes after injection compared with vehicle-treated animals (25 minutes: 20.4 g±0.5 vs. 11.6 g±0.6, 45 minutes: 18.7 g±0.4 vs. 11.9 g±0.5; Fig. 2C). In minocycline-treated animals, the antiallodynic effect of DAMGO (1 µg) was potentiated at both times as shown in the von Frey test (25 min: 22.6 g±0.7 vs. 20.4 g±0.5 for DAMGO-treated rats, 45 min: 21. 4 g±1.0 vs. 18.7 g±0.4 for DAMGO-treated rats; Fig. 2C). DAMGO at a dose of 1 µg did not influence thermal hyperalgesia but in minocycline- and DAMGO-treated group the antyhiperalgesic effect occurred at both time points but the better effect we observed 50 min after injection (21.2 s±1.8 vs. 16.4 s±1.7 for DAMGO-treated rats; Fig. 2D). The higher dose of DAMGO (2 µg) was effective in reducing mechanical allodynia 25 and 45 minutes after injection compared with vehicle-treated animals (25 min: 21.3 g±0.9 vs. 11.6 g±0.6, 45 min: 20.6 g±1.1 vs. 11.9 g±0.5; Fig. 2C). As shown in the von Frey test, repeated minocycline administration potentiated effect of DAMGO at a dose of 2 µg at both times, but a better effect was present after 45 minutes (24.9 g±0.5 vs. 20.6 g±1.1; Fig. 2C). In opposite to the lower dose, DAMGO at a dose of 2 µg showed antihyperalgesic effect at both time points (30 min: 18.0 s±2.9 vs. 7.6 s±0.9, 50 min: 16.9 s±1.5 vs. 8.2 s±0.8; Fig. 2D). We also observed increased effect of DAMGO in minocycline-treated

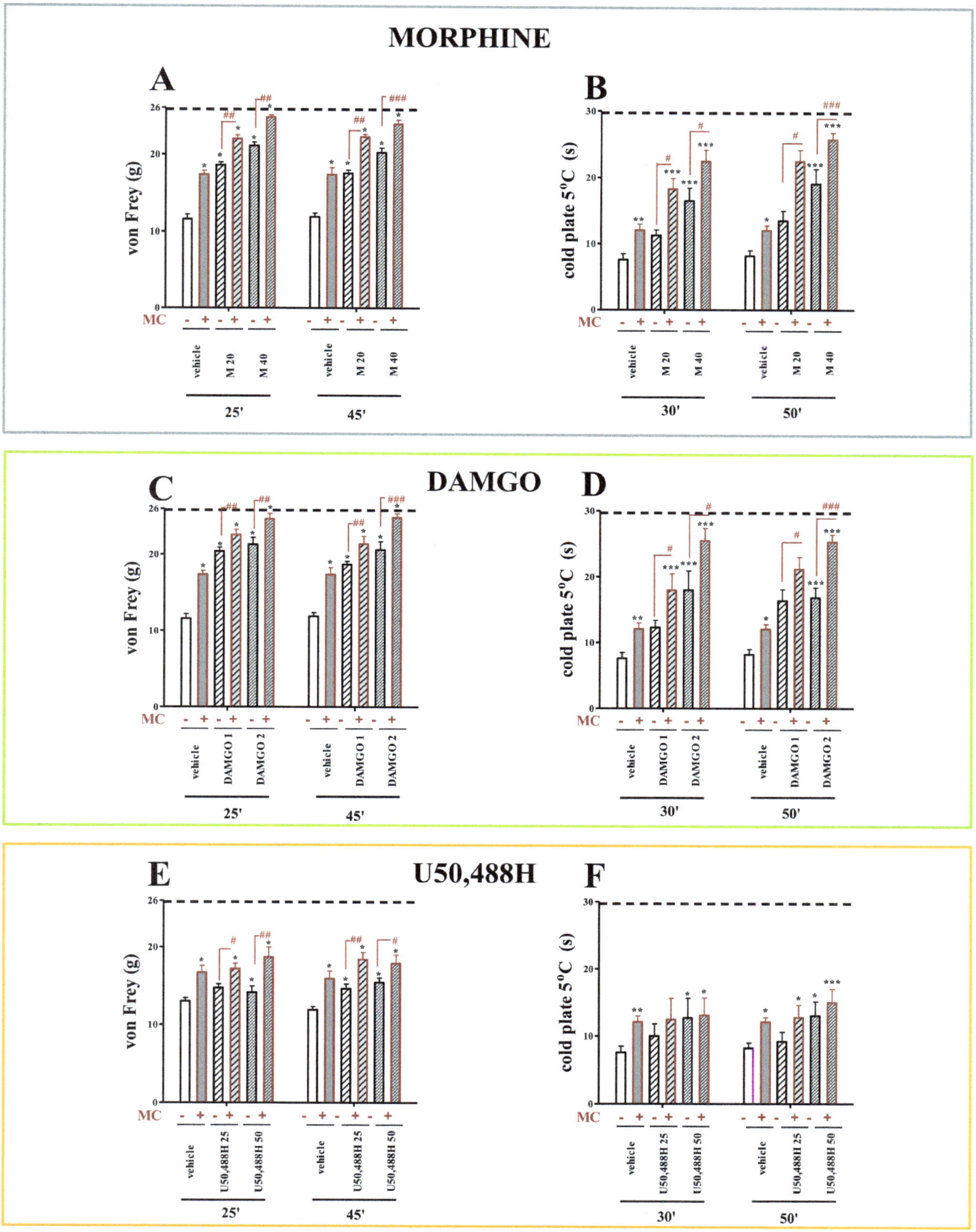

Figure 2. The effects of morphine, DAMGO and U50,488H on vehicle- and minocycline-treated CCI-exposed rats. The response to morphine, DAMGO and U50,488H was measured 25 and 45 minutes after administration by the von Frey test (A, C, E) and 30 and 50 minutes after

administration by the cold plate test (B, D, F). Minocycline (MC; 30 mg/kg; i.p.) was administered intraperitoneally pre-emptively 16 h and 1 h before CCI, and then repeatedly twice daily for 7 days. Vehicle-treated and minocycline-treated rats received intrathecal morphine (M; 20; 40 μg/5 μl), DAMGO (1; 2 μg/5 μl) or U50,488H (25; 50 μg/5 μl) one hour after the last morning administration on day 7 after CCI. The data are presented as the mean response ± S.E.M. (8–16 rats per group). The results of the experiments were statistically evaluated using One-way Analyses of Variance (ANOVA). The differences between the treatment groups throughout the study were further analysed with Bonferroni's *post-hoc* tests. *$P<0.05$, **$P<0.01$ and ***$P<0.001$ indicate significant differences compared with vehicle-treated CCI-exposed rats; #$P<0.05$, ##$P<0.01$ and ###$P<0.001$ indicate significant differences between vehicle-treated CCI-exposed rats that received a single dose of morphine and minocycline-treated CCI-exposed rats that received a single dose of morphine, DAMGO or U50,488H. Dotted line is a value for naïve animals (for von Frey test 25.8 g; for cold plate test 29.7 s).

group 30 minutes after opioid injection, however, this effect was more significant after 50 minutes (25.3 s±1.1 vs.16.9 s±1.5; Fig. 2D).

During neuropathy, the antiallodynic effect of U50,488H appeared after doses of 25 μg i.t. only 45 minutes after injection (14.6 g±0.6 vs. 11.9 g±0.5; Fig. 2E). The effect of this dose of U50,488H was potentiated in minocycline-treated group as shown in the von Frey test at both times, but at 45 minutes after injection the effect was more pronounced (18.4 g±0.9 vs. 14.6 g±0.6; Fig. 2E). U50,488H at a dose of 25 μg did not influence hyperalgesia and minocycline did not change this action (Fig. 2F). The higher dose (50 μg; i.t.) diminished allodynia at both times (25 min: 14.1 g±0.8 vs. 11.6 g±0.6, 45 min: 15.4 g±0.6 vs. 11.9 g±0.5; Fig. 2E). In minocycline-treated rats, the antiallodynic effect of U50,488H at a dose of 50 μg was potentiated at both times, but it potentiation was higher after 25 minutes (18.7 g±1.3 vs. 14.1 g±0.8; Fig. 2E). This dose of U50,488H slightly diminished hyperalgesia at 30 (12.7 s±2.9 vs. 7.6 s±0.9; Fig. 2F) and 50 (13.0 s±2.1 vs. 8.2 s±0.8; Fig. 2F) minutes after injection. Repeated minocycline administration did not change the action of U50,488H at a dose of 50 μg (Fig. 2F).

Repeated administration of minocycline did not influence the effects of DOR agonists (DPDPE, Deltorphin II and SNC80) in neuropathic pain in rats

DPDPE at a dose of 10 μg diminished allodynia 25 and 45 minutes after injection compared with vehicle-treated animals (25 min: 19.8 g±2.1 vs. 11.6 g±0.6, 45 min: 16.6 g±2.4 vs. 11.9 g±0.5; Fig. 3A) and minocycline treatment did not change this effect (Fig. 3A). Higher dose of DPDPE (20 μg) was effective in reducing mechanical allodynia only 25 minutes after injection compared with vehicle-treated animals (20.3 g±1.9 vs. 11.6 g±0.6, Fig. 3A) and this antiallodynic effect was not changed by minocycline (Fig. 3A). As shown in the cold plate test, DPDPE significantly diminished thermal hyperalgesia after both doses of 10 and 20 μg (30 min: 16.1 s±2.3 vs. 7.6 s±0.9; 50 min: 17.50 s±1.9 vs. 8.2 s±0.8 and 30 min: 20.3 s±1.9 vs. 7.6 s±0.9; 50 min: 23.6 s±1.7 8.2 s±0.8; respectively; Fig. 3B) and minocycline did not modulate this action (Fig. 3B).

Deltorphin II at a dose of 1.5 μg slightly diminished allodynia 25 and 45 minutes after injection compared with vehicle-treated animals (25 min: 17.7±1.7 vs. 11.6 g±0.6, 45 min: 17.4 g±1.4 vs. 11.9 g±0.5; Fig. 3C) and no changes in deltorphin II action in minocycline-treated group were observed (Fig. 3C). The higher dose of Deltorphin II (15 μg) was effective in reducing mechanical allodynia 25 (17.8 g±1.5 vs. 11.6 g±0.6; Fig. 3C) and 45 (17.2 g±2.1 vs. 11.9 g±0.5; Fig. 3C) minutes after injection compared with vehicle-treated animals. Repeated minocycline injection did not change the antiallodynic effect of deltorphin II (Fig. 3D). Deltorphin II at a dose of 1.5 μg did not influence hyperalgesia in CCI-exposed rats and minocycline also did not change this effect (Fig. 3D). As shown in the cold plate test, deltorphin II at a dose of 15 μg diminished thermal hyperalgesia only 50 minutes after injection (11.3 s±2.8 vs. 8.2 s±0.8; Fig. 3D) and minocycline did not change the antihyperalgesic action of the higher dose of Deltorphin II (Fig. 3D).

SNC80 at a dose of 10 μg slightly diminished allodynia 25 and 45 minutes after injection compared with vehicle-treated animals (25 min: 16.4 g±0.8 vs. 11.6 g±0.6, 45 min: 17.9 g±1.7 vs. 11.9 g±0.5; Fig. 3E). The higher dose of SNC80 (20 μg) was effective in reducing mechanical allodynia 25 (19.9 g±0.6 vs. 11.6 g±0.6; Fig. 3E) and 45 (19.0 g±1.2 vs. 11.9 g±0.5; Fig. 3E) minutes after injection compared with vehicle-treated animals. Repeated minocycline injection did not change the antiallodynic effect of both doses of SNC80 (Fig. 3E). As shown in the cold plate test, SNC80 at a dose of 10 μg influenced hyperalgesia in CCI-exposed rats (30 min: 19.5 s±2.8 vs. 7.6 s±0.9; 50 min: 13.0 s±2.3 vs. 8.2 s±0.8; Fig. 3F) SNC80 at a dose of 20 μg diminished thermal hyperalgesia 30 (24.2 s±2 vs. 7.6 s±0.9; Fig. 3F) and 50 (20.8 s±4.0 vs. 8.2 s±0.8; Fig. 3F) minutes after injection. Minocycline did not change the antihyperalgesic action of both doses of SNC80 (Fig. 3F).

Repeated administration of minocycline did not influence *MOR*, *DOR* and *KOR* mRNAs during neuropathic pain in rats

In the spinal cord the downregulation of *MOR* mRNA from 1±0.05 to 0.7±0.07 (Fig. 4A) and in the DRG from 1±0.03 to 0.5±0.06 (Fig. 4B) was observed compared to the naïve rats. Minocycline not influence the level of *MOR* mRNA in the spinal cord and in the DRG (Fig. 4A and B, respectively).

In the spinal cord the downregulation of *KOR* mRNA from 1±0.06 to 0.8±0.05 (Fig. 4C) and in the DRG from 1±0.06 to 0.6±0.04 (Fig. 4D) was observed compared to the naïve rats. Minocycline not influence the level of *KOR* mRNA in the spinal cord and in the DRG (Fig. 4C and D, respectively).

In the spinal cord the downregulation of *DOR* mRNA from 1±0.1 to 0.67±0.05 (Fig. 4E) and in the DRG from 1±0.1 to 0.3±0.07 (Fig. 4F) was observed compared to the naïve rats. Minocycline not influence the level of *KOR* mRNA in the spinal cord and in the DRG (Fig. 4E and F, respectively).

Opioid receptor expression in primary microglial cell cultures

Using a reverse transcriptase-polymerase chain reaction, we found that mRNA for *MOR* and *KOR*, but not for *DOR*, is expressed in rat primary microglial cell cultures (Fig. 5A). In the Western blot analysis, we found that protein for MOR and KOR is present in microglia (Fig. 5B). The protein for DOR was undetectable (Fig. 5B). The expression of MOR and KOR, but not DOR, in microglial cells was confirmed by immunocytochemistry (Fig. 5C).

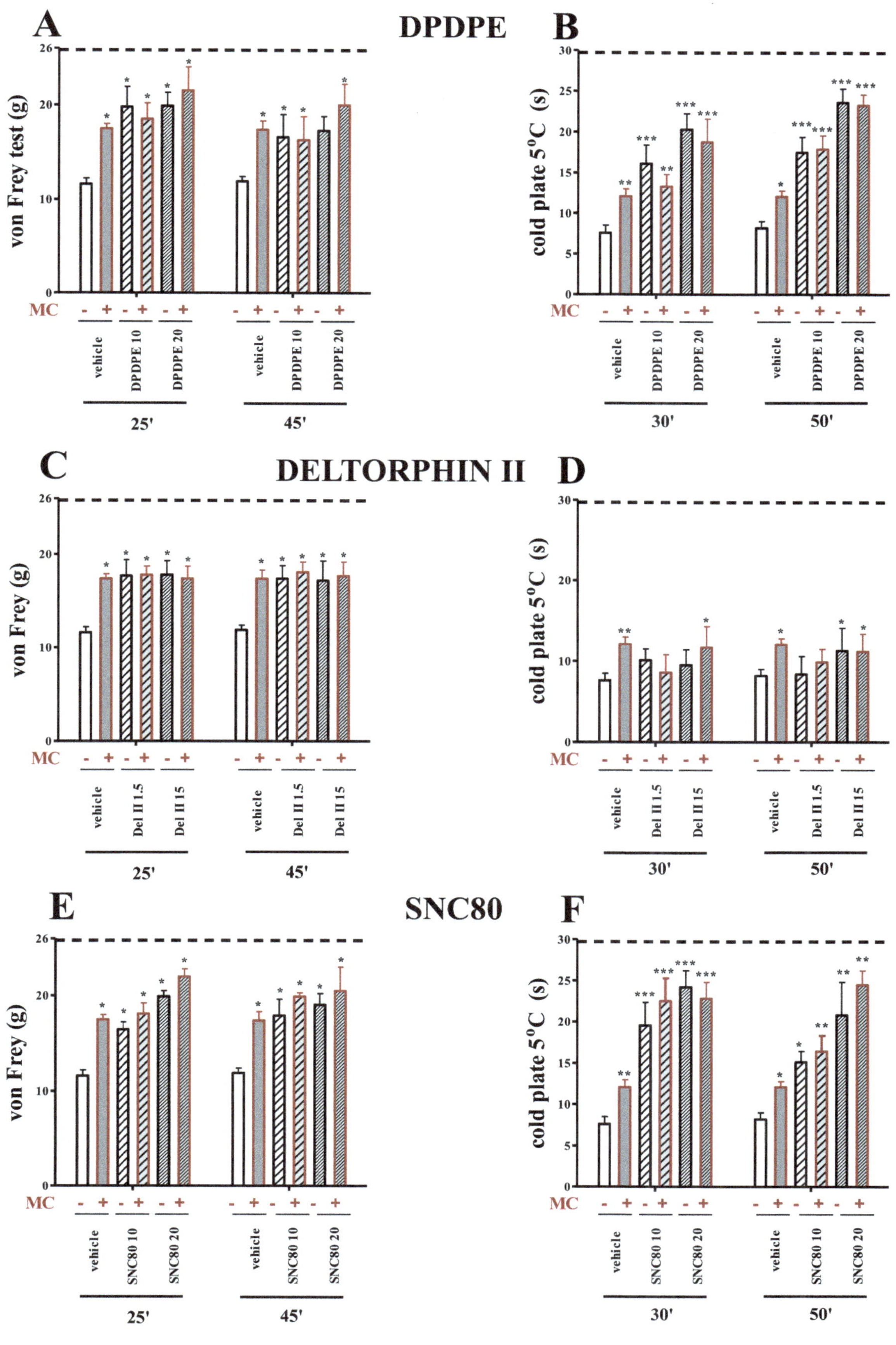
A
DPDPE
B
von Frey test (g)
cold plate 5°C (s)
MC
vehicle
DPDPE 10
DPDPE 20
25'
45'
30'
50'
C
DELTORPHIN II
D
von Frey (g)
Del II 1.5
Del II 15
E
SNC80
F
SNC80 10
SNC80 20

Figure 3. The effects of DPDPE, deltorphin II and SNC80 on vehicle- and minocycline-treated CCI-exposed rats. The response to DPDPE, deltorphin II and SNC80 was measured 25 and 45 minutes after administration by the von Frey test (A, C, E) and 30 and 50 minutes after administration by the cold plate test (B, D, F). Minocycline (MC; 30 mg/kg; i.p.) was administered intraperitoneally pre-emptively 16 h and 1 h before CCI, and then repeatedly twice daily for 7 days. Vehicle-treated and minocycline-treated rats received intrathecal DPDPE (10; 20 μg/5 μl), deltorphin II (del II; 1.5; 15 μg/5 μl) or SNC80 (10; 20 μg/5 μl) one hour after the last morning administration on day 7 after CCI. The data are presented as the mean response ± S.E.M. (8–16 rats per group). The results of the experiments were statistically evaluated using ANOVAs. The differences between the treatment groups throughout the study were further analysed with Bonferroni's *post-hoc* tests. **P*<0.05, ***P*<0.01 and ****P*<0.001 indicate significant differences compared with vehicle-treated CCI-exposed rats. Dotted line is a value for naïve animals (for von Frey test 25.8 g; for cold plate test 29.7 s).

Discussion

Opioids are fundamental to the treatment of pain, but their efficacy is limited by side effects, including tolerance and hyperalgesia [63]. Some authors suggest that reduced sensitivity to opioids and the increases in their dosages that are necessary to obtain adequate analgesia heighten the risk of side effects [4,5,64]. It remains unclear why morphine is a less potent analgesic in clinical [65,66] and experimental [15,46,67] studies of neuropathic pain in contrast to inflammatory pain [15,67]. In many studies it was shown that selective DOR agonists do not lose their effectiveness in the treatment of neuropathic pain [13,15,68]. It has been suggested that the lesser effects of morphine on neuropathic pain are due to the reduced number of presynaptic opioid receptors that results from nerve damage-induced degeneration of primary afferent neurons [64,69] besides other effects, like upregulation of the anti-opioid system CCK, and the NMDA receptor-dependent central sensitization, between others. Obara *et al.* [15] used ED_{50} analysis to demonstrate in 2009 that much higher doses of MOR and KOR agonists injected intraplantarly are required to produce antinociception in neuropathic than in inflammatory pain. However, it remains unclear why the ED_{50} of DOR agonists, but not those of MOR and KOR agonists, is comparable in both neuropathic and inflammatory pain [15]. Our study showed that the expression of all types of opioid receptor mRNA in the spinal cord and DRG was decreased in neuropathic pain. Also Stone *et al.* [70], using three animals models of peripheral nerve injury (CCI, SNL and SNT), observed decreases in spinal DOR expression at day 10th after operations at the side of injury. Herradon *et al.* [71] compared two strains of rats, Fischer 344 and Lewis rats, in neuropathic pain model and found significant down-regulation of DOR mRNA 28 days after CCI in the DRG of Lewis rats and the same trend was observed in F344 rats. Those data correspond well with our results obtained at day 7th after CCI in Wistar rats. In the study of Obara *et al.* [15] biochemical experiments were conducted at 3rd and 14th day (but not day 7th) after CCI and showed a non-significant, downward trend in the expression of mRNA for *MOR*, *DOR* and *KOR* at the spinal cord level. At the DRG level of neuropathic rats these authors observed down-regulation of mRNA level for *MOR* in L4–L5 DRGs (at day 3rd) and in L5 DRG (at day 14th), for *DOR* in L5 DRG (at both days) and for *KOR* in L4 and L5 DRGs (at day 3rd) and in L5 DRG (at day 14th) in comparison with naive animals. Those data correspond well with our results obtained at day 7th after CCI, however, in our experiments we pooled L4–L6 DRGs [15]. In the paper of Kabli and Cahill [68] the up-regulation of DOR protein was observed 14 days after sciatic nerve injury at the DRG level. The authors suggest that the increase in DOR protein is correlated with DOR trafficking to the site of injury, which may explain the lower level of mRNA as shown by our results. Should be noted, however, that in some papers no decrease in opioid receptor expression was observed [71,72]. Those discrepant data may result from different animal species used in experiments or time of the tissue collection after injury as it is shown in the mentioned works.

However, minocycline does not affect the reduced levels of all opioid receptor mRNAs, although it potentiates analgesia after such opioid agonists as morphine, DAMGO and U50,488H. Therefore, we should consider other mechanisms of weakened analgesia in neuropathic pain that can be restored by minocycline administration. These mechanisms may be important for sustained analgesia after administration of DOR ligands.

Several studies have suggested that the activation of glia and the enhancement of proinflammatory cytokine levels in the spinal cord and DRG are responsible for the development of both neuropathic pain and morphine tolerance [73,74,75]. We have previously observed an attenuation of the development of neuropathic pain when we administered minocycline, which is a substance that inhibits microglial activation in CCI-exposed rats [45,46]. Although minocycline can influence some neuronal functions, its ability to reduce microglial activation [76] as well as its selectivity of the action has been recently demonstrated [49]. We show in the present paper that the antiallodynic and antihyperalgesic effects of morphine, DAMGO and U50,488H, but not of DPDPE, deltorphin II or SNC80, were significantly potentiated with minocycline in CCI-subjected rats. In many studies we may found pharmacological evidence of distinct subtypes of DOR [77]. It is known that DOR_1 is activated by DPDPE, DOR_2 by deltorphin II and SNC80 is a a highly selective agonist for DOR. We had demonstrated in our previous studies the occurrence of strong antiallodynic and antihyperalgesic effects of DOR_1 and DOR_2 agonists after their acute and chronic i.t. administration in a rat neuropathic pain model [13]. Analgesic effects of i.t. injected SNC80 was also shown in many pain models [77,78,79]. In the present paper we have shown that the effectiveness of DPDPE, deltorphin II and SNC80 is not enhanced by minocycline treatment. Our results suggest that DOR analgesia is not dependent on injury-induced microglial activation. DORs are therefore a promising target for the development of analgesics. Indeed as previously reported by Holdridge *et al.* [80,81] the prolonged morphine treatment-induced incensement in microglial cell size was not functionally relevant in DOR analgesia, which confirms our research concerning the presence of DOR on microglia.

In the *in vitro* study, we used qRT-PCR, Western blot and immunocytochemistry assays to confirm the presence of MOR and KOR in microglia, and we have shown for the first time that those microglial cells do not express DOR. Our results are in agreement with other studies that have shown that microglia express MOR and KOR [82,83,84]. Chao *et al.* [85] first reported in 1996 that KOR was present in human microglia using qRT-PCR and a ligand-binding assay. The expression of KOR in microglial cells was also confirmed by the membrane binding of selective ligand [^{3}H]U69,593. Additionally, Chao *et al.* 1997 [86] have shown that morphine and DAMGO suppressed human microglia chemotaxis in a dose-dependent fashion and this effect is significantly attenuated by β-funaltrexamine (a MOR selective

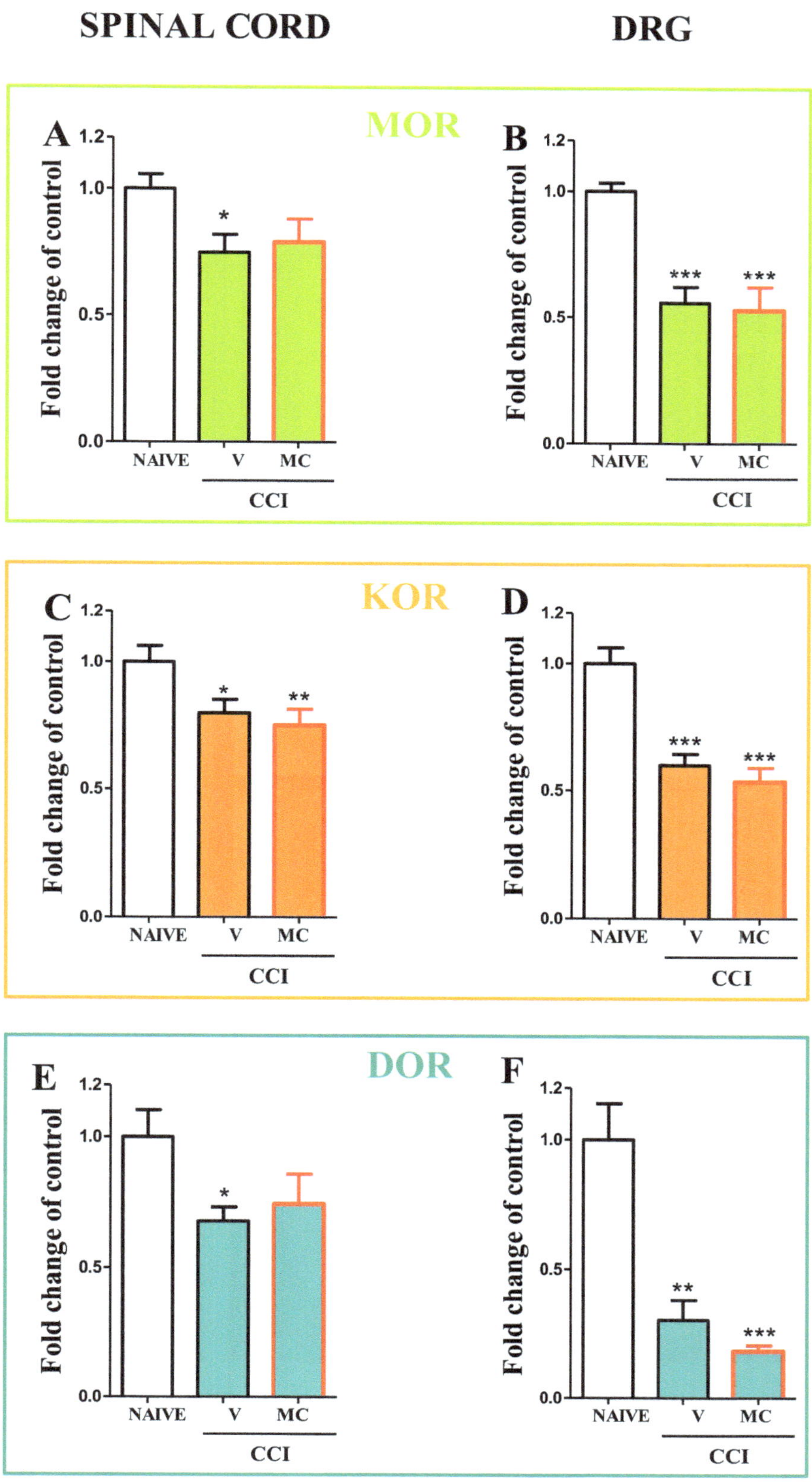

Figure 4. *MOR, DOR, KOR* mRNAs in spinal cord and DRGs in vehicle- and minocycline-treated CCI-exposed rats. Minocycline (MC; 30 mg/kg; i.p.) was administered intraperitoneally pre-emptively 16 h and 1 h before CCI, and then repeatedly twice daily for 7 days. On the seventh day, spinal cords (L4–L6) and DRG were collected for the qRT-PCR analysis of *MOR* (A, B), *KOR* (C, D) and *DOR* (E, F) gene expression. The data are presented as the means ± SEM and represent the normalised averages derived from the threshold qRT-PCR cycles from four to eight samples for each group. Intergroup differences were analysed using ANOVAs followed by Bonferroni's multiple comparison tests. *$P<0.05$; **$P<0.01$; ***$P<0.001$ indicate significant differences compared with naïve rats.

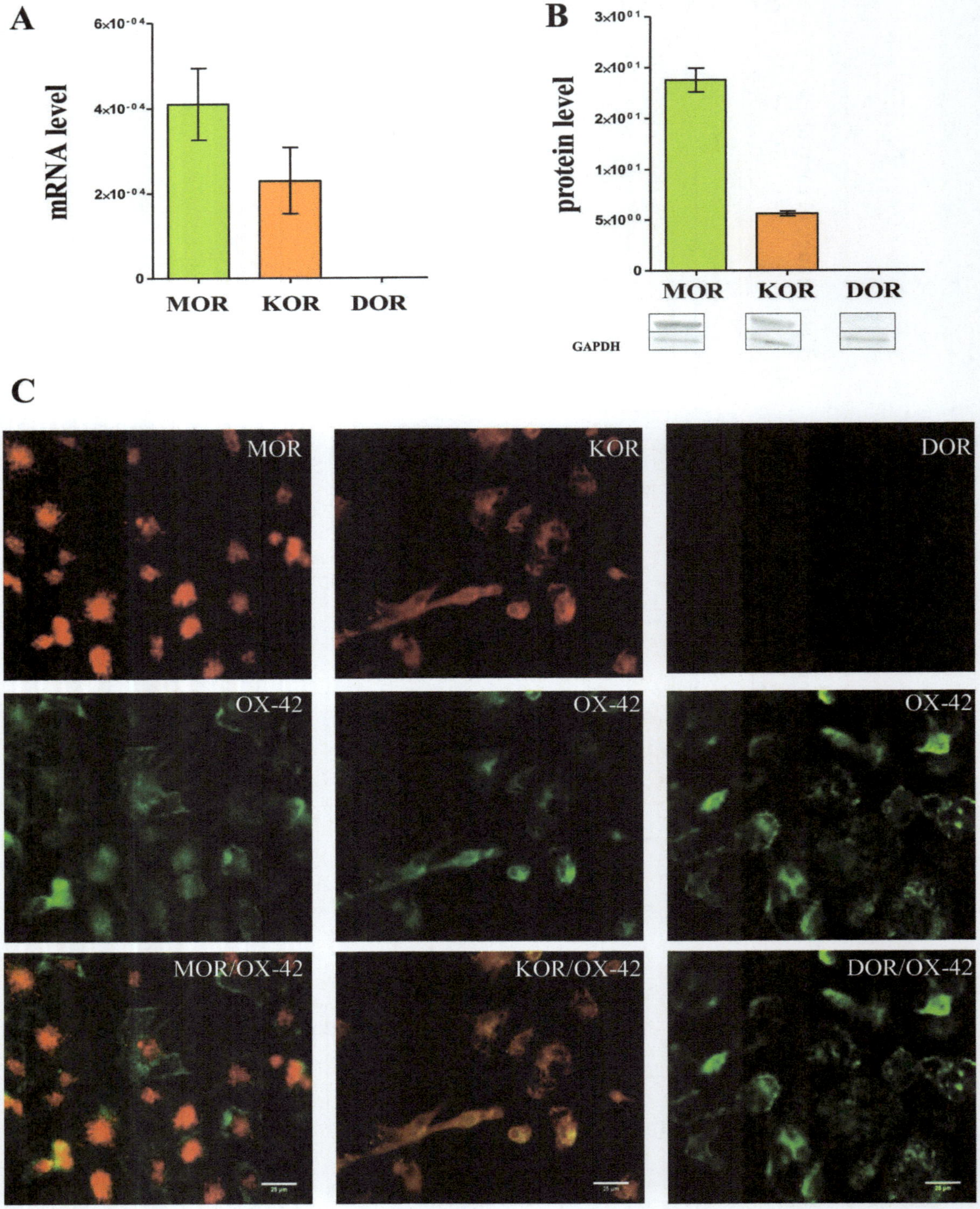

Figure 5. The presence of opioid receptors on microglia cells - *in vitro* studies. We analysed the presence of opioid receptors in primary microglial cell cultures. Using reverse transcriptase-polymerase chain reaction, we found that mRNA for *MOR* and *KOR*, but not *DOR*, is expressed in rat primary microglial cells cultures (A). Western blot analysis (B) detected proteins for MOR and KOR, but not DOR, in microglia. The presence of MOR and KOR, but not DOR, were confirmed by immunocytochemistry (C), and we show the colocalisation of MOR (left panel) and KOR (middle panel) antibodies (red) with OX/42 antibodies (green). The scale bar for all microphotographs is 25 μm. The data from 3–10 cell cultures are presented.

antagonist), which is consistent with our confirmation of the presence of MOR in microglial cells. The occurrence of DOR in microglial cells is still controversial. Our results strongly suggest that there is no DOR in rat primary microglial cells, although the studies of Turchan-Chlewo *et al.* [87] suggest their presence. However, Turchan-Chlewo *et al.* [87] used the PCR method (Sybr

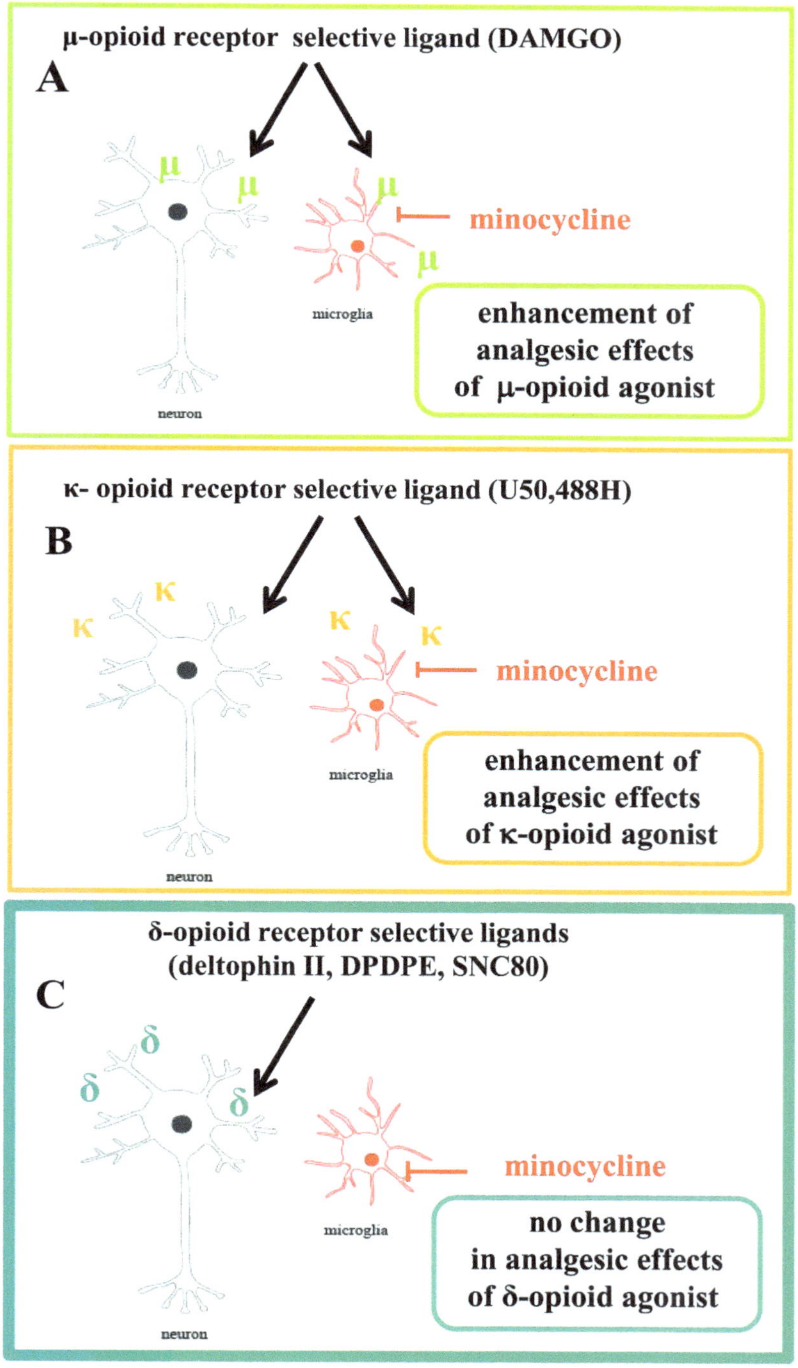

Figure 6. The possible influence of minocycline on analgesia after opioid receptors ligands. In our opinion, activated spinal microglia are key factors in the development of neuropathic pain and play a major role in the antagonizing of some opioids effectiveness. The results of our paper show for the first time that that DOR, in contrast to MOR and KOR, is not present in microglial cells. This phenomenon might be responsible for the different analgesic effects of MOR, KOR and DOR ligands (Fig. 2 and 3). We provide evidence that minocycline (a potent inhibitor of microglial activation and proliferation) enhances the effects of selective MOR (DAMGO; Fig. 2C,D) and selective KOR (U50,488H; Fig. 2E,F) agonists by inhibition of microglial cell activation. The effectiveness of DOR agonists (DPDPE, deltorphin II and SNC80) is not changed by minocycline (Fig. 3A–F). Our results indicate that an important element of the effectiveness of opioid drugs in neuropathic pain is the activation of microglia. The lack of DOR receptors in these cells causes that DOR receptor-mediated analgesia is not weaker under neuropathic pain, in which there is a strong activation of microglia. Earlier inhibition of microglial activation by minocycline administration therefore did not influence the effect of DOR selective agonists. The above results indicate not only that minocycline potentiates analgesia after MOR and KOR agonists but also that DOR is a potentially important target in the search for new drugs that would be effective against neuropathic pain.

Green), which is not sufficiently selective and can give false positive results. The TaqMan assay that we used is standardised and highly specific, and we confirmed the lack of DOR in microglia cell cultures by using Western blot and immunocytochemistry, therefore, our results are not consistent with those that were obtained by immunostaining by Turchan-Cholewo *et al.* [87] and Thorlin *et al.* [88]. Moreover studies by Turchan-Cholewo *et al.* [87] used commercial antibodies against DOR, which are no longer recommended for such studies. Due to the lack of selective DOR antibody a unique genetic mouse model was developed in order to investigate the distribution of DOR in the nervous system [16,89]. Opioid receptors have high degrees of homology, and antibodies may recognise other subtypes within the same family. DOR expression has also been observed on glial-like cells in the dentate gyrus [90] and rat cervical spinal cord [91], but none of these authors distinguished between astrocytes and microglia. Our results concerning the absence of DOR in microglia are consistent with recently published results of pharmacological studies that were conducted by Merighi *et al.* [84]. These authors have shown in primary microglia cell cultures that DPDPE, a DOR agonist, does not change the level of protein for PKC after LPS stimulation, while morphine and DAMGO up-regulate this kinase. The ineffectiveness of DPDPE in this study may be explained by the lack of DOR receptors in microglial cells. Horvath and DeLeo, [92] showed that selective agonists of DOR_1 DPDPE had no effect on microglial migration, which confirms our results that DOR, in contrast to MOR and KOR, is not present in microglial cells. DOR shows a functional profile that is distinct from that of MOR or KOR [93] and plays an important role in chronic pain, for example DOR knockout mice showed augmented neuropathic pain [94,95]. DOR agonists are poor analgesics in acute pain [96], but are highly effective following inflammatory or neuropathic pain [13,96,97,98,99].

Happel *et al.* [100] suggested in 2008 that morphine and DAMGO influence the immune system. For example, opioids alter macrophage functions and they modulate cytokine production and chemokine and chemokine receptor expression. Activation of proinflammatory chemokine receptors is known to down-regulate the analgesic functions of opioid receptors, and this enhances the perception of pain [101]. Horvath *et al.* [102] showed that morphine increases microglial migration by means of an interaction between *MOR* and $P2X_4$ receptors. This interaction is dependent on PI3K/Akt pathway activation [102]. Under neuropathic pain, the phosphorylation of p38 MAPK in microglia results in increased synthesis of the proinflammatory cytokines IL-1β, IL-6, and TNF-α. Spinal blockade of these cytokines is known to attenuate neuropathic pain and morphine tolerance [74,103]. Therefore, in cases where MOR and KOR agonists target microglial signalling by inhibiting the actions of chemokines (fractalkine, CCL2), ATP receptors (P2X4, P2X7), MMP-9, p38 MAPK, or/and proinflammatory cytokines (IL-1β, IL-6, and TNF-α) improve their effectiveness. However, this is not the case with DOR agonists. This difference deserves future exploration.

MOR agonists, especially morphine, still remain the drugs of choice for the treatment of neuropathic pain, despite the side effects and limited efficacy. It was shown that DOR agonists were effective in persistent pain [13,68,81,104,105] and the mechanisms underlying this analgesic action was probably linked with trafficking to the cell membrane or better receptor coupling to signalling effectors [104]. Nadal *et al.* [95] demonstrated that neuropathic pain was enhanced in delta-opioid receptor knockout mice. Some authors suggest a delta opioid agonists as a promising alternative to mu analgesics in the treatment of chronic pain [13,95,104,106]. Currently, research is being conducted on analgesic effects of new DOR ligands [107] and some of these substances are being tested in clinical trials [108].

The results of the present study document for the first time that DOR, in contrast to MOR and KOR, are not present in microglial cells (Figure 6). In conclusion, we provide evidence that minocycline not only diminishes neuropathic pain-related behaviour but also enhances the effectiveness of morphine and selective MOR and KOR opioid ligands under neuropathic pain conditions. Our findings lend support to the view that neuroimmunological changes in the spinal cord and DRG are important for opioid effectiveness in neuropathic pain. In our opinion, activated spinal microglia are key factors in not only the development of neuropathic pain but also in the different efficacies of opioid analgesics. Our results also suggest that DOR analgesia is not dependent on injury-induced microglial activation. We therefore suggest that DOR is an interesting target for the development of new drugs that would be effective against neuropathic pain.

Acknowledgments

This work was supported by MNiSzW/NCN grant NN405375937, grant OPUS NCN 2011/03/B/NZ4/00042, grant PRELUDIUM NCN 2012/07/N/NZ3/00379, grant MAESTRO NCN 2012/06/A/NZ4/00028 and statutory funds. Katarzyna Popiolek-Barczyk, is a Ph.D. student and has a scholarship from the KNOW sponsored by the Ministry of Science and Higher Education, Republic of Poland.

Author Contributions

Conceived and designed the experiments: JM KP-B ER KS BP. Performed the experiments: JM KP-B ER WM KS BP. Analyzed the data: JM KP-B ER WM KS BP. Contributed reagents/materials/analysis tools: JM KP-B ER WM KS BP. Wrote the paper: JM KP-B ER KS BP.

References

1. Hirsch SJ, Dickenson AH (2014) Morphine sensitivity of spinal neurons in the chronic constriction injury neuropathic rat pain model. Neurosci Lett 562: 97–101.
2. Przewlocki R, Przewlocka B (2001) Opioids in chronic pain. Eur J Pharmacol 429:79–91.
3. Przewlocki R, Przewlocka B (2005) Opioids in neuropathic pain. Curr Pharm Des 11: 3013–3025.
4. Eisenberg E, McNicol ED, Carr DB (2005) Efficacy and safety of opioid agonists in the treatment of neuropathic pain of non- malignant origin: Systematic review and meta-analysis of randomized controlled trials. JAMA; 293:3043–3052.
5. McQuay HJ (2002) Neuropathic pain: evidence matters. Eur J Pain.;6:11–8.
6. Evans CJ, Keith DE Jr, Morrison H, Magendzo K, Edwards RH (1992) Cloning of a delta opioid receptor by functional expression. Science 258: 1952–1955.
7. Kieffer BL, Befort K, Gavériaux-Ruff C, Hirth CG (1992) The delta-opioid receptor: isolation of a cDNA by expression cloning and pharmacological characterization. Proc Natl Acad Sci U S A 89: 12048–12052.
8. Chen Y, Mestek A, Liu J, Yu L (1993) Molecular cloning of a rat kappa opioid receptor reveals sequence similarities to the mu and delta opioid receptors. Biochem J 295: 625–628.
9. Minami M, Hosoi Y, Toya T, Katao Y, Maekawa K, et al. (1993) In situ hybridization study of kappa-opioid receptor mRNA in the rat brain. Neurosci Lett 162: 161–164.
10. George SR, Fan T, Xie Z, Tse R, Tam V, et al. (2000) Oligomerization of mu- and delta-opioid receptors. Generation of novel functional properties. J Biol Chem 275: 26128–26135.
11. Gomes I, Jordan BA, Gupta A, Trapaidze N, Nagy V, et al. (2000) Heterodimerization of mu and delta opioid receptors: a role in opiate synergy. J Neurosci 20: RC110.
12. Gomes I, Gupta A, Filipovska J, Szeto HH, Pintar JE, et al. (2004) A role for heterodimerization of mu and delta opiate receptors in enhancing morphine analgesia. Proc Natl Acad Sci USA 101: 5135–5139.
13. Mika J, Przewlocki R, Przewłocka B (2001) The role of delta-opioid receptor subtypes in neuropathic pain. Eur J Pharmacol 415: 31–37.

14. Nozaki C, Le Bourdonnec B, Reiss D, Windh RT, Little PJ, et al. (2012) δ-Opioid mechanisms for ADL5747 and ADL5859 effects in mice: analgesia, locomotion, and receptor internalization. J Pharmacol Exp Ther 342: 799–807.
15. Obara I, Parkitna JR, Korostynski M, Makuch W, Kaminska D, et al. (2009) Local peripheral opioid effects and expression of opioid genes in the spinal cord and dorsal root ganglia in neuropathic and inflammatory pain. Pain 141: 283–291.
16. Gavériaux-Ruff C, Kieffer BL (2011) Delta opioid receptor analgesia: recent contributions from pharmacology and molecular approaches. Behav Pharmacol 22: 405–414.
17. Fenalti G, Giguere PM, Katritch V, Huang XP, Thompson AA, et al. (2014) Molecular control of δ-opioid receptor signalling. Nature 506: 191–196.
18. Somvanshi RK, Kumar U (2014) δ-Opioid Receptor and Somatostatin Receptor-4 Heterodimerization: Possible Implications in Modulation of Pain Associated Signaling. PLoS One 9: e85193.
19. Lee YW, Chaplan SR, Yaksh TL (1995) Systemic and supraspinal, but not spinal, opiates suppress allodynia in a rat neuropathic pain model. Neurosci Lett 199: 111–114.
20. Steele AD, Szabo I, Bednar F, Rogers TJ (2002) Interactions between opioid and chemokine receptors: heterologous desensitization. Cytokine Growth Factor Rev 13: 209–222.
21. Osikowicz M, Mika J, Przewlocka B (2013) The glutamatergic system as a target for neuropathic pain relief. Exp Physiol 98: 372–384.
22. Cui Y, Liao XX, Liu W (2008) A novel role of minocycline: attenuating morphine antinociceptive tolerance by inhibition of p38 MAPK in the activated spinal microglia. Brain Behav Immun 22: 114–123.
23. Makuch W, Mika J, Rojewska E, Zychowska M, Przewlocka B (2013) Effects of selective and non-selective inhibitors of nitric oxide synthase on morphine- and endomorphin-1-induced analgesia in acute and neuropathic pain in rats. Neuropharmacology 75: 445–447.
24. Mika J, Rojewska E, Makuch W, Przewlocka B (2010) Minocycline reduces the injury-induced expression of prodynorphin and pronociceptin in the dorsal root ganglion in a rat model of neuropathic pain. Neuroscience 165: 1420–1428.
25. Mika J, Zychowska M, Popiolek-Barczyk K, Rojewska E, Przewlocka B (2013) Importance of glial activation in neuropathic pain. Eur J Pharmacol 716: 106–119.
26. Watkins LR, Maier SF (2003) Glia: a novel drug discovery target for clinical pain. Nat Rev Drug Discov 2: 973–985.
27. Wieseler-Frank J, Maier SF, Watkins LR (2005) Central proinflammatory cytokines and pain enhancement. Neurosignals 14: 166–174.
28. Amin AR, Attur MG, Thakker GD (1996) A novel mechanism of action of tetracyclines: effects on nitric oxide synthases. Proc Natl Acad Sci U S A 93: 14014–14019.
29. Colovic M, Caccia S (2003) Liquid chromatographic determination of minocycline in brain-to-plasma distribution studies in the rat. Life Sci 791: 337–343.
30. Ledeboer A, Sloane EM, Milligan ED, Frank MG, Mahony JH, et al. (2005) Minocycline attenuates mechanical allodynia and proinflammatory cytokine expression in rat models of pain facilitation. Pain 115: 71–83.
31. Pinkernelle J, Fansa H, Ebmeyer U, Keilhoff G (2013) Prolonged minocycline treatment impairs motor neuronal survival and glial function in organotypic rat spinal cord cultures. PLoS One 8: e73422.
32. Tikka T, Fiebich BL, Goldsteins G, Keinanen R, Koistinaho J (2001) Minocycline, a tetracycline derivative, is neuroprotective against excitotoxicity by inhibiting activation and proliferation of microglia. J Neurosci 21: 2580–2508.
33. Niimi N, Kohyama K, Matsumoto Y (2013) Minocycline suppresses experimental autoimmune encephalomyelitis by increasing tissue inhibitors of metalloproteinases. Neuropathology 33: 612–616.
34. Machado LS, Kozak A, Ergul A, Hess DC, Borlongan CV, et al. (2006) Delayed minocycline inhibits ischemia-activated matrix metalloproteinases 2 and 9 after experimental stroke. BMC Neurosci 7: 56.
35. Liu X, Su H, Chu TH, Guo A, Wu W (2013) Minocycline inhibited the pro-apoptotic effect of microglia on neural progenitor cells and protected their neuronal differentiation in vitro. Neurosci Lett 542: 30–36.
36. Garcia-Martinez EM, Sanz-Blasco S, Karachitos A, Bandez MJ, Fernandez-Gomez FJ, et al. (2010) Mitochondria and calcium flux as targets of neuroprotection caused by minocycline in cerebellar granule cells. Biochem Pharmacol 79: 239–250.
37. Kim TH, Kim HI, Kim J, Park M, Song JH (2011) Effects of minocycline on Na+ currents in rat dorsal root ganglion neurons. Brain Res 1370: 34–42.
38. Jin SX, Zhuang ZY, Woolf CJ, Ji RR (2003) p38 mitogen-activated protein kinase is activated after a spinal nerve ligation in spinal cord microglia and dorsal root ganglion neurons and contributes to the generation of neuropathic pain. J Neurosci 23: 4017–4022.
39. Zhuang ZY, Wen YR, Zhang DR, Borsello T, Bonny C, et al. (2006) A peptide c-Jun N-terminal kinase (JNK) inhibitor blocks mechanical allodynia after spinal nerve ligation: respective roles of JNK activation in primary sensory neurons and spinal astrocytes for neuropathic pain development and maintenance. J Neurosci 26: 3551–3560.
40. Chang YW, Waxman SG (2010) Minocycline attenuates mechanical allodynia and central sensitization following peripheral second-degree burn injury. J Pain 11: 1146–1154.
41. Hains BC, Waxman SG (2006) Activated microglia contribute to the maintenance of chronic pain after spinal cord injury. J Neurosci 26: 4308–4317.
42. Hua XY, Svensson CI, Matsui T, Fitzsimmons B, Yaksh TL, et al. (2005) Intrathecal minocycline attenuates peripheral inflammation-induced hyperalgesia by inhibiting p38 MAPK in spinal microglia. Eur J Neurosci 22: 2431–2440.
43. Radad K, Moldzio R, Rausch WD (2010) Minocycline protects dopaminergic neurons against long-term rotenone toxicity. Can J Neurol Sci 37: 81–85
44. González JC, Egea J, Del Carmen Godino M, Fernandez-Gomez FJ, Sánchez-Prieto J, et al. (2007) Neuroprotectant minocycline depresses glutamatergic neurotransmission and Ca(2+) signalling in hippocampal neurons. Eur J Neurosci 26: 2481–2495.
45. Mika J, Osikowicz M, Makuch W, Przewlocka B (2007) Minocycline and pentoxifylline attenuate allodynia and hyperalgesia and potentiate the effects of morphine in rat and mouse models of neuropathic pain. Eur J Pharmacol 560: 142–149.
46. Mika J, Wawrzczak-Bargiela A, Osikowicz M, Makuch W, Przewlocka B (2009) Attenuation of morphine tolerance by minocycline and pentoxifylline in naive and neuropathic mice. Brain Behav Immun 23: 75–84.
47. Zychowska M, Rojewska E, Kreiner G, Nalepa I, Przewlocka B, et al. (2013) Minocycline influences the anti-inflammatory interleukins and enhances the effectiveness of morphine under mice diabetic neuropathy. J Neuroimmunol 262: 35–45.
48. Filipovic R, Zecevic N (2008) Neuroprotective role of minocycline in co-cultures of human fetal neurons and microglia. Exp Neurol 211: 41–51.
49. Kobayashi K, Imagama S, Ohgomori T, Hirano K, Uchimura K, et al. (2013) Minocycline selectively inhibits M1 polarization of microglia. Cell Death Dis 4: e525.
50. Zimmermann M (1983) Ethical guidelines for investigations of experimental pain in conscious animals. Pain 16: 109–110.
51. Bennett GJ, Xie Y (1988) A peripheral mononeuropathy in rat that produces disorders of pain sensation like those seen in man. Pain 33: 87–107.
52. Osikowicz M, Mika J, Makuch W, Przewlocka B (2008) Glutamate receptor ligands attenuate allodynia and hyperalgesia and potentiate morphine effects in a mouse model of neuropathic pain. Pain 139: 117–126.
53. Yaksh TL, Rudy TA (1976) Chronic catheterization of the spinal subarachnoid space. Physiol. Behav 17: 1031–10.
54. Zawadzka M, Kaminska B (2005) A novel mechanism of FK506-mediated neuroprotection: downregulation of cytokine expression in glial cells. Glia 49: 36–51.
55. Przanowski P, Dabrowski M, Ellert-Miklaszewska A, Kloss M, Mieczkowski J, et al. (2014) The signal transducers Stat1 and Stat3 and their novel target Jmjd3 drive the expression of inflammatory genes in microglia. J Mol Med (Berl) 92: 239–254.
56. Chomczynski P, Sacchi N (1987) Single-step method of RNA isolation by acid guanidinium thiocyanate-phenol-chloroform extraction. Anal Biochem 162: 156–159.
57. Mika J, Obara I, Przewlocka B (2011) The role of nociceptin and dynorphin in chronic pain: implications of neuro-glial interaction. Neuropeptides 45: 247–261.
58. Kerros C, Brood I, Sola B, Jauzac P, Allouche S (2010) Reduction of cell proliferation and potentiation of Fas-induced apoptosis by the selective kappa-opioid receptor agonist U50 488 in the multiple myeloma LP-1 cells. J Neuroimmunol 220: 69–78.
59. Abcam website. Available: http://www.abcam.com/delta-opioid-receptor-antibody-ab66317.html. Accessed 2014 May 20.
60. Neuromics website. Available: http://www.neuromics.com/ittrium/visit/A1x66x1y1x85b1x1x9cy1x6217x1x96y1x4fax1x82y1x510x1x7f. Accessed 2014 May 20.
61. Mansson E, Bare L, Yang D (1994) Isolation of a human kappa opioid receptor cDNA from placenta. Biochem Biophys Res Commun 202: 1431–1437.
62. Ko JL, Arvidsson U, Williams FG, Law PY, Elde R, et al. (1999) Visualization of time-dependent redistribution of delta-opioid receptors in neuronal cells during prolonged agonist exposure. Brain Res Mol Brain Res 69: 171–185.
63. Mayer DJ, Mao J, Holt J, Price DD (1999) Cellular mechanisms of neuropathic pain, morphine tolerance, and their interactions. Proc Natl Acad Sci U S A 96: 7731–7736.
64. Ossipov MH, Lopez Y, Nichols ML, Bian D, Porreca F (1995) The loss of antinociceptive efficacy of spinal morphine in rats with nerve ligation injury is prevented by reducing spinal afferent drive. Neurosci Lett 199: 87–90.
65. Rowbotham MC, Twilling L, Davies PS, Reisner L, Taylor K, et al. (2003) Oral opioid therapy for chronic peripheral and central neuropathic pain. N Engl J Med 13: 1223–1232.
66. Gilron I, Bailey JM, Dongsheng Tu ME, Holden RR, et al. (2005) Morphine, Gabapentin, or Their Combination for Neuropathic Pain. N Engl J Med 13: 1324–1334.
67. Przewlocka B, Mika J, Labuz D, Toth G, Przewlocki R (1999) Spinal analgesic action of endomorphins in acute, inflammatory and neuropathic pain in rats. Eur J Pharmacol 367: 189–196.
68. Kabli N, Cahill CM (2007) Anti-allodynic effects of peripheral delta opioid receptors in neuropathic pain. Pain 127: 84–93.

69. Porreca F, Tang QB, Bian D, Riedl M, Elde R, et al. (1998) Spinal opioid mu receptor expression in lumbar spinal cord of rats following nerve injury. Brain Res 795: 197–203.
70. Stone LS, Vulchanova L, Riedl MS, Williams FG, Wilcox GL, et al. (2004) Effects of peripheral nerve injury on delta opioid receptor (DOR) immunoreactivity in the rat spinal cord. Neurosci Lett 361: 208–211.
71. Herradon G, Ezquerra L, Nguyen T, Wang C, Siso A, et al. (2008) Noradrenergic and opioidergic alterations in neuropathy in different rat strains. Neurosci Lett 438: 186–189.
72. Pol O, Murtra P, Caracuel L, Valverde O, Puig MM, et al. (2006) Expression of opioid receptors and c-fos in CB1 knockout mice exposed to neuropathic pain. Neuropharmacology 50: 123–132.
73. Raghavendra V, Tanga F, Rutkowski MD, DeLeo JA (2003) Anti-hyperalgesic and morphine-sparing actions of propentofylline following peripheral nerve injury in rats: mechanistic implications of spinal glia and proinflammatory cytokines. Pain 104: 655–664.
74. Raghavendra V, Rutkowski MD, DeLeo JA (2002) The role of spinal neuroimmune activation in morphine tolerance/hyperalgesia in neuropathic and sham-operated rats. J Neurosci 22: 9980–9989.
75. Mika J, Korostynski M, Kaminska D, Wawrzczak-Bargiela A, Osikowicz M, et al. (2008) Interleukin-1alpha has antiallodynic and antihyperalgesic activities in a rat neuropathic pain model. Pain 13: 587–597.
76. Cunningham CL, Martínez-Cerdeño V, Noctor SC (2013) Microglia regulate the number of neural precursor cells in the developing cerebral cortex. J Neurosci 33: 4216–4233.
77. Quock RM, Burkey TH, Varga E, Hosohata Y, Hosohata K, et al. (1999) The delta-opioid receptor: molecular pharmacology, signal transduction, and the determination of drug efficacy. Pharmacol Rev 51: 503–532.
78. Scherrer G, Imamachi N, Cao YQ, Contet C, Mennicken F, et al. (2009) Dissociation of the opioid receptor mechanisms that control mechanical and heat pain. Cell 137: 1148–1159.
79. Sluka KA, Rohlwing JJ, Bussey RA, Eikenberry SA, Wilken JM (2002) Chronic muscle pain induced by repeated acid Injection is reversed by spinally administered mu- and delta-, but not kappa-, opioid receptor agonists. J Pharmacol Exp Ther 302: 1146–1150.
80. Holdridge SV, Cahill CM (2007a) Spinal administration of a delta opioid receptor agonist attenuates hyperalgesia and allodynia in a rat model of neuropathic pain. Eur J Pain 11: 685–693.
81. Holdridge SV, Armstrong SA, Taylor AM, Cahill CM (2007b) Behavioural and morphological evidence for the involvement of glial cell activation in delta opioid receptor function: implications for the development of opioid tolerance. Mol Pain 3: 7.
82. Chang AC, Chao CC, Takemori AE, Gekker G, Hu S, et al. (1996) Arylacetamide-derived fluorescent probes: synthesis, biological evaluation, and direct fluorescent labeling of kappa opioid receptors in mouse microglial cells. J Med Chem 39: 1729–1735.
83. El-Hage N, Dever SM, Podhaizer EM, Arnatt CK, Zhang Y, et al. (2013) A novel bivalent HIV-1 entry inhibitor reveals fundamental differences in CCR5-µ-opioid receptor interactions between human astroglia and microglia. AIDS 27: 2181–2190.
84. Merighi S, Gessi S, Varani K, Fazzi D, Stefanelli A, et al. (2013) Morphine mediates a proinflammatory phenotype via µ-opioid receptor-PKCε-Akt-ERK1/2 signaling pathway in activated microglial cells. Biochem Pharmacol 86: 487–496.
85. Chao CC, Gekker G, Hu S, Sheng WS, Shark KB, et al. (1996) Kappa opioid receptors in human microglia downregulate human immunodeficiency virus 1 expression. Proc Natl Acad Sci U S A 93: 8051–8056.
86. Chao CC, Hu S, Shark KB, Sheng WS, Gekker G, et al. (1997) Activation of mu opioid receptors inhibits microglial cell chemotaxis. J Pharmacol Exp Ther 281: 998–1004.
87. Turchan-Cholewo J, Dimayuga FO, Ding Q, Keller JN, Hauser KF, et al. (2008) Cell-specific actions of HIV-Tat and morphine on opioid receptor expression in glia. J Neurosci Res 86: 2100–2110.
88. Thorlin T, Persson PA, Eriksson PS, Hansson E, Rönnbäck L (1999) Delta-opioid receptor immunoreactivity on astrocytes is upregulated during mitosis. Glia 25: 370–378.
89. Scherrer G, Tryoen-Tóth P, Filliol D, Matifas A, Laustriat D, et al. (2006) Knockin mice expressing fluorescent delta-opioid receptors uncover G protein-coupled receptor dynamics in vivo. Proc Natl Acad Sci U S A 103: 9691–9696.
90. Commons KG, Milner TA (1996) Cellular and subcellular localization of delta opioid receptor immunoreactivity in the rat dentate gyrus. Brain Res 738: 181–195.
91. Cheng PY, Liu-Chen LY, Pickel VM (1997) Dual ultrastructural immunocytochemical labeling of mu and delta opioid receptors in the superficial layers of the rat cervical spinal cord. Brain Res 778: 367–380.
92. Horvath RJ, DeLeo JA (2009) Morphine enhances microglial migration through modulation of P2X4 receptor signaling. J Neurosci 29: 998–1005.
93. Kieffer BL, Gavériaux-Ruff C (2002) Exploring the opioid system by gene knockout. Prog Neurobiol 66: 285–306.
94. Gavériaux-Ruff C, Karchewski LA, Hever X, Matifas A, Kieffer BL (2008) Inflammatory pain is enhanced in delta opioid receptor-knockout mice. Eur J Neurosci 27: 2558–2567.
95. Nadal X, Baños JE, Kieffer BL, Maldonado R (2006) Neuropathic pain is enhanced in delta-opioid receptor knockout mice. Eur J Neurosci 23: 830–834.
96. Gallantine EL, Meert TF (2005) A comparison of the antinociceptive and adverse effects of the mu-opioid agonist morphine and the delta-opioid agonist SNC80. Basic Clin Pharmacol Toxicol 97: 39–51.
97. Cahill CM, Morinville A, Hoffert C, O'Donnell D, Beaudet A (2003) Up-regulation and trafficking of delta opioid receptor in a model of chronic inflammation: implications for pain control. Pain 101: 199–208.
98. Fraser GL, Gaudreau GA, Clarke PB, Ménard DP, Perkins MN (2000) Antihyperalgesic effects of delta opioid agonists in a rat model of chronic inflammation. Br J Pharmacol 129: 1668–1672.
99. Hurley RW, Hammond DL (2000) The analgesic effects of supraspinal mu and delta opioid receptor agonists are potentiated during persistent inflammation. J Neurosci 20: 1249–1259.
100. Happel C, Steele AD, Finley MJ, Kutzler MA, Rogers TJ (2008) DAMGO-induced expression of chemokines and chemokine receptors: the role of TGF-beta1. J Leukoc Biol 83: 956–963.
101. Szabo I, Chen XH, Xin L, Adler MW, Howard OM, et al. (2002) Heterologous desensitization of opioid receptors by chemokines inhibits chemotaxis and enhances the perception of pain. Proc Natl Acad Sci U S A 99: 10276–10281.
102. Horvath RJ, Romero-Sandoval EA, De Leo JA (2010b) Inhibition of microglial P2X4 receptors attenuates morphine tolerance, Iba1, GFAP and µ opioid receptor protein expression while enhancing perivascular microglial ED2. Pain 150: 401–413.
103. Hutchinson MR, Coats BD, Lewis SS, Zhang Y, Sprunger DB, et al. (2008) Proinflammatory cytokines oppose opioid-induced acute and chronic analgesia. Brain Behav Immun 22: 1178–1189.
104. Cahill CM, Holdridge SV, Morinville A (2007) Trafficking of delta-opioid receptors and other G-protein-coupled receptors: implications for pain and analgesia. Trends Pharmacol Sci 28: 23–31.
105. Bie B, Pan ZZ (2007) Trafficking of central opioid receptors and descending pain inhibition. Mol Pain 3: 37.
106. Zhang X, Bao L, Guan JS (2006) Role of delivery and trafficking of delta-opioid peptide receptors in opioid analgesia and tolerance. Trends Pharmacol Sci. 27:324–329.
107. Pradhan AA, Befort K, Nozaki C, Gavériaux-Ruff C, Kieffer BL (2011) The delta opioid receptor: anevolving target for the treatment of braindisorders. Trends Pharmacol Sci 32: 581–590.
108. Clinicaltrials website. Available: http://clinicaltrials.gov/ct2/results?term = delta+ opioid&Search = Search. Accessed 2014 May 20.

Spinal fMRI Reveals Decreased Descending Inhibition during Secondary Mechanical Hyperalgesia

Torge Rempe[1,2]*, Stephan Wolff[1], Christian Riedel[1], Ralf Baron[2,3], Patrick W. Stroman[4], Olav Jansen[1], Janne Gierthmühlen[1,3]

1 Dept of Neuroradiology, University Hospital of Kiel, Arnold-Heller-Strasse 3, Haus 41, 24105 Kiel, Germany, **2** Dept of Neurology, University Hospital of Kiel, Arnold-Heller-Strasse 3, Haus 41, 24105 Kiel, Germany, **3** Division of Neurological Pain Research and Therapy, University Hospital of Kiel, Arnold-Heller-Strasse 3, Haus 41, 24105 Kiel, Germany, **4** Centre for Neuroscience Studies, Dept of Diagnostic Radiology, Dept of Physics, 228 Botterell Hall, Queen's University, Kingston, Ontario, Canada

Abstract

Mechanical hyperalgesia is one distressing symptom of neuropathic pain which is explained by central sensitization of the nociceptive system. This sensitization can be induced experimentally with the heat/capsaicin sensitization model. The aim was to investigate and compare spinal and supraspinal activation patterns of identical mechanical stimulation before and after sensitization using functional spinal magnetic resonance imaging (spinal fMRI). Sixteen healthy subjects (6 female, 10 male, mean age 27.2±4.0 years) were investigated with mechanical stimulation of the C6 dermatome of the right forearm during spinal fMRI. Testing was always performed in the area outside of capsaicin application (i.e. area of secondary mechanical hyperalgesia). During slightly noxious mechanical stimulation before sensitization, activity was observed in ipsilateral dorsolateral pontine tegmentum (DLPT) which correlated with activity in ipsilateral spinal cord dorsal gray matter (dGM) suggesting activation of descending nociceptive inhibition. During secondary mechanical hyperalgesia, decreased activity was observed in bilateral DLPT, ipsilateral/midline rostral ventromedial medulla (RVM), and contralateral subnucleus reticularis dorsalis, which correlated with activity in ipsilateral dGM. Comparison of voxel-based activation patterns during mechanical stimulation before/after sensitization showed deactivations in RVM and activations in superficial ipsilateral dGM. This study revealed increased spinal activity and decreased activity in supraspinal centers involved in pain modulation (SRD, RVM, DLPT) during secondary mechanical hyperalgesia suggesting facilitation of nociception via decreased endogenous inhibition. Results should help prioritize approaches for further in vivo studies on pain processing and modulation in humans.

Editor: Theodore J. Price, University of Texas at Dallas, United States of America

Funding: The study was supported by the German Federal Ministry of Education and Research (BMBF, 01EM05/04). However, the authors received no specific funding for this work. The funders had no role in study design, data collection and analysis, decision to publish, or preparation of the manuscript.

Competing Interests: Ralf Baron reported grant/research support by: Pfizer, Genzyme, Grünenthal. Member of the IMI "Europain" collaboration and industry members of this are: Astra Zeneca, Pfizer, Esteve, UCB-Pharma, Sanofi Aventis, Grünenthal, Eli Lilly and Boehringer Ingelheim. German Federal Ministry of Education and Research (BMBF): German Research Network on Neuropathic Pain, Modelling Pain Switches. German Research Foundation (DFG). He received honoraria as a speaker from Pfizer, Genzyme, Grünenthal, Mundipharma, Sanofi Pasteur, Medtronic, Eisai, UCB BioSciences, Lilly, Boehringer Ingelheim, Astellas, Desitin and as a consultant from Pfizer, Genzyme, Grünenthal, Mundipharma, Allergan, Sanofi Pasteur, Medtronic, Eisai, UCB BioSciences, Lilly, Boehringer Ingelheim, Astellas, Novartis, Bristol-Myers Squibb, Biogenidec, AstraZeneca. Olav Jansen received honoraria as a speaker from Penumbra and as a consultant from Strykker, Philips and Boehringer Ingelheim. Janne Gierthmu¨hlen received honoraria as a speaker from Pfizer and travel grants from Gru¨nenthal. There are no conflicts of interests relevant to this article and none of the competing interests.

* Email: t.rempe@neurologie.uni-kiel.de

Introduction

Mechanical pinprick hyperalgesia is a very distressing symptom presented by approximately 29% of neuropathic pain patients [1]. During a state of hyperalgesia, an already nociceptive stimulus is perceived as even more painful [1]. Secondary hyperalgesia develops in the uninjured area surrounding a nerve injury and is caused by central sensitization, i.e. by modulation of the spinal and supraspinal nociceptive system [2,3]. It can be induced experimentally in healthy humans by the heat/capsaicin model [4].

Anatomically, the vast majority of the nociceptive second order neurons is located in the dorsal gray matter (dGM) of the spinal cord. From there they project to supraspinal nuclei in the brainstem and the thalamus before these afferent nociceptive impulses are transferred to further subcortical and cortical structures [5]. The nociceptive neurons in the spinal cord and in the brainstem have an important contribution in the transmission and modulation of pain. This knowledge is based mostly on animal experiments, observation of the effects of injury and disease as well as postmortem anatomical studies [3,6,7].

With the emergence of functional magnetic resonance imaging of the brain (fMRI) [8] and, to a lesser extent, of the brainstem [9,10], non-invasive methods have become available to provide insight into human pain processing in vivo. To investigate pain processing on the spinal level and in the brainstem, spinal fMRI is of great interest, however, its utilization is limited because of significant technical challenges such as cerebro-spinal fluid-pulsations, breathing/swallowing-motions, and the spinal cord's small cross-sectional dimension.

In order to address these challenges, recent spinal fMRI studies use a turbo spin-echo sequence with a relatively short echo time rather than the more conventional gradient echo imaging sequence sensitive to the blood oxygenation level-dependent (BOLD) effect [11–14]. It demonstrates BOLD contrast but also reveals a second contrast mechanism and important source of neuronal activity-related signal change in spinal fMRI termed "signal enhancement by extravascular water protons" (SEEP). This functionally induced signal is thought to originate from cellular swelling and thus changed extravascular water content due to increased intravascular pressure at sites of activity. This new technique is believed to localize sites of neuronal activity more precisely than conventional T_2*-weighted gradient echo imaging sequences, which have rather poor field homogeneity [11–14].

However, spinal fMRI studies of human pain processing are still rare [15–17]. While spinal fMRI has recently been used successfully to demonstrate signal intensity changes in the spinal cord and brainstem during innocuous and noxious thermal stimulation and heat allodynia/hyperalgesia [18], there is still no spinal fMRI study that examines spinal and supraspinal changes in activity during secondary mechanical hyperalgesia up to this point.

Therefore, the aims were (A) to investigate spinal and supraspinal processes occurring as a consequence of mechanical stimulation and (B) to compare activation patterns of identical mechanical stimuli before and after induction of sensitization with the heat/capsaicin model in healthy subjects in order to investigate the specific pain-related components of secondary mechanical hyperalgesia. Within this study we could successfully demonstrate (A) increased activity in ipsilateral dGM after induction of hyperalgesia, (B) decreased activity in nociceptive regions of the brainstem and (C) a correlation between these supraspinal deactivations and activations of ipsilateral dGM during secondary mechanical hyperalgesia suggesting a facilitation of nociception via decreased descending endogenous inhibition.

Materials and Methods

Subjects

Sixteen right-handed [19] healthy volunteers (6 females, 10 males, mean age 27.2±4.0 years, range 23–32 years) were included in the study. All subjects were free of any acute or chronic pain conditions. Comorbidities such as diseases of the peripheral or central nervous system were ruled out. None of the subjects were on drugs that might have interfered with itch or pain sensations and flare responses. The study was in accordance with the Declaration of Helsinki and was approved by the Ethical Committee of the Faculty of Medicine at Christian-Albrechts-University of Kiel. Written informed consent was obtained from all participants.

Psychophysics

On the right (= ipsilateral) lateral volar forearm approximately 3 cm distal to the elbow in the C6 dermatome a 3×3 cm square area [area A, site of sensitization] and an adjacent 2×5 cm area directly distal to it [area B, for mechanical stimulation] were marked (figure 1).

Experimental set-up

All subjects underwent two identical MRI sessions back-to-back on the same day with mechanical stimulation in the same area before and after sensitization.

fMRI data acquisition. All scans were performed in a 3T human MRI scanner (Philips Achieva 3T). For acquisition of functional image data, a half-Fourier, single-shot turbo spin-echo sequence with a phased-array head-neck receiver coil (TE = 38 ms, TR = 9000 ms, 288×144×20 mm FOV, 192×96 matrix) was used [17,21]. At TE = 38 ms, this sequence is about equally sensitive to contributions of both BOLD and SEEP [14,22,23]. With this configuration 10 contiguous 2 mm thick sagittal slices were acquired, spanning from above the thalamus to below the C7/T1 intervertebral disc with a resulting voxel size of 1.5×1.5×2 mm^3. To reduce sources of motion artefacts (e.g. heart, lungs and throat), a spatial saturation pulse was applied to the region anterior to the vertebral column.

Mechanical stimulation. In order to enable the stimulation of a larger dermatomal area (possibly leading to a higher signal in the spinal cord) mechanical stimulation was performed using a self-made brush consisting of 15 stiff von-Frey-hairs (166 mN). Care was taken that the site of stimulation was always within the area of secondary hyperalgesia [area B]. The mechanical stimulation paradigms consisted of 8 stimulation periods of 40 seconds alternating with eight baseline periods (64 volumes). After each session, subjects were asked to rate the stimulus intensity on the numerical rating scale (NRS, ranging from 0 to 10 with 0 representing "no pain" and 10 being the "maximum pain that can be imagined") by verbal response.

Heat/Capsaicin sensitization model. The heat/capsaicin sensitization model was used to induce secondary mechanical hyperalgesia [4]. Therefore, area A was stimulated with a computer-controlled Peltier thermode (Medoc TSA-2001, Haifa, Israel) at 45°C for 5 minutes. Afterwards a gauze pad with 1 ml solution of 0.6% capsaicin in 45% ethanol was placed on area A for 30 minutes. During capsaicin-application, the subjects were asked once a minute for NRS ratings of perceived pain intensity and temperature sensation at the application site. The temperature sensation was quantified on the NRS with 0 representing "neutral temperature" and −10/+10 representing "the maximum cold/warmth that can be imagined". After patch removal and at the end of the second fMRI block the borders of the area of punctate mechanical hyperalgesia were assessed by a stiff von-Frey-hair (166 mN). The dimensions of flare and mechanical hyperalgesia were then determined by the calculation: $(D/2)\times(d/2)\times\pi$ (D = horizontal diameter, d = vertical diameters of the area) to assess the stability of the pain model throughout the experiment.

Analysis and Statistics

For the analysis of the resulting 3D fMRI image data a general linear model (GLM) was used. The basis set consists of a boxcar model paradigm convolved with the tissue response function [12] and models of cardiac-related spinal cord motion as confounds [17,21]. Its results demonstrate the weighting factors $\beta 1$ (magnitude of the pattern matching the stimulation paradigm convolved with the tissue response function) and $\beta 0$ (average voxel intensity). Corrections for bulk motion and a normalization to a consistent coordinate space of the brainstem and spinal cord were then performed as described previously [21]. A random-effects analysis by McGonigle et al. was used to determine combined group results [24]. This consists of the calculation of the mean and standard deviation of the ratio of $\beta 1/\beta 0$ representing the relative signal intensity response across studies. T values of >2.5 or <-2.5 were assumed as significant activity as they correspond with $p<0.0075$ [17]. Contrast calculations between mechanical stimulation before and after sensitization were performed on a voxel-by-voxel basis by the partial least squares (PLS) method [25]. A bootstrap ratio of

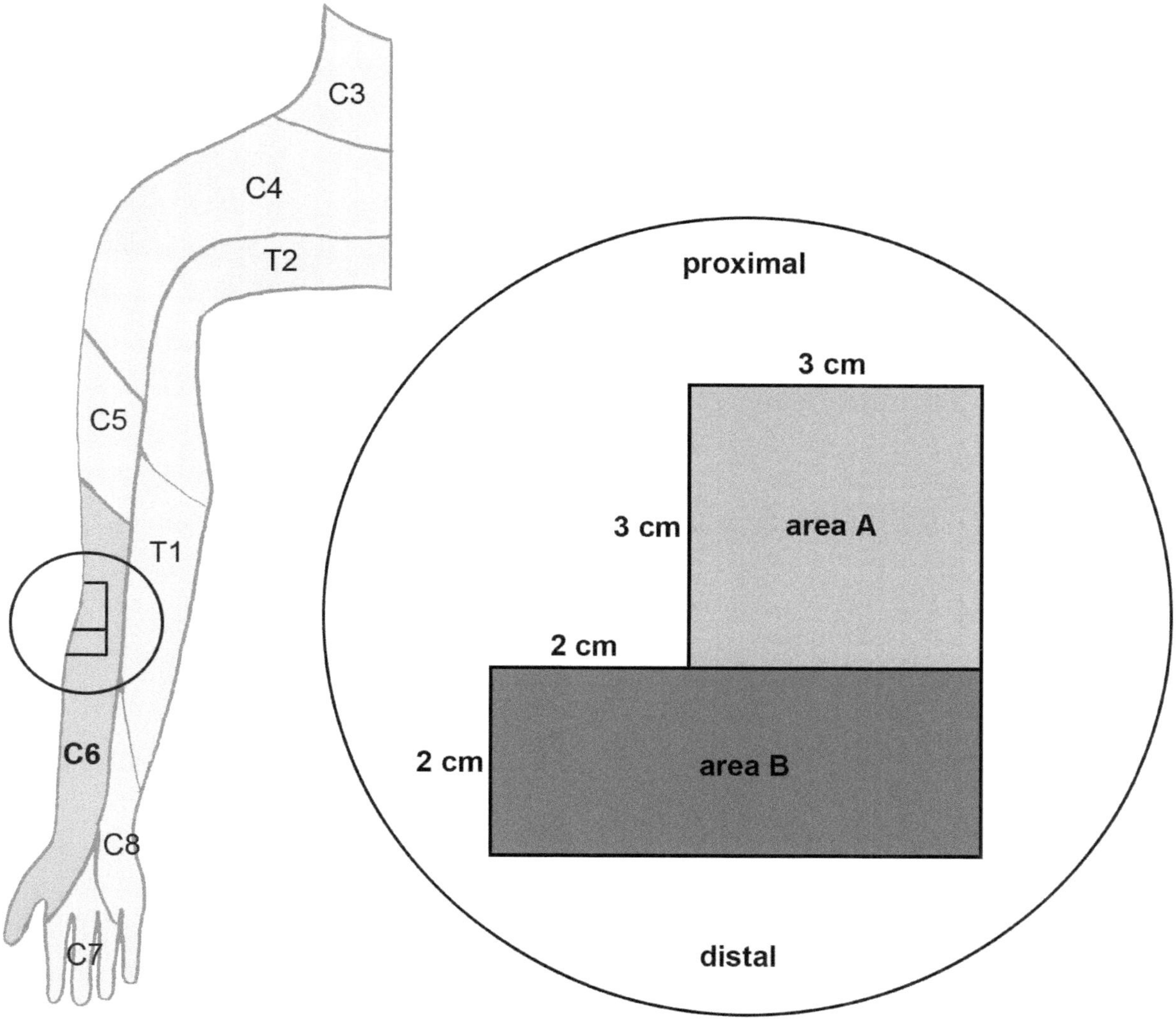

Figure 1. Areas of sensitization and stimulation on the right lateral volar forearm. For orientation, the schematic drawing on the left shows a dermatome map of the right upper extremity (redrawn and modified from [20]). The area of testing (marked by the circle) is situated on the right lateral volar forearm in the C6 dermatome. *Area A:* Site of sensitization with the heat/capsaicin model (3×3 cm square area 3 cm distal to the elbow in the C6 dermatome). *Area B:* Site of mechanical stimulation corresponding to the area of secondary mechanical hyperalgesia (2×5 cm area distal to area A).

≥5 was chosen for differences between two contrasted responses to be significant [17].

Spinal cord segments adjacent to C6 were included in the analysis since (A) primary afferent fibers split up into longitudinal collaterals innervating the bordering segments and (B) slightly individual anatomical dermatome-borders with a coincidental stimulation of surrounding dermatomes (i.e. C5, T1) were respected.

Psychophysical data are presented as mean ± standard deviation (SD) unless otherwise specified. Wilcoxon matched pairs test was used for calculation of psychophysical intragroup differences and Spearman rank test for correlation calculations using the numbers of voxels ($n_{(v)}$), signal change ($\Delta_{(S)}$) and % signal change ($\Delta_{(S/S)}$) across all volunteers provided by the fMRI data. P values <0.05 were considered to be statistically significant.

Results

Psychophysics

Capsaicin-application induced painful and warm sensations in all subjects (figure 2A). The capsaicin-induced flare decreased in size throughout testing (82.0 ± 18.8 cm^2 after patch removal vs. 67.0 ± 16.8 cm^2 at the end of testing, $p=0.002$). However, the dimension of secondary mechanical hyperalgesia was stable (77.1 ± 24.5 cm^2 after removal of capsaicin vs. 89.5 ± 35.7 cm^2 at the end of scanning, $p=0{,}125$) and included the area of stimulation [area B] at all times, thus ensuring the stability of the pain model throughout the experiment. Corresponding to mechanical hyperalgesia, the subjects' mean ratings of pain intensity for the mechanical stimulus were higher compared to those before sensitization (3.4 ± 2.2 vs. 2.1 ± 1.8, $p=0.003$; figure 2B).

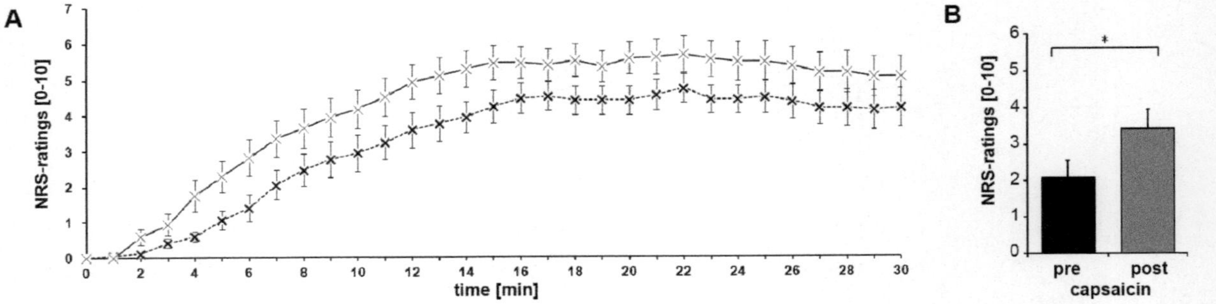

Figure 2. Psychophysical data. (A) Mean ratings of pain intensity (dashed line) and temperature perception (solid line) during capsaicin application. Capsaicin was applied at time 0. Mean ± standard error of the mean (SEM). (B) Mean pain ratings for the mechanical stimulus before and after application of capsaicin. Capsaicin induced secondary mechanical hyperalgesia. Mean ± SEM. *: $p<0.05$.

fMRI

Spinal group activation patterns and contrast maps. During mechanical stimulation prior to sensitization, spinal deactivations i.e. decreased signal intensity during stimulation were observed in deep dGM layers of C6 and C8 bilaterally and C7 contralaterally. After capsaicin exposure, mechanical stimulation in the area of secondary hyperalgesia lead to activations (increased signal intensity during stimulation) in T1 and deactivations in C7 in ipsilateral superficial dGM. Ventral activations were observed in ipsilateral ventral gray matter (vGM) of C4 before and after sensitization (figures 3, 4).

Activations in ipsilateral vGM of C7 correlated positively to the subjects' NRS-ratings before ($\Delta_{(S)}$: $R = 0.513$; $p = 0.042$) and after sensitization ($\Delta_{(S)}$: $R = 0.533$; $p = 0.041$), i.e. the higher the perceived pain intensity, the higher were activations in vGM of C7.

Contrast calculations between mechanical stimulation before and after sensitization with the heat/capsaicin model revealed activations in superficial ipsilateral (C7, C8) dGM. The observed lateral deviation of superficial dGM-activations might arise from BOLD-contributions in signal change located in superficial draining veins [14]. Contralateral activations were observed in deep dGM of C8 and vGM of C7. Deactivations were found in C4 in ipsilateral vGM and contralateral dGM (figures 3, 4).

Supraspinal group activation patterns and contrast maps. Prior to sensitization, supraspinal activity was observed in the ipsilateral dorsolateral pontine tegmentum (DLPT) (figure 5A). The activity in the ipsilateral dorsal pons correlated positively to activity in ipsilateral dGM of C4 ($n_{(v)}$: $R = 0.611$; $p = 0.012$) and C5 ($n_{(v)}$: $R = 0.613$; $p = 0.012$).

In contrast to measurements prior to sensitization, deactivations in contralateral DLPT were observed during secondary mechanical hyperalgesia (figure 5A). These deactivations correlated with activations in ipsilateral dGM of C5 ($n_{(v)}$: $R = 0.546$; $p = 0.035$) and T1 ($n_{(v)}$: $R = 0.621$; $p = 0.012$). Deactivations in the ipsilateral pons correlated with activations in ipsilateral dGM of C4 ($n_{(v)}$: $R = 0.595$; $p = 0.019$) and T1 ($n_{(v)}$: $R = 0.555$; $p = 0.039$; $\Delta_{(S/S)}$: $R = -0.538$; $p = 0.047$), i.e. the higher the deactivations in the dorsal pons, the higher were activations in ipsilateral dGM (note that R in $n_{(v)}$ is positive because $n_{(deactivated\ voxels)}$ correlates positively to $n_{(activated\ voxels)}$ while $\Delta_{(S/S)}$ is negative because activations, i.e. positive $\Delta_{(S/S)}$-values are correlating to deactivations, i.e. negative $\Delta_{(S/S)}$-values).

After sensitization, deactivations were also visible in the ipsilateral and median caudal pons/rostral medulla most likely corresponding to the area of the rostral ventromedial medulla (RVM, figure 5A). Deactivations in the ipsilateral rostral ventral medulla correlated with ipsilateral dGM activations (C4: $n_{(v)}$: $R = 0.699$; $p = 0.004$; $\Delta_{(S)}$: $R = -0.827$; $p<0.001$; $\Delta_{(S/S)}$: $R = -0.770$; $p = 0.001$; C6: $\Delta_{(S)}$: $R = -0.537$; $p = 0.039$). Deactivations in midline RVM correlated with deactivations in ipsilateral dGM (C5: $n_{(v)}$: $R = 0.556$; $p = 0.031$; C7 = $n_{(v)}$: $R = 0.599$; $p = 0.018$; $\Delta_{(S)}$: $R = 0.608$; $p = 0.016$). Visible deactivations in the caudodorsal contralateral medulla corresponded to the localization of the subnucleus reticularis dorsalis (SRD, figure 5B) and correlated with spinal activations in ipsilateral dGM (C4: $\Delta_{(S/S)}$: $R = -0.560$; $p = 0.030$; C8: $\Delta_{(S/S)}$: $R = -0.578$; $p = 0.024$; T1 = $n_{(voxels)}$: $R = 0.554$; $p = 0.040$).

Supraspinal calculations of contrast maps showed deactivations in the RVM (figure 5A).

Discussion

The present study shows spinal and supraspinal signal intensity changes during mechanical stimulation and secondary mechanical hyperalgesia in healthy subjects. The main findings are (A) increased activity in ipsilateral dGM after induction of hyperalgesia, (B) decreased activity in supraspinal centers of pain processing and modulation (DLPT, RVM, SRD) and (C) a correlation between supraspinal deactivations and activations of ipsilateral dGM during secondary mechanical hyperalgesia induced by the heat/capsaicin model. Results suggest a facilitation of nociception via decreased descending endogenous inhibition during secondary mechanical hyperalgesia.

Spinal cord

Ipsilateral dGM. Anatomically, the vast majority of primary nociceptive afferent fibers projects to the ipsilateral dGM. Therefore, application of noxious stimuli should lead to activation of projection neurons located in the marginal layer of the dorsal horn [27]. Supportingly, this study showed superficial dGM-activations during painful stimulation after sensitization. Animal experiments suggest a higher activation of spinal nociceptive projection neurons by the same noxious stimulus during experimental pain states [3,6]. For example, Simone et al. showed an increase of monkey spinothalamic tract neuron responses to punctate mechanical stimuli during capsaicin-induced secondary hyperalgesia [2]. The current study is now the first one to reproduce such findings from animal experiments in human subjects in vivo as contrast maps revealed activations in superficial dGM that may correspond with increased activity during central sensitization.

Mechanical hyperalgesia and increased dGM activity can also be due to deficient inhibitory interneuron (ININ)-mediated

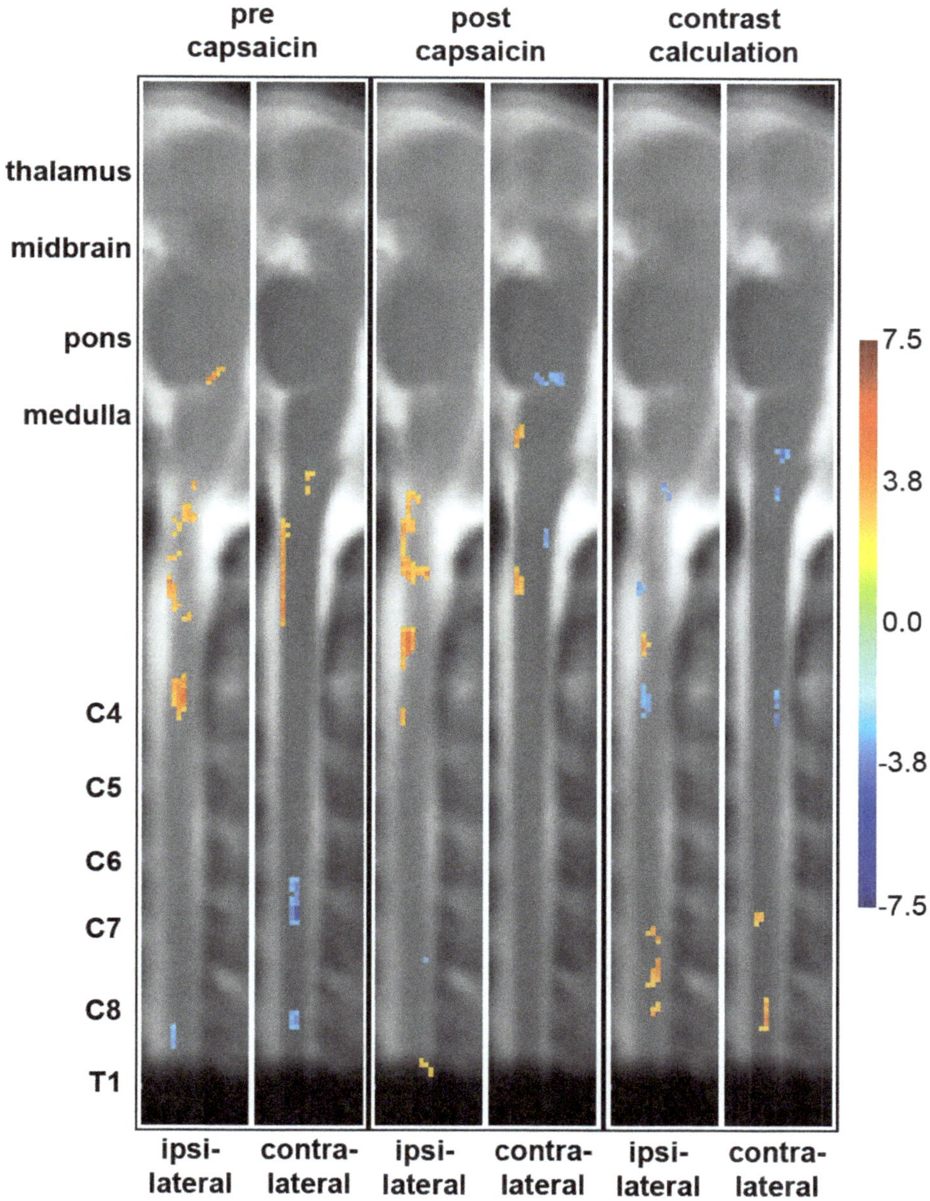

Figure 3. Sagittal slices of group activation patterns and contrast maps. Columns 1 to 4 show areas of activity across brain stem and cervical spinal cord before (1st and 2nd column) and after (3rd and 4th column) sensitization with the heat capsaicin model representing the significance (T-value) of each active voxel across the 16 subjects. Columns 5 and 6 show partial-least squares (PLS) results of contrast calculations on a voxel-by-voxel basis. The left column of each 2 columns (e.g. 1st, 3rd and 5th) corresponds to the ipsilateral side of the stimulus, the right column to the contralateral side. The color bar on the right indicates the corresponding significance, i.e. T-value (columns 1–4) or bootstrap-ratio (columns 5–6) for each color.

inhibition of projection neurons [28,29]. Interestingly, deactivations in deep dGM in C6 and C8 were observed prior to sensitization but disappeared during secondary mechanical hyperalgesia.

Contralateral dGM. Signal intensity changes were also observed in contralateral dGM during both conditions, consistent with a previous study using tactile stimuli [16]. These observations could be explained by primary afferent fibers ending in the contralateral dorsal horn [30] as well as by interneurons of ipsilateral dGM that cross the midline [17]. Our results also show differences during mechanical hyperalgesia compared to mechanical stimulation prior to sensitization suggesting a participation of the contralateral dGM in the development of central sensitization. It would be important for future studies to focus on such changes in contralateral dGM as contralateral somatosensory abnormalities have been observed in human unilateral neuropathic pain states [31].

vGM. Pain stimuli lead to withdrawal reflexes, i.e. the activation of ipsilateral motor neurons via spinal interneurons or supraspinal reticular nuclei [32]. Because mechanical stimuli were perceived as (slightly) painful, vGM-activity can be expected and was accordingly observed in both fMRI sessions. The positive correlation between the subjects' NRS-ratings and the activity in ipsilateral vGM of C7 suggests that stronger pain stimuli lead to

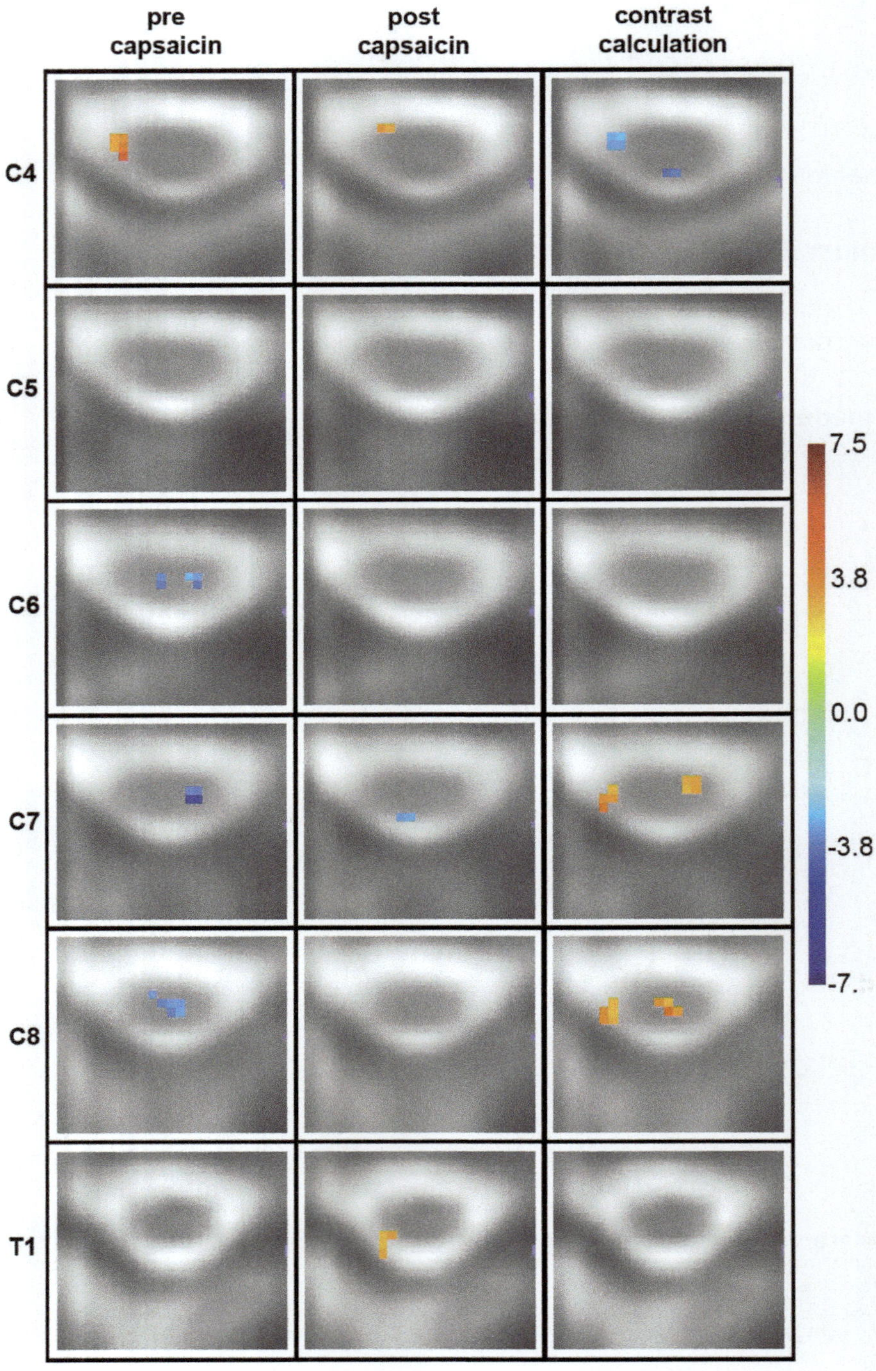

Figure 4. Spinal group activation patterns before (left column) and after (middle column) sensitization and contrast maps (right column). The transverse slices are in radiological orientation with the left side corresponding to the right body side and approximate the corresponding spinal cord segment for a rostral-caudal span from C4 to T1. They show spinal regions of signal intensity change before (left column) and after (middle column) sensitization with the heat/capsaicin model representing the significance (T-value) of each active voxel across the 16 subjects. The right column shows partial-least squares (PLS) results of contrast calculations on a voxel-by-voxel basis. The color bar in figure 3 indicates the corresponding significance, i.e. T-value (left and middle column) or bootstrap-ratio (right column) for each color. *Left Column:* Activations in ipsilateral vGM of C4. Deactivations in bilateral deep dGM of C6 and C8 and contralateral deep dGM of C7. *Middle column:* Ipsilateral activations in superficial dGM of T1 and vGM of C4. Deactivations in ipsilateral superficial dGM of C7. *Right column:* Activations in ipsilateral superficial dGM (C7, C8) and in contralateral vGM (C7) and deep dGM (C8). Deactivations in ipsilateral vGM and contralateral dGM of C4.

higher reflex answers. The C7 segment innervates both M. pronator teres and M. pronator quadratus. As the arm was held in a supine position throughout noxious stimulation, the activation of these muscles would be needed to escape the stimulus.

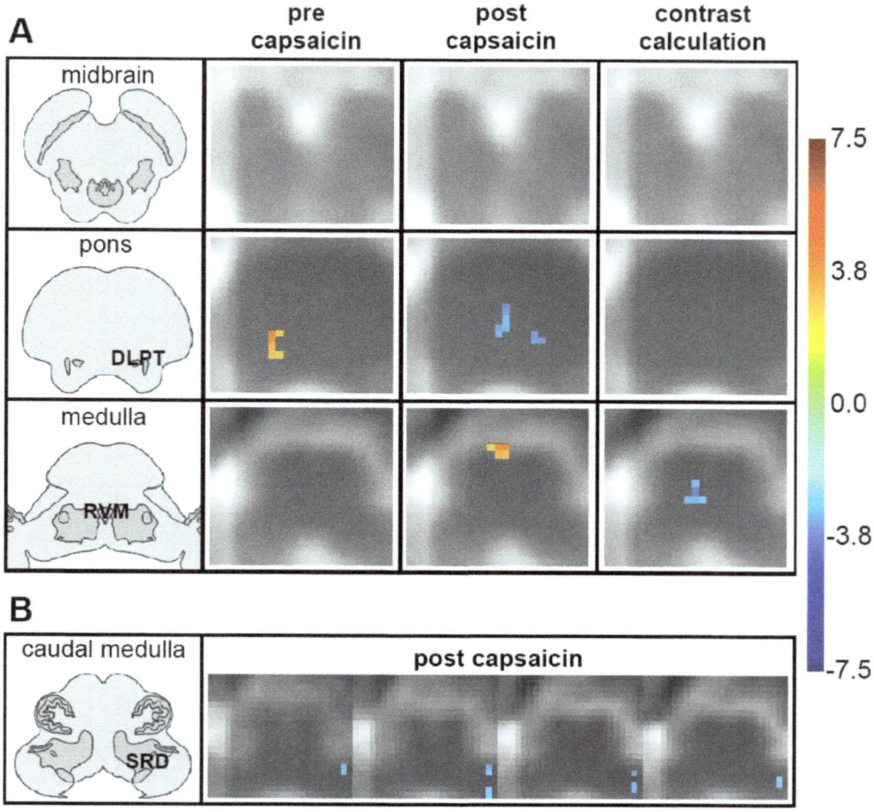

Figure 5. Supraspinal group activation patterns and contrast maps. Slices are in radiological orientation with the left side corresponding to the right body side. The color bar in figure 3 indicates the corresponding significance, i.e. T-value (combined group results pre/post capsaicin) or bootstrap-ratio (contrast calculation) for each color. Anatomical transverse sections on the left were modified from [26]. (A) The transverse slices approximate the corresponding brainstem region (midbrain, pons, medulla) for a rostral-caudal span. They show supraspinal regions of signal intensity change before (left column) and after (middle column) sensitization with the heat/capsaicin model representing the significance (T-value) of each active voxel across the 16 subjects. The right column shows partial-least squares (PLS) results of contrast calculations on a voxel-by-voxel basis. *Left column:* Activations in the ipsilateral DLPT (dorsolateral pontine tegmentum) during mechanical stimulation prior to application of capsaicin. *Middle column:* Deactivations in the contralateral DLPT and in the RVM (rostral ventromedial medulla) during secondary mechanical hyperalgesia (note that visible medial pontine deactivations are situated in the caudal pons/rostral medulla and therefore most likely correspond to the location of the RVM). *Right column:* Deactivations in the RVM. (B) The adjacent 1 mm thick transverse slices in consecutive arrangement located in the medulla show signal intensity changes during secondary mechanical hyperalgesia. Deactivations are observed in contralateral subnucleus reticularis dorsalis (SRD).

Brainstem

DLPT. Animal testing shows that the DLPT plays a central role in the modulation of nociception. With its noradrenergic fibers to the dGM, it mediates a negative feedback loop triggered by noxious stimuli to prevent excessive pain sensation [7,33]. This descending inhibition is for the most part mediated by the ipsilateral DLPT [34]. Accordingly, this study showed activations in the ipsilateral DLPT during painful mechanical stimulation prior to sensitization. Moreover these activations correlated with activations in ipsilateral dGM, possibly reflecting either an augmented activation of endogenous inhibition by higher activation of projection neurons [7] or a noradrenergic activation of spinal ININs (indirect inhibition of projection neurons) as it has been shown in animal studies [35]. Similarly, previous fMRI studies also showed activations of the DLPT during painful stimuli in healthy humans [15,36].

An absence of this noradrenergic inhibition by the DLPT is thought to be a mechanism for the development of neuropathic pain [3,37]. Interestingly, a bilateral decrease of DLPT-activation was seen during secondary mechanical hyperalgesia which correlated with ipsilateral dGM-activations. Compatibly, Becerra et al. showed bilaterally decreased DLPT-activity during mechanical hyperalgesia/allodynia in neuropathic pain patients [38]. Our results could thus correspond to a reduced descending noradrenergic inhibition with consecutive higher activation of spinal projection neurons.

Besides decreased inhibition, central sensitization is also thought to be mediated by coexisting excitatory descending facilitation [3,6,39]. Two earlier fMRI studies investigating secondary mechanical hyperalgesia demonstrated activity in rostral brainstem regions (midline-periaqueductal gray, contralateral cuneiform nucleus [10], contralateral mesencephalic pontine reticular formation [9]) that could be a correlate for excitatory nociceptive facilitation. Why did the current study not show these activations? Possible explanations could be overlapping processes of activation and simultaneous suppression of anti-nociceptive descending pathways in the very limited space of these brainstem nuclei or the different experimental set ups (MRI sequences or devices).

RVM. Based on current concepts of pain modulation, OFF-cells, a specific cell-type of the RVM, physiologically mediate antinociception [39,40]. In the condition of central sensitization, this OFF-cell activity is decreased [41]. Compatibly, this study shows decreased activity in the RVM during secondary mechanical hyperalgesia. A deactivation of OFF-cells would lead to a decreased inhibition of spinal projection neurons. Supportingly, this study shows correlations between deactivation of ipsilateral RVM and activations in ipsilateral dGM during secondary mechanical hyperalgesia. However, it has to be kept in mind that spinal inhibition can also be caused by the activation of ININs [29]. The observed correlation between deactivations in median RVM and ipsilateral dGM could therefore correspond to decreased OFF-cell mediated activation of ININs during secondary mechanical hyperalgesia.

SRD. The SRD is believed to play a major role in the mechanism of diffuse noxious inhibitory control (DNIC) [42]. An absence of this control is thought to be a reason for the development of neuropathic pain [39]. Accordingly, this study shows deactivations in contralateral SRD during secondary mechanical hyperalgesia which correlated with activations in the ipsilateral dGM. This could correspond to a facilitation of nociception via decreased endogenous inhibition by SRD and consequently higher dGM-activations - a similar and additional mechanism to nociceptive modulation by DLPT and RVM.

Limitations

Even though spin-echo spinal cord fMRI is a new reliable and non-invasive method to show functional processes in the spinal cord [15–18], its spatial resolution is still limited. Thus, an exact localization of the anatomical area corresponding to the observed activity is extremely difficult and can sometimes be only speculative. Furthermore, interpretation of results is complicated due to interconnections and often dichotomous roles of areas involved in pain processing/modulation, i.e. excitatory and inhibitory roles.

Conclusion

Using spin-echo spinal cord fMRI, it was possible to investigate pain modulatory processes during secondary mechanical hyperalgesia in the brainstem and spinal cord of healthy subjects. This study is the first one to show an increase of ipsilateral dGM-activity during secondary mechanical hyperalgesia in human subjects in vivo. Furthermore, this study succeeds in showing decreased activity in areas of the brainstem that have been proven important for processes of central sensitization in animal experiments (DLPT, RVM, SRD). Moreover, those deactivations correlated with dGM-activity. With these findings, this study gives new insights in human pain processing in vivo. Since findings of animal experiments and results of previous fMRI studies could be reproduced, spin-echo spinal cord fMRI has been shown to be a reliable method for the examination of spinal and supraspinal pain processing and modulation. Herewith, it qualifies for further investigations including treatment of neuropathic pain.

Acknowledgments

We are indebted to the subjects who participated in the study for their consent and co-operation.

Author Contributions

Conceived and designed the experiments: JG. Performed the experiments: TR SW. Analyzed the data: TR PWS JG. Contributed reagents/materials/analysis tools: PWS. Contributed to the writing of the manuscript: TR CR RB PWS OJ JG.

References

1. Baron R, Binder A, Wasner G (2010) Neuropathic pain: diagnosis, pathophysiological mechanisms, and treatment. Lancet Neurol 9: 807–819.
2. Simone DA, Sorkin LS, Oh U, Chung JM, Owens C, et al. (1991) Neurogenic hyperalgesia: central neural correlates in responses of spinothalamic tract neurons. J Neurophysiol 66: 228–246.
3. Westlund KN (2006) The dorsal horn and hyperalgesia. In: Cervero F, Jensen TS, editors. Handbook of Clinical Neurology, Vol 81 (3rd series): Pain. Amsterdam: Elsevier B.V. pp. 178–186.
4. Petersen KL, Rowbotham MC (1999) A new human experimental pain model: the heat/capsaicin sensitization model. Neuroreport 10: 1511–1516.
5. Villanueva L, Lopez-Avila A, Le Bars D (2006) Ascending nociceptive pathways. In: Cervero F, Jensen TS, editors. Handbook of Clinical Neurology, Vol 81 (3rd series): Pain. Amsterdam: Elsevier B.V. pp. 93–102.
6. Ossipov MH, Porreca F (2006) Descending excitatory systems. In: Cervero F, Jensen TS, editors. Handbook of Clinical Neurology, Vol 81 (3rd series): Pain. Amsterdam: Elsevier B.V. pp. 193–210.
7. Pertovaara A, Almeida A (2006) Descending inhibitory systems. In: Cervero F, Jensen TS, editors. Handbook of Clinical Neurology, Vol 81 (3rd series): Pain. Amsterdam: Elsevier B.V. pp. 179–192.
8. Baron R, Baron Y, Disbrow E, Roberts TP (1999) Brain processing of capsaicin-induced secondary hyperalgesia: a functional MRI study. Neurology 53: 548–557.
9. Lee MC, Zambreanu L, Menon DK, Tracey I (2008) Identifying brain activity specifically related to the maintenance and perceptual consequence of central sensitization in humans. J Neurosci 28: 11642–11649.
10. Zambreanu L, Wise RG, Brooks JC, Iannetti GD, Tracey I (2005) A role for the brainstem in central sensitisation in humans. Evidence from functional magnetic resonance imaging. Pain 114: 397–407.
11. Stroman PW (2005) Magnetic resonance imaging of neuronal function in the spinal cord: spinal FMRI. Clin Med Res 3: 146–156.
12. Stroman PW, Kornelsen J, Lawrence J, Malisza KL (2005) Functional magnetic resonance imaging based on SEEP contrast: response function and anatomical specificity. Magn Reson Imaging 23: 843–850.
13. Stroman PW, Krause V, Malisza KL, Frankenstein UN, Tomanek B (2002) Extravascular proton-density changes as a non-BOLD component of contrast in fMRI of the human spinal cord. Magn Reson Med 48: 122–127.
14. Stroman PW, Wheeler-Kingshott C, Bacon M, Schwab JM, Bosma R, et al. (2014) The current state-of-the-art of spinal cord imaging: methods. Neuroimage 84: 1070–1081.
15. Cahill CM, Stroman PW (2011) Mapping of neural activity produced by thermal pain in the healthy human spinal cord and brain stem: a functional magnetic resonance imaging study. Magn Reson Imaging 29: 342–352.
16. Ghazni NF, Cahill CM, Stroman PW (2010) Tactile sensory and pain networks in the human spinal cord and brain stem mapped by means of functional MR imaging. AJNR Am J Neuroradiol 31: 661–667.
17. Stroman PW (2009) Spinal fMRI investigation of human spinal cord function over a range of innocuous thermal sensory stimuli and study-related emotional influences. Magn Reson Imaging 27: 1333–1346.
18. Rempe T, Wolff S, Riedel C, Baron R, Stroman PW, et al. (2014) Spinal and supraspinal processing of thermal stimuli: An fMRI study. J Magn Reson Imaging DOI:10.1002/jmri.24627.
19. Oldfield RC (1971) The assessment and analysis of handedness: the Edinburgh inventory. Neuropsychologia 9: 97–113.
20. Trepel M (2008) Neuroanatomie: Struktur und Funktion. Munich: Elsevier GmbH, Urban & Fischer Verlag.
21. Stroman PW, Figley CR, Cahill CM (2008) Spatial normalization, bulk motion correction and coregistration for functional magnetic resonance imaging of the human cervical spinal cord and brainstem. Magn Reson Imaging 26: 809–814.
22. Figley CR, Stroman PW (2012) Measurement and characterization of the human spinal cord SEEP response using event-related spinal fMRI. Magn Reson Imaging 30: 471–484.
23. Stroman PW, Bosma RL, Beynon M, Dobek C (2012) Removal of synergistic physiological motion and image artefacts in functional MRI of the human spinal cord. 20th Annual Meeting of the International Society for Magnetic Resonance in Medicine. Melbourne, Australia.
24. McGonigle DJ, Howseman AM, Athwal BS, Friston KJ, Frackowiak RS, et al. (2000) Variability in fMRI: an examination of intersession differences. Neuroimage 11: 708–734.
25. McIntosh AR, Lobaugh NJ (2004) Partial least squares analysis of neuroimaging data: applications and advances. Neuroimage 23 Suppl 1: S250–263.
26. Naidich TP, Duvernoy HM, Delman BN, Sorensen AG, Kollias SS, et al. (2009) Duvernoy's Atlas of the Human Brain Stem and Cerebellum. Wien New York: Springer. pp. 53–93.

27. Millan MJ (1999) The induction of pain: an integrative review. Prog Neurobiol 57: 1–164.
28. Meisner JG, Marsh AD, Marsh DR (2010) Loss of GABAergic interneurons in laminae I–III of the spinal cord dorsal horn contributes to reduced GABAergic tone and neuropathic pain after spinal cord injury. J Neurotrauma 27: 729–737.
29. Millan MJ (2002) Descending control of pain. Prog Neurobiol 66: 355–474.
30. Light AR, Perl ER (1979) Spinal termination of functionally identified primary afferent neurons with slowly conducting myelinated fibers. J Comp Neurol 186: 133–150.
31. Huge V, Lauchart M, Forderreuther S, Kaufhold W, Valet M, et al. (2008) Interaction of hyperalgesia and sensory loss in complex regional pain syndrome type I (CRPS I). PLoS One 3: e2742.
32. Morgan MM (1998) Direct comparison of heat-evoked activity of nociceptive neurons in the dorsal horn with the hindpaw withdrawal reflex in the rat. J Neurophysiol 79: 174–180.
33. Fields HL, Basbaum AI (1994) Central nervous system mechanisms of pain modulation. In: Wall PD, Melzack R, editors. Textbook of Pain. 3 ed. Edinburgh: Churchill Livingstone. pp. 243–257.
34. Clark FM, Proudfit HK (1991) The projection of noradrenergic neurons in the A7 catecholamine cell group to the spinal cord in the rat demonstrated by anterograde tracing combined with immunocytochemistry. Brain Res 547: 279–288.
35. Gassner M, Ruscheweyh R, Sandkuhler J (2009) Direct excitation of spinal GABAergic interneurons by noradrenaline. Pain 145: 204–210.
36. Dunckley P, Wise RG, Fairhurst M, Hobden P, Aziz Q, et al. (2005) A comparison of visceral and somatic pain processing in the human brainstem using functional magnetic resonance imaging. J Neurosci 25: 7333–7341.
37. Xu M, Kontinen VK, Kalso E (1999) Endogenous noradrenergic tone controls symptoms of allodynia in the spinal nerve ligation model of neuropathic pain. Eur J Pharmacol 366: 41–45.
38. Becerra L, Morris S, Bazes S, Gostic R, Sherman S, et al. (2006) Trigeminal neuropathic pain alters responses in CNS circuits to mechanical (brush) and thermal (cold and heat) stimuli. J Neurosci 26: 10646–10657.
39. Ossipov MH, Dussor GO, Porreca F (2010) Central modulation of pain. J Clin Invest 120: 3779–3787.
40. Gebhart GF (2004) Descending modulation of pain. Neurosci Biobehav Rev 27: 729–737.
41. Kincaid W, Neubert MJ, Xu M, Kim CJ, Heinricher MM (2006) Role for medullary pain facilitating neurons in secondary thermal hyperalgesia. J Neurophysiol 95: 33–41.
42. Villanueva L, Bouhassira D, Le Bars D (1996) The medullary subnucleus reticularis dorsalis (SRD) as a key link in both the transmission and modulation of pain signals. Pain 67: 231–240.

19

Persistent At-Level Thermal Hyperalgesia and Tactile Allodynia Accompany Chronic Neuronal and Astrocyte Activation in Superficial Dorsal Horn following Mouse Cervical Contusion Spinal Cord Injury

Jaime L. Watson, Tamara J. Hala, Rajarshi Putatunda, Daniel Sannie, Angelo C. Lepore*

Department of Neuroscience, Farber Institute for Neurosciences, Sidney Kimmel Medical College at Thomas Jefferson University, Philadelphia, Pennsylvania, United States of America

Abstract

In humans, sensory abnormalities, including neuropathic pain, often result from traumatic spinal cord injury (SCI). SCI can induce cellular changes in the CNS, termed central sensitization, that alter excitability of spinal cord neurons, including those in the dorsal horn involved in pain transmission. Persistently elevated levels of neuronal activity, glial activation, and glutamatergic transmission are thought to contribute to the hyperexcitability of these dorsal horn neurons, which can lead to maladaptive circuitry, aberrant pain processing and, ultimately, chronic neuropathic pain. Here we present a mouse model of SCI-induced neuropathic pain that exhibits a persistent pain phenotype accompanied by chronic neuronal hyperexcitability and glial activation in the spinal cord dorsal horn. We generated a unilateral cervical contusion injury at the C5 or C6 level of the adult mouse spinal cord. Following injury, an increase in the number of neurons expressing ΔFosB (a marker of chronic neuronal activation), persistent astrocyte activation and proliferation (as measured by GFAP and Ki67 expression), and a decrease in the expression of the astrocyte glutamate transporter GLT1 are observed in the ipsilateral superficial dorsal horn of cervical spinal cord. These changes have previously been associated with neuronal hyperexcitability and may contribute to altered pain transmission and chronic neuropathic pain. In our model, they are accompanied by robust at-level hyperaglesia in the ipsilateral forepaw and allodynia in both forepaws that are evident within two weeks following injury and persist for at least six weeks. Furthermore, the pain phenotype occurs in the absence of alterations in forelimb grip strength, suggesting that it represents sensory and not motor abnormalities. Given the importance of transgenic mouse technology, this clinically-relevant model provides a resource that can be used to study the molecular mechanisms contributing to neuropathic pain following SCI and to identify potential therapeutic targets for the treatment of chronic pathological pain.

Editor: Guglielmo Foffani, Hospital Nacional de Parapléjicos, Spain

Funding: This work was funded by the NIH (1R01NS079702 to A.C.L.) and the Craig H. Neilsen Foundation (#190140 to A.C.L.). The funders had no role in study design, data collection and analysis, decision to publish, or preparation of the manuscript.

Competing Interests: The authors have declared that no competing interests exist.

* Email: Angelo.Lepore@jefferson.edu

Introduction

Spinal cord injury (SCI) is a debilitating condition with widespread symptoms that affect patient quality of life. As many as 327,000 SCI patients are currently living in the United States, and approximately 12,000 new cases are reported each year [1]. Clinical studies propose that 64–82% of SCI patients experience some form of pathological pain following injury, and this pain has been associated with mood changes as well as difficulty with work and social activities [2]. Neuropathic pain constitutes a significant percentage of pain resulting from SCI; 41% of patients encounter at-level and 34% experience below-level neuropathic pain [3] following injury. Although SCI most often involves an acute injury to the spinal cord, the resulting pathological pain is often chronic and can increase in severity over time [4]. Thus, SCI-related neuropathic pain and its treatment is an important focus of spinal cord research.

In this study, we wanted to identify the molecular changes accompanying the alterations of at-level pain sensitivity in a mouse model of cervical contusion SCI. We induced SCI in the mouse and measured changes in pain behavior, specifically thermal hyperalgesia and tactile allodynia. Additionally, we studied the expression of various proteins in the dorsal horn of the spinal cord that may contribute to neuropathic pain and the cell types expressing these proteins. Importantly, we chose to utilize a mouse model of SCI that is clinically relevant but has not previously been used to study neuropathic pain.

Currently, mouse models of SCI-induced neuropathic pain are available, but do not address cervical contusion injury. According to the National Spinal Cord Injury Statistical Center, the majority of SCI patients in the United States experience injury to the cervical regions of the spinal cord [1], but most rodent SCI models involve injury to thoracic regions. Therefore, we chose to target our SCI to the cervical region of the spinal cord.

Additionally, contusion-type injury is most common in human patients [5] and is a popular model of SCI in rodents [6]. The respiratory and other dysfunctions that commonly accompany cervical contusion injuries make this model difficult to study [7]. To date, our group [8], [9], [10] and others [11] have used models of cervical contusion SCI in the mouse and rat to study motor deficits following injury. In the study of neuropathic pain, however, contusive injury to the cervical regions of the spinal cord has not been utilized in mice. Instead, transection, compression, contusion and other procedures are used primarily at thoracic levels to induce SCI in mice for studying neuropathic pain [6]. Here, we designed a model of moderate hemicontusive injury to the cervical spinal cord in the mouse that does not develop significant respiratory or other life-threatening complications for the study of neuropathic pain.

The development of neuropathic pain following SCI involves the disruption of neurons involved in nociception in the dorsal horn of the spinal cord. Under normal circumstances, neurons in the superficial laminae of the dorsal horn are responsible for pain transmission from peripheral nociceptors to the thalamus and, ultimately, the sensory cortex. Upon injury to the spinal cord, however, local changes can occur that alter how nociceptive neurons respond to peripheral stimuli [12]. These changes, termed central sensitization, can underlie pathological pain behaviors such as allodynia and hyperalgesia [12], [13].

One mechanism involved in central sensitization is the hyperexcitability of pain transmission neurons. Neuronal hyperexcitability results in an increase in the response of neurons to electrical input or even the firing of neurons in the absence of input. Hyperexcitability is characterized by spontaneous neuronal activity, aberrant responses to subthreshold stimuli, and increased transmission of suprathreshold input [12], [13]. In SCI, pain projection neurons in the dorsal horn can become more easily excited by noxious as well as non-noxious stimuli, resulting in pathological pain transmission. Changes to the neuron itself, as well as to its extracellular environment, can alter the neuron's electrophysiological profile, increasing its resting membrane potential and/or decreasing its action potential threshold. As one example of a mechanism underlying central sensitization, increased activity of transcription factors can trigger changes in gene expression that lead to long-term alterations in neuronal function and excitability. For instance, ΔfosB, a commonly used marker of persistent neuronal activation, has been associated with plasticity of pain transmission circuits in inflammatory pain, possibly through downstream targets such as CDK5 [14], [15].

Underlying hyperexcitability and central sensitization in SCI are changes in glial activation and glutamate transporter function. Astrocytes play an essential role in the central nervous system, providing support to neurons, regulating the uptake of glutamate and other factors from the extracellular space, and modulating synapse formation and function [13], [16]. Soon after insult, astrocytes can become activated (marked by glial fibrillary acidic protein (GFAP)) and possibly even proliferative and act to minimize the effects of the injury by reestablishing the blood brain barrier, releasing antioxidants, and protecting the lesion site from detrimental molecules. Activation of astrocytes, however, can also be harmful to neighboring neurons; when persistently active, astrocytes can contribute to neuronal hyperexcitability through the release of factors such as proinflammatory molecules, nitric oxide, and ATP [13], [17], [18].

The loss of glutamate transporters by activated astrocytes and the resulting imbalance in glutamate homeostasis may also contribute to the development of post-SCI neuropathic pain. Under normal conditions, glutamate is cleared from the synapse via glutamate transporters, such as GLT1 and GLAST, located in the plasma membrane of neurons and, more often, astrocytes. However, elevated release of glutamate from presynaptic neurons and/or injured neurons and glia or from damage to the glutamate transporter system can cause an excess of glutamate to linger in synaptic and extra-synaptic locations [13]. This disruption in glutamate homeostasis leads to overactivation of glutamate receptors, which can in some instances result in increased Ca^{2+} concentrations in the postsynaptic neuron. These changes can have negative impacts on cell health and function and alter the activation state of the neuron [19], [20], [21]. In SCI, glutamate excitotoxic damage to inhibitory interneurons can also indirectly boost the excitability of nociceptive neurons in the dorsal horn [18]. In this way, the loss of GLT1 in astrocytes observed following injury by our group [22], [23], [24] and others [25], [26] may contribute to central sensitization and neuropathic pain.

Recently published data from our group showed changes in neuronal and astrocyte activation as well as GLT1 expression in the superficial dorsal horn following cervical contusion SCI-induced hyperalgesia in the rat [24]. The study characterized a moderate hemicontusion injury to cervical regions of the rat spinal cord, which resulted in ipsilateral hyperalgesic behavior. Accompanying hyperalgesia were chronic increases in ΔfosB expression in neurons, astrocyte activation and proliferation in addition to a loss of GLT1 both at the site of the injury and in intact spinal cord caudal to the contusion site [24].

In the current study we characterize increases in pain sensitivity in a mouse model of cervical contusion SCI and the accompanying molecular alterations in the dorsal horn of the spinal cord. Our model exhibits at-level thermal hyperalgesia and tactile allodynia in addition to increases in neuronal and astrocyte activation and a decrease in astrocyte glutamate transporter expression in the superficial dorsal horn. Alterations in pain behavior, as well as neuronal and glial activation and glutamate transport expression in the dorsal horn, have not previously been characterized in mice receiving cervical contusion SCI. Thus, this study provides an observation of the molecular and behavioral changes that occur following cervical SCI in the mouse that can be used to further study the mechanisms underlying neuropathic pain in SCI.

Methods

Animal Studies

Ethics Statement. All animal care and treatment were conducted in strict accordance with the *European Communities Council Directive* (2010/63/EU, 86/609/EEC and 87-848/EEC) and the *NIH Guide for the Care and Use of Laboratory Animals*. Experimental protocols were approved by the Thomas Jefferson University Institutional Animal Care and Use Committee.

Animals. Fifty-six male C57BL/6 mice (25–30 g; The Jackson Laboratory, USA) and 26 transgenic BAC-GLT1-eGFP reporter mice [27] were used. The BAC-GLT1-eGFP reporter mice were created by Regan et al. [27]. The transgene in these mice involves cDNA for eGFP inserted into the start codon of a mouse BAC encompassing the entire GLT-1 gene. Thus, in these mice, eGFP expression is driven by the GLT1 promoter. Mice were housed 5 per cage in a controlled light-dark environment in the Thomas Jefferson University Animal Facility and were given food and water *ad libitum*. To prevent suffering, a combination of ketamine/xylazine and isofluorane was used to anesthetize animals during surgical procedures.

SCI Models. We chose to utilize two models in the C57BL/6 mice in this study; one with injury at the C5 level and another with injury at the C6 level. We did this to show that contusion injury to various levels of the cervical spinal cord has the potential to produce at-level neuropathic pain. Mice were anesthetized initially with ketamine (100 mg/kg) and xylazine (5 mg/kg) injected intraperitoneally, and the anesthetic plane was maintained with 1% isofluorane for the duration of the surgery. The body was immobilized by taping the forelegs to a fixation plate, and the head was immobilized by the isofluorane nose cone. The skin and muscle overlying the spinal column were retracted from levels C3 to T1, and spinal cord was exposed by unilateral laminectomy from the midline blood vessel to the lateral edge of the vertebral lamina at the level of C5 or C6. The spinal column was stabilized at the C3 and T1 spinous processes by microforceps attached to the fixation plate and the far right and left corners. C57BL/6 mice received unilateral contusion injuries at the exposed portion of the spinal cord using the Infinite Horizon Impactor (Precision Systems and Instrumentation; Lexington, KY) with an impactor tip of 0.7 mm in diameter, a force of 40 kilodynes, two seconds of dwell time, and an approximately perpendicular impact angle, parameters similar to our previously published cervical contusion SCI paradigms [8], [9], [10]. Injury parameters for BAC-GLT1-eGFP mice included a 1.0 mm diameter tip, 50 kilodyne force, and no dwell time at the C5 level. Control animals received unilateral laminectomy but not contusion injury to the spinal cord. Following injury, the forceps were removed and the muscle layers were secured with a sterile 4-0 silk suture. Sterile wound clips were used to close the skin, and 1 ml of lactated Ringers solution and 0.1 mg/kg of buprenorphine-HCl were administered subcutaneously.

Unilateral Hargreaves Thermal Test. A modified version of the Hargreaves test for thermal hyperaglesia, based on previously established methods [28], was conducted for the forepaws of each animal. This test detects sensitivity to thermal nociceptive stimuli by determining the latency to withdrawal of the paw from an infrared stimulus of a particular intensity. Prior to surgery, baseline measures were collected once weekly for two weeks. Following contusion SCI or laminectomy, each animal was tested weekly for six weeks. Before the first baseline test, the animals were acclimated to the testing room for an hour each day for five days. Prior to each session, mice were also acclimated to the testing room for an hour. Individually, the mice were restrained manually by the scruff only and placed on a thin glass pane, with one of the forepaws directly above the source of the infrared stimulus (UgoBasile; Comerio, VA). The animals continued to be restrained, but movement of the forepaw was unimpeded. The stimulus was initiated, and a fiber optic sensor on the movable infrared heat source measured the time to forepaw withdrawal. Forepaw withdrawal was defined as a quick movement of the paw away from the infrared stimulus often accompanied by licking of the forepaw. Spontaneous movements of the forepaw were not considered forepaw withdrawal and resulted in discarding the data and repeating the trial. Three trials were conducted for each forepaw of each animal, alternating the left and right forepaws, with an inter-trial interval of 120 seconds.

von Frey Filament Test. Semmes-Weinstein monofilaments (Stoetling Company; Dale, IL) ranging from 1.65 grams to 4.56 grams of force were utilized to measure tactile allodynia using the up-down method. Testing occurred twice prior to surgery to obtain baseline data and once weekly for six weeks after injury. Acclimation procedures were the same as those used for the Hargreaves test. Each mouse experienced ten trials per testing day with an inter-trial interval of 120 seconds. The first trial of each testing day utilized a filament of 3.84 grams. A single trial involved directing a monofilament at the center of the plantar surface of the forepaw of interest and application until the filament buckled. Mice were not restrained for this testing. The response of the mouse was then recorded as a positive or negative withdrawal response. The filament application was considered to produce a positive response if the mouse rapidly withdrew its forepaw, which was mostly accompanied by vocalization and/or licking of the forepaw. If the response was positive, the filament used in the next trial would be the next smaller filament. If instead the response was negative, the next larger filament would be used in the next trial. Withdraw threshold was determined as the lowest filament/force that evoked a positive withdrawal response in greater than 50% of the trials with that particular filament.

Grip Strength Testing. Grip strength was measured by the DFIS-2 Series Digital Force Gauge (Columbus Instruments, OH) [26], used previously by our group [8]. Attached to the force gauge is a triangular metal pull bar that allows for the transduction of force from the mouse to the gauge. The Digital Force Gauge measures the strength with which the mouse is able to grasp and hold onto a thin metal bar. Three baseline measures spread across two weeks were obtained prior to surgery, and mice were tested once weekly for six weeks following injury. In each trial, the mouse was allowed to grab the bar with one forepaw and was then quickly pulled away from the gauge so its grip was released, providing a measurement of the force with which the mouse gripped the bar. During each testing session, three trials for each forepaw were performed with an inter-trial interval of at least 60 seconds.

Histological Analyses

Tissue Processing. Mice were sacrificed at two days or two or six weeks following injury or laminectomy by anesthetic overdose and transcardial perfusion with 0.9% saline followed by 4% paraformaldehyde. The spinal cord was harvested following perfusion, fixed in 4% paraformaldehyde at room temperature for 24 hours, washed in 0.1M phosphate buffer at 4°C for 24 hours and then cryoprotected in 30% sucrose in 0.1M phosphate buffer at 4°C for three days. The cervical/rostral thoracic spinal cord was dissected from the rest of the cord, embedded in freezing medium, and flash-frozen with dry ice. Embedded tissue was cut transversely by cryostat at a thickness of 30 μm and mounted directly onto slides. Slides were stored at −20°C.

Motor Neuron Counts. A representative sample (i.e. every fifth section) of spinal cord tissue was used to locate the injury epicenter. Slides were thawed at room temperature for an hour and stained with 0.5% Cresyl violet acetate/Eriochrome cyanine. For each section, large motor neurons ventral to the central canal in the grey matter were counted for the ipsilateral and contralateral sides [9]. The motor neuron cell bodies were identified by their size and characteristic morphology. The injury epicenter was defined as the section with the fewest large motor neurons in the ipsilateral ventral grey matter.

Immunohistochemistry. Immunohistochemical analysis was performed both ipsilaterally and contralaterally to the unilateral injury at the injury epicenter as well as 1.05 mm caudal to the epicenter (Figure 1A–B). Sectioned tissue was thawed and dried at room temperature for an hour and then washed in TBS. Sections were blocked in 10% normal goat serum/0.2% Triton/TBS at room temperature for one hour followed by primary antibody incubation in 2% goat serum/0.5% Triton/TBS at 4°C overnight. Secondary antibody was incubated in 2% goat serum/0.5% Triton/TBS at room temperature for two hours. Primary and secondary antibodies used were rabbit polyclonal ΔfosB (IHC 1:100; Santa Cruz, USA) [30], rabbit polyclonal Ki67 (IHC 1:200; Abcam, USA) [31], mouse monoclonal GFAP (IHC 1:400, Sigma Aldrich, USA) [32], rabbit polyclonal GLT1 (IHC 1:800, kindly

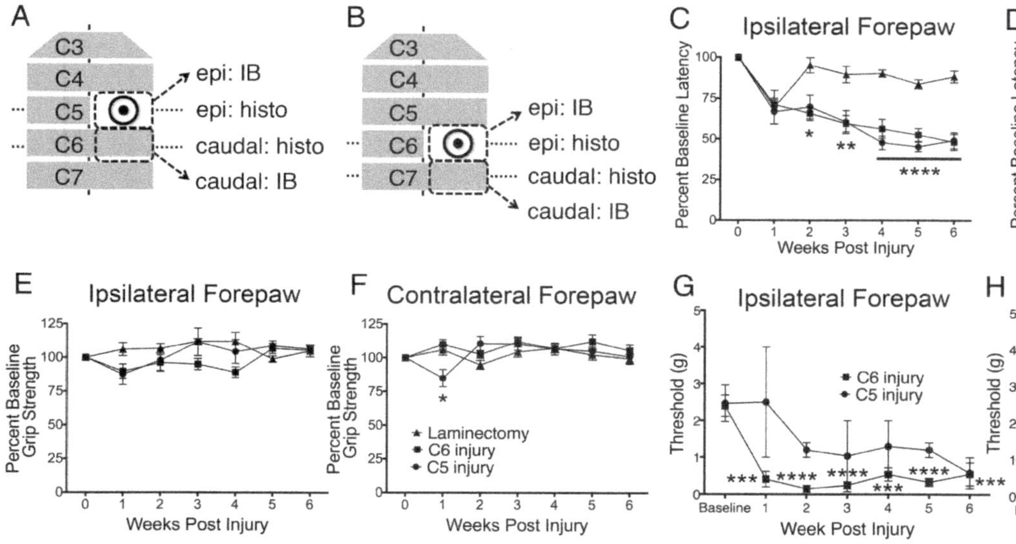

Figure 1. Animals receiving unilateral cervical contusion SCI exhibited persistent thermal hyperalgesia and tactile allodynia in the forepaw. Cervical contusion SCI was administered at the C5 or C6 level of the spinal cord while uninjured control animals received only laminectomy at the C6 level. Tissue from the level of laminectomy or epicenter of the injury and from the region immediately caudal was harvested for either immunoblotting or histology (A–B). Thermal hyperalgesia was measured using a modified version of the Hargreaves test. Animals receiving contusion injury showed a decrease in latency to withdrawal in the ipsilateral forepaw, measured as a percentage of baseline latency, compared to control animals (C). This difference was first observed at two weeks after injury and persisted until the animals were sacrificed at six weeks after injury. No change in withdrawal latency was seen in injured vs. uninjured animals in the contralateral forepaw (D). Animals receiving SCI were also tested for tactile allodynia using von Frey filament testing. In animals receiving C6 injury, but not C5 injury, a significant decrease compared to pre-injury baseline in the force threshold required to elicit a withdrawal response was evident both ipsilaterally (E) and contralaterally (F) for each of the six weeks following injury. The decrease in ipsilateral forepaw withdrawal latency and bilateral force threshold in injured animals occurred in the absence of changes in grip strength in either forepaw (G–H). Epi = epicenter; IB = immunoblotting; histo = histology; * = $p<0.05$; ** = $p<0.01$; **** = $p<0.0001$.

provided by Jeffrey Rothstein's lab at Johns Hopkins University) [29],, mouse monoclonal CD11b (IHC 1:4,000, AbD Serotec, USA), rhodamine-conjugated goat-anti-rabbit IgG (1:100; Jackson Immuno, USA) and FITC-conjugated goat-anti-mouse IgG (1:100; Jackson Immuno, USA).

Fluorescence Imaging and Quantification. Imaging and quantification of fluorescence immunostaining and BAC-GLT1-eGFP tissue were performed using a Zeiss Imager M2 upright fluorescence microscope [23]. Images were taken and analyses performed on saved PNG images for analyses. All immunostaining was quantified in the most superficial laminae (I–II) or lamina III of the spinal cord dorsal horn (Figure 2F–G). Laminae I–III were delineated by beginning at the most lateral portion of the dorsal horn, drawing a horizontal line across the gray matter, and following the outline of the gray matter back to the lateral extension of the dorsal horn. The border between laminae I–II and lamina III was identified by the change in tissue morphology represented by darker tissue in laminae I–II and lighter tissue in lamina III. Quantification analyses were performed using Metamorph software (Molecule Devices; Sunnyvale, CA). ΔfosB- and Ki67-positive cells were quantified by counting the stained nuclei in the superficial laminae. GFAP and GLT1 staining was more diffusely distributed and was therefore quantified in laminae I–II as an integrated intensity, or the sum of the intensity of pixels over a region, at constant exposure, brightness, and contrast. In BAC-GLT1-eGFP tissue, quantification was performed for laminae I–II and lamina III. eGFP-positive cells were counted separately for these regions [23].

Biochemical Analyses

Tissue Harvesting. Sacrifice occurred at two or six weeks after injury or laminectomy. Following anesthetic overdose, animals were perfused with 0.9% saline and the cervical spinal cord removed, dissected, and flash-frozen in dimethylbutane. The spinal cord was sub-dissected to collect the ipsilateral cord at the level of the injury and the segment directly caudal to the injury (Fig. 1A–B). To identify the regions of interest, the muscles were first removed to expose the spinal column. The laminectomy area was located, and the contralateral vertebral lamina was removed. Microdissection scissors were used to cut the spinal cord along the midline, and a 1.0 mm piece of tissue between the remaining laminae was collected. Flash-frozen tissue was stored at −80°C.

Western Blotting. Tissue samples were homogenized on ice in 50 μl of RIPA buffer containing 50 mM TRIS-HCl pH 7.6, 150 mM NaCl, 2 mM EDTA, 0.1% SDS, 0.01% NP-40, and Protease Inhibitor Cocktail (Roche Diagnostics, Indianapolis, IN). Protein concentration was determined by the Bradford assay, and equal amounts of protein were run on 4–12% Bis-Tris gels and transferred to nitrocellulose membranes. Odyssey blocking buffer (Li-Cor; Lincoln, NE) was used to block the membranes at room temperature for one hour. Primary antibodies for GLT1 (1:2,000) and actin (1:2,000; Abcam) were diluted in Odyssey blocking buffer and membranes were incubated at 4°C overnight. The membranes were then probed with IRDye-conjugated goat anti-rabbit or goat anti-mouse IgG (1:20,000; Li-Cor) at room temperature for one hour. Imaging was performed by the Li-Cor Odyssey infrared imaging system, and GLT1 band intensity was measured and normalized to actin band intensity using ImageJ software [22].

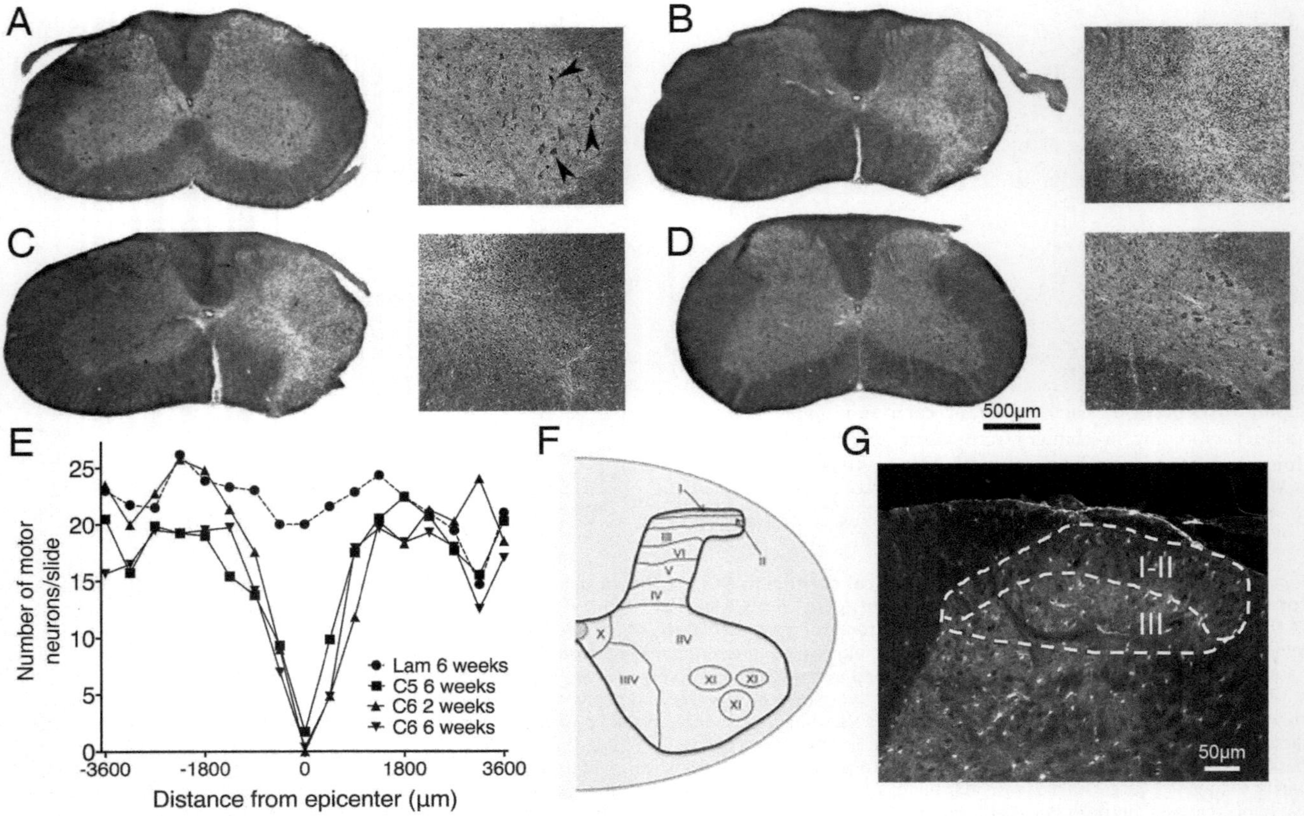

Figure 2. Unilateral contusion SCI induced a loss of ventral horn motor neurons at the injury epicenter. Harvested tissue was stained with Cresyl violet and Eriochrome cyanine. At the level of the laminectomy, uninjured control animals (A) exhibited large motor neurons in the ventral horn (arrowheads). At six weeks post-injury, animals receiving unilateral C5 (B) or C6 (C) contusion SCI showed a loss of these motor neurons at the injury epicenter but not 1.0 mm caudal to the injury (D). The spread of ventral horn motor neuron loss was approximately 1.0 mm rostrally and 1.0 mm caudally (2.0 mm total) from the epicenter (E). Immunohistochemical analyses of the injury models were performed in laminae I–II and lamina III of the cervical spinal cord dorsal horn (F–G). Lam = laminectomy.

Statistical Analyses

All data are presented as mean ± SEM. Statistical analyses were performed using GraphPad Prism (GraphPad Software, Inc.; La Jolla, CA). Bar graphs are presented as averages with error bars representing standard error. The Hargreaves test and von Frey threshold data were analyzed using a two-way ANOVA with repeated measured to compare the means within each group (laminectomy, C5 injury, or C6 injury) at each time point. The immunohistochemical and biochemical data were assessed with one-way ANOVA, comparing each group (laminectomy, C6 2 weeks, or C6 6 weeks) to one another. Statistical significance is defined as $p<0.05$ for all analyses.

Results

Robust and persistent forepaw thermal hyperalgesia and tactile allodynia were observed following unilateral cervical contusion SCI

Here we present a model of unilateral cervical contusion SCI in the mouse that exhibits persistent changes in pain behavior in the absence of motor deficits. Following baseline behavior testing, animals received unilateral laminectomy and contusion injury of 40 kilodyne of force with two seconds of dwell time at either the C5 (Fig. 1A) or C6 (Fig. 1B) level of the spinal cord. Control animals underwent laminectomy without injury. In both injury models, no grossly observable deficits in respiratory or other vital functions were present.

Beginning one week after injury, thermal hyperalgesia, tactile allodynia and grip strength were measured in laminectomy (n = 8) and injured animals (C5: n = 8; C6: n = 10) for six weeks. A modified version of the Hargreaves test was utilized to measure sensitivity to noxious thermal stimuli in the ipsilateral and contralateral forepaws. In both injured and uninjured animals, forepaw withdrawal upon noxious thermal stimulation was deliberate and was often accompanied by licking or scratching of the paw. Two-way ANOVA was used to compare withdrawal latency between animals with C5 injury, C6 injury, and laminectomy only at each time point. Post-injury measurements of latency to forepaw withdrawal are reported as a percentage of the baseline average for each animal. In laminectomy-only animals, withdrawal latency non-significantly decreased in the ipsilateral forepaw at one week post-injury but returned to and persisted at baseline levels until six weeks after injury (Fig. 1C). Beginning two weeks after injury and persisting for the length of testing, ipsilateral forepaw withdrawal latencies for animals receiving unilateral contusion SCI at the C5 or C6 level were significantly reduced compared to uninjured laminectomy animals (Fig. 1C). In the contralateral forepaw, no significant changes amongst the three experimental groups were seen (Fig. 1D).

In addition, tactile allodynia was assessed in C5 injured and C6 injured animals. The threshold force required to elicit a withdrawal response in each of the forepaws was measured by the von Frey test. In the C6 injury group, but not as robustly in the C5 injury group, tactile allodynia was evident (Fig. 1E–F). Animals were tested prior to injury to obtain baseline data and were then assessed for six weeks following injury. When values for each testing week were compared to pre-injury baseline data, animals receiving C6 injury exhibited a significant decrease in threshold force both ipsilaterally (Fig. 1E) and contralaterally (Fig. 1F). Although the data were not significant for animals receiving C5 injury, there was a similar trend in decreased response threshold.

While thermal and mechanical sensitivity increased in injured animals, this was not associated with changes in grip strength. Grip strength results were analyzed by two-way ANOVA to identify significance between each group at each time point. For the ipsilateral forepaw, no changes were observed between injured and uninjured animals for the six weeks following surgery (Fig. 1G). A significant decrease in contralateral grip strength for animals receiving injury at the C5 level was seen one week after injury compared to laminectomy or C6 injury (Fig. 1H). However, because the change occurred so soon after surgery and grip strength recovered to baseline levels by the next testing session, a spinal shock mechanism may be responsible for this unexpected change.

Together, the Hargreaves, von Frey, and grip strength data suggest hypersensitivity to noxious thermal and tactile stimuli in the absence of altered grip strength, indicating that the observed changes in forepaw withdrawal resulted from aberrant pain processing rather than motor deficits.

Unilateral cervical contusion SCI produced an injury characterized by a focal loss of ventral horn motor neurons

The animals that received unilateral contusion SCI exhibited loss of large motor neurons in the ventral grey matter as well as a disruption of lateral grey matter, dorsolateral funiculus, and ventrolateral funiculus of the ipsilateral hemicord (Fig. 2B–C). In laminectomy-only animals (n = 8), large motor neurons of distinct morphology were present throughout the ipsilateral ventral horn (Fig. 2A). These motor neurons were absent or their numbers were greatly reduced, however, at the injury site in animals receiving C5 (Fig. 2B; n = 8) or C6 (Fig. 2C; 2 weeks: n = 8; 6 weeks: n = 10) injury. This effect was limited to the injury site, as motor neuron populations and white matter were intact in regions rostral and caudal to the injury (Fig. 2D). Additionally, no loss of motor neurons was observed on the contralateral side of the spinal cord at any point along the rostral-caudal axis (data not shown). Thus, the anatomical disruption sustained by injured animals was restricted to the injury site ipsilaterally.

In order to quantify the contusion injury sustained by the animals and identify the injury epicenter along the rostral-caudal axis, sections were stained with Cresyl violet acetate/Eriochrome cyanine and motor neurons in the ventral horn were counted. The epicenter of the injury was determined by the extent of motor neuron loss, and the motor neuron counts were plotted by distance from this site (Fig. 2E). Significance was determined using one-way ANOVA to compare motor neuron counts between each group. Compared to laminectomy animals, a significant decrease in ventral horn motor neurons was observed for animals receiving injury at either cervical level and at both time points. The spread of both C5 and C6 injuries was approximately 2.0 mm (1.0 mm rostrally and 1.0 mm caudally from the epicenter) with a gradual decrease in motor neurons immediately rostral and caudal to the epicenter. The epicenter identified by this method was used for further immunohistochemical analyses of the neuronal and glial populations of the spinal cord dorsal horn, which were performed in laminae I–II and laminae III (Fig. 2F–G).

Chronic neuronal activation in the superficial laminae of the dorsal horn resulted from contusion SCI

Because injury at either the C5 or C6 level produced thermal hyperalgesia and tissue damage to a similar extent, we chose to move forward with a single model, the C6 injury, for further analyses. ΔfosB, a truncated splice version of the immediate early gene c-fos, is a transcription factor and marker of persistent neuronal activation. Chronic upregulation of this gene has been implicated in plasticity and inflammatory pain [14], [15] and has the potential to contribute to neuropathic pain. To study the extent of ΔfosB expression in our SCI model, we sacrificed animals at two weeks and six weeks after injury (n = 7–10) or six weeks after laminectomy (n = 8). Immunohistochemistry for ΔfosB was performed at the injury epicenter and 1.0 mm caudal to the injury in laminae I–II.

We found that ΔfosB-positive cells exhibited a defined pattern of nuclear staining in the superficial laminae. In our SCI model, we observed a persistent increase in the number of Δfos-expressing cells, suggesting chronic neuronal activation following cervical contusion injury. One-way ANOVA was used to compare the number of ΔfosB-positive cells between each group. Following laminectomy, limited-to-no ΔfosB expression was seen in the dorsal horn (Fig. 3A). Two weeks after injury (Fig. 3B), there was an increase in ΔfosB-positive cells on the ipsilateral side at and caudal to the injury epicenter. At six weeks (Fig. 3C), ΔfosB was upregulated bilaterally in the superficial laminae at the injury epicenter and 1.0 mm caudal. These changes are quantified in Figure 3D. The greatest increase in ΔfosB expression was observed at six weeks, suggesting that its expression was persistent and cumulative over time. Additionally, the expression of ΔfosB in the injured animals was specific to the dorsal horn of the spinal cord. There were few to no ΔfosB-positive cells in other regions of the spinal cord, including the ventral horn. This suggests that the effects of our injury paradigm on chronic neuronal activation were focal to the dorsal horn, an important region of the spinal cord for pain transmission and modulation.

Astrocytes were activated and proliferated in the dorsal horn of the spinal cord following cervical contusion SCI

Astrocytes play important protective and homeostatic roles in both the immediate and delayed response to CNS injury. Chronic activation in the spinal cord, however, can contribute to neuronal hyperexcitability of pain transmission neurons that underlies neuropathic pain [12], [13]. When astrocytes become activated, they express distinct proteins and in some cases proliferate [21]. In order to measure the spatial and temporal change in astrocyte activation in our model of SCI, we used immunohistochemistry to stain for GFAP, expressed by activated astrocytes, and Ki67, a marker of cellular proliferation. As in the previous immunohistochemical analyses, animals were studied two or six weeks after injury (n = 7–10) or six weeks after laminectomy (n = 8). For each analysis, one-way ANOVA was utilized to identify significance between the three groups.

Figure 4B shows the distinct morphology of activated astrocytes observed following injury compared to uninjured control (Fig. 4A). We found that injury induced diffuse GFAP expression throughout the gray matter of the spinal cord; therefore, we quantified astrocyte expression in laminae I–II by measuring GFAP intensity.

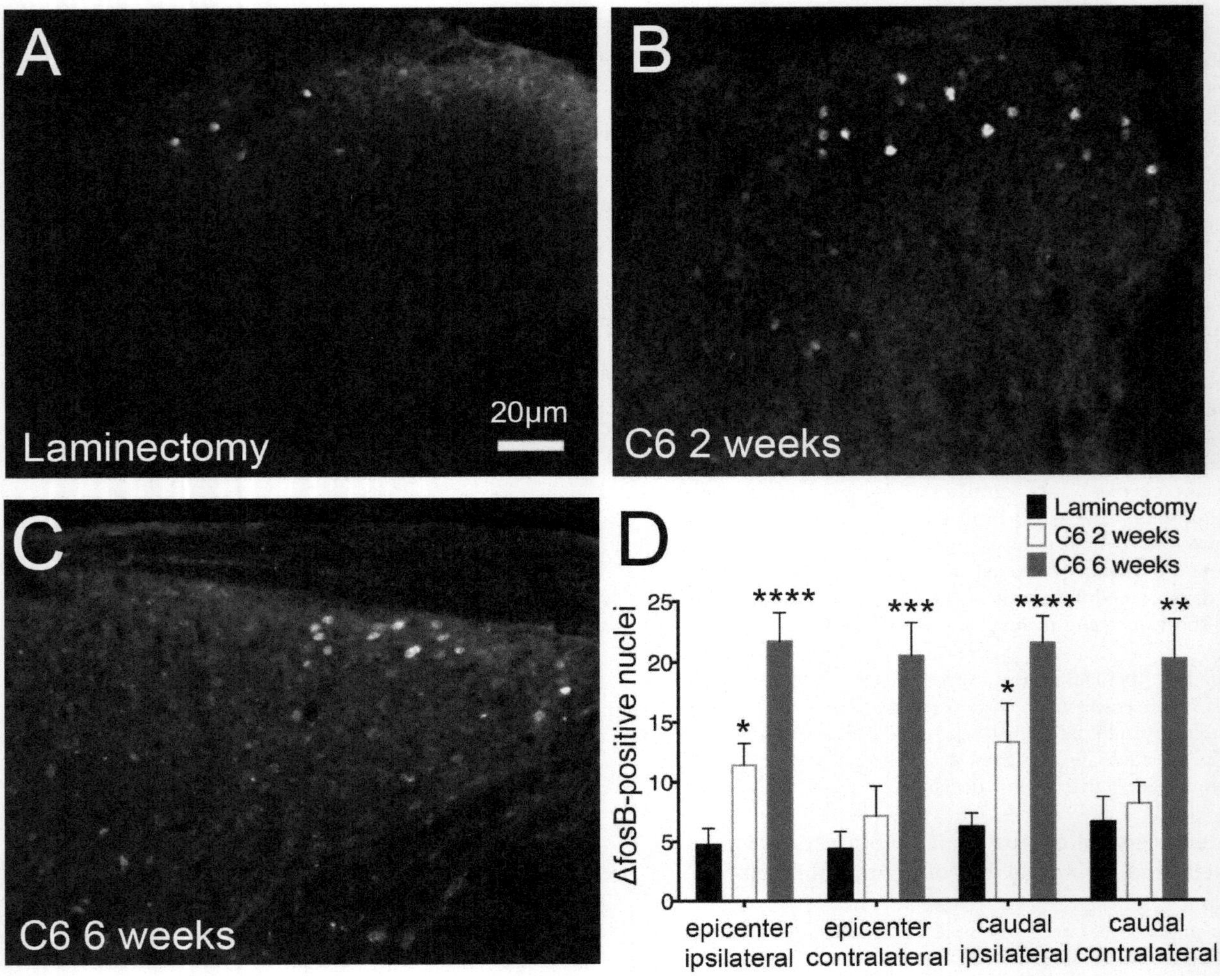

Figure 3. Chronic neuronal activation in the dorsal horn resulted from cervical contusion SCI. ΔfosB staining was used to measure the extent of persistent neuronal activation in the spinal cord. Following injury, ΔfosB-positive nuclei (arrowheads) were evident in laminae I–II (A–C). At all regions, laminectomy control animals (A) showed little-to-no ΔfosB expression (D). Two weeks after C6 injury (B), a significant increase in numbers of ΔfosB expressing cells in the superficial laminae of the ipsilateral dorsal horn was observed at the injury epicenter and caudal to the injury (D). ΔfosB levels were further increased at all regions in animals sacrificed six weeks post-injury (C, D). * = $p<0.05$; ** = $p<0.01$; *** = p 0.001; **** = $p<0.0001$.

Compared to laminectomy (Fig. 4C), GFAP intensity was significantly greater at both time points in animals receiving contusion SCI (Fig. 4D–E). These changes were observed ipsilaterally at the injury epicenter, with no alterations in GFAP expression at the other regions analyzed (Fig. 4F). GFAP expression was highest two weeks after injury, which suggests that, while post-injury astrocyte activation is chronic, it may lessen over time.

We next sought to study the extent of astrocyte proliferation in the dorsal horn to further support our assertion that astrocytes respond to the spinal cord insult we induced. We confirmed using confocal microscopy that, after injury, the majority of Ki67-expresing cells in the superficial were GFAP-positive astrocytes (Fig. 5A). Basally, proliferating cell numbers, and thus Ki67 expression, in the spinal cord were low (Fig. 5B). Two weeks following injury (Fig. 5C), the superficial laminae expressed a robust increase in bilateral Ki67 that was also seen in the ipsilateral dorsal horn caudal to the injury (Fig. 5E). At six weeks (Fig. 5D), an increase in Ki67 was also observed but did not reach the levels seen at two weeks.

We identified the phenotypes of these Ki67-positive proliferative cells. First, we quantified microglial activation in the superficial dorsal horn by immunostaining for CD11b (Fig. 5G–I). Like astrocytes, microglia play a role in both immediate and delayed responses to injury to the spinal cord and may contribute to the development of pathological pain (13). Compared to laminectomy (Fig. 5G), the intensity of CD11b expression was greater in animals with C6 SCI at both two (Fig. 5H–I) and six (Fig. 5I) weeks after injury. This increase was significant at the injury site both ipsilaterally and contralaterally, as well as caudal to the injury on the ipsilateral side (Fig. 5I).

We also quantified the percentage of Ki67-positive cells that were either GFAP-positive or CD11b-positive. This allowed us to determine if the proliferative cells are, in fact, astrocytes (GFAP-positive) or microglia (CD11b-positive). One-way ANOVA was used to identify significance in Ki67 and GFAP or CD11b colocalization. In laminectomy animals, the percentage of cells

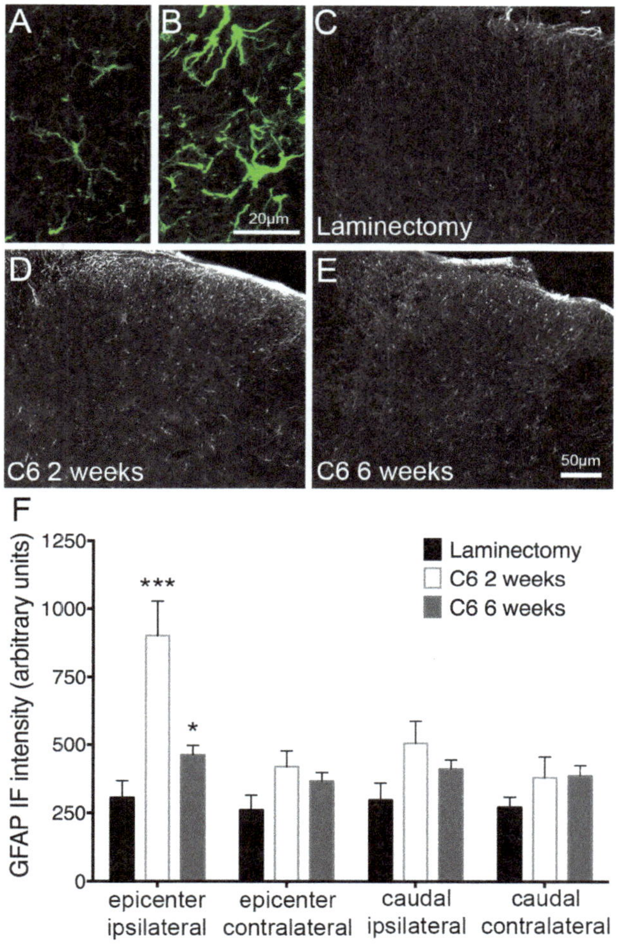

Figure 4. Astrocytes were activated and proliferated in the dorsal horn following cervical contusion SCI. Astrocyte activation in the superficial dorsal horn was characterized by quantification of GFAP expression in laminae I–II. (A) and (B) show representative images of dorsal horn GFAP expression at high magnification in laminectomy and injured animals, respectively. At the injury epicenter, compared to uninjured control animals (C), an increase in GFAP expression in the ipsilateral dorsal horn was evident at two (D) and six weeks (E) following injury. No significant changes in GFAP expression were observed at the other regions studied (F). IF = immunofluorescence; * = $p<0.05$; *** = $p<0.001$.

that are positive for both Ki67 and GFAP or CD11b is zero because there are no Ki67-positive cells present (Fig. 5F). At both two weeks and six weeks after C6 injury, there is a significant increase in the percentage of Ki67-positive cells that are also GFAP-positive or CD11b-positive (Fig. 5F). No significant difference exists between the percentage of Ki67-positive cells that are GFAP-positive or those that are CD11b-positive (Fig. 5F). Thus, both astrocytes and microglia are proliferative following cervical contusion SCI. These data further support the notion that activated astrocytes are present in the spinal cord following injury but retreat over time and/or that proliferation is mostly an early process of astrocyte activation post-SCI. The effects of astrocyte activation can be lasting, however, through the release of factors, for example, that can contribute to hyperexcitability.

Cervical contusion SCI led to reduced expression of GLT1 in the superficial dorsal horn of the spinal cord

The most abundant glutamate transporter in the CNS is GLT1, and its greatest expression is in astrocytes [33]. Through GLT1 and other glutamate transporters, astrocytes clear excitatory amino acids from the synapse after they are released, regulating glutamate's duration of action, controlling normal synaptic communication, and protecting cells from excitotoxic effects [33]. After SCI, we and others [23], [24], [25], [26] have reported a loss in astrocyte GLT1 expression. In this study, we utilized two animal models to study localized decreases in GLT1 in the context of neuropathic pain in the superficial dorsal horn.

In BAC-GLT1-eGFP reporter mice, the GLT1 promoter drives expression of eGFP [27]. Following injury, we sacrificed animals at two days ($n = 7$), two weeks ($n = 9$), and six weeks ($n = 8$) and quantified eGFP-positive cells separately in laminae I–II and lamina III. We used one-way ANOVA to compare the number of eGFP-positive cells at each time point. In uninjured animals (Fig. 6D; $n = 6$), eGFP expression was robust and widespread throughout the grey and white matter. Furthermore, almost all of the GFAP-expressing astrocytes in these regions co-localized with eGFP-positive cells (Fig. 6A–B). eGFP-positive cells were decreased, however, at two days, two weeks, and six weeks (Fig. 6E) at various regions in the spinal cord. Despite the increase in GFAP expression after injury, there were few cells co-expressing eGFP and GFAP, suggesting a loss of GLT1 expression in activated astrocytes (Fig. 6C). At the injury epicenter, eGFP expression was downregulated at two days ipsilaterally (Fig. 6F) and at all time points contralaterally in laminae I–II (Fig. 6G). In lamina III, a decrease in eGFP-positive cells was observed bilaterally at the injury epicenter (Fig. 6F–G). Caudal to the injury, we report a decrease in eGFP at all time points in laminae I–II and at two days and six weeks in lamina III (Fig. 6H). No changes in the contralateral dorsal horn caudal to the injury were observed (Fig. 6I).

In wild-type C57BL/6 animals, we employed immunohistochemical staining for GLT1 after C6 injury ($n = 7–10$) or laminectomy ($n = 8$). One-way ANOVA was used to identify significant differences in GLT1 staining between laminectomy, injured animals at 2 weeks, and injured animals at six weeks. Compared to laminectomy-only animals (Fig. 7A), animals receiving injury two weeks (Fig. 7B) or six weeks (Fig. 7C) prior to analysis showed a decrease in diffuse GLT1 protein expression in laminae I–II. These changes were seen at all regions analyzed (Fig. 7D). We further quantified the extent of GLT1 protein expression in injured ($n = 7–8$) and uninjured animals ($n = 7$) using immunoblotting techniques. At the injury epicenter, we observed a decrease in GLT1 protein in the ipsilateral hemicord at both time points after injury (Fig. 7E). Caudal to the injury, however, this glutamate transporter loss was not observed (Fig. 7F).

These data seem to contradict the immunohistochemical results we reported above. Thus, we performed immunohistochemical quantifications in regions outside of the superficial dorsal horn to try to identify the source of these contradictory results. At six weeks after injury, there is a significant loss of GLT1 expression in the ventral horn ipsilaterally at the epicenter compared to laminectomy animals (Fig. 7G). No significant change is seen in the ventral horn or white matter ipsilaterally caudal to the injury (Fig. 7G). These data suggest that, focally at the injury site, GLT1 loss occurs in multiple anatomical regions. However, caudal to the injury, the decrease in GLT1 expression may be more specific to the superficial dorsal horn (Fig. 7G). The changes in GLT1 from the immunoblotting data may not be evident due to the lack of anatomical specificity.

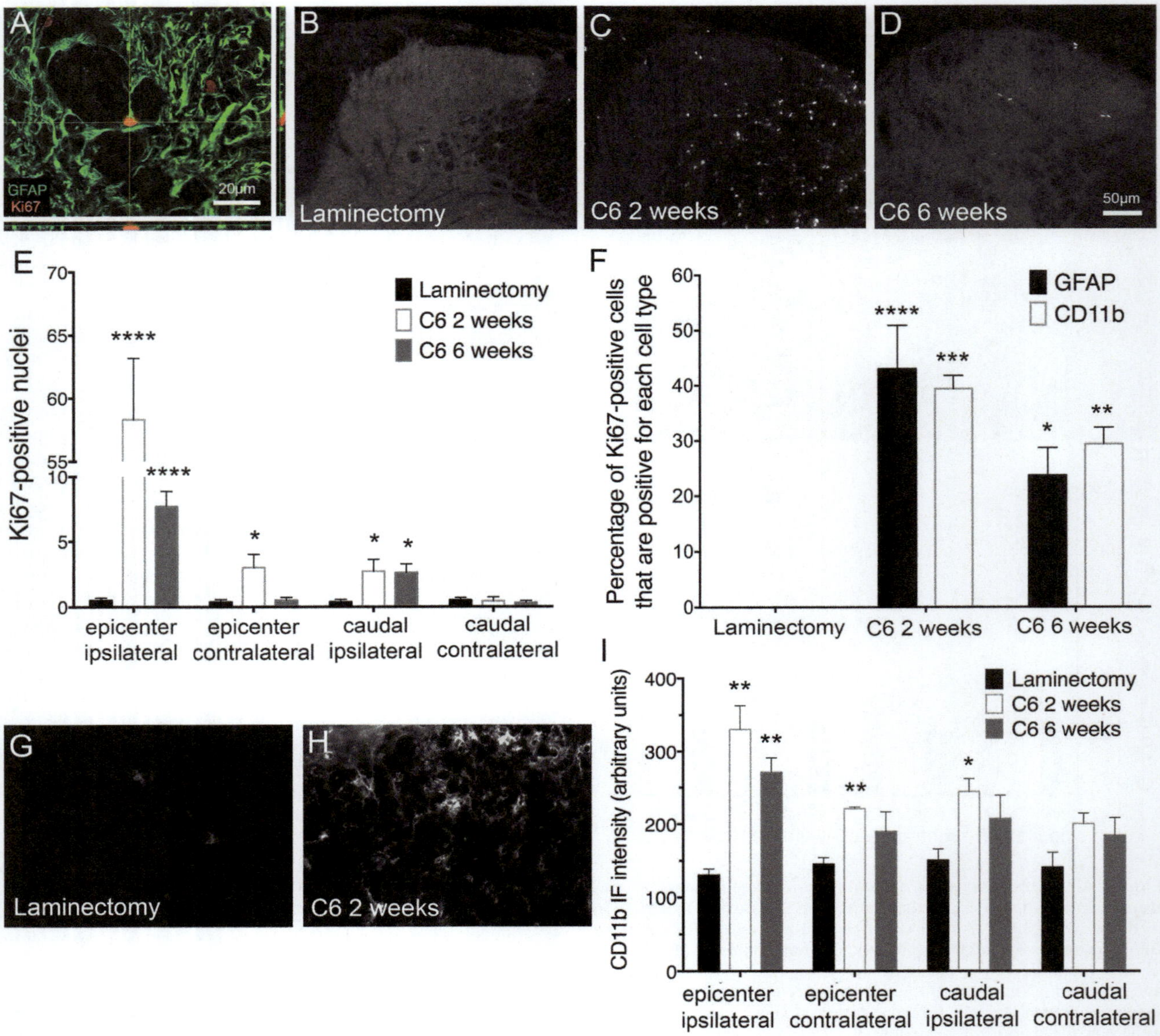

Figure 5. Enhanced cell proliferation, including proliferation of astrocytes, was evident after cervical contusion SCI. In the superficial laminae of the injured ipsilateral dorsal horn, we observed cells co-expressing GFAP and Ki67 (A), representing activated and proliferating astrocytes. In laminectomy control animals, little to no cell proliferation was evident (B). However, the number of Ki67-positive cells was significantly increased at two weeks (C) and six weeks (D) after injury on the ipsilateral side both at the level of and caudal to the injury (E). Additionally, at two weeks, there was a significant increase in proliferating cells contralaterally at the injury site (E). At both two and six weeks, a significant percentage of Ki67-positive cells were also either GFAP-positive or CD11b-positive (F). Compared to laminectomy (G), the intensity of CD11b expression in the superficial dorsal horn was greater in animals with C6 SCI at both two (H–I) and six (I) weeks after injury. This increase was significant at the injury site both ipsilaterally and contralaterally, as well as caudal to the injury on the contralateral side (I). * = $p<0.05$; ** = $p<0.01$; **** = $p<0.0001$.

Discussion

Here we describe changes in neuronal, astrocyte and microglial activation and GLT1 expression accompanying at-level thermal hyperalgesia in a cervical contusion SCI mouse model. In our model, robust and persistent thermal hyperalgesia and tactile allodynia are evident beginning one-two weeks after injury. Additionally, cervical contusion SCI induces an upregulation of ΔfosB, a marker of neuronal activity, in the superficial laminae of the dorsal horn. Astrocyte and microglial activation and proliferation, as measured by increases in GFAP, CD11b and Ki67 immunostaining, are also increased in these regions. We also observe a decrease in GLT1 expression and the number of GLT1-expressing cells in this model. These molecular changes that accompany hyperalgesia and allodynia in this study may contribute to the development of this aberrant pain response and represent important targets for better understanding the development of and treating neuropathic pain in SCI.

Hyperalgesia, defined as an increase in sensitivity to noxious stimuli, whether due to a decrease in pain threshold or an increase in response to stimuli above the pain threshold [36], is common in humans and is associated with sensory changes resulting from

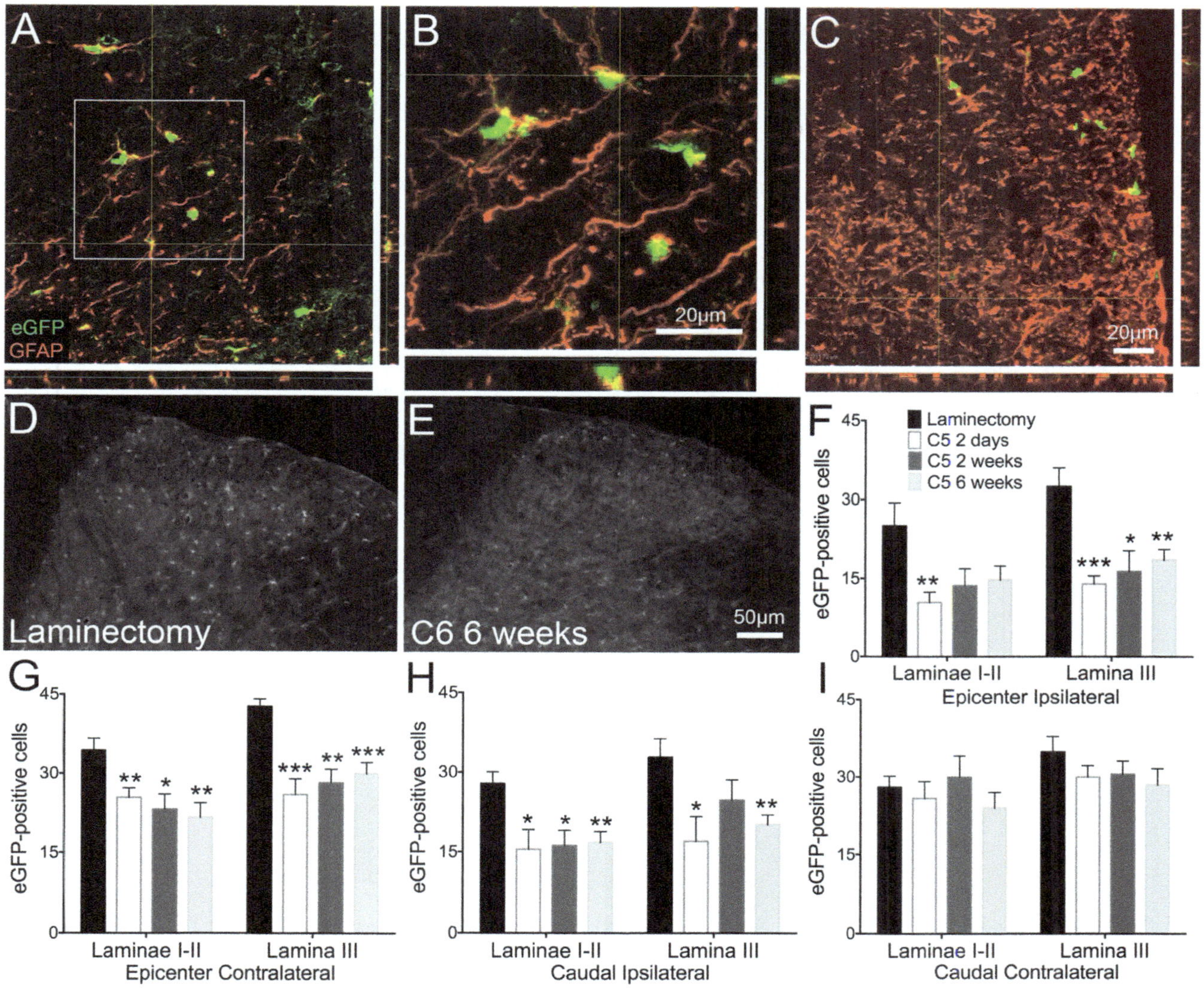

Figure 6. Astrocyte GLT1 promoter activity was reduced in injured BAC-GLT1-eGFP transgenic reporter mice. Following cervical contusion SCI, GLT1 expression/promoter activity, represented by eGFP-positive cells, was decreased in the superficial dorsal horn. In laminectomy animals, there were low levels of GFAP, although many of the cells that were GFAP-positive also expressed GLT1 (A–B). Following injury, however, an increase in GFAP was observed, but fewer of these activated astrocytes co-expressed GLT1 (C). Laminectomy control animals (D) had greater numbers of eGFP-positive cells compared to animals that received contusion injury two days, two weeks, or six weeks (E) prior to analysis. This decrease in GLT1 expression was observed at the injury epicenter in both the ipsilateral (F) and contralateral (G) superficial laminae as well as caudal to the injury on the ipsilateral side (H). No change in the number of eGFP-positive cells was found caudal to the injury on the contralateral side (I). * = $p<0.05$; ** = $p<0.01$; *** = p 0.001.

neuronal hyperexcitability [34], [35]. In mice, hyperalgesia in response to thermal stimuli can be measured using the Hargreaves test, in which a noxious infrared heat stimulus is placed under the paw and the paw withdrawal is recorded. In the models presented here, we observe thermal hyperalgesia in the ipsilateral forepaw beginning two weeks following cervical contusion SCI and persisting for the duration of the experiment. This is consistent with data from other groups, which report the development of hyperalgesia between two and three weeks after contusion SCI at various spinal levels in the mouse [37], [38] [39]. In the rat, our group and others observed thermal hyperalgesia as early as one week after cervical contusion injury [24], [40].

Like injured animals, laminectomy control animals show a decrease in withdrawal latency one week after surgery in the ipsilateral forepaw. This finding was unexpected, but not previously unreported. The development of post-laminectomy pain has been studied in the context of the extent of laminectomy, spinal deformation, and the loss of spinal stability following surgery [41], [42]. Researchers also showed that minimal laminectomy can induce transient hyperalgesic behavior at about one week after surgery [41]. While the cause of this pain behavior is unknown, it could reflect peripheral changes or spinal deformity rather than central sensitization or only transient central sensitization.

The ipsilateral development of thermal hyperalgesia in the mouse after SCI is consistent with the injury we see histologically. At the site of the injury, we observe a loss of ventral horn motor neurons and a disruption of normal tissue anatomy on the ipsilateral but not contralateral side. This suggests a disruption of

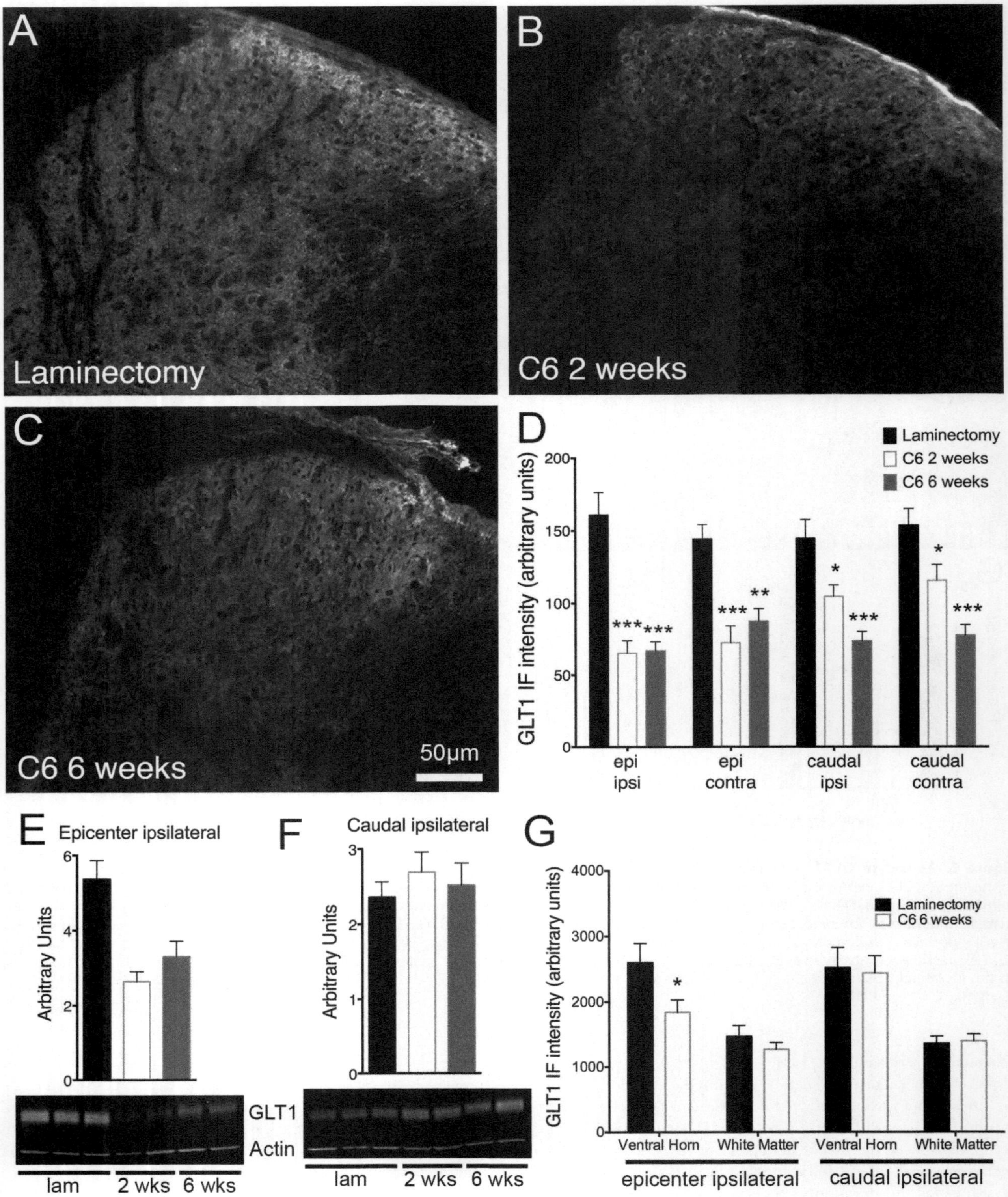

Figure 7. Cervical contusion SCI resulted in decreased astrocyte GLT1 expression in the dorsal horn. Immunohistochemical analysis revealed a decrease in GLT1 protein expression two (B) and six weeks (C) after cervical contusion SCI compared to laminectomy (A). This downregulation of the glutamate transporter was seen in the superficial dorsal horn on both sides of the spinal cord both at the injury site and caudal to the injury (D). Immunoblots of spinal cord tissue also showed a significant loss of GLT1 expression on the ipsilateral side at both time points following injury. However, this difference was seen only at the epicenter (E) and not caudal to the injury (F). Representative immunoblots are shown for each region (E–F). Analysis of GLT1 levels in regions of the spinal cord other than the superficial laminae at six weeks after injury reveal a loss of GLT1 expression in the ventral horn at the epicenter with no changes caudal to the injury (G). IF = immunofluorescence; epi = epicenter; ipsi = ipsilateral; contra = contralateral; lam = laminectomy; * = $p<0.05$; ** = $p<0.01$; *** = p 0.001.

pain transmission circuitry on the side of the injury, which may contribute to the hyperalgesia in the ipsilateral forepaw displayed by injured animals. The unilateral extent of the injury is also consistent with previous findings from our group; we previously reported damage to the ipsilateral dorsolateral and ventrolateral funiculi that did not extend bilaterally following moderate unilateral cervical SCI [10].

Unlike other studies [40], [44], we observe thermal hyperalgesia ipsilaterally but not contralaterally to the site of the injury. This discrepancy may reflect the modified version of the Hargreaves test that we utilized compared to these other groups. The Hargreaves test is most often used to measure thermal hyperalgesia in the hindpaw rather than the forepaw. Despite attempts to perform the Hargreaves test without restraint, including changes to the environment and longer acclimation times, we were unable to obtain reliable results. To overcome these difficulties, we restrained the mice in a way that did not impede forepaw movement but ensured that the mice remained still long enough to respond to the thermal stimulus. This method was introduced previously by Menendez, Lastra, Hidalgo, and Baamonde [28] for the study of hyperalgesia in the mouse forepaw. While the restraint improved the reliability of our thermal hyperalgesia measures, however, it may have affected the sensitivity of the mice to pain, which could have influenced the results we observed contralaterally.

Interestingly, while the hyperalgesia behavior changes we see are limited to the injured side of the spinal cord, we observe some molecular changes both ipsilaterally and contralaterally. ΔfosB and Ki67 expression is increased and GLT1 levels are decreased contralaterally after injury. The one alteration that is present ipsilaterally but not contralaterally is the activation of astrocytes. One possible explanation for the lack of hyperalgesic behavior in the contralateral forepaw is that the molecular changes we see are all required to elicit changes in pain behavior. There may be some interaction between activated neurons and glia that can disrupt pain transmission in the superficial laminae of the spinal cord following injury. Without activation of glia, pain transmission may continue normally.

Using von Frey filament testing, we assessed tactile allodynia following SCI. Allodynia, defined as a pain response to a previously non-noxious stimulus, is a common form of neuropathic pain [34]. In our model, we were able to identify allodynia following injury compared to baseline in the C6 injury group, but a similar significant effect was not observed in animals receiving C5 injury. We observed persistent tactile allodynia in both forepaws, which unlike the thermal testing results coincides with the anatomy of the histological findings.

Both hyperalgesia and allodynia are evoked pain behaviors in that they require a stimulus, whether noxious or non-noxious. We did not, however, study spontaneous pain, meaning pain that occurs in the absence of an external stimulus [43]. Spontaneous pain could potentially result, for example, from spontaneous activity in dorsal horn nociceptive neurons. Furthermore, while we measured at-level pain in the forepaw, we did not investigate below-level pain, which describes pain in dermatomes caudal to the level of injury and has been observed in the hindpaws of rats receiving cervical contusion SCI [40].

In this study, changes in pain behavior are exhibited in the absence of changes in motor behavior, as measured by grip strength. Because measures of evoked pain, such as the Hargreaves test and von Frey test, rely on motor activity (i.e. forepaw withdrawal) as a response, any dysfunction in motor behavior could affect test outcomes. The decrease in grip strength seen in the contralateral forepaw of C5 injury animals at one-week post injury was unexpected and could reflect transient local changes to the cervical spinal cord rather than a global alteration of pain transmission circuitry. Importantly, grip strength returns to baseline levels after this first week, at which point hyperalgesia and allodynia have developed.

Despite the maintenance of forepaw grip strength, we observed a significant loss of ventral horn motor neurons at the injury epicenter on the ipsilateral side following injury. One likely explanation for this disconnect is that our current injury model is milder and results in less motor neuron loss compared to our previous unilateral cervical contusion model in the mouse [9], which did produce persistent forelimb motor dysfunction. There is presumably some level of motor neuron loss necessary to result in quantifiable motor deficits.

At the molecular level, changes in ΔfosB and GLT1 were observed in the superficial dorsal horn of the injured spinal cord of our SCI model. Alterations in the expression of these proteins may contribute to central sensitization of pain transmission neurons in the cervical spinal cord. Central sensitization, including post-translational and transcriptional changes to dorsal horn neurons, affects the output of nociceptive neurons and the way in which peripheral stimuli are perceived. Thus, the observed changes may contribute to the hyperalgesic and allodynic phenotypes seen in our cervical contusion SCI.

C-fos is a member of the Fos family of transcription factors, which are induced quickly and transiently by a variety of stimuli. Because its expression is stimulated by an influx of calcium into neurons, c-fos acts as a marker of neuronal activity [45]. Previously, researchers have shown an induction of c-fos expression in the dorsal horn of the spinal cord following exposure to noxious stimuli in various forms [46],[47], [48], [49], [50]. ΔfosB is a truncated splice variant of the Fos family member, FosB. Unlike c-fos, which is expressed quickly but returns to basal levels within hours after stimulation, ΔfosB is induced gradually and is stable, so it accumulates over time and persists on the order of weeks or months [50]. ΔfosB has been implicated in a number of processes in the nervous system, including addiction, plasticity, and stress [45], [50] but may also play a role in neuronal changes associated with pain [14], [15].

In our SCI model, we see long-term elevation in the levels of ΔfosB in the superficial dorsal horn of the spinal cord, suggesting persistently increased activation of these neurons. These results are in accordance with another study that reported an increase in ΔfosB expression following pain induction, specifically carrageenan-induced inflammation [14]. Additionally, we previously reported an increase in ΔfosB expression in the rat following cervical contusion SCI [24]. While ΔfosB expression is significantly increased ipsilaterally at two weeks after injury, there is an even greater increase that spreads bilaterally at the six-week time point. This is consistent with the protein's stability and tendency to accumulate over time [46]. Furthermore, this persistent expression of the protein in the dorsal horn suggests an increase in the activity of these nociceptive neurons, possibly due to an increase in spontaneous firing and/or synaptic input, which may contribute to central sensitization. Thus the expression of ΔfosB that we see in our injury model is likely in accordance with its role in pain and plasticity.

In the nucleus accumbens and cortex, identified targets of ΔfosB include GluA2 and GluN1. In these regions, ΔfosB has been shown to upregulate these two proteins [50]. These targets are subunits of the glutamate receptors AMPAR and NMDAR, and their upregulation may contribute to increased glutamatergic transmission. Excessive stimulation of glutamate receptors can lead to hyperexcitability directly by increased activation of dorsal horn neurons and indirectly via glutamate excitotoxic loss of inhibitory interneurons [18]. It is unknown whether ΔfosB also targets these AMPAR and NMDAR subunits in the spinal cord following SCI. However, researchers have reported changes in GluA1 trafficking and expression in spinal neurons following central and peripheral injury and pain [51], [52], [53] as well as an upregulation of GluN1 and GluN2A in the ventral horn as a result of contusion SCI [54]. Despite this potential connection between ΔfosB and glutamate receptor subunits, ΔfosB does not definitively measure hyperexcitability. Instead, a continuation of this experiment to provide more conclusive evidence of the hyperexcitability could include electrophysiological measures of dorsal horn neurons.

Also following injury, we observe an increase in GFAP, a protein upregulated in activated astrocytes, in the dorsal horn of the spinal cord. We see this change at both time points, but it is more pronounced two weeks after injury. These data are in accordance with our group and others who have shown localized increases in markers of astrocyte activation following SCI [23], [24], [55], [56]. The observed increase in GFAP is seen only at the injury epicenter on the ipsilateral side, suggesting that this change is region-specific and may not play a role in potential above- or below-level changes, at least in our model.

The increase in activated astrocytes in our model of SCI could potentially have negative effects on the injured spinal cord and pain transmission circuitry. Often, activated astrocytes in the context of SCI and other injuries are considered detrimental because of their role in the formation of the glial scar, which can inhibit axon regeneration and plasticity, and the release of pro-inflammatory and other harmful molecules that can alter the excitability of neurons. Astrocytes, however, play many beneficial roles in the CNS, such as maintaining extracellular ion and neurotransmitter homeostasis, providing neurotrophic factor support, aiding in metabolic functions, and regulating the formation and maintenance of synapses [57].

Interestingly, while at-level thermal hyperalgesia is maintained through six weeks after injury, GFAP levels decrease slightly by this time point. Activated astrocytes play a significant role in the structural and molecular maintenance of the injury site [13], [17], [18], [57], [58]. The repair process following spinal cord injury, however, occurs in various phases, including acute, sub-acute, and chronic. While the effects of the glial scar and other repair processes can last months or years, not all of the molecules contributing to post-injury repair may be present at all stages. Thus, some astrocytes may return to the basal state in the days or weeks following injury, explaining the decrease in GFAP we see at six weeks compared to two weeks. Another explanation for the persistence of thermal hyperalgesia and tactile allodynia despite GFAP levels decreasing is that the loss of GLT1 also persists and contributes more strongly to the development of neuropathic pain after SCI. Alternatively, there may be irreversible damage to the spinal cord at this point that the inactivation of astrocytes may have no effect on.

Considering the various roles that astrocytes play following injury, it is important not only to study the reactive state of astrocytes in our model but also the effects of our injury on important homeostatic and protective functions of astrocytes. In light of this, we decided to investigate how our injury paradigm alters a centrally important function of astrocytes in the CNS, the uptake of glutamate through GLT1. Several groups have reported decreases in GLT1 levels following SCI [22], [23], [24], [25], [26], but the role of such changes has not been studied extensively in the context of neuropathic pain. To study GLT1 expression, we utilized both C57BL/6 wild-type and BAC-GLT1-eGFP reporter mice as well as both immunohistochemistry and western blotting. In our mouse cervical contusion SCI model, GLT1 levels are diminished in the dorsal horn at both time points at the epicenter and caudally on the ipsilateral side, suggesting a significant compromise in glutamate clearance in the injured spinal cord. Unlike with wild-type mice, in BAC-GLT1-eGFP mice, we see no change in the caudal contralateral region of the dorsal horn. This is likely due to a slightly different injury used in these two mouse paradigms.

Western blotting reveals that GLT1 protein levels are decreased ipsilaterally at the epicenter. However, no change in GLT1 levels is observed at the caudal ipsilateral region, which is contrary to the results we report using immunohistochemistry. This discrepancy likely reflects the difference in spatial resolution between these two techniques. Using immunohistochemistry, analyses of very specific regions, such as the superficial dorsal horn, are possible. For western blotting, however, we use a piece of tissue that encompasses an entire spinal cord level, including both the dorsal and ventral horn and surrounding white matter tracts. For our immunohistochemical analyses of the injured spinal cord, we examined the most superficial laminae of the dorsal horn, laminae I–II, as well as laminae III.

Importantly, co-localization analyses of GFAP and GLT1-eGFP at high-magnification reveal that, in control animals, most of the GLT1-positive cells are also GFAP-positive astrocytes. However, after injury, while the number of GFAP-positive cells is increased, the number and percentage of these astrocytes also expressing GLT1 is greatly reduced. This suggests that the loss of GLT1 that is observed in our animals occurs mostly in astrocytes, supporting our proposal that astrocytes activated after injury are deficient in glutamate clearance.

Like astrocytes, microglia play a major role in both immediate and delayed responses to injury to the spinal cord and may contribute to the development of pathological pain [13]. We also noted significant microglial activation in the superficial dorsal horn following cervical contusion SCI. Unlike astrocyte reactivity, we observed microglial activation not just at the ipsilateral epicenter region, but also at contralateral epicenter and caudal ipsilateral locations. Though we focused mostly on astrocyte changes, including down-regulation of GLT1 expression, it is likely that microglial activation also played a significant role in the persistent neuropathic pain phenotype observed in this study.

Here we present a model of unilateral cervical contusion SCI in the mouse that is representative of typical injury seen clinically in humans [1], [5]. The model exhibits at-level neuropathic pain accompanied by relevant molecular changes in the superficial dorsal horn. The protein expression changes suggest the presence of activated and proliferating astrocytes and a loss of GLT1 function, which may contribute to central sensitization, and underlie the development of neuropathic pain. We have identified a number of proteins that are altered by SCI and accompany thermal hyperalgesia and tactile allodynia, but their roles in the development of neuropathic pain have yet to be fully elucidated. Further research with the model may include identifying the factors and processes underlying the formation and maintenance of neuropathic pain in the spinal cord as well as recognizing targets for the treatment of chronic pathological pain resulting from SCI and similar injuries. Importantly, the availability of this model in the mouse allow for the use of valuable transgenic tools.

Acknowledgments

We would like to thank Drs. Luis Menéndez and Ana Baamonde for their assistance in the thermal testing procedures. We would also like to thank Dr. Jeannie Chin, Dr. Anupam Hazra and Brain Corbett for their advice and technical help with ΔFosB immunohistochemistry. Additionally, J.W.

would like to thank the members of her thesis committee, Dr. Piera Pasinelli and Dr. Lorraine Iacovitti, for their guidance and support.

Author Contributions

Conceived and designed the experiments: JLW ACL. Performed the experiments: JLW TJH RP DS ACL. Analyzed the data: JLW TJH RP DS ACL. Wrote the paper: JLW ACL.

References

1. National Spinal Cord Injury Statistical Center, University of Birmingham, Alabama (2013) Spinal cord injury facts and figures at a glance. Available: https://www.nscisc.uab.edu/PublicDocuments/fact_figures_docs/Facts%202013.pdf.
2. de Miguel M, Kraychete DC (2009) Pain in patients with spinal cord injury: A review. Rev Bras Anestheiol 59: 350–357.
3. Siddall PJ, McClelland JM, Rutkowski SB, Cousins MJ (2003) A longitudinal study of the prevalence and characteristics of pain in the first 5 years following spinal cord injury. Pain 103: 249–257.
4. Ravenscroft A, Ahmed YS, Burnside IG (2000) Chronic pain after SCI: A patient survey. Spinal Cord 38: 611–614.
5. McDonald JW, Becker D (2003) Spinal cord injury: Promising interventions and realistic goals. Am J Phys Med Rehabil 82: S38–S49.
6. Nakae A, Nakai K, Yano K, Hosokawa K, Shibata M, et al. (2011) The animal model of spinal cord injury as an experimental pain model. J Biomed Biotechnol 2011: 939023.
7. Kundi S, Bicknell R, Ahmed Z (2013) Spinal cord injury: Current mammalian models. Am J Neurosci 4: 1–12.
8. Nicaise C, Hala TJ, Frank DM, Parker JL, Authelet M, et al. (2012) Phrenic motor neuron degeneration compromises phrenic axonal circuitry and diaphragm activity in a unilateral cervical contusion model of spinal cord injury. Exp Neurol 235: 539–552.
9. Nicaise C, Putatunda R, Hala TJ, Regan KA, Frank DM, et al. (2012) Degeneration of phrenic motor neurons induces long-term diaphragm deficits following mid-cervical spinal contusion in mice. J Neurotrauma 29: 2748–2760.
10. Nicaise C, Frank DM, Hala TJ, Authelet M, Pochet R, et al. (2013) Early phrenic motor neuron loss and transient respiratory abnormalities after unilateral cervical spinal cord contusion. J Neurotrauma 30: 1092–1099.
11. Streijger F, Beernink TM, Lee JH, Bhatnagar T, Park S, et al. (2013) Characterization of a cervical spinal cord hemicontusion injury in mice using the infinite horizon impactor. J Neurotrauma 30: 869–883.
12. Latremoliere A, Woolf CJ (2009) Central sensitization: A generator of pain hypersensitivity by central neural plasticity. J Pain 10: 895–926.
13. Hulsebosch CE, Hains BC, Crown ED, Carlton SM (2009) Mechanisms of chronic central neuropathic pain after spinal cord injury. Brain Res Rev 60: 202–213.
14. Luis-Delgado OE, Barrot M, Rodeau JL, Ulery PG, Freund-Mercier MJ, et al. (2006) The transcription factor deltafosB is recruited by inflammatory pain. J Neurochem 98: 1423–1431.
15. Pareek TK, Kulkarni AB (2006) Cdk5: A new player in pain signaling. Cell Cycle 5: 585–588.
16. Clarke LE, Barres BA (2013) Emerging roles of astrocytes in neural circuit development. Nat Rev Neurosci 14: 311–321.
17. Karimi-Abdolrezaee S, Billakanti R (2012) Reactive astrogliosis after spinal cord injury: Beneficial and detrimental effects. Mol Neurobiol 46: 251–264.
18. Nakagawa T, Kaneko S (2010) Spinal astrocytes as therapeutic targets for pathological pain. J Pharmacol Sci
19. Chen CJ, Liao SL, Kuo JS (2000) Gliotoxic action of glutamate on cultured astrocytes. J Neurochem 74: 1557–1565.
20. Mark LP, Prost RW, Ulmer JL, Smith MM, Daniels DL, et al. (2001) Pictorial review of glutamate excitotoxicity: Fundamental concepts for neuroimaging. AJNR Am J Neuroradiol 22: 1813–1824.
21. Doble A (1999) The role of excitotoxicity in neurodegenerative disease: Implications for therapy. Pharmacol Ther 81: 163–221.
22. Lepore AC, O'Donnell J, Kim AS, Yang EJ, Tuteja A, et al. (2011) Reduction in expression of the astrocyte glutamate transporter, GLT1, worsens functional and histological outcomes following traumatic spinal cord injury. Glia 59: 1996–2005.
23. Lepore AC, O'Donnell J, Bonner JF, Paul C, Miller ME, et al. (2011) Spatial and temporal changes in promoter activity of the astrocyte glutamate transporter GLT1 following traumatic spinal cord injury. J Neurosci Res 89: 1001–1017.
24. Putatunda R, Hala TJ, Chin J, Lepore AC (2014) Chronic at-level thermal hyperalgesia following rat cervical contusion spinal cord injury is accompanied by neuronal and astrocyte activation and loss of the astrocyte glutamate transporter, GLT1, in superficial dorsal horn. Brain Res: in press.
25. Vera-Portocarrero LP, Mills CD, Ye Z, Fullwood SD, McAdoo DJ, et al. (2002) Rapid changes in expression of glutamate transporters after spinal cord injury. Brain Res 927: 104–110.
26. Olsen ML, Campbell SC, McFerrin MB, Floyd CL, Sontheimer H (2010) Spinal cord injury causes a wide-spread, persistent loss of Kir4.1 and glutamate transporter 1: Benefit of 17 beta-oestradiol treatment. Brain 133: 1013–1025.
27. Regan MR, Huang YH, Kim YS, Dykes-Hoberg ML, Jin L, et al. (2007) Variations in promoter activity reveal a differential expression and physiology of glutamate transporters by glia in the developing and mature CNS. J Neurosci 27: 6607–6619.
28. Menendez L, Lastra A, Hidalgo A, Baamonde (2002) Unilateral hot plate test: a simple and sensitive method for detecting central and peripheral hyperalgesia in mice. J Neurosci Methods 113: 91–97.
29. Lepore AC, Rauck B, Dejea C, Pardo AC, Rao MS, et al. (2008) Focal transplantation-based astrocyte replacement is neuroprotective in a model of motor neuron disease. Nat Neurosci 11: 1294–1301.
30. Perrotti LI, Weaver RR, Robison B, Renthal W, Maze I, et al. (2008) Distinct patterns of DeltaFosB induction in brain by drugs of abuse. Synapse 62: 358–369.
31. Lepore AC, Dejea C, Carmen J, Rauck B, Kerr DA, et al. (2008). Selective ablation of proliferating astrocytes does not affect disease outcome in either acute or chronic models of motor neuron degeneration. Exp Neurol 211: 423–432.
32. Lepore AC, Fischer I. (2005) Lineage-restricted neural precursors survive, migrate, and differentiate following transplantation into the injured adult spinal cord. Exp Neurol 194: 230–242.
33. Maragakis NJ, Rothstein JD (2001) Glutamate transporters in neurologic disease. Arch Neurol 58: 365–370.
34. Jorum E, Warncke T, Stubhaug A (2003) Cold allodynia and hyperalgesia in neuropathic pain: The effect of N-methyl-D-aspartate (NMDA) receptor antagonist ketamine–double-blind, cross-over comparison with alfentanil and placebo. Pain 101: 229–235.
35. Gwak YS, Hulsebosch CE (2011) Neuronal hyperexcitability: A substrate for central neuropathic pain after spinal cord injury. Curr Pain Headache Rep 15: 215–222.
36. Sandkuhler J (2009) Models and mechanisms of hyperalgesia and allodynia. Physiol Rev 89: 707–758.
37. Hoschouer EL, Basso DM, Jakeman LB (2010) Aberrant sensory responses are dependent on lesion severity after spinal cord contusion injury in mice. Pain 148: 328–342.
38. Mesiner JG, Marsh AD, Marsh DR (2010) Loss of GABAergic interneurons in laminae I–III of the spinal cord dorsal horn contributes to reduced GABAergic tone and neuropathic pain after spinal cord injury. J Neurotrauma 27: 729–737.
39. Hoschouer EL, Yin FQ, Jakeman LB (2009) L1 cell adhesion molecule is essential for the maintenance of hyperalgesia after spinal cord injury. Exp Neurol 216: 22–34.
40. Detloff MR, Wade ER Jr, Houle JD (2013) Chronic at- and below-level pain after moderate unilateral cervical spinal cord contusion in rats. J Neurotrauma 30: 884–890.
41. Kosta V, Kojundzic SL, Sapunar LC, Sapunar D (2012) The extent of laminectomy affects pain-related behavior in a rat model of neuropathic pain. Eur J Pain 13: 243–248.
42. Busic Z, Kostic S, Kosta V, Carija R, Puljak L, et al. (2012) Postlaminectomy stabilization of the spine in a rat model of neuropathic pain reduces pain-related behavior. Spine 15: 1874–1882.
43. Djouhri L, Koutsikou S, Fang X, McMullan S, Lawson SN (2006) Spontaneous pain, both neuropathic and inflammatory, is related to frequency of spontaneous firing in intact C-fiber nociceptors. J Neurosci 26:1281–1292.
44. Christensen MD, Everhart AQ, Pickelman JT, Hulsebosch CE (1996) Mechanical and thermal allodynia in chronic central pain following spinal cord injury. Pain 68: 97–107.
45. Bullitt E (1990) Expression of c-fos-like protein as a marker for neuronal activity following noxious stimulation in the rat. J Comp Neurol 296: 517–530.
46. Abbadie C, Honore P, Besson JM (1994) Intense cold noxious stimulation of the rat hindpaw induces c-fos expression in lumbar spinal cord neurons. Neuroscience 59: 457–468.
47. Jinks SL, Simons CT, Dessirier JM, Carstens MI, Antognini JF, et al. (2002) C-fos induction in rat superficial dorsal horn following cutaneous application of noxious chemical or mechanical stimuli. Exp Brain Res 145: 261–269.
48. Yi DK, Barr GA (1995) The induction of Fos-like immunoreactivity by noxious thermal, mechanical and chemical stimuli in the lumbar spinal cord of infant rats. Pain 60: 257–265.
49. Bester H, Beggs S, Woolf CJ (2000) Changes in tactile stimuli-induced behavior and c-Fos expression in the superficial dorsal horn and in parabrachial nuclei after sciatic nerve crush. J Comp Neurol 428: 45–61.
50. McClung CA, Ulery PG, Perrotti L, Zachariou V, Berton O, et al. (2004) DeltaFosB: A molecular switch for long-term adaptation in the brain. Brain Res Mol Brain Res 132: 146–154.
51. Galan A, Laird JM, Cervero F (2004) In vivo recruitment by painful stimuli of AMPA receptor subunits to the plasma membrane of spinal cord neurons. Pain 112: 315–323.
52. Katano T, Furue H, Okuda-Ashitaka E, Tagaya M, Watanabe M, et al. (2008) N-ethylmaleimide-sensitive fusion protein (NSF) is involved in central sensitization in the spinal cord through GluR2 subunit composition switch after inflammation. Eur J Neurosci 27: 3161–3170.

53. Larsson M, Broman J (2008) Translocation of GluR1-containing AMPA receptors to a spinal nociceptive synapse during acute noxious stimulation. J Neurosci 28: 7084–7090.
54. Grossman SD, Wolfe BB, Yasuda RP, Wrathall JR (2000) Changes in NMDA receptor subunit expression in response to contusive spinal cord injury. J Neurochem 75: 174–184.
55. Iwasaki R, Matsuura Y, Ohtori S, Suzuki T, Kuniyoshi K, et al. (2013) Activation of astrocytes and microglia in the C3-T4 dorsal horn by lower trunk avulsion in a rat model of neuropathic pain. J Hand Surg Am 38: 841–846.
56. Cho DC, Cheong JH, Yang MS, Hwang SJ, Kim JM, et al. (2011) The effect of minocycline on motor neuron recovery and neuropathic pain in a rat model of spinal cord injury. J Korean Neurosurg Soc 49: 83–91.
57. Pekny M, Nilsson M (2005) Astrocyte activation and reactive gliosis. Glia 50: 427–434.
58. Rolls A, Schechter R, Schwartz M (2009) The bright side of the glial scar in CNS repair. Nat Rev Neurosci 10: 235–241.

Surgical Decompression of Painful Diabetic Peripheral Neuropathy: The Role of Pain Distribution

Chenlong Liao, Wenchuan Zhang*, Min Yang, Qiufeng Ma, Guowei Li, Wenxiang Zhong

Department of Neurosurgery, XinHua Hospital, affiliated to Shanghai JiaoTong University School of Medicine, Shanghai, P. R. China

Abstract

Objective: To investigate the effect of surgical decompression on painful diabetic peripheral neuropathy (DPN) patients and discuss the role which pain distribution and characterization play in the management of painful DPN as well as the underlying mechanism involved.

Methods: A total of 306 patients with painful diabetic lower-extremity neuropathy were treated with Dellon surgical nerve decompression in our department. Clinical evaluation including Visual analogue scale (VAS), Brief Pain Inventory Short Form for diabetic peripheral neuropathy (BPI-DPN) questionnaire, two-point discrimination (2-PD), nerve conduction velocity (NCV) and high-resolution ultrasonography (cross-sectional area, CSA) were performed in all cases preoperatively, and at 6 month intervals for 2 years post-decompression. The patients who underwent surgery were retrospectively assigned into two subgroups (focal and diffuse pain) according to the distribution of the diabetic neuropathic pain. The control group included 92 painful DPN patients without surgery.

Results: The levels of VAS, scores in BPI-DPN, 2-PD, NCV results and CSA were all improved in surgical group when compared to the control group ($P<0.05$). More improvement of VAS, scores in BPI-DPN and CSA was observed in focal pain group than that in diffuse group ($P<0.05$).

Conclusions: Efficacy of decompression of multiple lower-extremity peripheral nerves in patients with painful diabetic neuropathy was confirmed in this study. While both focal and diffuse group could benefit from surgical decompression, pain relief and morphological restoration could be better achieved in focal group.

Editor: Massimo Pietropaolo, University of Michigan Medical School, United States of America

Funding: This study was supported by the grant from the National Science Foundation of China. The grant number: 81371373. The URL of the funder's website: http://isisn.nsfc.gov.cn/egrantindex/funcindex/prjsearch-list.

Competing Interests: The authors have declared that no competing interests exist.

* Email: zhangwench88@hotmail.com

Introduction

There are over 250 million people in the world with type 1 and 2 diabetes mellitus. [1] Neuropathy is one of the most common complications of diabetes mellitus and leads to increasingly high morbidity and mortality, resulting in a huge economic burden for diabetes care. [2] Diabetic neuropathy is a heterogeneous condition containing symmetrical neuropathies and focal neuropathies, [3] presenting diverse clinical manifestations. Of all the neuropathies in diabetes, chronic diabetic peripheral neuropathy (DPN) is the commonest. [4] Of all the symptoms in DPN, pain is the most distressing and is the main factor that prompts the patients to seek medical advice. [5] One-third of diabetic patients have symptoms of neuropathic pain according to a recent community-based study [6] and up to 15–20% of patients with DPN may experience painful symptoms. [7] Therefore, a high proportion of patients are suffering from neuropathic pain as well as the relative depression, anxiety and sleep deprivation.

The management of neuropathic pain in diabetes still remains challenging mainly due to its various clinical features, wide spectrum severity and different distribution involved. Descriptions of pain can be burning, prickling, lancinating, shooting, cramping, aching, and also contact hypersensitivity (allodynia) and "dead feeling" (numbness) in their legs. [5] The severity may range from mild symptoms in one toe or two to continuous painful symptoms involving both legs and may even extend to the upper limbs. The extent involved may be focal or diffuse. One additional factor that contributes to the treatment dilemma of neuropathic pain is the varied response to the currently different treatments. The diverse manifestations of neuropathic pain in diabetes and various responses to current interventions imply that a number of mechanisms could contribute. Therefore, the management of painful DPN may not be one single intervention and a series of factors should be taken into consideration, one of which, as Vinik, A. and his colleagues put it in one guideline, [8] may be the distribution of pain. According to our clinical experience with management of painful diabetic neuropathy, features and severity of pain may change during the course of diabetic neuropathy while the distribution of pain is relatively invariable, which may be of some value for patient selection for surgical decompression. Thus we carry out this retrospective study to investigate the effects of surgical decompression on the outcome of painful diabetic patients and discuss the role which pain distribution plays in the management of painful diabetic neuropathy as well as the underlying mechanism involved.

Aside from traditional management including glucose control, lifestyle modification and pharmacological treatment, surgical decompression is recommended for pain relief in the recent reports [9–15] based on the "double crush" hypothesis. [16] Clinical observations revealed that many of the symptoms of diabetic neuropathy, including pain, are similar to those of chronic nerve compression, suggesting that entrapment of nerves may happen in the patients with diabetic neuropathy. Allowing for the currently traditional treatment dilemma on pain relief in patients with diabetic neuropathy, surgical decompression targeting superimposed compression, as an newly emerging promising approach, should be impartially taken into account.

Methods

This study is approved by the Xinhua Hospital Ethics Review Board and the forms of consent were obtained from all patients involved in this study.

Patients

A consecutive series of 306 patients (108 males and 198 females) with painful diabetic lower-extremity neuropathy, who underwent Dellon surgical nerve decompression [17] in our department from January 2008 to December 2011 was collected in this study. The control group included 92 painful DPN patients (38 males and 54 females) without surgery. The control group was mainly made up of the outpatients who refused hospitalization for surgical intervention owing to various personal reasons, most of which included fear of surgery and economic issues. Patients in the control group were all qualified for the inclusion criteria described below. According to the Wagner classification, 77 patients in surgical group (25.2%) and 26 patients in control group (28.3%) were rated as class 1 (surface ulcers and no clinical infection) before surgery. All patients had a history of type II diabetes mellitus according to 1999 WHO diagnostic criteria and showed symptoms of neuropathic pain, with high Toronto clinical scoring system (TCSS) scores. According to the definition proposed by the International Association for the Study of Pain, neuropathic pain in diabetes is "pain arising as a direct consequence of abnormalities in the somatosensory system in people with diabetes". [18] After reviewed the histories, we retrospectively defined the focal pain (the pain mainly confined to one to three scattered areas of the legs, dorsum of feet, the heels, the toes, or the plantar aspect of feet) and the diffuse pain (the pain is so dispersed along the affected extremities that exactly position can not be localized) and then divide the surgical group into two subgroups according to this definition. The focal pain was observed in 145 patients and the diffuse pain in the remaining 161 patients. The baseline characteristics of patients are displayed in Table 1.

Inclusion criteria include (1) history of pain in the distribution of the posterior tibial (medial and lateral plantar surface), common and superficial peroneal (lateral calf and dorsum of the foot), or deep peroneal nerves (dorsum of the foot, first web space), (2) positive Tinel sign presented at a known site of nerve entrapment including the fibular tunnel at the lateral side of the knee, for the common peroneal nerve, the tarsal tunnel at the ankle for the tibial nerve, and the junction between the first and second metatarsals and the cuneiforms for the deep peroneal nerve, (3) Decreased two-point discrimination: the big toe pulp two-point discrimination was greater than 9 mm [19].

Exclusion criteria include (1) presence of defined risk factors such as alcohol, nutrition, uremia and peripheral vascular disease, as demonstrated by absence of a palpable pulse, (2) previous history of cervical and lumbar spondylosis, (3) radiculopathy, (4) pedal edema.

Surgical Technique

The decompression surgery adopting Dellon triple procedures [17] were performed by the same senior surgeon (Zhang WC), with the use of microscope under continuous epidural anesthesia.

A 3 cm-long incision was made below the fibular head and the skin, superficial and deep fascia was cut. After excision of fascia above the common peroneal nerve and the peroneus longus muscle tendon, the common peroneal nerve trunk was exposed and decompressed.

A 6 cm-long curved incision was made along the medial malleolus and the skin, superficial and deep fascia was cut. After excision of the flexor retinaculum, the posterior tibial artery and veins and the tibal nerve were indentified and decompressed. Following this, the abductor halluces brevis was cut and spread to expose and divide the roof of the medial and of the lateral plantar tunnels. The medial calcaneal tunnel was then identified and decompressed. Epineurium decompression was performed if there was evidence of epineurial thickening.

A 2 cm-long incision was made longitudinally between the first and second metatarsal heads and the skin, superficial and deep fascia were cut to expose the tendon of the extensor hallucis brevis muscle. This tendon was then excised to decompress the deep peroneal nerve.

During the perioperative period, blood glucose was controlled at 6.2–8.0 mmol/L. After the patients were discharged, they were required to monitor their fasting plasma glucose every week and control their blood glucose levels to <8.0 mmol/L.

Clinical evaluation

Careful history taking and peripheral neurological/vascular examination were completed in all patients at admission. Aside from pain as a chief complaint, some of them simultaneously presented with other sensory symptoms including numbness, tingling and so forth. Patients were additionally inquired about their functional status, normal activities, ability to work, walking distance, family history of diabetes and the use of medications.

Assessment of pain including visual analogue scale (VAS) and Brief Pain Inventory Short Form for diabetic peripheral neuropathy (BPI-DPN), of sensation including plantar big toe and small toe two-point discrimination (2-PD), of morphological changes of nerves employing high-resolution ultrasound, of electrophysiological changes performing nerve conduction velocity (NCV) on admission prior to surgery and then at 6 months intervals for two years after surgery. The follow-up was conducted mainly on an outpatient basis.

Pre and post operative evaluations were performed by two clinical residents (in charge of history taking and peripheral neurological/vascular examination), one sonographer (undertaking high-resolution ultrasound of peripheral nerves) and one technician of electrophysiology (performing the NCV tests).

The visual analogue scale (VAS) [20], which is one of the oldest and best validated measurement (0 = no pain to 10 = worst possible pain), was used to assess the severity of diabetic neuropathic pain. All patients were asked to complete Brief Pain Inventory Short Form for diabetic peripheral neuropathy (BPI-DPN) to assess pain severity and pain interference with daily functioning. The BPI-DPN includes the four-item pain Severity scale (Worst Pain, Least Pain, Average Pain, and Pain Now) and

Table 1. Baseline of characteristics of patients.

	Control(n = 92)	Focal(n = 145)	Diffuse(n = 161)	P(a, b)*
Patient characteristics				
Median age(yr) (%)	57±13.62(36–86)	60±11.59(34–86)	58±11.36(36–85)	0.08, 0.93
Age in years, n (%)				
<40	9(9.7)	7(4.8)	11(6.8)	
40–49	21(22.8)	26(17.9)	31(19.3)	
50–59	25(27.1)	36(24.8)	39(24.2)	
60–69	22(23.9)	62(42.8)	67(41.6)	
>70	15(16.3)	14(9.7)	13(8.1)	
Sex, n (%)				0.29, 0.84
Male	38(41.3)	52(35.9)	56(34.8)	
Female	54(58.7)	93(64.1)	105(65.2)	
Course of DM(yr)	7.2±1.62	7.7±2.72	8.1±1.85	0.83, 0.78
Course of pain(mo)	47±5.38	43±5.61	57±6.32	0.80, 0.74

All variables were expressed in mean ± SD.
DM = Diabetes Mellitus.
*a: control group vs. focal & diffuse (surgical group), b: focal group vs. diffuse group.

the seven-item pain Interference scale (General Activity, Mood, Walking Ability, Normal Work, Relations with Others, Sleep, Enjoyment of Life). Each items of BPI uses a 0 to 10 numeric rating scale anchored at "no pain," and 10 for "pain as bad as you can imagine" for Severity, and "does not interfere" to "completely interferes" for Interference [21].

Neurosensory examination mainly included percussion over a distribution of the affected peripheral nerve (Tinel sign) and two-point discrimination (2-PD) using the Disk-Criminator at the big and small toes for medial and lateral plantar nerves, respectively. A positive Tinel sign was taken to be a positive response that indicated either a tingling or radiating electriclike perception either into the heel, the arch, or the toes (the most common responses), or proximally up the inside of the ankle (the least common response) [22].

Nerve conduction velocity was detected with the employment of a Denmark Medtronic EMG (DK 1 2740). The testing was performed under a quiet indoor environment with a room temperature of 25°C and skin temperature of 30°C, using surface electrodes for stimulation and recording. Bilateral motor NCVs of tibial nerve and sensory NCVs of the common peroneal nerve and superficial peroneal nerve were recorded in all patients.

High-resolution ultrasound of peripheral nerves was performed employing a Sequoia 512 ultrasound device (Siemens) with a 8–14 MHz transducer. Multislice, longitudinal, and transverse scans were made through the common peroneal nerve and the posterior tibial nerve to observe the continuity and echogeneity of the nerves. The anteroposterior diameter (Da) and transverse diameter (Dt) of the nerves were measured at the cross-section of 1.5 cm below the distal tip of fibular head (common peroneal nerve) and distal tip of medial malleolus (posterior tibial nerve). And then cross-sectional area (CSA) was calculated by the formula of $S = \pi(Da*Dt/4)$ [23].

Statistical Methods

Analysis was performed separately for patients comparing the change from preoperative levels to that of last visit (BPI-DPN, 2-PD, NCV, CSA). Data were expressed as the mean ± standard deviation. Pearson's χ^2 test and student's t-test were used with the employment of SPSS 18.0. A P value <0.05 was considered statistically significant.

Results

Twenty-five patients in surgical groups and six patients in control group were lost during the follow-up. The differences of age, sex, course of diabetes and pain symptom between the two groups were not statistically significant ($P>0.05$). The average courses of diabetes mellitus were longer than the average courses of pain symptom in all groups. In some individuals, however, the onset of pain symptom came before the diagnosis of diabetes, some may even lead to the diagnosis of diabetes, in which situation other potential diseases had been excluded before the diagnosis of diabetic neuropathy. There is no statistically significant difference between surgical and control groups and, also no statistically significant difference among the three groups (focal pain group, diffuse pain group and control group) after dividing the surgical group into two subgroups regarding to the initial VAS level, 2-PD, scores in BPI-DPN, NCV and CSA ($P>0.05$).

Visual Analogue Scales

The VAS levels in different time points were recorded and comparison was made among the three groups to assess the outcome of surgery. (Figure 1) In focal pain group, the average score of VAS was 8.20 on admission and at 6 months after surgery decreased to 2.28 ($P<0.01$). The average pain level remained between 2 and 1 for the remainder of the study. The mean VAS pain level of patients with diffuse pain was 8.32 and decreased to 3.43 ($P<0.01$) 6 months after surgery, higher than that of patients with focal pain ($P<0.05$). The mean pain level of diffuse pain group remained between 4 and 2 with fluctuation for the remainder of the study. The average VAS of patients in control group was 8.03 at first visit and remained around 8.0 during the two-year follow-up ($P>0.05$). There was a statistically significant difference as to VAS level between surgical and control groups after surgery ($P<0.01$). The results show pain relief can be achieved through surgical decompression, especially in the patients with focal pain.

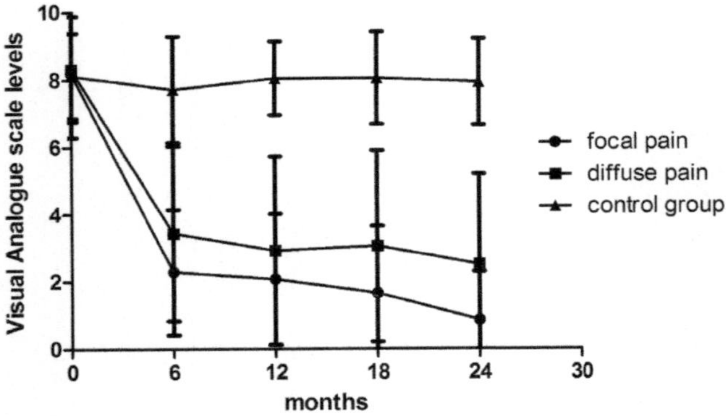

Figure 1. The figure displays the records of VAS levels at different time points. The VAS scores in both surgical groups showed notable decline with the time course while no changes occurred in control group during the follow-up. The overall postoperative VAS levels of focal pain group were much lower than that of diffuse pain group ($P<0.01$).

Two-point discrimination

In focal pain group, the postoperative (two years later) average big toe 2-PD (6.43±1.46 mm) and small toe 2-PD (6.24±1.72 mm) showed a statistically significant improvement ($P<0.05$) comparing to those before surgery (17.4±1.86 mm, 16.7±1.71 mm). Analogously, markedly improvement can also be observed when comparison was made between preoperative (18.7±1.68 mm, 19±1.34 mm) and postoperative (7.34±1.54 mm, 10.24±1.94 mm) big toe and small toe 2-PD in diffuse pain group ($P<0.05$). There is no statistically significant difference between two groups with regard to both big toe 2-PD ($P = 0.73$) and small 2-PD ($P = 0.77$) after decompression. In control group, no statistically significant difference could be seen between preoperative and postoperative 2-PD of big toe (pre: 16.3±1.77 mm, post: 17.8±1.72 mm, $P>0.05$) and small toe (pre: 16.3±1.77 mm, post: 16.8±1.57 mm, $P>0.05$). A statistically significant improvement in both small toe and big toe 2-PD could be observed between surgical and control groups ($P<0.05$) (Figure 2 A, B).

BPI-DPN questionnaire

The scores of all items in BPI-DPN were recorded, and the "Mean severity" as well as the "Mean interference" was compared in this study. (Figure 2 C, D) In the focal pain group, the preoperative scores of "Mean severity" (5.56±1.14) decreased greatly after two years (0.52±0.78) ($P<0.05$). There is also an observable decline (5.64±1.07, 1.12±1.01) in "Mean severity" two years after surgery in the diffuse pain group ($P<0.05$). Initial "Mean interference" of focal and diffuse pain group is 4.75±0.86 and 4.73±0.82, which decreased to 1.88±1.15 ($P<0.05$) and 2.00±1.07 ($P<0.05$) respectively. Statistically significant difference existed between the two groups regarding both postoperative "Mean severity" ($P<0.05$) and "Mean interference" ($P<0.05$). As respect to "Mean severity" (preoperative: 5.77±1.05, postoperative: 5.37±0.83) and "Mean interference" (preoperative: 4.69±0.88, postoperative: 4.36±0.83), there was almost no changes in control group.

Nerve conduction velocity (NCV) study

Two years after surgery, NCVs of all the patients increased significantly compared to that before surgery ($P<0.05$) while NCVs of patients in control group remained almost unchanged. Statistically significant difference could be observed between the surgical and control groups ($P<0.05$) while no statistically significant difference existed between the focal and diffuse pain group ($P = 0.84$) two years after surgery (Table 2).

High-resolution ultrasonography

In all groups, fusiform swelling of the nerves, intraneural hypoecho and, disappearance of intraneural parallel and linear structure were observed by high-resolution ultrasonography. Two years after surgery, the restoration of nerve structure can be seen in both focal and diffuse pain group. More decrease of CSA was seen in patients with focal pain ($P<0.05$). (Figure 3) The CSA of patients in control group remained larger than that of both focal ($P<0.05$) and diffuse ($P<0.05$) pain group after surgery (Table 3).

All patients underwent surgical decompression recovered well except that three patients suffered from surgical complications. Wound dehiscence in two patients healed within 2 months after strict blood glucose control, antibiotics administration and daily dressing change. One patient with extensive lower-leg subcutaneous hemorrhage was treated by surgical incision and drainage. In the control group, ten patients developed superficial ulcers in the lower-limb and two underwent surgical amputation during this period. None of the operated patients had developed new ulcer, ulcer progression or amputation in two-year follow-up.

Discussion

Diabetic neuropathy has traditionally been considered as an irreversible condition and the treatments are mostly symptomatic aiming to prevent the development of complications rather than to target the underlying pathologic mechanisms. [24] However, the proposal of "double crush" hypothesis contributed by the combination of increase endoneurial water content [25,26] and consequent slow axoplasmic flow [27–29] offers hope to people with diabetic neuropathy and superimposed nerve compression since neurolysis of these entrapped nerves may give symptomatic relief and possess potential for reversibility. As such, over the past two decades, surgical decompression of peripheral nerves has become an increasingly popular method for treating patients suffering from painful diabetic neuropathy.

Painful DPN can be divided into two varieties: acute and chronic painful DPN. Here we mainly focus on chronic painful DPN due to its highly prevalence and the facts that acute painful DPN is relatively rare and the acute symptoms may resolve within a year. [30,31] According to our clinical experience with management of painful diabetic neuropathy, pain is a heterogeneous sensation and patients may describe their symptoms in markedly different ways. Features and severity of the pain may change with the development of diabetic neuropathy while the extent of pain is relatively invariable, which may be of somewhat value. We observed that some patients with painful DPN localized their pain mainly to the scattered areas of the legs, dorsum of feet, the heels, the toes, or the plantar aspect of feet while some others complained the pain was so dispersed that it even involved the whole lower limbs and the exact position could not be localized. Inspired by one previous guideline [8], we retrospectively defined the former as focal pain and the later as diffuse pain, and divided a series of 306 painful diabetic patients who underwent decompression surgery into two subgroups in the light of this definition. In this study we firstly compared the surgical result between surgical group and control group and, confirmed the efficacy of these decompression surgeries. Then we compared the surgical result of pain relief in patients of surgical group, revealing different responses of patients with focal and diffuse pain to the surgical decompression: people with focal painful DPN show a greater

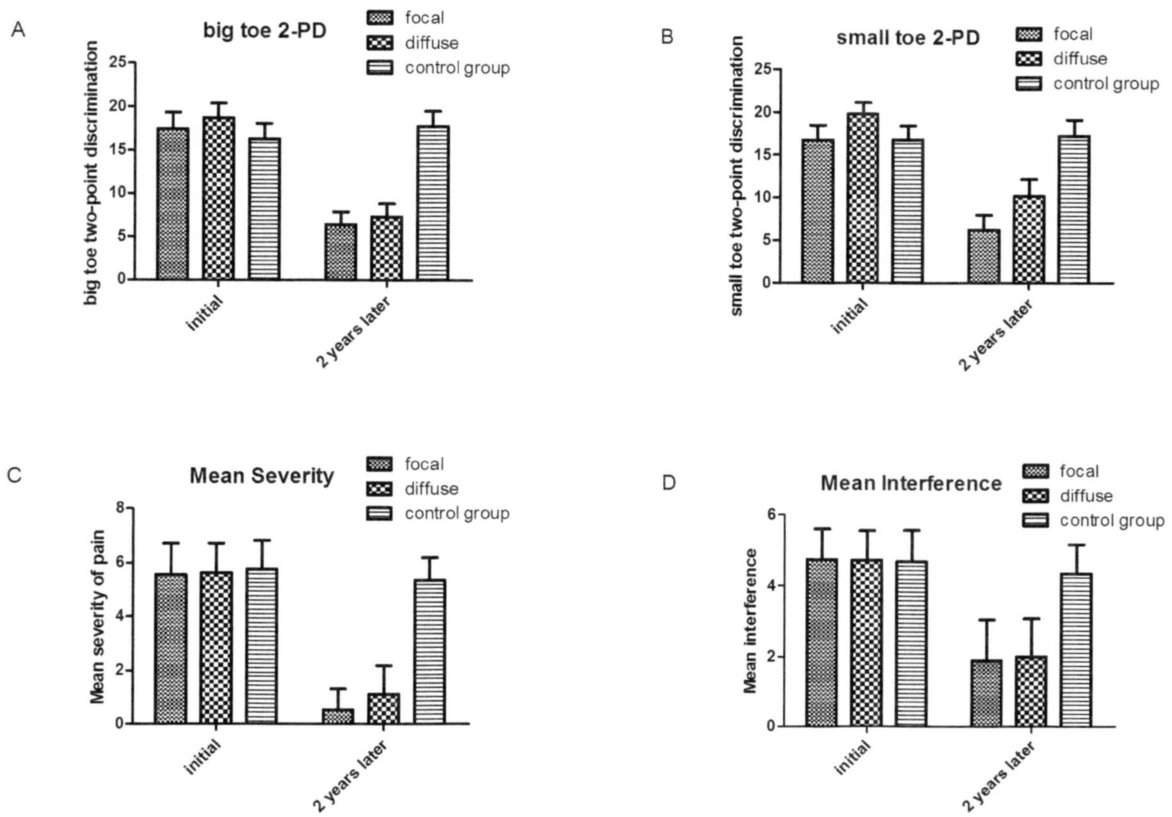

Figure 2. Graphs illustrate results of two-point discrimination and BPI-DPN in all groups. A, B, both surgical groups show marked decline in plantar big toe and small toe 2-PD while no apparent improvement can be observed in the control group; C, both surgical groups exhibit significant alleviation in pain severity through surgery while the control group remained at nearly the same level of mean severity of pain; D, decrease in the mean activity interference was displayed in both surgical groups and almost no changes existed in the control group.

potential to achieve pain relief. Morphologically, in addition, better ultrasound restoration could be observed in focal pain group than diffuse pain group.

The answer to the question of "what is the pathophysiology behind the distinct reaction to the decompression between patients with focal or diffuse painful DPN" should be started with the mechanisms of neuropathic pain in diabetes. Although the exact pathophysiological mechanisms of neuropathic pain in diabetes remain enigmatic, several mechanisms including peripheral and central mechanisms have been postulated based on the result of experiments in animal model of neuropathic pain. [32–36] It is suggested that all levels of the nervous system, from peripheral nerve to the brain, were affected by the diabetic neuropathy. [37] Both metabolic and mechanical (compressive) mechanism may be the source of the painful symptom.

Diabetes causes deposition of collagen in the small arteries that supply the peripheral nerves, hypothetically resulting in a length-dependent sensorimotor neuropathy. Increased aldose reductase

Table 2. Pre and post operative NCVs of DPN patients ($\overline{x}\pm S$).

	Preoperative NCV(ms)			Postoperative NCV(ms)		
	Control Group	**Focal Group**	**Diffuse Group**	**Control Group**	**Focal Group**	**Diffuse Group**
Posterior tibial nerve	36.7±3.4	33.5±3.1	35.5±3.6	31.6±3.5	41.8±2.6	42.0±2.8
Common peroneal nerve	33.8±2.8	37.8±3.4	36.8±1.9	28.6±3.3	42.5±2.4	42.2±2.9
Superficial peroneal nerve	38.6±3.7	35.8±2.5	37.6±2.9	34.4±3.6	42.2±3.1	43.6±2.3
Sural nerve	37.4±2.8	37.8±3.4	37.7±3.9	37.0±2.5	43.6±2.7	43.2±3.6

All variables were expressed in mean ± SD.
NCV: nerve conduction velocity.
Nerve decompression increases NCV in operated cases by 15–20%.

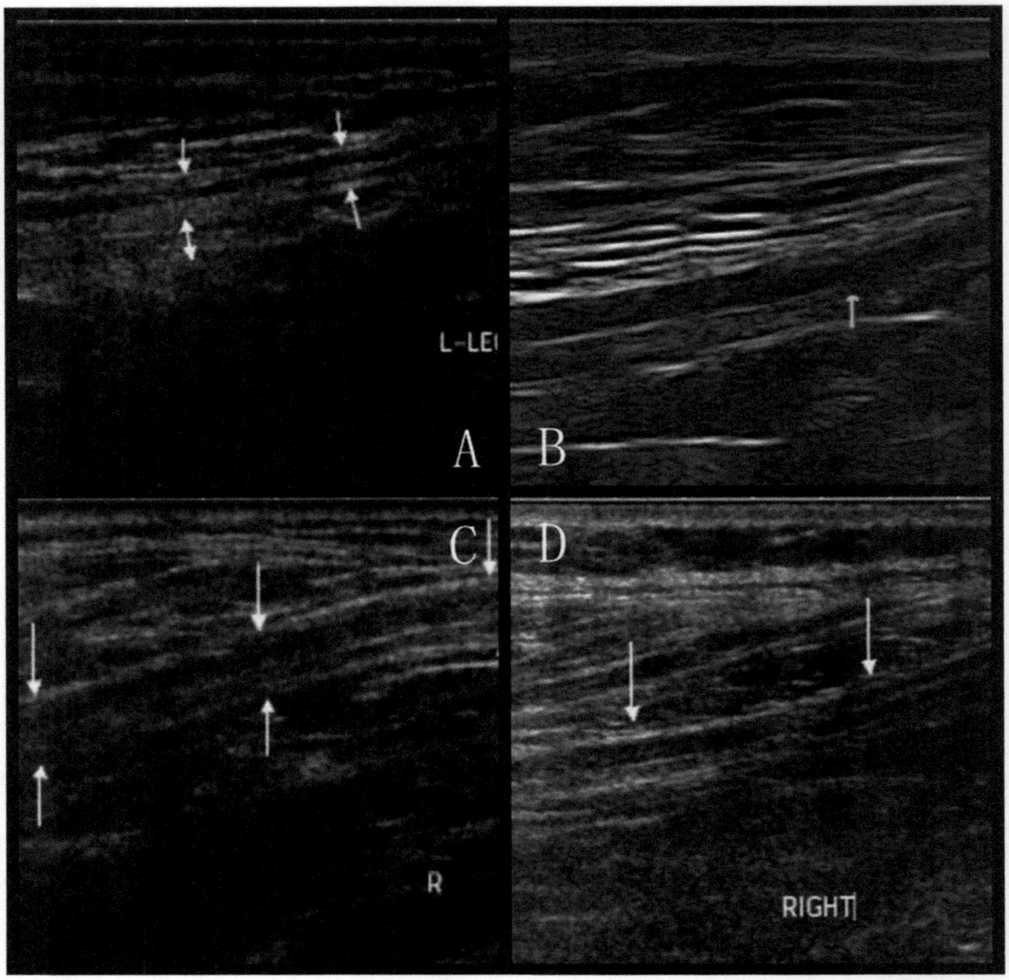

Figure 3. Longitudinal sonograms showing difference of morphological changes after surgical decompression between two patients with focal and diffuse painful DPN. A and B represent the preoperative (Da: 4.4 mm, Dt: 7.6 mm) and postoperative (Da: 2.9 mm, Dt: 6.3 mm) sonograms of the common peroneal nerve at the level of knee joint of patient with focal painful DPN. C and D represent the preoperative (Da: 4.2 mm, Dt: 7.0 mm) and postoperative (Da: 3.7 mm, Dt: 6.8 mm) sonograms of the common peroneal nerve at the level of knee joint of patient with diffuse painful DPN.

activity in diabetes converts glucose to sorbitol, which is hydrophilic and draws water into the nerve, rendering the peripheral nerve susceptible to mechanical compression and decreasing the slow axoplasmic transport in the diabetic nerve. As a consequence, proteins for structural repairs could not be transported to the impaired site within the diabetic nerve. [38] Injured peripheral nerve fibers give rise to the intense and prolonged input of ectopic activity to the central nervous system. After that, neurons in the spinal and the brain may change their response characteristics and exhibit signs of hyperexcitability in a fashion, mimicking that presented after peripheral nerve injury [39].

Table 3. Pre and post operative CSA of DPN patients ($\bar{x}\pm$s).

	Preoperative CSA			Postoperative CSA		
	Control Group	**Focal Group**	**Diffuse Group**	**Control Group**	**Focal Group**	**Diffuse Group**
Tibial nerve CSA(mm^2)	24.4±4.2	25.3±3.5	25.1±4.1	25.1±3.6	16.9±3.2	19.7±3.8
Common peroneal nerve CSA(mm^2)	21.6±3.7	20.8±3.5	21.2±4.0	21.9±3.2	14.6±2.8	15.9±3.5

All variables were expressed in mean ± SD.
CSA: cross-sectional area.

Given all that above, in the early stage of some cases, nerve thickening is suggested to play a fundamental role in the pathophysiology of painful diabetic neuropathy, with a manifestation of focal pain. As such, it is conceivable that entrapment of affected nerves at sites of anatomic narrowness may occur, which could be treated through surgical decompression. As the compression continues, however, neuroplastic changes in central nervous system happen after reorganization of structures participating in the processing of noxious information, which may present with diffuse pain in certain patients. The management is rather complicated. Aside from the current medical therapies including tricyclic antidepressants, the serotonin and noradrenaline re-uptake inhibitor and anti-convulsants, and so forth, an unmet need still exists for pharmacological agents targeting the underlying mechanisms due to the ineffectiveness and the side effects of the available drugs. In this study, the severity of pain, two-point discrimination, NCV results and morphological changes (SCA) of compressed nerve were all improved in surgical group when compared to the control group. Furthermore, there is no significant difference between the focal and diffuse pain groups regarding the results of two-point discrimination and NCV testing, which was increased by 15–20% after nerve decompression. (Table 2) Therefore, surgical decompression is also encouraged among the patients with diffuse painful DPN when the Tinel sign is positive, which indicates the existence of entrapment and regeneration of axons [40].

The limitations in our study include: (1) although being queried on admission, non-surgical treatment such as pharmacotherapy of neuropathic pain was not precisely measured among all the patients due to the retrospective nature of this study. For this reason, preoperative evaluation including pain levels was performed with both VAS and BPI-DPN and no significant difference was observed. (2) The specific definition of the focal and diffuse pain. Although extent of pain in most patients is relatively invariable, parts of patients would experience both focal and diffuse pain during the course of painful DPN. The phenotype of pain was decided on admission prior to surgery. Further prospective, randomized and controlled trial with blinded study executers and observers is needed to verify the role of peripheral nerve decompression in patients with painful DPN and further elucidate the role which pain distribution and characterization play in managing painful diabetic neuropathy as well as the underlying mechanism involved.

Allowing for the mixed results reported and the continuing controversy among researchers as to the effectiveness of nerve decompression surgery on DPN, [9,10,12,13,15,17,41–46] patient selection for surgery becomes increasingly critical through the long march to definitely delineate and confirm the place for nerve decompression. Distribution of pain indeed plays a practical role in predicting the response of painful DPN to the surgery according to the result of this study.

Conclusions

The results of this study continue to support the efficacy of decompression of multiple lower-extremity peripheral nerves in patients with painful diabetic neuropathy who presented with a positive Tinel sign. Favorable outcomes could be achieved in treating focal painful DPN through surgical decompression, which would also be helpful and should not be abandoned in diffuse painful DPN in the presence of Tinel sign.

Author Contributions

Conceived and designed the experiments: CLL WCZ. Performed the experiments: CLL MY. Analyzed the data: CLL QFM GWL WXZ. Contributed reagents/materials/analysis tools: MY WXZ QFM. Contributed to the writing of the manuscript: CLL.

References

1. Shaw JE, Sicree RA, Zimmet PZ (2010) Global estimates of the prevalence of diabetes for 2010 and 2030. Diabetes Res Clin Pract 87: 4–14.
2. Vinik AI, Park TS, Stansberry KB, Pittenger GL (2000) Diabetic neuropathies. Diabetologia 43: 957–973.
3. Thomas PK (1973) Metabolic neuropathy. J R Coll Physicians Lond 7: 154–160.
4. Boulton AJ, Malik RA, Arezzo JC, Sosenko JM (2004) Diabetic somatic neuropathies. Diabetes Care 27: 1458–1486.
5. Quattrini C, Tesfaye S (2003) Understanding the impact of painful diabetic neuropathy. Diabetes Metab Res Rev 19 Suppl 1: S2–8.
6. Abbott CA, Malik RA, van Ross ER, Kulkarni J, Boulton AJ (2011) Prevalence and characteristics of painful diabetic neuropathy in a large community-based diabetic population in the U.K. Diabetes Care 34: 2220–2224.
7. Tesfaye S, Boulton AJ, Dickenson AH (2013) Mechanisms and management of diabetic painful distal symmetrical polyneuropathy. Diabetes Care 36: 2456–2465.
8. Vinik AI, Casellini CM (2013) Guidelines in the management of diabetic nerve pain: clinical utility of pregabalin. Diabetes Metab Syndr Obes 6: 57–78.
9. Wieman TJ, Patel VG (1995) Treatment of hyperesthetic neuropathic pain in diabetics. Decompression of the tarsal tunnel. Ann Surg 221: 660–664; discussion 664–665.
10. Aszmann O, Tassler PL, Dellon AL (2004) Changing the natural history of diabetic neuropathy: incidence of ulcer/amputation in the contralateral limb of patients with a unilateral nerve decompression procedure. Ann Plast Surg 53: 517–522.
11. Biddinger KR, Amend KJ (2004) The role of surgical decompression for diabetic neuropathy. Foot Ankle Clin 9: 239–254.
12. Rader AJ (2005) Surgical decompression in lower-extremity diabetic peripheral neuropathy. J Am Podiatr Med Assoc 95: 446–450.
13. Siemionow M, Alghoul M, Molski M, Agaoglu G (2006) Clinical outcome of peripheral nerve decompression in diabetic and nondiabetic peripheral neuropathy. Ann Plast Surg 57: 385–390.
14. Karagoz H, Yuksel F, Ulkur E, Celikoz B (2008) Early and late results of nerve decompression procedures in diabetic neuropathy: a series from Turkiye. J Reconstr Microsurg 24: 95–101.
15. Wood WA, Wood MA (2003) Decompression of peripheral nerves for diabetic neuropathy in the lower extremity. J Foot Ankle Surg 42: 268–275.
16. Upton AR, McComas AJ (1973) The double crush in nerve entrapment syndromes. Lancet 2: 359–362.
17. Dellon AL (1992) Treatment of symptomatic diabetic neuropathy by surgical decompression of multiple peripheral nerves. Plast Reconstr Surg 89: 689–697; discussion 698–689.
18. Treede RD, Jensen TS, Campbell JN, Cruccu G, Dostrovsky JO, et al. (2008) Neuropathic pain: redefinition and a grading system for clinical and research purposes. Neurology 70: 1630–1635.
19. Bril V, Perkins BA (2002) Validation of the Toronto Clinical Scoring System for diabetic polyneuropathy. Diabetes Care 25: 2048–2052.
20. Scott J, Huskisson EC (1976) Graphic representation of pain. Pain 2: 175–184.
21. Zelman DC, Gore M, Dukes E, Tai KS, Brandenburg N (2005) Validation of a modified version of the Brief Pain Inventory for painful diabetic peripheral neuropathy. J Vasc Nurs 23: 97–104.
22. Lee CH, Dellon AL (2004) Prognostic ability of Tinel sign in determining outcome for decompression surgery in diabetic and nondiabetic neuropathy. Ann Plast Surg 53: 523–527.
23. Zhang W, Zhong W, Yang M, Shi J, Guowei L, et al. (2013) Evaluation of the clinical efficacy of multiple lower-extremity nerve decompression in diabetic peripheral neuropathy. Br J Neurosurg.
24. Melenhorst WB, Overgoor ML, Gonera EG, Tellier MA, Houpt P (2009) Nerve decompression surgery as treatment for peripheral diabetic neuropathy: literature overview and awareness among medical professionals. Ann Plast Surg 63: 217–221.
25. Gabbay KH (1973) The sorbitol pathway and the complications of diabetes. N Engl J Med 288: 831–836.
26. Jakobsen J (1978) Peripheral nerves in early experimental diabetes: expansion of the endoneurial space as a cause of increased water content. Diabetologia 14: 113–119.
27. Medori R, Autilio-Gambetti L, Monaco S, Gambetti P (1985) Experimental diabetic neuropathy: impairment of slow transport with changes in axon cross-sectional area. Proc Natl Acad Sci U S A 82: 7716–7720.
28. Dahlin LB, Meiri KF, McLean WG, Rydevik B, Sjostrand J (1986) Effects of nerve compression on fast axonal transport in streptozotocin-induced diabetes

mellitus. An experimental study in the sciatic nerve of rats. Diabetologia 29: 181–185.

29. Fink DJ, Purkiss D, Mata M (1987) Alterations in retrograde axonal transport in streptozocin-induced diabetic rats. Diabetes 36: 996–1000.
30. Tesfaye S, Malik R, Harris N, Jakubowski JJ, Mody C, et al. (1996) Arterio-venous shunting and proliferating new vessels in acute painful neuropathy of rapid glycaemic control (insulin neuritis). Diabetologia 39: 329–335.
31. Vinik A (2010) The approach to the management of the patient with neuropathic pain. J Clin Endocrinol Metab 95: 4802–4811.
32. Tesfaye S, Kempler P (2005) Painful diabetic neuropathy. Diabetologia 48: 805–807.
33. Ueda H (2006) Molecular mechanisms of neuropathic pain-phenotypic switch and initiation mechanisms. Pharmacol Ther 109: 57–77.
34. DeJong RN (1977) CNS manifestations of diabetes mellitus. Postgrad Med 61: 101–107.
35. Suzuki C, Ozaki I, Tanosaki M, Suda T, Baba M, et al. (2000) Peripheral and central conduction abnormalities in diabetes mellitus. Neurology 54: 1932–1937.
36. Eaton SE, Harris ND, Rajbhandari SM, Greenwood P, Wilkinson ID, et al. (2001) Spinal-cord involvement in diabetic peripheral neuropathy. Lancet 358: 35–36.
37. Kapur D (2003) Neuropathic pain and diabetes. Diabetes Metab Res Rev 19 Suppl 1: S9–15.
38. Barrett SL, Dellon AL, Fleischli J, Gould JS, Wang C (2010) Metabolic and compressive neuropathy. Foot Ankle Spec 3: 132–139.
39. Jensen TS, Baron R (2003) Translation of symptoms and signs into mechanisms in neuropathic pain. Pain 102: 1–8.
40. Dellon AL, Muse VL, Scott ND, Akre T, Anderson SR, et al. (2012) A positive Tinel sign as predictor of pain relief or sensory recovery after decompression of chronic tibial nerve compression in patients with diabetic neuropathy. J Reconstr Microsurg 28: 235–240.
41. Valdivia Valdivia JM, Weinand M, Maloney CT Jr, Blount AL, Dellon AL (2013) Surgical treatment of superimposed, lower extremity, peripheral nerve entrapments with diabetic and idiopathic neuropathy. Ann Plast Surg 70: 675–679.
42. Hollis Caffee H (2000) Treatment of diabetic neuropathy by decompression of the posterior tibial nerve. Plast Reconstr Surg 106: 813–815.
43. Aszmann OC, Kress KM, Dellon AL (2000) Results of decompression of peripheral nerves in diabetics: a prospective, blinded study. Plast Reconstr Surg 106: 816–822.
44. Therapeutics, Technology Assessment Subcommittee of the American Academy of N, Chaudhry V, Stevens JC, Kincaid J, et al. (2006) Practice Advisory: utility of surgical decompression for treatment of diabetic neuropathy: report of the Therapeutics and Technology Assessment Subcommittee of the American Academy of Neurology. Neurology 66: 1805–1808.
45. Cornblath DR, Vinik A, Feldman E, Freeman R, Boulton AJ (2007) Surgical decompression for diabetic sensorimotor polyneuropathy. Diabetes Care 30: 421–422.
46. Chaudhry V, Russell J, Belzberg A (2008) Decompressive surgery of lower limbs for symmetrical diabetic peripheral neuropathy. Cochrane Database Syst Rev: CD006152.

Permissions

All chapters in this book were first published in PLOS ONE, by The Public Library of Science; hereby published with permission under the Creative Commons Attribution License or equivalent. Every chapter published in this book has been scrutinized by our experts. Their significance has been extensively debated. The topics covered herein carry significant findings which will fuel the growth of the discipline. They may even be implemented as practical applications or may be referred to as a beginning point for another development.

The contributors of this book come from diverse backgrounds, making this book a truly international effort. This book will bring forth new frontiers with its revolutionizing research information and detailed analysis of the nascent developments around the world.

We would like to thank all the contributing authors for lending their expertise to make the book truly unique. They have played a crucial role in the development of this book. Without their invaluable contributions this book wouldn't have been possible. They have made vital efforts to compile up to date information on the varied aspects of this subject to make this book a valuable addition to the collection of many professionals and students.

This book was conceptualized with the vision of imparting up-to-date information and advanced data in this field. To ensure the same, a matchless editorial board was set up. Every individual on the board went through rigorous rounds of assessment to prove their worth. After which they invested a large part of their time researching and compiling the most relevant data for our readers.

The editorial board has been involved in producing this book since its inception. They have spent rigorous hours researching and exploring the diverse topics which have resulted in the successful publishing of this book. They have passed on their knowledge of decades through this book. To expedite this challenging task, the publisher supported the team at every step. A small team of assistant editors was also appointed to further simplify the editing procedure and attain best results for the readers.

Apart from the editorial board, the designing team has also invested a significant amount of their time in understanding the subject and creating the most relevant covers. They scrutinized every image to scout for the most suitable representation of the subject and create an appropriate cover for the book.

The publishing team has been an ardent support to the editorial, designing and production team. Their endless efforts to recruit the best for this project, has resulted in the accomplishment of this book. They are a veteran in the field of academics and their pool of knowledge is as vast as their experience in printing. Their expertise and guidance has proved useful at every step. Their uncompromising quality standards have made this book an exceptional effort. Their encouragement from time to time has been an inspiration for everyone.

The publisher and the editorial board hope that this book will prove to be a valuable piece of knowledge for researchers, students, practitioners and scholars across the globe.

List of Contributors

Cleverton K. F. Lima, Bruna L. R. Santos, Rafaela V. Silva and Ana L. P. Miranda
Laboratório de Estudos em Farmacologia Experimental (LEFEx), Faculdade de Farmácia, Universidade Federal do Rio de Janeiro, Rio de Janeiro, RJ, Brazil

Rafael M. Silva, Luciana S. Amaral, Luís E. M. Quintas and Marília Z. P. Guimaraes
Instituto de Ciências Biomédicas, Universidade Federal do Rio de Janeiro, Rio de Janeiro, RJ, Brazil

Renata B. Lacerda and Eliezer J. Barreiro
Laboratório de Avaliac¸ão e Síntese de Substâncias Bioativas (LASSBio), Faculdade de Farmácia, Universidade Federal do Rio de Janeiro, Rio de Janeiro, RJ, Brazil

Carlos A. M. Fraga
Instituto de Ciências Biomédicas, Universidade Federal do Rio de Janeiro, Rio de Janeiro, RJ, Brazil
Laboratório de Avaliac¸ão e Síntese de Substâncias Bioativas (LASSBio), Faculdade de Farmácia, Universidade Federal do Rio de Janeiro, Rio de Janeiro, RJ, Brazil

Martin Kaczocha, Mario J. Rebecchi and William Galbavy
Department of Anesthesiology, Stony Brook University, Stony Brook, New York, United States of America

Brian P. Ralph, Matthew W. Elmes, Liqun Wang and Dale G. Deutsch
Department of Biochemistry and Cell Biology, Stony Brook University, Stony Brook, New York, United States of America

Yu-Han Gary Teng, William T. Berger and Iwao Ojima
Department of Chemistry and the Institute of Chemical Biology and Drug Discovery, Stony Brook University, Stony Brook, New York, United States of America

Sherrye T. Glaser
Department of Biological Sciences, Kingsborough Community College, Brooklyn, New York, United States of America

Robert C. Rizzo
Department of Applied Mathematics and Statistics, Stony Brook University, Stony Brook, New York, United States of America

Ji Young Kim and Young-Jin Ko
Department of Preventive Medicine, Seoul National University College of Medicine, Seoul, Republic of Korea

Joongyub Lee and Nam-Kyong Choi
Medical Research Collaborating Center, Seoul National University Hospital, Seoul, Republic of Korea

Ju-Young Shin and Sun-Young Jung
Korea Institute of Drug Safety and Risk Management, Seoul, Republic of Korea

Byung-Joo Park
Department of Preventive Medicine, Seoul National University College of Medicine, Seoul, Republic of Korea
Korea Institute of Drug Safety and Risk Management, Seoul, Republic of Korea

Glenn-Marie Le Coz, Fernand Anton and Ulrike Hanesch
Laboratory of Neurophysiology & Psychobiology, University of Luxembourg, Luxembourg, Luxembourg

Nobuhiro Ogawa, Hiromichi Kawai, Tomoya Terashima and Hiroshi Maegawa
Department of Medicine, Molecular Genetics in Medicine, Shiga University of Medical Science, Otsu, Shiga, Japan

Hideto Kojima
Department of Molecular Genetics in Medicine, Shiga University of Medical Science, Otsu, Shiga, Japan

Kazuhiro Oka and Lawrence Chan
Departments of Medicine and Molecular and Cellular Biology, Baylor College of Medicine, Houston, Texas, United States of America

Vincent Cibert-Goton, Guanglu Yuan, Anna Battaglia, Sarah Fredriksson, Thomas Sears and Isabella Gavazzi
Wolfson Centre for Age-Related Diseases, The Wolfson Wing, King's College London, Guy's Campus, London, United Kingdom

Mark Henkemeyer
Department of Developmental Biology, Kent Waldrep Center for Basic Research on Nerve Growth and Regeneration, University of Texas Southwestern Medical Center, Dallas, Texas, United States of America

Chia-shu Lin
Department of Dentistry, School of Dentistry, National Yang-Ming University, Taipei, Taiwan (ROC)

Aleksandar Lj. Obradovic
Department of Anesthesiology, University of Virginia Health System, Charlottesville, Virginia, United States of America
Department of Physiology, Faculty of Pharmacy University of Belgrade, Belgrade, Serbia

Sung Mi Hwang
Department of Anesthesiology, University of Virginia Health System, Charlottesville, Virginia, United States of America
Department of Anesthesiology and Pain Medicine, Chuncheon Sacred Heart Hospital, College of Medicine, Hallym University, Chuncheon, South Korea

Joseph Scarpa
Department of Anesthesiology, University of Virginia Health System, Charlottesville, Virginia, United States of America

Sung Jun Hong
Department of Anesthesiology, University of Virginia Health System, Charlottesville, Virginia, United States of America
Department of Anesthesiology and Pain Medicine, Kangdong Sacred Heart Hospital, College of Medicine, Hallym University, Seoul, South Korea

Slobodan M. Todorovic and Vesna Jevtovic-Todorovic
Department of Anesthesiology, University of Virginia Health System, Charlottesville, Virginia, United States of America.
Department of Neuroscience, University of Virginia Health System, Charlottesville, Virginia, United States of America
Neuroscience Graduate Program, University of Virginia Health System, Charlottesville, Virginia, United States of America

Elaine G. Boland
Academic Unit of Radiology, Faculty of Medicine, Dentistry & Health, University of Sheffield, Sheffield, United Kingdom
Academic Unit of Supportive Care, Department of Oncology, University of Sheffield, Sheffield, United Kingdom

Dinesh Selvarajah and Solomon Tesfaye
Department of Diabetes, Sheffield Teaching Hospitals NHS Foundation Trust, Sheffield, United Kingdom

Mike Hunter
Academic Clinical Psychiatry, Department of Neuroscience, University of Sheffield, Sheffield, United Kingdom

Yousef Ezaydi and John A. Snowden
Department of Haematology, Sheffield Teaching Hospitals NHS Foundation Trust, Sheffield, United Kingdom

Sam H. Ahmedzai
Academic Unit of Supportive Care, Department of Oncology, University of Sheffield, Sheffield, United Kingdom

Iain D. Wilkinson
Academic Unit of Radiology, Faculty of Medicine, Dentistry & Health, University of Sheffield, Sheffield, United Kingdom

Zhiyou Peng, Huiling Li, Zhiying Feng and Shengmei Zhu
Department of Anesthesiology, First Affiliated Hospital, School of Medicine, Zhejiang University, Hangzhou, Zhejiang Province, China

Chong Zhang
Department of Thoracic Surgery, First Affiliated Hospital, School of Medicine, Zhejiang University, Hangzhou, Zhejiang Province, China

Xiang Qian
Department of Anesthesiology, Perioperative and Pain Medicine, Stanford University School of Medicine, Stanford, California, United States of America

Qi-Liang Mao-Ying
Neuroimmunology Laboratory, Department of Symptom Research, University of Texas M.D. Anderson Cancer Center, Houston, Texas, United States of America
Department of Integrative Medicine and Neurobiology, State Key Laboratory of Medical Neurobiology, School of Basic Medical Sciences, Fudan University, Shanghai, People's Republic of China

Annemieke Kavelaars, Karen Krukowski, Xiao-Jiao Huo, Wenjun Zhou and Cobi J. Heijnen
Neuroimmunology Laboratory, Department of Symptom Research, University of Texas M.D. Anderson Cancer Center, Houston, Texas, United States of America

Theodore J. Price
School of Behavioral and Brain Sciences, University of Texas at Dallas, Richardson, Texas, United States of America

Charles Cleeland
Department of Symptom Research, University of Texas M.D. Anderson Cancer Center, Houston, Texas, United States of America

Asha R. Kallianpur
Department of Genomic Medicine, Lerner Research Institute, Cleveland Clinic Foundation, Cleveland, Ohio, United States of America
Department of Molecular Medicine, Cleveland Clinic Lerner College of Medicine of Case Western Reserve University, Cleveland, Ohio, United States of America

Peilin Jia and Zhongming Zhao
Department of Biomedical Informatics, Vanderbilt University School of Medicine, Nashville, Tennessee, United States of America

Ronald J. Ellis
Department of Neurology, University of California San Diego, San Diego, California, United States of America

Cinnamon Bloss
Scripps Genomic Medicine, Scripps Translational Science Institute, and Scripps Health, La Jolla, California, United States of America

Wanqing Wen and Todd Hulgan
Department of Medicine, Vanderbilt University School of Medicine, Nashville, Tennessee, United States of America

Christina M. Marra
Department of Neurology, University of Washington, Seattle, Washington, United States of America

David M. Simpson and Susan Morgello
Department of Neurology, Icahn School of Medicine of Mt. Sinai, New York, New York, United States of America

Justin C. McArthur
Department of Neurology, Johns Hopkins University, Baltimore, Maryland, United States of America

David B. Clifford
Department of Neurology, Washington University, St. Louis, Missouri, United States of America

Ann C. Collier
Department of Medicine, University of Washington, Seattle, Washington, United States of America

Benjamin B. Gelman
Department of Pathology, University of Texas Medical Branch, Galveston, Texas, United States of America

J. Allen McCutchan and Scott Letendre
Department of Medicine, University of California San Diego, San Diego, California, United States of America

Donald Franklin and Debralee Rosario
HIV Neurobehavioral Research Center & CHARTER Center, University of California San Diego, San Diego, California, United States of America

David C. Samuels, Emily Holzinger and Deborah G. Murdock
Department of Molecular Physiology and Biophysics and Center for Human Genetics Research, Vanderbilt University School of Medicine, Nashville, Tennessee, United States of America

Igor Grant
Department of Psychiatry, University of California San Diego, San Diego, California, United States of America

Xiaoyan Zhu, Qian Li, Zongbing Song, Qulian Guo and Changsheng Huang
Department of Anesthesiology, Xiangya Hospital of Central South University, Changsha, China

Ruimin Chang
Liver Cancer Laboratory, Xiangya Hospital of Central South University, Changsha, China

Dong Yang
Department of Anesthesiology, Union Hospital, Tongji Medical College, Huazhong University of Science and Technology, Wuhan, China

Katarzyna Starowicz, Wioletta Makuch, Natalia Malek, Magdalena Zychowska and Barbara Przewlocka
Dept. of Pain Pharmacology, Institute of Pharmacology, Polish Academy of Sciences, Smetna, Krakow, Poland

Michal Korostynski and Michal Slezak
Dept. of Molecular Neuropharmacology, Institute of Pharmacology, Polish Academy of Sciences, Smetna, Krakow, Poland

Stefania Petrosino and Vincenzo Di Marzo
Endocannabinoid Research Group, Istituto di Chimica Biomolecolare, CNR, Pozzuoli (Naples), Italy

Luciano De Petrocellis and Luigia Cristino
Endocannabinoid Research Group, Istituto di Cibernetica, CNR, Pozzuoli (Naples), Italy

Valéria Martinez
Anesthésiologie-Réanimation, Hôpital Raymond-Poincaré , Garches, France

Nadine Attal and Didier Bouhassira
INSERM U-987, Centre d'Evaluation et de Traitement de la Douleur, CHU Ambroise Paré, Boulogne-Billancourt, France
Université Versailles-Saint-Quentin, Versailles, France

Bertrand Vanzo
General Practitioner, Athis Mons, France

Eric Vicaut
Unité de Recherche Clinique – Hôpital Fernand Widal, Paris, France

Jean Michel Gautier
Réseau InterCLUD Languedoc Roussillon, CHRU Montpellier, Montpellier, France

Michel Lantéri-Minet
CHU de Nice, Centre d'Evaluation et Traitement de la Douleur, Nice, France
INSERM/UdA, U1107, Neuro-Dol, Université de Clermont-Ferrand, Clermont-Ferrand, France

Ihsan Ekin Demir, Stephan Schorn, Elisabeth Schremmer-Danninger, Timo Kehl, Helmut Friess and Güralp O. Ceyhan
Department of Surgery, Klinikum rechts der Isar, Technische Universität München, Munich, Germany

Kun Wang
Key laboratory of Carcinogenesis and Translational Research (Ministry of Education), Department of Hepatic, Biliary and Pancreatic Surgery, Peking University School of Oncology, Beijing Cancer Hospital and Institute, Beijing, China

Nathalia A. Giese
Department of General Surgery, University of Heidelberg, Heidelberg, Germany

Hana Algül
Department of Internal Medicine II, Klinikum rechts der Isar, Technische Universität München, Munich, Germany

Joanna Mika, Katarzyna Popiolek-Barczyk, Ewelina Rojewska, Wioletta Makuch, Katarzyna Starowicz and Barbara Przewlocka
Department of Pain Pharmacology, Institute of Pharmacology, Polish Academy of Sciences, Krakow, Poland

Torge Rempe
Dept of Neuroradiology, University Hospital of Kiel, Arnold-Heller-Strasse 3, Haus 41, 24105 Kiel, Germany
Dept of Neurology, University Hospital of Kiel, Arnold-Heller- Strasse 3, Haus 41, 24105 Kiel, Germany

Stephan Wolff, Christian Riedel and Olav Jansen
Dept of Neuroradiology, University Hospital of Kiel, Arnold-Heller-Strasse 3, Haus 41, 24105 Kiel, Germany

Ralf Baron
Dept of Neurology, University Hospital of Kiel, Arnold-Heller- Strasse 3, Haus 41, 24105 Kiel, Germany
Division of Neurological Pain Research and Therapy, University Hospital of Kiel, Arnold-Heller-Strasse 3, Haus 41, 24105 Kiel, Germany

Patrick W. Stroman
Centre for Neuroscience Studies, Dept of Diagnostic Radiology, Dept of Physics, 228 Botterell Hall, Queen's University, Kingston, Ontario, Canada

Janne Gierthmühlen
Dept of Neuroradiology, University Hospital of Kiel, Arnold-Heller-Strasse 3, Haus 41, 24105 Kiel, Germany.
Division of Neurological Pain Research and Therapy, University Hospital of Kiel, Arnold-Heller-Strasse 3, Haus 41, 24105 Kiel, Germany

Jaime L. Watson, Tamara J. Hala, Rajarshi Putatunda, Daniel Sannie and Angelo C. Lepore
Department of Neuroscience, Farber Institute for Neurosciences, Sidney Kimmel Medical College at Thomas Jefferson University, Philadelphia, Pennsylvania, United States of America

Chenlong Liao, Wenchuan Zhang, Min Yang, Qiufeng Ma, Guowei Li and Wenxiang Zhong
Department of Neurosurgery, XinHua Hospital, affiliated to Shanghai JiaoTong University School of Medicine, Shanghai, P. R. China

Index

S

T